AF898531

CRITICAL CARE MEDICINE

Prof. (Dr.) Sujata K. Das

ALLIED
HEALTH
PRESS

Critical Care Medicine

Author: **Prof. (Dr.) Sujata K. Das**

Allied Health Press
4164 Lakeshore Road
Burlington ON L7L 1A4
Canada
www.alliedhealthpress.com
Email: orders@arclereducation.com

© 2026 Allied Health Press
ISBN: 978-1-77956-799-4

This book contains information obtained from highly regarded resources. Reprinted material sources are indicated and copyright remains with the original owners. Copyright for images and other graphics remains with the original owners as indicated. A Wide variety of references are listed. Reasonable efforts have been made to publish reliable data. Authors or Editors or Publishers are not responsible for the accuracy of the information in the published chapters or consequences of their use. The publisher assumes no responsibility for any damage or grievance to the persons or property arising out of the use of any materials, instructions, methods or thoughts in the book. The authors or editors and the publisher have attempted to trace the copyright holders of all material reproduced in this publication and apologize to copyright holders if permission has not been obtained. If any copyright holder has not been acknowledged, please write to us so we may rectify.

General Disclaimer:
This book is a summation of information from different sources and encompasses a wide range of medical conditions, the latest therapy methods, principals and techniques that are used in current practice, at the time of publication. This book offers general information with educational purposes, it is not to be applied or relied on for any diagnostic or treatment purposes. Please do not use the data/matter as a substitute for professional diagnosis and treatment. Please consult your healthcare provider or a licensed physician before making any healthcare queries or treatment choices. The medical information and research findings presented in this book are for educational purposes only and should not be used for the treatment of specific individual patients, as individual cases may vary. The author(s), editors(s) and publisher cannot be held accountable and make no guarantees that the information provided in this book will apply to each and individual patient. This book is meant to serve as a basic guideline and other relevant literature sources should be used for more specific information. This text can be a vital resource for students, trainees, and practitioners, covering essential topics. This book encompasses a wide range of medical conditions and the latest therapy options used in current practice. Through the utilization of many different medical studies this book provides the basics of different medical conditions, which can be used as a basic guide from where medical students, trainees and practitioners can extract necessary information. Further, some of the books have graphic images to explain anatomy for medical/educational purposes only. Hence, the book is intended for students or teachers/staff or individuals with a mature outlook looking to learn or enhance their knowledge.

Notice: Registered trademark of products or corporate names are used only for explanation and identification without intent of infringement.

Allied Health Press publishes wide variety of books and eBooks. For more information about Allied Health Press and its products, visit our website at www.alliedhealthpress.com

ABOUT THE AUTHOR

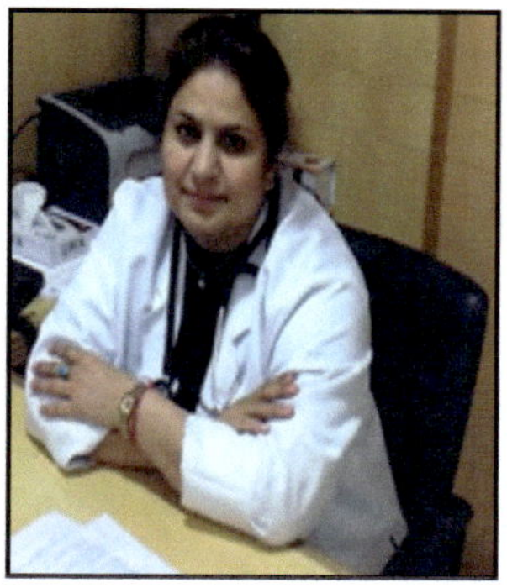

Prof (Dr) Sujata K. Dass, M.B.B.S, D.N.B, Ph.D. (Medicine) is a distinguished neuro-physician and academician, currently serving as an Attending Consultant in the Department of Neurology, B.L. Kapur Hospital, a renowned super-specialty medical institution in the New Delhi. Her illustrious career in medicine and research spans over three decades, characterized by her profound contributions to neurology and her unwavering commitment to medical education.

Dr. Dass began her educational journey at Flushing High School in New York, USA, and completed her High School Diploma thereafter she joined Queens College of the City University of New York as an undergrad student. With a passion for medicine, she pursued her MBBS degree at King George Medical College, Lucknow, U.P., India. Her academic prowess and dedication to medicine were evident early on, setting the stage for a remarkable career. Dr Dass worked under the supervision of Dr M.S. Bains, M.D. as a Visiting Fellow in cardio-thoracic surgery at Memorial Sloan Kettering Cancer Research Center, New York, USA. Dr. Dass furthered her medical training by obtaining a D.N.B. (Family Medicine) and conducted significant research on hematological changes in malaria. Her quest for knowledge and excellence led her back to New York, where she completed her Ph.D. (Medicine) at the Department of Obstetrics & Gynecology, The New York Hospital-Cornell University Medical Center under the mentorship of Prof. Brij B. Saxena. Her groundbreaking work on Sn-Proto and Sn-Mesoporphyrin and the chemoprevention of neonatal jaundice culminated in the award of her D.Sc. (Medicine). Dr. Sujata Dass joined as the BR Ambedkar Chair Professor in July 2002 in the Institute of Biomedical Sciences, Faculty of Medicine, Bundelkhand University, Jhansi. Her tenure was marked by her dedication to advancing medical research and education. She also served as UGC National Research Award (Professor) at V.P. Chest Institute, University of Delhi. Throughout her career, Dr. Dass has received numerous awards and accolades on a global level. Notable among these are the UGC Research Award, the Fast Track Young Scientist Award from the Department of Science and Technology (DST), and the Women's Award of Highest Honour from Soka University, Japan. She has also received numerous research grants from DST, DBT and ICMR, UGC etc. These awards and grants underscore her exceptional contributions to medical science and research.

Dr. Dass is a respected member of various scientific and administrative bodies like Planning Board (IGNOU), Executive Council - Bhagat Phool Singh Mahila Vishwavidhlaya, Haryana (2008-2011) where she continues to influence the medical community with her insights and expertise. Her commitment to guiding and mentoring students in their master's and doctoral thesis highlights her dedication to nurturing the next generation of medical professionals. Dr. Dass remains a beacon of excellence and a role model for aspiring medical professionals worldwide.

Brief Table of Contents

Getting Started with This Book

Chapter Openers

A list of Chapter Outline is presented providing a brief Introduction to what will be covered in the chapter.

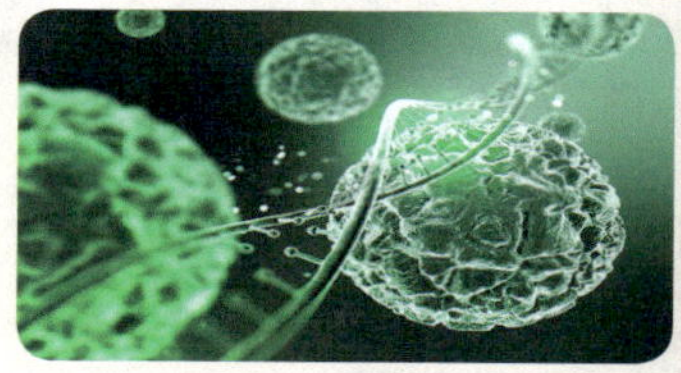

Introduction

Often referred to as the science of life, biology is a broad field of study aimed at comprehending the several kinds of life on Earth, from tiny creatures to sophisticated multicellular entities. Comprising several subfields, including molecular biology, ecology, and evolutionary biology, each of which advances our knowledge of living systems, this field clarifies the mechanisms controlling life events, including development, reproduction, and interaction with the surroundings, which is the central goal of biology. Moreover, biology fills in the void between the natural sciences and medicine by offering a necessary understanding of health, illness, and the interactions between organisms and their environments. Dealing with urgent global issues such as climate change, biodiversity loss, and new diseases depends on an awareness of these complex biological interactions, therefore highlighting the critical part biology plays in modern civilization. Fundamentally, biology explores and tests ideas about the living world using the scientific method. Through methodical observation and experimentation,

LEARNING OBJECTIVES

After studying this chapter, you will be able to:

1. Discuss the scientific method in biology;
2. Explain the cell theory;
3. Discuss the genetics and heredity;
4. Evolution and natural selection;
5. Focus on ecology and ecosystems;
6. Learn about human biology;
7. Evaluate the plant biology;
8. Explain the microbiology;
9. Focus on current trends in biology.

1.1. The Scientific Method in Biology

Learning Outcome

1. Describe the steps of the scientific method;
2. Focus on hypothesis formation;
3. Learn about experimental design.

Learning Outcomes

The beginning of each section of every chapter contains a set of Learning Outcomes that inform students of concepts they should understand. These outcomes help students understand what they should be able to do if they have mastered the material in that section.

Test Your Knowledge

Throughout each chapter, Test Your Knowledge cues you to note which topics have been covered and to self-test your understanding of the material presented.

Test Your Knowledge

1. Explain why correlation does not imply causation in scientific experiments.
2. How does the scientific method help reduce the influence of personal opinions in research?

Chapter Summary

The Summary Section appear at the end of each chapter and summarize main concepts covered throughout the chapter. These points provide key concepts in an engaging and meaningful way.

Summary

The investigation of biological principles highlights the importance of a comprehensive view of life by reflecting the intricate interactions that occur within living systems. The complexity of biology goes beyond individual species or systems, as this essay highlights; it also includes the interactions that mold ecosystems and affect biodiversity. Researchers can conduct in-depth analyses of metabolomic data using sophisticated technologies like MetaboAnalyst, which offer insights into the molecular mechanisms underlying these interactions. As demonstrated by the developments in MetaboAnalyst, for example, the integration of diverse omics data promotes a thorough understanding of metabolic pathways and helps identify important biological markers necessary for research on development and disease (Chong et al., 2018). Additionally, the phenomenon of ecological invasions is a key component of biological research and a vital field of study. The introduction of non-native species into unfamiliar habitats has significant ramifications and calls for multidisciplinary management strategies. Examining the origins and effects of these biological incursions, invasion science has become a crucial field that highlights the need to comprehend ecological dynamics and community interactions. As interest in biological invasions increases, new findings are emerging that put conventional ecological theories and practices to the test. The importance of incorporating various scientific viewpoints is shown by this developing discipline, which also highlights how invasive species shape ecosystems and advances our knowledge of ecological resilience (David et al., 2013). When taken as a whole, these discoveries from invasion science and metabolomics highlight the value of multidisciplinary biology research. Fostering cross-disciplinary collaboration and utilizing technological breakthroughs to improve our comprehension of intricate biological interactions are crucial as we look to the future of biological research. In addition to deepening our understanding of the complexities of life, this method lays the groundwork for tackling urgent environmental issues. Future studies can ensure the continued relevance of biology in a world that is constantly changing by acknowledging the interconnection of biological systems and opening the door to creative solutions that support sustainability and biodiversity conservation. We might imagine a thorough comprehension of life that serves both academia and society at large through ongoing investigation and integration of scientific knowledge.

Knowledge Assessment

The chapter includes material designed to review and reinforce each content. It includes Critical Thinking Questions to help test of your understanding of information presented in the chapter and Short answer Questions to review your understanding of the key concepts presented in the chapter.

Critical Thinking Questions

1. **Who is known as the "Father of Modern Biology"?**
   a. Aristotle
   b. Charles Darwin
   c. Gregor Mendel
   d. Louis Pasteur
2. **What is the basic unit of life?**
   a. Atom
   b. Molecule
   c. Cell
   d. Organism
3. **Which branch of biology studies the interaction of organisms with their environment?**
   a. Genetics
   b. Ecology
   c. Physiology
   d. Botany
4. **Which macromolecule is the main source of energy for living organisms?**
   a. Proteins
   b. Lipids
   c. Carbohydrates
   d. Nucleic acids
5. **DNA is primarily responsible for which function in living organisms?**
   a. Energy production
   b. Protein synthesis
   c. Storing genetic information
   d. Regulating body temperature

Short Answer Questions

1. What is biology, and why is it important to study biology?
2. What are the three main domains of life, and how are they different from one another?
3. Define homeostasis and give an example of how it works in living organisms.
4. What is the cell theory, and why is it fundamental to biology?
5. How do autotrophs and heterotrophs differ in the way they obtain energy?
6. What is the scientific method, and how is it applied in biological research?
7. Discuss how biology helps address global challenges such as climate change, disease, and food security.
8. Explain the levels of biological organization from the smallest unit to the largest. Provide examples at each level.
9. Describe the relationship between structure and function in biology, giving specific examples from cells or organs.
10. How has the discovery of genetics shaped our understanding of inheritance and variation among organisms?

Supplementary Materials

Key Terms: A list of key terms is given for quick reference

KEY TERMS FROM THIS CHAPTER

Annotation enrichment analysis	Biological structure	Cell
Cell theory	Cellular structure	Ecology
Ecosystems	Genetics	Human biology
Microbiology	Natural selection	Organism
Plant biology		

Further Resources: Recommendations for additional readings, websites, and multimedia resources.

References

1. Argelaguet, R., Velten, B., Arnol, D., Dietrich, S., Zenz, T., Marioni, J. C., Buettner, F., et al. (2018). Multi-omics factor analysis—A framework for unsupervised integration of multi-omics data sets. *Molecular Systems Biology, 14*. https://doi.org/10.15252/msb.20178124.
2. Bacher, S., Blackburn, T. M., Essl, F., & Genovesi, P. (2017). *Socio-Economic Impact Classification of Alien Taxa (SEICAT)*. https://core.ac.uk/download/286567949.pdf (accessed on 8th March 2025).
3. Barnett, R., Brace, S., Cucchi, T., & Dobney, K. (2013). *Divergent Evolutionary Processes Associated with Colonization of Offshore Islands*. https://core.ac.uk/download/20664364.pdf (accessed on 8th March 2025).

Detailed Table of Contents

CHAPTER 3

Airway Management and Respiratory Support 65

CHAPTER 4

Hemodynamic Monitoring and Management 101

CHAPTER 5

Shock Management 137

CHAPTER 6

Sepsis and Multi-Organ Dysfunction 169

CHAPTER 7

Acute Respiratory Distress Syndrome (ARDS) 203

CHAPTER 8

Acute Renal Failure and Renal Replacement Therapy 237

CHAPTER 9

CHAPTER 10

CHAPTER 11

Nutritional Support in Critical Illness 329

CHAPTER 12

End-of-Life Care and Palliative Medicine in the ICU 359

CHAPTER 13

LIST OF FIGURES

PREFACE

Critical care medicine has an essential role in today's healthcare, dealing with the critically ill patient with life-threatening illness who needs constant surveillance and prompt intervention. Critical care medicine combines advanced physiological understanding with technical proficiency to support failing organ systems and stabilize critically ill patients whose survival depends on timely, evidence-based therapies. In intensive care units worldwide, teams of physicians, nurses, respiratory therapists, and other specialists collaborate to monitor critical functions, interpret complex hemodynamic data, and adjust treatment in real time. The environment is that of high acuity, ethical complexity, and need for precision in assessment and management.

Over the past few decades, advances in monitoring technology, mechanical ventilation, hemodynamic support, and renal replacement therapies have transformed the outcomes of critically ill patients. What is now possible with simple observation and symptom relief is made available through advanced modalities such as extracorporeal membrane oxygenation, continuous renal replacement therapy, and targeted temperature management. Evidence-based recommendations and large clinical trials govern sepsis treatment protocols, shock resuscitation, and acute respiratory distress syndrome, but tailored approaches recognize unique physiological responses of each patient. Within this fast-paced setting, an understanding of the organ failure pathophysiology and the mechanisms of therapeutic actions is essential to improve survival and reduce long-term morbidity.

This book, *Critical Care Medicine*, has been written with the aim of developing a wide and accessible reference for practicing clinicians, trainees, and allied healthcare providers who manage critically ill patients. It combines basic science, clinical guidelines and pragmatic information to guide decision-making at the bedside and in multidisciplinary team discussions. By combining the best practice approach with patient safety and quality improvement, the book aims to equip readers with the knowledge as well as critical thinking skills necessary to tackle the whole spectrum of critical illnesses.

Chapter 1: Introduction to Critical Care Medicine provides a historical perspective on the development of critical care medicine and delineates the organizational models of modern intensive care units. It addresses the historical evolution of critical care as a specialty, significant milestones in technology and research, and team members' roles. The chapter addresses primary ethical principles, resource allocation, and measures for assessing quality of care.

Chapter 2: Assessment and Diagnosis in Critical Care revolves around rigorous patient assessment, such as history, physical examination skills adapted for sedated or ventilated patients, and interpretation of imaging and laboratory results. Emphasis is placed on early detection of deterioration, differential diagnosis of shock states, and correct bedside use of ultrasound.

Chapter 3: Airway Management and Respiratory Support covers indication for endotracheal intubation, rapid sequence induction approaches, and alternatives such as high-flow nasal cannula. It provides mechanical modes for ventilation, weaning approaches, and noninvasive ventilation approaches. Key topics include lung-protective ventilation, strategies to minimize ventilator-associated events and difficult airway management.

Chapter 4: Hemodynamic Monitoring and Management describes invasive and non-invasive techniques for the quantitation of cardiac output, preload, afterload, and systemic vascular resistance. Arterial lines, central venous catheters, pulmonary artery catheters, and more recent modalities such as pulse contour analysis are addressed. The chapter continues to address vasoactive drug selection, fluid responsiveness evaluation, and the principles of goal-directed therapy.

Chapter 5: Shock Management outlines the diagnosis and management of hypovolemic, distributive, cardiogenic, and obstructive shock. It discusses fluid resuscitation strategies, including the use of crystalloid verses colloid, dosing and timing of vasopressors and inotropes, and the application of advanced therapies with devices such as mechanical circulatory support.

Chapter 6: Sepsis and Multi-Organ Dysfunction outlines pathogenesis of sepsis, including dysregulated host responses and microvascular derangements. It provides recommendations for sepsis bundles, antimicrobial stewardship and supportive therapy to avert sepsis progression to multi-organ failure.

Chapter 7: Acute Respiratory Distress Syndrome (ARDS) addresses the diagnostic criteria, the inflammatory mechanisms and the scientific evidence supporting lung-protective therapies. It also addresses adjunctive treatments such as prone positioning, neuromuscular blockade and extracorporeal support when standard ventilation is insufficient.

Chapter 8: Acute Renal Failure and Renal Replacement Therapy addresses the spectrum of acute kidney injury in critical illness, including risk and prevention factors. Intermittent hemodialysis, slow low-efficiency dialysis and continuous renal replacement modalities are contrasted and advice is given on the timing of initiation and anticoagulation management.

Chapter 9: Neurological Monitoring and Management addresses how to assess and care for brain function in comatose or neurologically brain-injured individuals. Topics addressed include intracranial pressure monitoring, electroencephalography, sedation management, and techniques to manage elevated intracranial pressure or secondary brain injury.

Chapter 10: Infection Control and Management of the ICU focuses on prevention of healthcare-associated infections through hand hygiene, catheter care bundles and environmental control. The diagnosis and management of common ICU infections, antimicrobial stewardship principles, and strategies to minimize the spread of multidrug-resistant organisms are also managed.

Chapter 11: Nutritional Support in Critical Illness offers recommendations on caloric and protein requirements, the timing of enteral versus parenteral nutrition, and monitoring tolerance and metabolic complications. The chapter focuses on the impact of early nutrition interventions on outcomes and the role of dietitian.

Chapter 12: End-of-Life Care and Palliative Medicine in the ICU addresses communication competencies for goals-of-care conversations, ethical decision-making, and symptom management when curative therapy is not indicated. It provides guidelines for family meetings, withdrawal of life-sustaining therapies, and integration of palliative services into critical care.

Chapter 13: Trauma and Burn Management in the Context of the ICU discusses first and second survey principles in polytrauma, resuscitation strategies such as damage-control strategies, and specialized burn patient management such as fluid resuscitation protocols, wound care, and infection prevention.

Chapter 14: Cardiovascular Critical Care Emergencies addresses acute coronary syndromes, arrhythmias, cardiogenic shock, and advanced cardiac life support practice updates. It provides algorithms for immediate treatment and identification, as well as integration with cardiac catheterization and surgical intervention as appropriate.

Chapter 15: Pharmacology in Critical Care provides an overview of the commonly encountered drug classes, organ failure dosing, interactions, and toxicity monitoring. It also provides pragmatic guidance on antimicrobial dosing, sedation, analgesia, and the use of novel therapies.

This text is directed to training critical care residents, practicing intensivists in need of a concise yet comprehensive reference, as well as critical care nurses, respiratory therapists, and other allied health professionals dedicated to the care of critically ill patients. Medical students and residents rotating through intensive care units will find the foundational chapters helpful in establishing clinical competence. Besides trainees, the book will be a valuable resource for multidisciplinary teams who work to achieve the highest patient safety standards, promote clinical outcomes, and advance intensive care medicine practice.

INTRODUCTION TO CRITICAL CARE MEDICINE

1

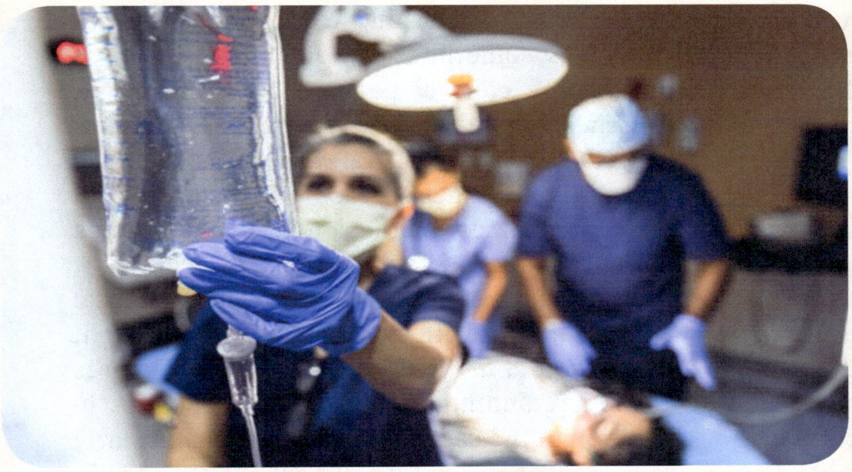

LEARNING OBJECTIVES

After studying this chapter, you will be able to:

1. Define the history and evolution of critical care medicine.
2. Discuss the common conditions treated in critical care.
3. Describe the role of the critical care team.
4. Identify the diagnostic tools and techniques.
5. Explain the treatment modalities in critical care.

Introduction

Critical care medicine is a branch of medicine aimed at diagnosing and treating dangerous conditions that require a lot of monitoring and treatment. It is a multidisciplinary approach that incorporates an assembly of professionals comprising intensivists, nurses, respiratory therapists, and pharmacists who all come together to render specialized care for the critically ill. The core mission of critical care medicine is to stabilize patients and promote recovery from acute illnesses such as severe infection, traumatic injury, or respiratory failure. This specialty demands the use of advanced technologies and interventions aimed at monitoring vital functions as well as the control of complex physiological imbalances, which play a crucial role in optimizing patient outcomes in high-risk environments like intensive care units (ICUs) (Kochanek *et al.*, 2019). In establishing the breadth of critical care medicine, there is to be recognition of its multi-faceted application beyond merely the resolution of acute illness. It is also applied in preoperative and postoperative settings, where patients are scrutinized closely for anesthesia and operative complications before and after operations. Furthermore, critical care medicine also deals with the management of chronic diseases that have the potential to lead to acute exacerbation. It thus focuses on prevention and long-term interventions in addition to immediate interventions. Research and guideline development continue, evolving with advances in evidence-based practices that will steer the management of conditions like severe traumatic brain injury (Kochanek *et al.*, 2019). The specialty is thus ever-evolving, reacting to newly developing challenges as they arise in modern medicine. The ethical challenges of critical care medicine are profound and at the heart of its practice. Given the inherent uncertainty of treatment outcomes and the complexity of delivering care in circumstances of life and death, practitioners are often confronted with difficult choices regarding patient autonomy, consent, and allocation of limited resources. A requirement for good communication with patients and families regarding prognosis and therapeutic options further complicates the setting. For instance, discussing end-of-life care and palliative options is a crucial aspect that highlights why caring counts in critical settings. As the practice continues to develop, constant regard for ethical matters counts in offering respectful and dignified care for patients with critical health conditions. Ultimately, critical care medicine is that complex assemblage of high-tech medicine and the human touch of caring that characterizes patient-focused practice.

Overview of Critical Care Medicine

Critical care medicine is a specialty of medicine aimed at treating the complicated conditions of life-threatening patients. It deals with the diagnosis, management, and treatment of critically ill patients with equal emphasis on medical and surgical treatment. The physicians who specialize in this discipline are professionally referred to as intensivists and work in ICUs, utilizing advanced technology and clinical pathways to treat patients. Critical care is an interdisciplinary strategy, interfacing with a variety of healthcare professionals, including nurses, respiratory therapists, and pharmacists, to deliver comprehensive patient-centered care. Critical care medicine has increased in recent health care settings due to the aging patient population and increased prevalence of chronic illnesses requiring intensive monitoring and intervention. The complexity in critical care also manifests in the moral challenges posed by decisions concerning treatment. Decision-making is sometimes a weighing of the pros against the cons of particular interventions, especially where the patient's prognosis remains uncertain. Besides, critical care medicine is also confronted by issues of resource allocation. With scarce resources, medical teams must decide upon the most effective lines of treatment that take into consideration both the medical efficacy and cost-effectiveness, an issue brought up in April *et al.* (2017). This balance requires an understanding of healthcare economics in addition to the capacity of systems, particularly in emergency rooms where spontaneous decisions require the promptest response available. As a critical component of providing healthcare, ethical aspects and the costs of providing care in critical settings require an in-depth understanding of the guidelines that govern such care. Globalization and the merging of many medical practices also influence the evolving landscape of critical care medicine. As medical practices grow more pluralistic, patients and providers tend to navigate through several treatment approaches, such as complementary and alternative medicine (CAM) treatments in addition to standard care. This is called medical pluralism, and it undermines the accepted model of care delivery in critical environments, raising the need for an expanded concept of patient health that includes multiple practices and beliefs. The appreciation of these nuances plays a key role in the establishment of efficacious treatment programs respecting patient values and maximizing clinical outcomes, as discussed in Penkala-Gawęcka *et al.* (2016). This multifaceted approach to critical care not only optimizes case-by-case patient treatment but also solidifies the entire medical community through the encouragement of a culture of inclusivity and responsiveness to patients' varied ideologies of health (Figure 1.1).

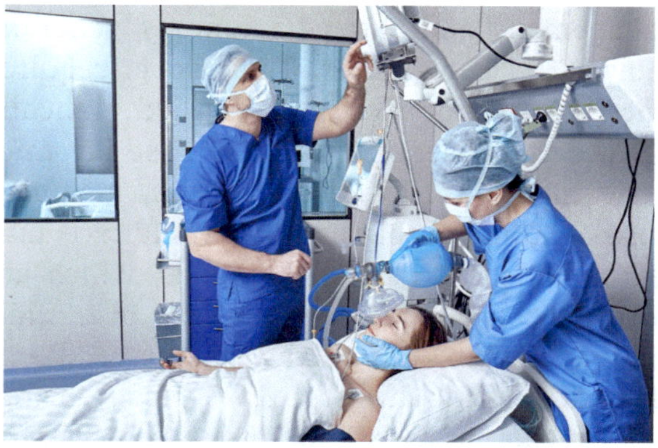

Figure 1.1. Medical and surgical treatment.

Source: https://asterhealthacademy.com/wp-content/uploads/2024/03/shutterstock_2262211833-1-scaled-2559x1693-1-2558x1692.jpg.

Importance in the Healthcare System

The importance of specialized care in the healthcare system is particularly evident in the case of critical care medicine, when timely and targeted intervention may significantly impact patient outcomes. Critical care environments, such as ICUs, are explicitly designed to address patients with life-threatening injuries or illnesses that necessitate ongoing medical attention. The complexity of such conditions typically demands similarly complex technological intervention along with a multidisciplinary approach by healthcare professionals. In this context, the contribution of the integration of cutting-edge digital systems cannot be exaggerated. The United States Pharmacopeia Expert Panel identifies the imperative need for accurate electronic transmission of prescriptions, particularly compounded nonsterile preparations (CNSPs), to minimize drug errors during critical transitions of care. This alludes to the paradigmatic contribution that effective communication plays in healthcare, particularly in ensuring patient safety in high-stakes environments like critical care (Parrish *et al.*, 2022). Also, the increased focus on personalized medical markers, including magnesium levels, signifies the broader applications for systematic health screening in critical settings. Magnesium, although often underemphasized, plays a vital role in numerous cellular processes and is a participant in more than 600 enzymatic reactions necessary for optimal physiological function. Hypomagnesemia, where there are low magnesium levels, has been determined to be a predictive determinant of unfavorable outcomes in critically ill patients, impacting conditions of cardiovascular and renal disease (Salinas *et al.*, 2020). Detection and treatment of hypomagnesemia, particularly in vulnerable populations such as the elderly or chronic disease patients, is critical to successful patient management. This highlights the necessity of vigilance in monitoring as well as intervention procedures within the healthcare system because underserved deficits can have serious complications, particularly in intensive care units. Lastly, the value of a properly formulated healthcare system lies in its capacity to address effectively the challenges posed by critical care situations. The ability to rapidly detect and treat specific medical conditions can influence not only the path of care but also the ultimate fate of intensive care patients. Strategies towards the creation of interoperable platforms for the sharing of clinical data, as demonstrated by initiatives by the United States Pharmacopeia, are critical in ensuring that all interested stakeholders, from physicians to pharmacists, run smoothly in harmony with one another (Parrish *et al.*, 2022). Further, integration of assessment of typically ignored markers, such as serum magnesium, into routine clinical practice has profound effects on the quality of care. By focusing on these fields, the health system fortifies its pillar, hence promoting patient safety, alleviating complications, and ultimately enhancing health outcomes in critical care medicine.

Distinction from Other Medical Specialties

Critical care medicine is unique among all other specialties due to its sole focus on life-threatening disease and the involved management of critically ill patients. Unlike most specialties dealing with elective or chronic diseases, critical care necessitates immediate intensive care, primarily in an ICU setting. Within this environment, clinicians are frequently forced to deal with patients who require advanced decision-making and instant reactions to dynamic clinical instability. This urgency is a hallmark of critical care, distinguishable from those specialties in which preplanning of care is the norm and follow-up care extends over years. Critical care also embraces a multidisciplinary approach that integrates the talents of all of the healthcare professionals—nurses, pharmacists, and respiratory therapists—highlighting the team effort characteristic of this specialty versus more single-discipline ones. Besides, the specialty of critical care medicine is necessarily characterized by reliance on advanced technology and continuous monitoring. ICU patients are often connected to an assortment of life-sustaining machines, which closely monitor vital organs and body processes, allowing healthcare professionals to make timely and informed decisions. This is a special feature that distinguishes critical care from the rest of medicine, where monitoring intensity or necessity is not necessarily high. The role of data interpretation in critical care cannot be overestimated since clinicians have to synthesize immediate information to modify treatment protocols adeptly. It centers on evidence-based practice, which is of most tremendous significance to patient success, separating critical care from other specialties of medicine that may not entail such emergent, technologically driven interventions (McGain, 2018). Also, the ethical concerns at the heart of critical care practice provide yet another lens through which to perceive its separation from other medical domains. Critical care practitioners are continually confronted with dilemmas in end-of-life care, resource management, and patient autonomy, generally in urgent circumstances. This aspect requires practitioners not just to be skilled clinically but also to possess an intimate base in ethics and compassion. Other specialties, including those handling outpatient or chronic care, may involve different ethical dilemmas, which are more concerned with patient care over time. The emphasis placed on the making of life-or-death decisions with urgency typically brings a moral climate that is unique to critical care, featuring a complexity that sets it apart from other specialty domains of medicine. Tackling such challenges in the proper manner demands a balanced perspective to both the medical and philosophical aspects of the discipline, with special emphasis on the richness and depth of critical care (Elsner, 2022).

1.1. History and Evolution of Critical Care Medicine

Learning Outcome

1. Define early practices in critical care
2. Understand the development of intensive care units (ICUs)
3. Explain the advances in technology and treatment protocols

The development of critical care medicine relies on the advancement of medical science and technology, particularly in the 20th century. The advancement began with a response to the polio epidemic of the 1950s, with iron lungs developing, and intensive care units (ICUs) being given priority to manage respiratory failure (Smith, 2019). With the realization of the requirement for specialized care came the theory of a coordinated response to critically ill patients that reoriented the response of healthcare systems to serious illness. It facilitated multi-disciplinary practice, whereby specialists working together became a prerequisite for successful care. With the growing emphasis on critical care, the demand for standardized protocols also emerged, which, ever since, have been instrumental in shaping training and education among healthcare professionals within this specialty. The subsequent years saw technology and monitoring devices take an entirely new dimension, further shaping the concept of critical care medicine. The presence of sophisticated machinery such as ventilators, cardiac monitors, and dialysis equipment also made a big difference in the outcome of the patient and transformed the job of intensivists. Evidence-based medicine, which emerged in the 1990s, took critical care to the next level, where bedside decision-making was founded on systematic research and facts rather than anecdotal application (Kruk *et al.*, 2018). This transition highlighted the specific challenges that critically ill patients presented and underscored the necessity of personalized interventions. With increasing recognition on the part of the healthcare systems worldwide of these needs, guidelines and protocols have been developed, so critical care teams have adopted best practices to improve survival and quality of life for the patient. Critical care medicine has also evolved with growing awareness of the ethical considerations and inequities inherent in healthcare delivery. The history of critical care is a narrative intricately woven around issues of access, equity, and quality, most applicable to low- and middle-income nations (LMICs) where the health system cannot keep up with expanding demands against scarce resources (Kruk *et al.*, 2018). It is in the acknowledgment that high-quality care is not an amenity of affluent societies that has prompted a broader debate on the social determinants of health and calls for reform in the global health system. As critical care continues its development, there remains a responsibility to sort out systemic inequalities and hold out a vision for delivering holistic, high-quality care to all patients regardless of how affluent or deprived their socio-economic status or geographical location (Figure 1.2).

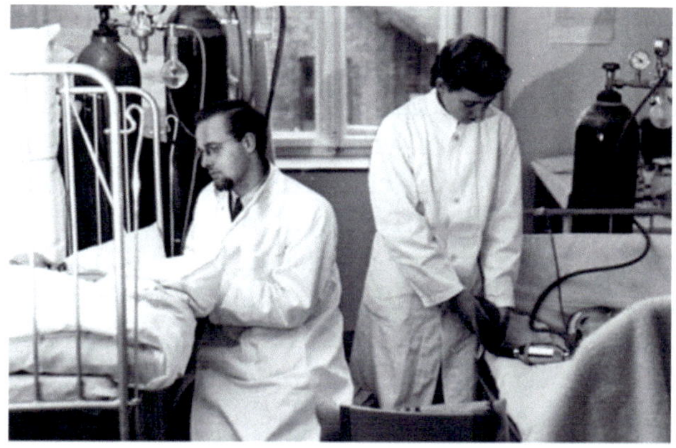

Figure 1.2. History of intensive care units (ICUs).

Source: https://ics.ac.uk/static/49071775-2e1c-4a2a-8fbb82c1ce17fcf1/500x335_highestperformance__4a7c7e45a350/History-hand-venting.png.

1.1.1. Early Practices in Critical Care

The evolution of critical care medicine can be traced back to trailblazing procedures that paved the way for modern patient management of acute disease. Observation and management of symptoms were the physician's primary reliance in ancient times, with a rare complete picture of the underlying disease. With advances in medical science over time, milestone progress was made, with the majority taking place between the 19th and early 20th centuries. Pathfinders such as Florence Nightingale emphasized the importance of hygiene and environmental control within the medical profession, knowing that the environment through which patients convalesced was a critical factor in their destiny. This initial comprehension of patient-centered care was revolutionary, uncovering the very origins of what would ultimately become critical care medicine (Medetalibeyoğlu *et al.*, 2024). These procedures emphasized rigorous attention to observation and the proper application of nursing principles to develop a critical connection between basic care and more immediate treatment. With the evolution of critical care, practitioners started recognizing the need for even more specialized intervention against acute medical crises, most importantly, the regulation of vital organ function. The post-WWII era was characterized by improved management and treatment of trauma, which culminated in the establishment of ICUs that cared for critically ill patients. In the ICUs, the care providers utilized an interdisciplinary model of care that combined medical knowledge with nursing care to facilitate healing. Also, the early experiments in respiratory monitoring and support, such as the application of positive pressure ventilation in patients with respiratory failure, stressed the need for technological innovation to maximize patient outcomes. These pioneering practices set the stage for the sweeping paradigms that evolved to become present-day critical care practices, where continuous monitoring and proactive management of critically endangered patients (Ullah *et al.*, 2023). The concept of critical care kept advancing as physicians understood the intricacy of multi-organ failure and the requirement for comprehensive intervention. Initial sepsis and shock management guidelines included evidence of evolving appreciation of requirements for intensive management practices. Pharmacotherapy advances, fluid resuscitation, and advances in monitoring technology made it possible for clinicians to more effectively administer focused interventions in a timely manner. With time, the role of critical care changed from just survival to entire treatment, including rehabilitation and long-term care. This is because with time, there was more understanding of psychosocial recovery due to early practice having included emotional and psychological as well as physical care. The legacy of these first critical care practices still impacts medicine today, maintaining patient care global and multidirectional (Medetalibeyoğlu *et al.*, 2024).

1.1.2. Development of Intensive Care Units (ICUs)

The evolution of the ICU is a landmark in the history of critical care medicine, changing the treatment delivery to critically ill patients. Taking up a new role for the first time in the mid-20th century, ICUs were established to provide specialized care to patients requiring intensive observation and highly advanced medical interventions. The development of such units has addressed the sophistication of medicine today, wherein many patients with extreme illness or injury require constant and instantaneous monitoring. With the advancement of healthcare technology, the demand for structured environments with skilled professionals and advanced monitoring devices came into being, a deviation from general medical wards to specialized centers of life-sustaining care. The development of ICUs has reflected the growing recognition of the notion that some patients require more intensive therapy and, therefore, has raised survival rates as well as the overall quality of care in critical illness. A significant part of the development of ICUs has been the evolution of nursing and medical practice specifically for critically ill patients. The interdisciplinarity of ICU care has facilitated coordination among physicians, nurses, respiratory therapists, and other experts toward enhancing patient outcomes. Today's ICUs utilize several technologies in monitoring vital functions and sustaining organ function, emphasizing ongoing education and training in critical care procedures. Particular protocols, such as those addressing sedation, pain relief, and infection prevention, have been formulated systematically to optimize patient care. Besides, teamwork strategies cannot be overstated because research shows that multidisciplinary teaming improves communication and awareness of context among clinicians and, therefore, leads to better decision-making in high-risk environments. Focus on integrative approaches to care is essential to providing an integrated response to problems presented by critically ill patients. Over the recent couple of years, the unyielding demands of international health crises, the most recent of which has been the COVID-19 pandemic, have emphasized on the need for efficient and responsive ICU systems. When hospitals were faced with unprecedented tidal waves of severely ill patients, the worth of prepared ICUs was best demonstrated. These steps such as the two-track strategy of peace and war policy facilitated proactive investment in intensive care units ensuring that resources would be kept available to handle shifting needs in case of public health emergencies (Wang *et al.*, 2022). The need for proper training of the health workforce has also been questioned, considering the reality that the majority of the members were redeployed in times of emergencies, where the acquisition of new skills, such as the transfer of patients in infectious statuses, was an urgent need (Glasbey *et al.*, 2021). These lessons emphasize the importance of ongoing improvement of critical care systems that maintain pace with emerging challenges with a guarantee of quality, safety, and teamwork in patient care.

1.1.3. Advances in Technology and Treatment Protocols

The terrain of critical care medicine has been dramatically altered by advances in technology and improved treatment modalities. New technologies like newer imaging methods and bedside ultrasound have transformed diagnosis, enabling clinicians to obtain timely and accurate diagnoses of critically ill patients. These technologies provide real-time monitoring and assessment of patient status, thus permitting the timely initiation of appropriate therapy modalities. For instance, the use of biomolecular techniques has enhanced rapid pathogen identification in ventilator-associated pneumonia, as highlighted in the study by Kollef and Burnham, with a focus on early implementation of targeted antimicrobial therapy. By diminishing the presumptive use of broad-spectrum antibiotics, the innovations enhance patient outcomes while reducing by a wide margin the likelihood of acquiring antimicrobial resistance. Further, treatment guidelines in intensive care units have been shaped by an increasing understanding of the complexities involved in treating hospital-acquired infections. Particularly, guidelines for treating hospital-acquired pneumonia (HAP) have been much refined as more information is gathered regarding the efficacy of existing treatment protocols. Ongoing debate among experts has necessitated reconsideration of established protocols, particularly the timing of the commencement of antibiotic therapy. While it's critical to initiate early treatment in patients with HAP symptoms, recent evidence now advocates for limited use of therapy, as emphasized by Hassinger and Sawyer. This shift towards a culture of specificity in using antibiotics is now attempting to address the issue of resistance in multidrug-resistant organisms and mitigate the adverse impact of broad-spectrum antibiotic therapy, all for the improvement in patient safety and quality of care. The advances in critical care also extend to primary immunodeficiency diseases (PIDs) with revolutionary progress in diagnosis and therapy. Over the past decades, developments such as improved immunoglobulin substitution therapies, enzyme replacement therapy, and improvements in stem cell transplantation protocols have changed the treatment paradigm for patients with PIDs. The historical context of these advances is significant because it illustrates the growing understanding of immunological disease that enables clinicians to manage genetic features and patient-dependent parameters more effectively. Furthermore, the introduction of gene therapy for certain PIDs represents a significant advancement, with future treatments available and expanding the armamentarium available to critical care practitioners managing these complex disorders, as detailed in the review by Ochs and Hitzig. These advances not only highlight the potential for improved patient outcomes but also portray the dynamic nature of critical care interventions as they adapt to new knowledge and technology.

Test Your Knowledge

1. What were some key features of early practices in critical care medicine?
2. How did the development of intensive care units (ICUs) transform patient management?

1.2. Common Conditions Treated in Critical Care

Learning Outcome

1. Explain the respiratory failure
2. Define sepsis and septic shock
3. Understand the cardiac arrest and arrhythmias

In intensive care, there is a broad range of conditions that need immediate and complex medical attention. Respiratory failure and sepsis are among the most prevalent conditions treated in ICUs. Respiratory failure is a condition in which the lungs are not able to oxygenate the blood or remove carbon dioxide, which typically needs to be supported by mechanical ventilation. COPD, pneumonia, and acute respiratory distress syndrome (ARDS) are diseases that frequently admit patients to ICUs. Early treatment and diagnosis of respiratory failure are life-saving, since if untreated, it can lead to multi-organ dysfunction rapidly. Sepsis, or a potentially lethal reaction to infection producing organ dysfunction, is another risk. Early recognition, coupled with early antibiotic treatment and supportive therapy, is the most significant factor in improving the outcomes in patients with sepsis who are being treated in the ICU, and this once again underscores the importance of specialized care in these complex cases. Another common condition frequently encountered in intensive care units is acute heart failure. This is a clinical emergency that presents when the heart's pumping ability is inadequate, leading to congestion and decreased perfusion of vital organs. The patients may present with clinical findings such as dyspnea, weakness, and edema and require immediate management. The management of acute heart failure is usually a combination of medication therapy and aggressive supportive treatment like diuretics, vasodilators, and, in some cases, mechanical circulatory support. Further, adjunct therapy like acetazolamide has emerged as a valuable option in some situations. As highlighted in Giamello *et al.* (2024), this carbonic anhydrase inhibitor may decrease fluid overload and alleviate respiratory distress, and as such is a valuable tool for critically ill patients with end-stage cardiac disease being treated by clinicians. Finally, therapeutic plasma exchange (TPE) has emerged as a useful modality of care for numerous disparate indications within the critical care setting. As discussed in the case of 105 patients, TPE is frequently applied in the treatment of conditions such as thrombotic microangiopathies, transplant complications, and vasculitis, among others, proving its effectiveness. TPE is generally needed as a result of severe, drug-resistant disease where traditional therapy is ineffective, demonstrating the need for patient-oriented treatment in the ICU. However, with some risks in relation, such as anaphylaxis, stringent patient selection and intra-procedure monitoring are necessary to avoid complications (Ring *et al.*, 2023). In general terms, TPE is but one of the many specialist treatments that illustrate the gravity of intensive care patient management, a correlate of the heterogeneity and complexity of these conditions to be managed within this field (Figure 1.3).

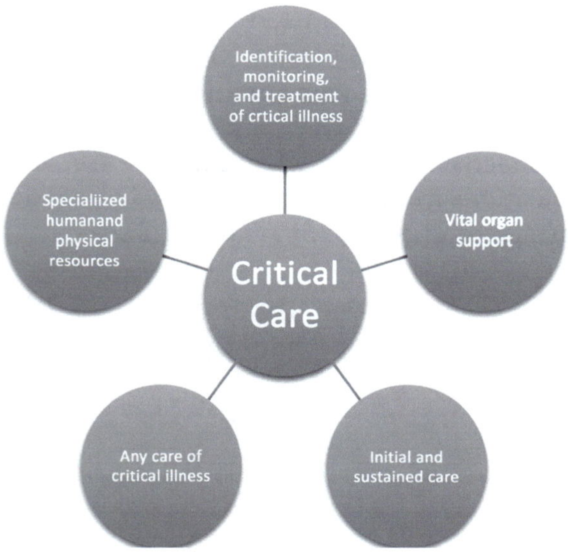
Identification, monitoring, and treatment of crtical illness
Specialiized humanand physical resources
Critical Care
Vital organ support
Any care of critical illness
Initial and sustained care

Figure 1.3. The defining attributes of critical care.

Source: https://bmjopen.bmj.com/content/12/9/e060972.

1.2.1. Respiratory Failure

In critical medicine, respiratory failure is a significant clinical challenge, where the respiratory system cannot maintain adequate gas exchange. Such a deficiency can lead to hypoxemia, with compromised oxygen delivery to tissues, or hypercapnia, in which carbon dioxide removal from the body fails. The pathogenesis of respiratory failure is diverse and can be classified into two types broadly: type I respiratory failure, which usually occurs in the form of hypoxemia without hypercapnia, and type II respiratory failure with both hypoxemia and hypercapnia. Identification of the type of respiratory failure and the etiology is critical for its effective management since the treatment protocols are significantly different based on the underlying pathophysiology. of the most essential conditions for respiratory failure, ARDS is particularly noteworthy because it can quite often present in the context of severe disease such as pneumonia, sepsis, or trauma. Not only does ARDS compromise respiratory function, but it meaningfully affects patient morbidity and mortality (Figure 1.4).

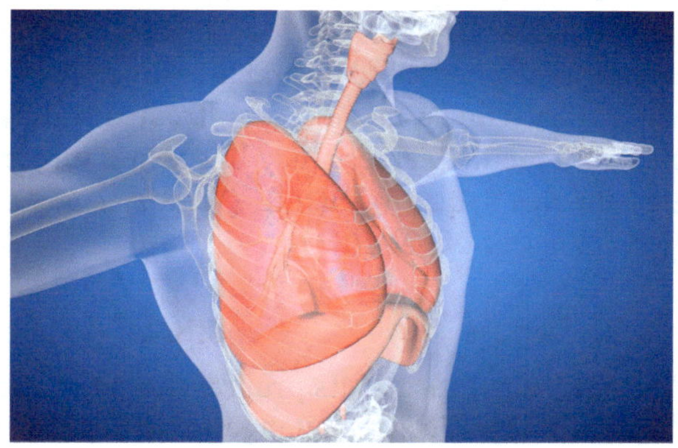

Figure 1.4. Respiratory failure.

Source: https://anmj.org.au/wp-content/uploads/2021/09/Respiratory-failure-scaled-1.jpg.

Clinical progression of ARDS is characterized by increasing dyspnea, hypoxemia, and bilateral chest imaging infiltrates. In light of this, early recognition and prompt management, including mechanical ventilation strategies and supportive care, are essential to improve patient outcomes. Importantly, existing knowledge concerning the pathophysiology of conditions like ARDS has also pointed to an understanding of the role of inflammation processes and their importance in guiding therapeutic intervention. With increasingly common viral infections, such as those due to COVID-19, the incidence of respiratory failure has escalated enormously, highlighting once more the importance of successful critical care. COVID-19 patients frequently experience severe respiratory complications, and the implementation of specific respiratory rehabilitation measures to avoid long-term dysfunction is indicated. Critically ill patients' respiratory rehabilitation guidelines are evolving and focus on interdisciplinary management strategies involving physiotherapy and psychological support to assist in coping with both physical and psychological issues faced by patients. Healthcare providers need to integrate these physical rehabilitation techniques into the overall care plan, as highlighted in current best practice to optimize recovery from respiratory failure and thereby treat not only the acute medical emergency but also improve the survivor's quality of life (Węgrzyn *et al.*, 2017; Zhao *et al.*, 2020).

1.2.2. Sepsis and Septic Shock

The state of sepsis and its progression to septic shock is a significant challenge in critical care medicine practice. Sepsis is characterized by a systemic inflammatory response syndrome as a result of infection, leading to critical organ dysfunction and, in the majority of cases, death if not recognized immediately and treated appropriately. Patients who present with signs of infection and an abrupt deterioration of their physiological status require early intervention. Such demand is further augmented by sepsis's heterogeneous clinical presentation and is hence of vital significance that physicians in ICUs value in pursuing in-depth comprehension of its treatment and pathophysiology modalities. Timely diagnosis and early initiation of therapeutic interventions enable healthcare professionals to improve patient outcomes. Treatment of septic shock demands a multi-dimensional approach, focusing primarily on hemodynamic instability that accompanies this syndrome as a rule. The cornerstones of treatment are fluid resuscitation and vasoactive support, used to restore the perfusion and oxygenation of the organ systems. However, trouble lies in the administration of fluid therapy. Fluid boluses, while essential to hypovolemia management, may cause complications, including edema of tissues, particularly when administered in high volumes without vigilant monitoring. The application of personalized therapy, including the proposed Resuscitation, Equilibrium, and De-escalation (RED) protocol, seeks to enhance outcomes for patients by individually tailored intervention, thus highlighting the dynamic aspect of cardiovascular support in sepsis and septic shock. This paradigm shift towards precision medicine warrants more research into its effectiveness in varied clinical cases as it transitions from theory to practice (Fernández-Sarmiento *et al.*, 2025) (Figure 1.5).

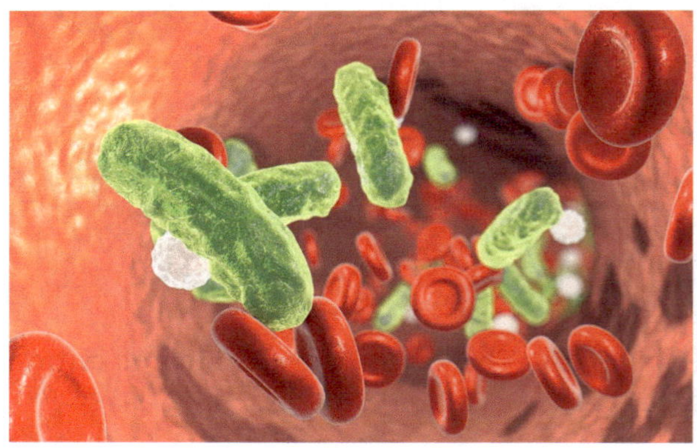

Figure 1.5. Sepsis remains a common and deadly condition that occurs when the body reacts to an infection in the bloodstream.

Source: https://sbpdiscovery.org/wp-content/uploads/2018/10/Sepsis-press-release.jpg-.jpg.

The instructional component with respect to the management of septic shock is as important for intensivists as it is for the surgical teams, and emphasizing the utilization of simulation-based education is a priority. Simulated clinical scenarios can effectively educate healthcare providers on dealing with the complexity of real emergencies in sepsis. Evidence also shows that even experienced clinicians may overlook critical steps, such as the need for timely fluid resuscitation, administration of timely antibiotics, and vigilant monitoring for invasive line placement under intraoperative management. Ongoing enhancement of simulation education not only enhances knowledge but also enhances skills required to handle septic shock effectively under pressure conditions (Webb *et al.*, 2020). As the profile of critical care continues to change, there is a greater appreciation of the need for continuous training and education of practitioners, in a bid to reduce the morbidity and mortality from this lethal disease (Figure 1.6).

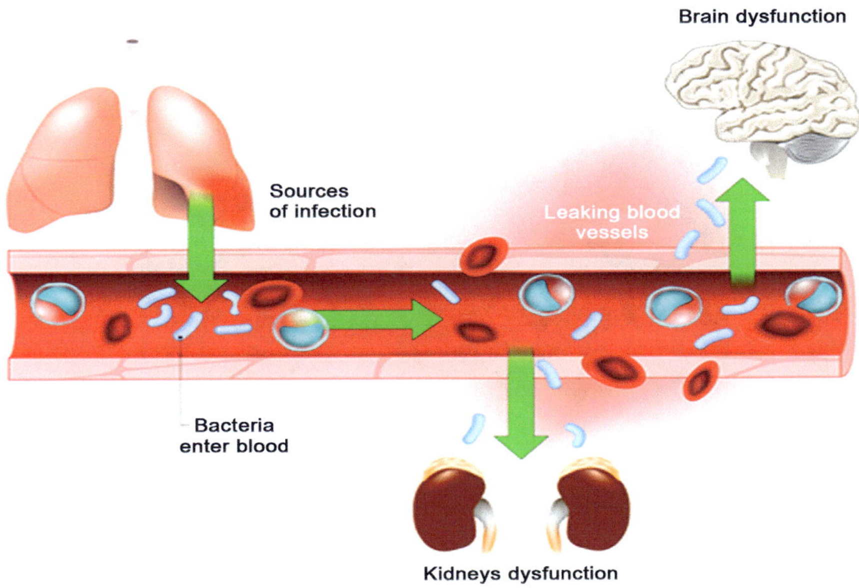

Figure 1.6. Septic shock.

Source: https://external-content.duckduckgo.com/iu/?u=https%3A%2F%2Fi.ytimg.com%2Fvi%2FfZBDRxdc3AU%2Fmaxresdefault.jpg&f=1&nofb=1&ipt=0010e0ec7ffe8c806b4ec5a8084d4162c54d4e80dc803684a6127b51afbebd50.

1.2.3. Cardiac Arrest and Arrhythmias

Cardiac arrest is a potentially lethal medical occurrence characterized by an abrupt loss of practical heart function, which causes systemic circulation to fail. The cornerstone of understanding cardiac arrest relies on the frequency of cardiac arrhythmias that can occur before or with its onset. Arrhythmias are, by definition, aberrant heartbeats whose etiologies and physiological effects are exceedingly variable. For instance, ventricular fibrillation and pulseless electrical activity are two of the most fatal arrhythmias due to their direct diminishment of the heart's capacity for blood circulation. Critical care professionals must be able to easily identify these rhythms on electrocardiogram (ECG) monitoring because immediate intervention is essential in optimizing patient prognosis in such life-threatening cases. Moreover, understanding the pathophysiological basis of such arrhythmias becomes paramount in making effective therapeutic decisions aimed at the restoration of normal rhythm and function. During cardiac arrest, arrhythmias are most often caused by situations such as ischemic heart disease, electrolyte imbalance, and congenital heart defects. Acute coronary ischemia, for example, is a common cause of potentially lethal rhythms because damage to the myocardium will lead to significant conduction abnormalities. of note, complete heart block is a severe arrhythmia, in which there is a total dissociation of ventricular and atrial activity resulting in the reduction of heart rate and poor cardiac output. In the context of myocardial infarction (MI), up to an incidence of 8% complete heart block in patients can occur, and the earliest intervention and detection should be obtained to prevent progression to cardiac arrest. Effective management protocols involve proper interpretation of 12-lead ECGs and proper pharmacologic interventions, and therefore, clinician preparedness is of paramount significance in the case of such emergencies (Meloy *et al.*, 2022) (Figure 1.7).

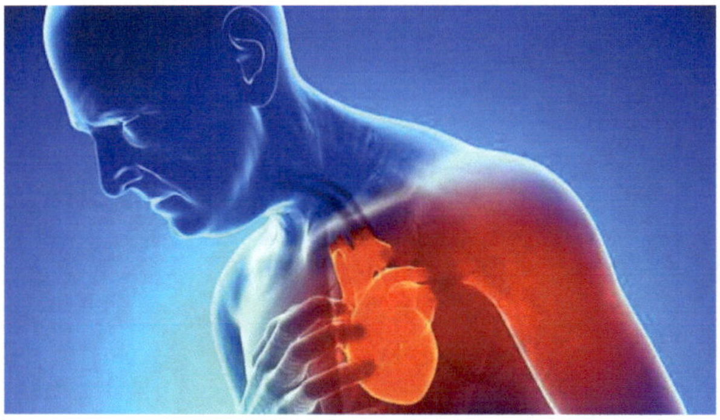

Figure 1.7. Cardiac arrest.

Source: https://thefirstaidcoursesydney.com.au/wp-content/uploads/2021/10/Cardiac-arrest.jpeg.

The significance of early intervention becomes even more vital when considering particular patient populations affected by cardiac arrest and arrhythmias, such as children. In this population, special obstacles are present that demand a specific approach for management according to the variation in metabolic and anatomical elements. Younger pediatric patients who are below the age of five, for example, will have complications with respiratory acidosis and coagulopathy that differ from those in adults. In addition, they are also at risk for lethal bradyarrhythmia that can be prodromal to cardiac arrest. Their evolution demands in-depth insight into how physiology related to aging and possible cardiac derangements interact, underscoring again the requirement of extensive training in critical care environments. Implementation of evidence-based protocols taking these variables into account can enhance outcomes and enable emergency responders to be better able to deliver good care during emergencies (Mojtabaee *et al.*, 2017).

Test Your Knowledge

1. What are the common causes and types of respiratory failure in critical care?
2. How is septic shock differentiated from sepsis in terms of clinical presentation and management?

1.3. Role of the Critical Care Team

Learning Outcome

1. Define composition of the critical care team
2. Describe the responsibilities of critical care physicians
3. Define importance of interdisciplinary collaboration

The critical care team plays a core role in the care of patients who have complex medical needs, particularly in environments of high risk such as ICUs. The critical care team is commonly a multidisciplinary group of intensivists, nurses, respiratory therapists, pharmacists, and other specialist healthcare professionals (HCPs). This collaboration is required to manage the diverse issues of critically ill patients. Every individual within the team brings unique competencies and knowledge, thereby enhancing clinical decision-making processes that can translate into improved patient outcomes. Through building synergistic relationships between team members, the critical care environment becomes a dynamic workplace where evidence-based care is at the forefront, hence elevating the quality of care provided to patients with critical conditions. Effective communication and well-structured protocols within the critical care team provide a framework to deliver high-quality care. Regular team meetings, huddles, and rounds permit the sharing of crucial information among the team members to ensure all members of the team are aligned with patient management goals. Such collaborative practice also enables the team to better react to changing clinical conditions prevalent in critical care settings. Furthermore, the application of standardized instruments in measurement promotes enhanced outcome measurements, which allow for consistent tracking and evaluation of the efficacy of care. Through these measures, the critical care team will be able to deal with complications in a proactive way and forecast healthcare needs ahead of time, hence minimizing threats associated with critical illness. Uniformity of the team as a whole thus finds expression in enhanced resilience in dealing with challenges presented by patients presenting life-threatening conditions.

The critical care team is likewise a motivation for education and innovation in critical care practice. Through regular training, case discussion, and continuous education initiatives, the team members can be updated with the latest developments in critical care medicine, including new modes of therapy and advances in technology. Assuming that the team is highly educated about innovative approaches, this goes beyond enabling single providers to complete gaps in care because it boosts the potential of the health system as a whole. Moreover, the recognition of psychosocial dimensions of critical care works to emphasize the need for incorporating comprehensive patient management. Understanding the emotional and psychological needs of patients and their families is fundamental in critical care environments, providing an integrative model of care that is nurturing and compassionate (Becker *et al.*, 2020; Srivastava *et al.*, 2020) (Figure 1.8).

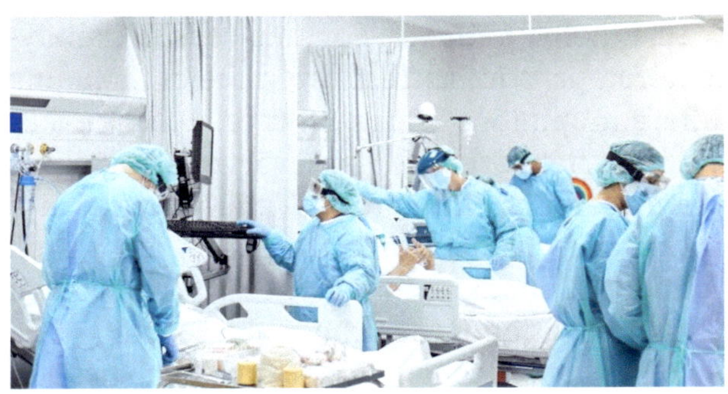

Figure 1.8. The critical care team.

Source: https://www.sriramakrishnahospital.com/wp-content/uploads/2022/04/ICU.jpg.

1.3.1. Composition of the Critical Care Team

How the critical care team is formed is the key to providing good care for patients in intensive care units. There are usually critical care physicians, nurses, respiratory therapists, pharmacists, social workers, and several other specialists working together in this unit. Every member of the team is essential; doctors are in-charge of diagnosing and planning treatment, and nurses provide ongoing care and emotional help to patients. Because everyone on the team works together, healthcare quality improves, and patients and their families are better supported. Having teams collaborate is very important, especially when treating severe medical conditions, since fast decisions and personalized care are necessary to help patients with various medical issues. Family-centered care practices have significantly changed how the critical care team works together. More and more, it is understood that including families in making decisions is vital for better care. Family-centered rounds, which involve both the medical team and the patient's family, are a good example of this new approach. Having families in daily rounds has helped healthcare providers and families communicate better, so the care plan is understood and carried out well. It has been found that working together like this improves the satisfaction of both families and staff, which in turn helps patients. For this reason, family-centered practices stress the value of including different opinions in patient care, which makes the experience better for everyone. Bringing rhetorical and humanities approaches into critical care teams can make patient care even better. The medical humanities try to prevent dehumanization in healthcare by teaching and encouraging reflection. If rhetorical scholars and medical professionals work together, they can improve the curriculum by increasing skills in communication, empathy, and ethical choices in critical care. This area of study highlights the value of patient experiences and stories, supporting a more caring approach to care. With this approach, the critical care team to address all the needs of patients, both medical and emotional, which highlights the importance of complete care that suits each patient's situation.

1.3.2. Responsibilities of Critical Care Physicians

The responsibilities of critical care physicians are multifaceted, encompassing a broad range of clinical and administrative tasks that work to provide the best possible patient outcomes in intensive care settings. Perhaps most prominently, these physicians are responsible for the diagnosis and treatment of life-threatening conditions, which can include complex decision-making maneuvers that require the integration of sophisticated medical knowledge and immediate assessment of patient states. They must communicate well with interprofessional teams to develop and implement holistic care plans tailored to patients' needs. Moreover, in the face of uncertainty that characterizes critical illness, the ability to carry out intricate procedures under pressure is an essential one. This skill set not only emphasizes technical skill, but also the need for effective communication with families of patients and in team settings to establish the foundation for well-informed decision-making within high-stakes decision-making. Beyond care for direct patient needs, critical care physicians are also responsible for the management of ICU resources, a key area for optimizing the provision of care. This administrative aspect involves the management of nursing staff, the regulation of medical supplies, and ensuring institutional rules and clinical guidelines are obeyed. All these need practical leadership skills because these doctors are likely to be the cornerstone of acute care facilities. Furthermore, even with continued challenges such as physician shortages and variations in staffing models, effective strategic planning is critical to maintaining the quality of care in often high-demand environments, as underscored by the recent Iowa ED staffing patterns study findings (Boone *et al.*, 2025). In so doing, physicians navigate the complexity of both patient and institutional logistics; their commitment to ongoing improvement and evidence-based practice must stay strong. The COVID-19 pandemic further emphasized the humongous responsibilities of critical care physicians, compelling them to adapt very quickly in the face of unprecedented issues. As the healthcare scenario transformed dramatically, many physicians were confronted with a knowledge vacuum, and it became very challenging for them to bank on tested medical strategies (Härgestam *et al.*, 2023). In this environment, critical care professionals had to recreate their medical rationality to respond to clinical imperatives and reaffirm their professional ethical responsibilities to patients. They were required to improvise in the provision of care as well as deal with intensified patient loads and resource shortages. The pandemic not only highlighted their clinical skills but also placed a focus on maintaining resilience and flexibility within high-pressure settings, indicating a shift in the scope of their work that will continue to shape critical care medicine in the coming years (Figure 1.9).

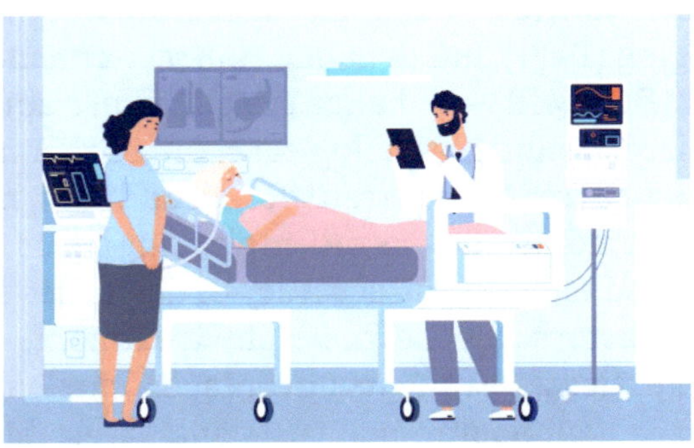

Figure 1.9. Critical care physicians spend their days juggling a myriad of responsibilities while experiencing the roller-coaster ups and downs of both challenges and triumphs.

Source: https://www.healthecareers.com/career-resources/on-the-job/daily-responsibilities-critical-care.

1.3.3. Importance of Interdisciplinary Collaboration

Nowadays, critical care medicine relies more on healthcare professionals working together from various backgrounds. This way of working improves patient outcomes are and also enhances the quality of care given in intensive care units. A team of physicians, nurses, pharmacists, social workers, and spiritual care providers usually forms an interdisciplinary team, each one bringing their skills to patient care. Sharing various opinions helps healthcare workers understand a patient's needs well, so all health issues are handled completely. Collaborating in this way allows different skills and knowledge to come together, which helps improve the way patients are managed. For instance, the integration of spiritual care specialists and mental health professionals has been shown to support both the emotional and psychological dimensions of patient recovery, emphasizing how interdisciplinary teamwork can effectively respond to complex health issues facing critically ill patients (Johnson *et al.*, 2025). Also, working together across different fields and using advanced technology makes critical care even more important. It has been shown by recent studies that tools such as machine learning are now being used to improve clinical diagnostics and help with decision-making. Wang and Long's study demonstrates how artificial intelligence is used to predict the risks of intensive care unit-acquired weakness which is becoming more common in people who are critically ill. The correct use of such technology depends on strong teamwork among different experts to help clinicians use the insights gained. Health professionals must join forces to analyze data and take into account the various needs of patients related to health, emotions, and spirituality. This partnership facilitates the development of tailored therapeutic interventions that lead to better health outcomes and more responsive care environments (Dragonieri, 2024). How healthcare professionals cooperate in critical care medicine affects both patients and their families. When families experience medical difficulties, they often go through emotional and psychological stress, and they need support from many areas to handle these problems. Together, members of an interdisciplinary team can build care plans that address physical health and also take care of patients' spiritual and emotional needs. As noted in reflections on team-based care attempts in pediatric critical care settings, the communication and partnership between chaplains and pediatric psychologists exemplify how interdisciplinary collaboration can enhance patient care (Johnson *et al.*, 2025). By fostering an inclusive atmosphere that values contributions from all disciplines, critical care can be transformed into a more holistic practice that effectively aids patients and their families during their most vulnerable moments (Figure 1.10).

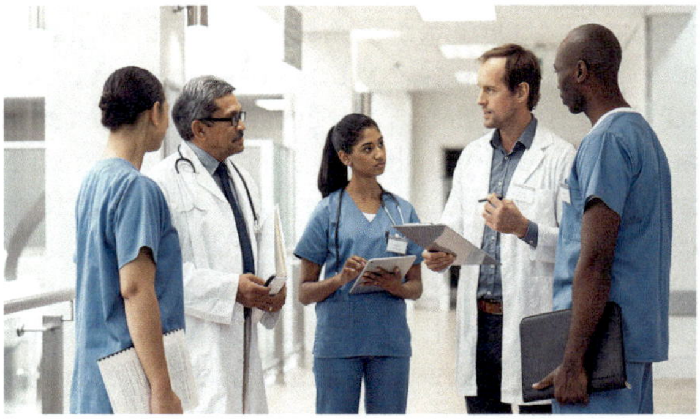

Figure 1.10. Healthcare professionals working together.

Source: https://blog.wcei.net/wp-content/uploads/2024/06/collaborationinhealthcare.jpg.

Test Your Knowledge

1. What are the primary responsibilities of critical care physicians in the ICU?
2. Why is interdisciplinary collaboration essential in delivering effective critical care?

1.4. Diagnostic Tools and Techniques

Learning Outcome

1. Understand the monitoring vital signs and hemodynamics
2. Explain the imaging studies in critical care
3. Define laboratory tests and their significance

Having access to advanced diagnostic tools is very important in managing patients in critical care medicine. Among these tools, Magnetic Resonance Imaging (MRI) offers a sophisticated ability to assess conditions requiring precise imaging. Being able to show high-quality images of soft tissues is very important for spotting and managing medical conditions, mainly those that are malignant. MRI's advanced functionalities—such as diffusion-weighted imaging (DWI) and dynamic contrast-enhanced MRI (DCE-MRI)—enhance the clinician's ability to discern subtle pathological changes that may influence treatment strategies. In addition, new developments such as AI in reading MRIs are expected to boost the accuracy of diagnoses and help doctors choose the right treatments for each patient. Despite its advantages, challenges such as high operational costs and accessibility issues must be addressed to leverage MRI's potential within critical care settings fully (AlHarbi *et al.*, 2024). In addition to MRI, point-of-care ultrasound (POCUS) has emerged as a versatile diagnostic tool, especially relevant in critical care environments. It allows doctors to quickly see and assess patients at the bedside, which helps with fast decision-making in urgent situations. Critical care ultrasound (CCUS) encompasses a range of applications, from cardiac assessments to lung evaluations, underscoring its effectiveness in diverse clinical scenarios. Educators and governing bodies, such as the Accreditation Council for Graduate Medical Education (ACGME), recognize the importance of training fellows in these imaging techniques but have yet to establish comprehensive guidelines. The European Society of Intensive Care Medicine has recently tried to create a common framework for what practitioners should know and how they are assessed. This evolution in training practices highlights the growing recognition of POCUS as a vital component in the armamentarium of critical care diagnostics (Kassutto *et al.*, 2023). Using advanced tools like MRI and POCUS helps healthcare professionals do their job better and also dramatically affects the results for patients in critical care. Working together, imaging and clinical judgment help healthcare providers decide quickly and correctly in serious situations. Also, it is essential to create training courses that teach people how to use these tools, as research continues to find effective ways to measure competence in CCUS. As the area grows, using new imaging tools and updating teaching approaches will help critical care clinicians become experts in using these techniques. Ultimately, these efforts aim to improve patient care protocols and ensure that innovations in diagnostic tools translate into better therapeutic outcomes in critical care medicine (Kassutto *et al.*, 2023).

1.4.1. Monitoring Vital Signs and Hemodynamics

Hemodynamic and vital sign monitoring in critical care medicine is essential to patient safety and successful treatment. These signs, such as heart rate, blood pressure, respiratory rate, and temperature, are all real-time measures of a patient's physiologic status. Monitoring of these parameters in the acute setting allows clinicians to identify possible complications, follow the response to therapy, and intervene promptly. For instance, acute changes in blood pressure may reveal hemorrhage or cardiodynamic malfunction. Monitoring is thus generally continuous with the aid of advanced technology to provide real-time data, which is of the essence in making judicious clinical decisions. Hemodynamic monitoring supplements the assessment of vital signs by providing information concerning the function of the circulatory system, particularly cardiac output and fluid status. It is extremely necessary to properly evaluate hemodynamics, especially in patients with severe illness or patients suffering from diseases like Acute Heart Failure (AHF). Presently, guidelines emphasize the necessity of proper evaluation of hemodynamics to initiate appropriate treatment early.

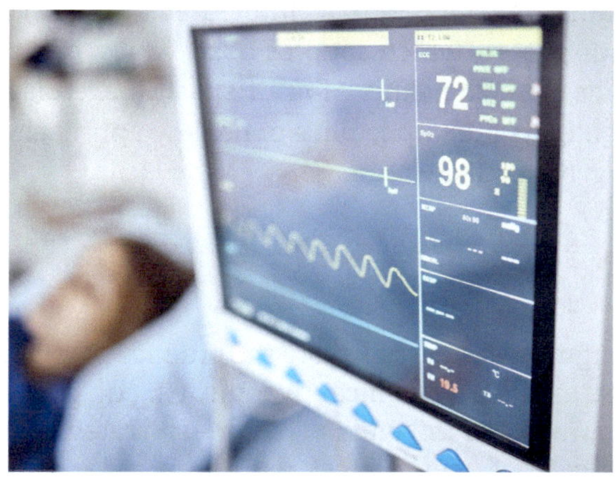

Figure 1.11. Vital signs monitoring.

Source: https://nhcps.com/wp-content/uploads/2024/08/hemodynamic-instability-patient-vital-signs.jpg.

In our current practice, routine methods of hemodynamic status evaluation are largely invasive, which poses a risk to the patient. Therefore, there is a growing demand for precise noninvasive devices that offer continuous monitoring of cardiac hemodynamics and fluid load to facilitate the individualization of interventions based on patients' particular requirements (Somma *et al.*, 2021) (Figure 1.11).

Furthermore, the implementation of formalized nursing guidelines alongside hemodynamic monitoring has proven beneficial in optimizing patient outcomes. Evidence indicates that the implementation of exercise protocols by nurses will optimize hemodynamic values and functional capacity among patients after cardiac surgery. These protocols generally emphasize respiratory physiotherapy, ambulation, and tailored exercise programs, all of which optimize patient recovery while taking great care of vital signs. Effective nursing interventions not only improve physiological parameters but also reduce complications and improve overall well-being in critical care units (Gamal *et al.*, 2019). This integrated approach to patient care, which couples observation of vital signs with the utilization of specific exercises, highlights the importance of holistic approaches to critical care medicine.

1.4.2. Imaging Studies in Critical Care

Imaging tests are central to the practice of critical care medicine, significantly improving diagnostic accuracy and informing treatment strategies. In the case of acute illness or trauma, timely and accurate imaging can demonstrate underlying pathology that is not necessarily evident on physical exam alone. Technologies like CT scans, MRIs, and ultrasounds enable doctors to see through organ structures, measure the severity of the injury, and track disease progression. The speed with which images are acquired is essentialin critical care, where time is of the essence. Adding these cutting-edge imaging technologies to everyday practice ensures that clinical decision-making is informed, ultimately producing better patient outcomes as well as more efficient use of healthcare system resources. As the technological environment continues evolving, the integration of artificial intelligence (AI) into imaging examinations is a potential that augurs well for the future of critical care practice. AI algorithms can assist in the analysis of vast amounts of imaging data, thereby improving the accuracy of the interpretation and reducing the time needed for diagnostic evaluation. This is particularly crucial in the emergency department, where advanced imaging technology can assist in the expedient diagnosis of conditions such as stroke, pulmonary embolism, and abdominal emergencies. In addition to this, AI-driven models can improve the imaging process itself, enabling quick provision of vital diagnostic information. Despite these advancements, medical imaging with AI necessitates careful consideration of ethical factors, regulatory contexts, and putting in place robust validation frameworks to demonstrate its effectiveness and safety in critical care settings (Biesheuvel *et al.*, 2024).

Furthermore, the increased complexity and volume of imaging data in critical care necessitate even more interdisciplinary coordination while managing patients. There should be close collaboration among radiologists, intensivists, and other clinicians to interpret imaging tests and make effective use of them in clinical care plans. Diagnostic accuracy is maximized, and optimal treatment plans tailored to individual patient needs are developed through the collaborative process. Ongoing education and training in the use of imaging modalities are also required so that healthcare providers are competent enough to operate these technologies in effective ways. As imaging examinations become increasingly seminal in shaping critical care medicine, ongoing contention regarding their application and ethics will be the hallmark of maximizing their potential benefit in patient care (Chen *et al.*, 2025) (Figure 1.12).

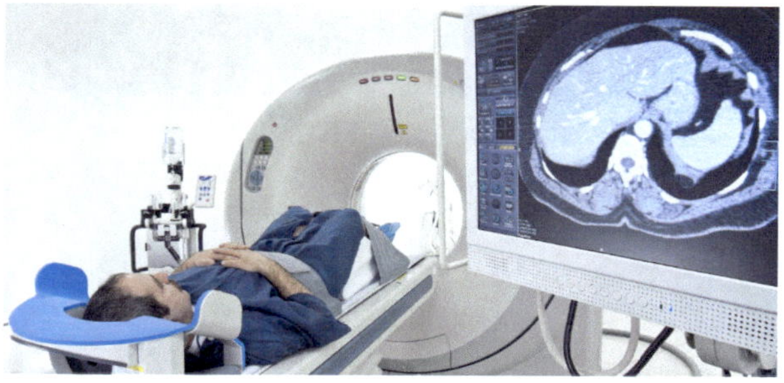

Figure 1.12. Advanced medical imaging has revolutionized critical health care.

Source: https://www.pbmchealth.org/news-events/blog/various-types-medical-imaging-explained.

1.4.3. Laboratory Tests and Their Significance

Laboratory studies form the core practice of critical care medicine, as necessary diagnostics, monitoring, and management devices for critically ill patients. Laboratory tests provide essential information about various physiological processes, enabling healthcare providers to make timely, evidence-based decisions. Specifically, systemic inflammatory marker quantification measured by the Neutrophil-to-Lymphocyte Ratio (NLR) and Systemic Immune-Inflammation Index (SII) has been emphasized for its prognostic value, notably in diseases like COVID-19. The significance of these laboratory values lies in their ability to detect the relationship between inflammation and nutrition, both of which are vital to measure the patient's risk for unfavorable outcomes throughout the process of hospitalization. As shown in research, inflammatory markers at the systemic level have the potential to provide critical information for mortality risk evaluation among acutely ill patients (Wani *et al.*, 2025). In critical care, laboratory tests are not only employed to aid in diagnosis but also as prognostic markers to guide treatment and management in patients. A good case in point is the Haemoglobin Albumin Lymphocyte Platelet (HALP) index that has been identified as a novel biomarker in predicting the prognosis of patients with COVID-19. Studies have established a low HALP index to be in line with higher hospital stay and in-hospital mortality, which speaks to its utility in the clinical setting. The HALP index integrates several laboratory variables, both indicative of a patient's inflammatory process and nutritional status, and thus gives a general picture of a patient's condition. This dual role of laboratory tests—both as markers of disease progression and predictors of treatment response—underscores their vital role in intensive care units (Wani *et al.*, 2025).

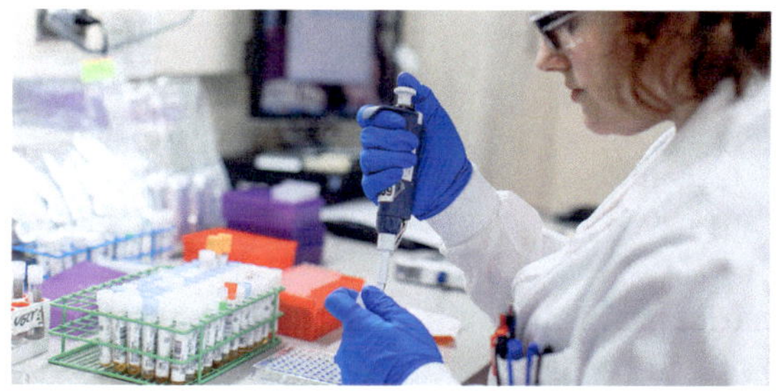

Figure 1.13. Laboratory tests play a pivotal role in critical care medicine.

Source: https://www.labtestingmatters.org/wp-content/uploads/2019/10/generic-8.jpg.

In addition, laboratory tests make ongoing monitoring of patients' conditions possible, making them indispensable in ICUs. For instance, the Acute Gastrointestinal Injury (AGI) score has been developed to describe and categorize gut dysfunction, a frequent occurrence among critically ill patients. Research has identified a close relationship between AGI and mortality rates, suggesting the prognostic relevance of gastrointestinal function in this population. Utilization of laboratory reports to monitor several parameters, such as fluid balance and creatinine, provides valuable information for clinicians that can guide therapy. Therefore, continuous monitoring via laboratory tests facilitates early interventions, eventually maximizing patient outcomes and reducing morbidity in critical care patients (Figure 1.13).

Test Your Knowledge

1. How does continuous monitoring of vital signs and hemodynamics guide critical care decisions?
2. What imaging studies are commonly used in critical care, and for what purposes?

1.5. Treatment Modalities in Critical Care

Learning Outcome

1. Discuss the pharmacological interventions
2. Define mechanical ventilation and respiratory support
3. Explain the nutritional support and management

In critical care medicine, patient treatment relies on a variety of treatment approaches tailored to address the various needs of the critically ill patient. Contemporary knowledge of combined medical care focuses on the requirement for a multidisciplinary treatment approach in managing problems such as facial palsy. For instance, a study highlighted that over 75% of traditional Korean medicine doctors have adopted integrated medical systems, utilizing modalities such as acupuncture, herbal medicine, and thermal therapy, alongside conventional treatments like corticosteroids and antivirals. This blending of traditional and contemporary practices suggests the necessity to create critical pathways that incorporate different types of therapeutic interventions for the advanced care of complex health conditions, thereby enhancing patient outcomes and enhancing the effectiveness of treatment plans in intensive care settings (Kim *et al.*, 2022). Apart from the integration of various medical modalities, management of some complications in critical care focuses on the importance of efficient treatment modalities. Among the most frequent issues is postextubation dysphagia, which affects patient recovery extensively and increases the risk of complications such as aspiration pneumonia. With approximately 517,000 patients receiving mechanical ventilation every year, the occurrence of postextubation dysphagia varies, recognizing the impact of the condition. Screening tests such as the water swallow test have been proven to reveal that about 12% of ICU patients experience aspiration after extubation, and hence, immediate interventions are necessary. Consequently, identification of the symptoms and implementation of effective care mechanisms are crucial in ensuring patient safety and the decrease of the burden on healthcare systems (Brodsky *et al.*, 2020). Furthermore, the establishment and application of evidence-based clinical pathways are critical in the process of simplifying treatment modalities in critical care.

The pathways incorporate best practice from conventional as well as complementary therapies to enable healthcare providers to deliver standardized and evidence-based care. By combining holistic assessments and interventions, as observed in studies into facial palsy treatments, critical care teams can enhance both the quality and efficiency of patient care. Creation of clinical practice guidelines using solid evidence also encourages continuous improvement in outcome measures, motivating critical care practitioners to remain alert and responsive amidst shifting patient demands. This harmony of multi-disciplinary care is the core of the nature of critical care medicine, essentially striving for optimal patient recovery and well-being while avoiding potential complications.

1.5.1. Pharmacological Interventions

Pharmacotherapy plays a critical role in the management of patients in critical care settings, where there may be an urgent need for a therapeutic response due to the nature of critical illness. The medications are supposed to yield a reaction to resulting pathophysiological conditions and to avoid further deterioration of patient health. However, the effectiveness of pharmacological therapy has been questioned in the last few years, with numerous clinical trials yielding inconclusive results. An important point of note is that pharmacologic therapies can fail to demonstrate overt advantages due to the uniformity of patient groups, such as in ARDS and sepsis, for instance, that are often grouped according to syndromic rather than their distinct biological underpinnings (Reddy *et al.*, 2021). Hence, an appeal for a more refined approach based on individual patient characteristics is gathering strength in the realm of critical care medicine. The identification of biologically relevant subphenotypes of critical illness syndromes is a vibrant field for enhancing the effectiveness of pharmacological treatments. Research has indicated that individuals who approach the clinic with the same clinical syndromes can have different biological markers and responses to treatment, and hence, there exists a requirement for individually oriented therapeutic approaches (Reddy *et al.*, 2021). This being the case, pharmacological treatments may be optimized for specific subgroups of patients more than following a uniform treatment strategy. For instance, more recent retrospective studies have shown that certain subphenotypes of ARDS are highly predictive of mortality, again supporting the hypothesis that these biological distinctions reflect significant predictors for targeted therapy (Reddy *et al.*, 2021). This kind of study points towards a paradigm shift in critical care, positioning pharmacologic treatments to address not only symptomatology but also more closely align with actual pathophysiologic disease mechanisms. In addition, non-pharmacological delirium therapies, in many respects the stepchild of pharmacologic therapy discussions, add an added level of intricacy in critical care management. A systematic review found that many studies on delirium interventions have systematically excluded palliative care patients despite having data showing these patients have similar characteristics that are pertinent to delirium. Such exclusion gives rise to serious concerns on the applicability and efficacy of pharmacological interventions among such a patient population. Moreover, few studies recruited palliative care patients, and none of these were clearly described or provided detailed results, which made it difficult to understand how pharmacologic therapy might function among these patient populations. It is thus of utmost importance to formulate models that include all patient populations in critical care so that pharmacologic interventions are both practical as well as justifiable in a variety of clinical settings (Figure 1.14).

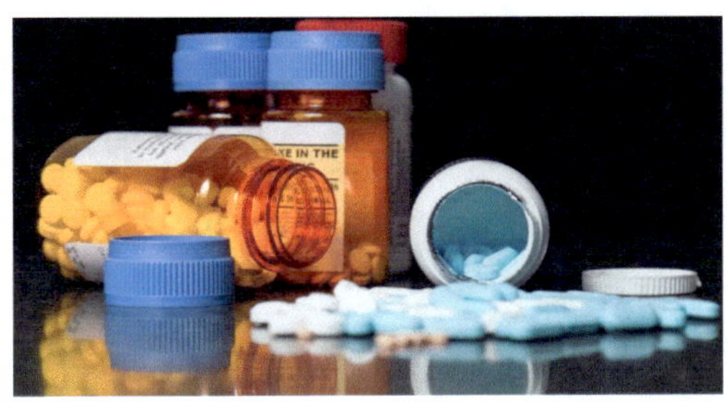

Figure 1.14. Pharmacological Interventions in critical care settings.

Source: https://www.findatopdoc.com/var/fatd/storage/images/_aliases/fb_thumb/healthy-living/medical-advancements-new-treatments-and-perspectives-on-fibromyalgia/pharmacological-treatments/3584078-1-eng-US/Pharmacological-treatments.jpg.

1.5.2. Mechanical Ventilation and Respiratory Support

The role of mechanical ventilation has increasingly been more essential in critical care medicine, particularly among critically ill patients with acute respiratory failure. Mechanical ventilation facilitates the exchange of gases in the lungs, hence delivering oxygen to essential organs while simultaneously eliminating carbon dioxide. This intervention is of much concern in conditions such as bronchiectasis, where patients may present with chronic bacterial infections and severe exacerbations that may lead to respiratory failure. As evidence supports, the failure of non-invasive ventilation (NIV) in the management of bronchiectasis exacerbations may be greater than 25%, and thus, strict assessment and immediate intervention are warranted in these circumstances. Although NIV is likely to reduce ICU stay, its limitations necessitate the aid of invasive mechanical ventilation in situations where patients do not stabilize or improve with NIV (Ranjan *et al.*, 2024) (Figure 1.15).

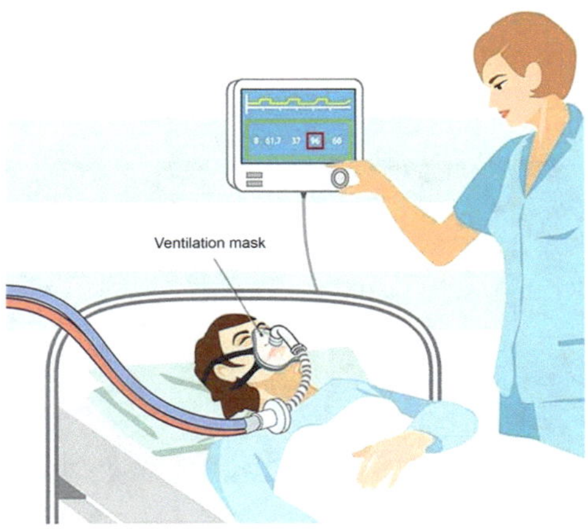

Figure 1.15. Managing the patient on mechanical ventilation.

Source: https://www.informedhealth.org/grafiken/en_lunge_beatmung_maske_replacement_image.jpg.

Furthermore, the evolution of respiratory support technology has also introduced the use of alternatives such as high-flow nasal cannula (HFNC) therapy, a less invasive form of therapy than traditional methods, including routine oxygen therapy. HFNC provides heated and humidified air at higher flow rates that eliminate upper airway dead space and may improve oxygenation without causing the risks of re-intubation or prolonged mechanical ventilation. During clinical trials comparing its efficacy with standard oxygen therapy, HFNC demonstrated a significant reduction in the rates of treatment failure, highlighting its application post-extubation in mechanically ventilated patients. This breakthrough has been a paradigm shift in the treatment of respiratory failure, with a focus on individualizing respiratory support based on the requirements of the patient (Angurana *et al.*, 2024). Finally, the decision-making process involved in choosing the proper mode of respiratory support demands a multi-faceted approach. Variables such as the underlying patient condition, the severity of the respiratory failure, and the response to early treatment all play essentialroles in determining the appropriateness of invasive versus non-invasive support. Ongoing monitoring is required to evaluate the effectiveness of the intervention strategy used, particularly in light of the risk for complications with each modality. Consequently, understanding the nuances of mechanical ventilation and respiratory support not only enhances patient outcomes but also helps to assist with the overall goals of critical care management—stabilizing the patient and allowing for recovery within an appropriate time span. Continued development of critical care medicine will realize greater benefit from research that will further refine these therapeutic strategies and improve the delivery of care within the ICU setting.

1.5.3. Nutritional Support and Management

In critical care medicine, nutrition support becomes a vital factor in the improvement of patient outcomes. Nutrition care is needed not just to sustain energy but also to aid in recovery and avoid complications. For critically ill children and adults, particularly, the complexity of the condition necessitates individualized nutritional strategies that consider underlying disease and the physiological insult of illness. Comprehensive nutritional support involves careful planning that may include specialized supplements and modifications based on the individual patient's needs. Notably, deficiencies in nutrients can yield huge adverse consequences, exacerbating a critically ill patient's already poor condition. Therefore, medical teams should have high priority in making timely assessments and interventions so that nutritional needs are adequately addressed for the duration of the patient's intensive care stay. Enteral nutrition (EN) plays a vital role in the administration of proper nutrition care in critical care, particularly in pediatric illnesses. It has been indicated in evidence that the initiation of EN early is associated with good clinical outcomes, but its delay results in prolonged fasting and inadequate energy intake, thus posing the risk of complications. Research has found that children undergoing surgery, particularly children with congenital heart defects, are more likely to exhibit immediate delays in EN advancement. In such patients, failure to meet energy and micronutrient requirements may significantly hinder healing and prolong hospital stay. To counteract these hindrances, caregivers should prioritize EN administration and implement strategies to minimize feeding breaks, thereby ensuring a maximum energy supply and enhancing the quality of care provided to critically ill children (Slater *et al.*, 2014). Multidisciplinary intervention is the cornerstone of efficient adoption of nutritional care in critical care medicine. Health practitioners from diverse specialties, including doctors, nurses, and nutritionists, must collaborate in devising and executing effective dietary strategies that overcome the particular problems of critically ill patients. For instance, in biliary atresia conditions, the curative process not only encompasses nutritional therapy but also ongoing medical observation and appropriately timed intervention strategies like liver transplantation (Hadzic *et al.*, 2012). This coordinated plan is required to optimize patient outcomes, since it encompasses supplementation with fat-soluble vitamins, regular assessments of nutritional needs, and continuous adjustment of nutritional therapy according to clinical courses. Finally, an orchestrated approach for nutritional care optimizes recovery patterns and highlights the importance of cohesive care in critical illness environments (Figure 1.16).

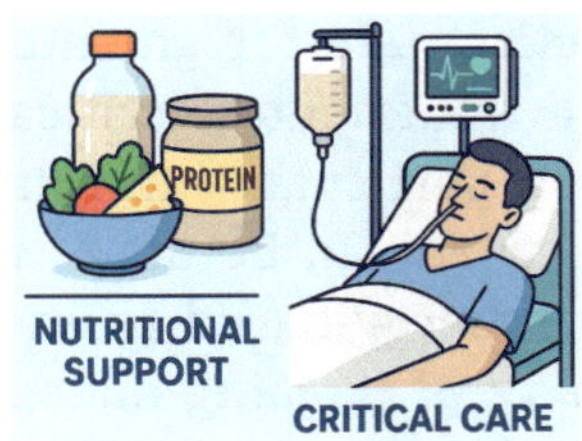

Figure 1.16. Nutritional Support and Management.

Source: https://sdmntprsouthcentralus.oaiusercontent.com/files/00000000-f9c4-61f7-9a87-5b3e1233bd2c/raw?se=2025-05-02T12%3A29%3A41Z&sp=r&sv=2024-08-04&sr=b&scid=f9184f9e-2ca0-5e33-b5e8-08d832076dc7&skoid=365eb242-95ba-4335-a618-2c9f8f766a86&sktid=a48cca56-e6da-484e-a814-9c849652bcb3&skt=2025-05-02T02%3A46%3A33Z&ske=2025-05-03T02%3A46%3A33Z&sks=b&skv=2024-08-04&sig=GhJF8zQD3sO9vvpFndcEZjDb2Tp6T8D517skdTZV2HE%3D.

Test Your Knowledge

1. What are common pharmacological interventions used in critical care settings?
2. When is mechanical ventilation indicated for respiratory support in ICU patients?

SUMMARY

A summary of a journey into Critical Care Medicine reveals the complexity and rapid evolution of this field of medicine. Technology progression, particularly the incorporation of artificial intelligence within ICUs, is challenging yet promising to health professionals. As indicated, although immense potential of AI in refining patient monitoring and decision-making, its application in critical practice, such as mechanical ventilation management, remains in its nascent stages. A guarded response is in order, prioritizing ethical implications, regulatory guidelines, and the need for extensive training, aligning AI functionalities with clinical practice. In the end, these advances highlight the need to enhance clinical results through judicious and responsible adoption of advancing technologies. The use of AI within critical care medicine is not just a case of mere monitoring; it is an arena for enhancing patient care as a whole and optimizing healthcare processes. As outlined, AI's potential to predict patient outcomes and augment clinical decision-making has the potential to make critical care settings more efficient. However, the success of AI technologies is contingent upon transparency and comprehension of suggestions generated by AI by healthcare professionals. Mitigating these pitfalls, e.g., ascertaining the dependability and robustness of AI systems, is integral in fostering trust in these technologies. In addition, with the advancement of AI, the integration of feedback from practice can help refine these tools for use in the critically ill patient's benefit. In conclusion, the future of Critical Care Medicine holds much promise anchored in technology and new practices. A strategic integration of AI has the potential to create a paradigm shift in the diagnosis and treatment of critically ill patients. Yet, research must fill the necessary gaps that currently exist, particularly in relation to safe and effective use of AI in patient care. Continuous research into what can be done with AI, coupled with solid training of healthcare professionals, will create a synergy-based relationship that optimizes critical care benefits. The findings point to the necessity of ongoing dialogue and research because the potential consequences of AI on the healthcare industry are multifarious and necessitate meticulous attention to patient safety as well as quality of care (Misseri *et al.*, 2024; Saqib *et al.*, 2023).

Technology, in critical care medicine, has revolutionized the management and outcome of patients to a great extent. One of the most critical advancements in this field is the application of AI, which holds the central position of emergency medical dispatch and triage. AI-based systems enhance patient assessment speed and accuracy, allowing interventions to be made in time, which could be lifesaving. Existing evidence indicates that such models not only employ huge patient data but also excel humans in retrospectively predicting outcomes. Thus, the application of AI in ICUs facilitates effective monitoring and early warning systems that can forecast complications, thereby simplifying clinical processes and improving care quality provided to critically ill patients (Biesheuvel *et al.*, 2024). Also, the role of laboratory medicine in critical care has evolved from that of a service organization to an active participant in clinical decision-making. With advances in automated systems, laboratory professionals are now directly involved in test ordering and results interpretation, phases which are known to carry a higher risk of error. By optimizing these processes through effective demand management interventions, healthcare professionals are in a position to facilitate prompt diagnosis of otherwise potentially undetected conditions. The focus on patient safety enhancement and adherence to clinical guidelines also underscores the increasing importance of laboratory contribution to critical care settings, illustrating how advancements result in better patient outcomes (Salinas *et al.*, 2024). Besides, the challenges in integrating new technology in critical care medicine cannot be overlooked. While AI and high-technology laboratory procedures hold bright promise, ethics, law, and technical issues present tremendous barriers to their acceptance worldwide. For instance, the challenge of verifying AI models remains a serious issue since it compromises decision-making processes in settings where stakes are as high as in the ICU. To overcome these challenges, joint action by healthcare professionals, policymakers, and technology innovators. A coordinated effort towards broad training, ethics-based practice, and patient-centric focus will be fundamental to unlocking the full potential of these innovations to revolutionize critical care medicine and make progress serve a purpose in enhancing patient care (Biesheuvel *et al.*, 2024; Salinas *et al.*, 2024).

KEY TERMS FROM THIS CHAPTER

- Acute care
- Critical care medicine
- Dialysis
- Early goal-directed therapy (EGDT)
- Ethical dilemmas in the ICU
- Hemodynamic monitoring
- ICU-Acquired Infections
- Inotropes
- Intensive care unit (ICU)
- Life support
- Mechanical ventilation
- Multidisciplinary team
- Oxygen therapy
- Patient-centered care
- Triage
- Vasopressors

CRITICAL THINKING QUESTIONS

1. **Which of the following best defines critical care medicine?**
   a. The long-term management of chronic illnesses
   b. The treatment of only cardiac-related emergencies
   c. The specialized care of patients with life-threatening conditions requiring comprehensive monitoring and support
   d. Basic first aid is provided in emergency rooms
2. **What is the primary goal of intensive care units (ICUs)?**
   a. To provide long-term rehabilitation
   b. To deliver general outpatient services
   c. To manage stable patients
   d. To support and stabilize critically ill patients with organ dysfunction
3. **Which of the following professionals is typically part of the critical care team?**
   a. Dermatologist
   b. Intensivist
   c. Pathologist
   d. Orthodontist
4. **Which of the following is a common indication for admission to an ICU?**
   a. Mild asthma
   b. Stable hypertension
   c. Septic shock
   d. Common cold
5. **What does the term "mechanical ventilation" refer to in critical care?**
   a. A method to treat broken bones
   b. Manual CPR performed continuously
   c. A machine-assisted process to help a patient breathe
   d. A nutritional support system

Short Answer Questions

1. What major medical and technological advances contributed to the development of modern critical care medicine?
2. Name three common conditions that often require critical care intervention.
3. Who are the key members of a critical care team, and what are their primary responsibilities?
4. What diagnostic tools are commonly used to monitor patients in critical care settings?
5. Describe two life-sustaining treatment modalities frequently used in critical care units.
6. How does effective teamwork and timely diagnostics impact patient outcomes in critical care medicine?

Answer to Critical Thinking Questions

1. (c); 2. (d); 3. (b); 4. (c); 5. (c)

REFERENCES

1. AlHarbi, N. M., AlHarbi, F. H., Al-Shalali, A. M. S., Alheary, W. E., Althbyani, B. M., Alaeinbawi, M. H., Alrehaili, H. A. S., *et al.* (2024). Advancing cancer care: A critical review of MRI imaging in pretherapeutic malignancy assessment. *Journal of Eco Humanism*. https://www.semanticscholar.org/paper/c9568d93158e1d4c36f812365837c018adbbe75c (accessed on 22 May 2025).

2. Amin, M. B., Greene, F. L., Edge, S. B., Compton, C. C., Shen, H., Brookland, R. K., Meyer, L., *et al.* (2017). The eighth edition AJCC cancer staging manual: Continuing to build a bridge from a population-based to a more "personalized" approach to cancer staging. *CA: A Cancer Journal for Clinicians, 67*, 93–99. https://doi.org/10.3322/caac.21388.

3. Angurana, S., Sudeep, K., Nallasamy, K., Bansal, A., & Jayashree, M. (2024). High flow nasal cannula vs conventional oxygen therapy and incidence of post extubation airway obstruction in PICU: An open-label randomized controlled trial (Hiflocot-PICU Trial). *Indian Journal of Critical Care Medicine, 28*(Suppl 1), S424–S426. https://www.semanticscholar.org/paper/395fcb4c5bf36aded23494c48e8ca03a944090c0 (accessed on 22 May 2025).

4. April, M., & Murray, B. (2017). Cost-effectiveness analysis appraisal and application: An emergency medicine perspective. *Academic Emergency Medicine, 24*, 754–768. https://www.semanticscholar.org/paper/c34dddd8cea13e3fbeb93e8c859a3034250623b9 (accessed on 22 May 2025).

5. Becker, W. C., & Fiellin, D. A. (2020). When epidemics collide: Coronavirus disease 2019 (COVID-19) and the opioid crisis. *Annals of Internal Medicine, 173*, 59–60. https://doi.org/10.7326/m20-1210.

6. Biesheuvel, L., Dongelmans, D., & Elbers, P. (2024). Artificial intelligence to advance acute and intensive care medicine. *Current Opinion in Critical Care, 30*, 246–250. https://www.semanticscholar.org/paper/790a5f0072d08fd7a133703f569be138e73ce5be (accessed on 22 May 2025).

7. Boone, N., Samuelson, T., Mohr, N., Whitaker, N., Jennett, B., & Kluesner, N. (2025). Iowa emergency departments lack board-certified emergency physicians: A comprehensive statewide emergency department workforce study. *Academic Emergency Medicine*. https://www.semanticscholar.org/paper/90d65304a1fbadfee429e5c9e63ca1797acfd0e2 (accessed on 22 May 2025).

8. Brodsky, M., Nollet, J. L., Spronk, P., & González-Fernández, M. (2020). Prevalence, pathophysiology, diagnostic modalities, and treatment options for dysphagia in critically ill patients. *American Journal of Physical Medicine & Rehabilitation, 99*, 1164–1170. https://www.semanticscholar.org/paper/66390cad3df803d4301607e91733e3c6a0a710c4 (accessed on 22 May 2025).

9. Campbell, L. (2017). The rhetoric of health and medicine as a "teaching subject": Lessons from the medical humanities and simulation pedagogy. https://core.ac.uk/download/213073246.pdf (accessed on 22 May 2025).

10. Chastre, J., & Luyt, C. (2017). Controversies and evolving concepts in hospital-acquired pneumonia. *Seminars in Respiratory and Critical Care Medicine, 38*(3), 235–236. https://www.semanticscholar.org/paper/0b6b7dbd14edab6c26bc0b5f918e803d13312e7f (accessed on 22 May 2025).

11. Chen, D., & Sami, A. (2025). Introduction to the 102st volume of the UTMJ issue on technology in medicine. *University of Toronto Medical Journal*. https://www.semanticscholar.org/paper/8659425df138ccc81168103161a428d8ad65bbec (accessed on 22 May 2025).

12. Di Somma, S. (2021). An update of armamentarium for non-invasive cardiac hemodynamics and congestion evaluation for acute heart failure patients. https://core.ac.uk/download/386962064.pdf (accessed on 22 May 2025).

13. Dragonieri, S. (2024). Pioneering role of machine learning in unveiling intensive care unit-acquired weakness. *World Journal of Clinical Cases, 12*, 2157–2159. https://www.semanticscholar.org/paper/a5e8f578a85491dc1d672938e1aa5463058b74e0 (accessed on 22 May 2025).

14. Elsner, R. (2022). A philosopher goes to the doctor: A critical look at philosophical assumptions in medicine, by Dien Ho. *Cambridge Quarterly of Healthcare Ethics, 31*(1), 141–143. https://www.semanticscholar.org/paper/835ceba750b8a528b8428bd37b3289087cc7aa00 (accessed on 22 May 2025).

15. Fernández-Sarmiento, J., Ranjit, S., Sanchez-Pinto, L. N., Nadkarni, V. M., Jabornisky, R., & Kissoon, N. (2025). The resuscitation, equilibrium and de-escalation (RED) strategy: A phased, personalized hemodynamic support in children with sepsis. *Frontiers in Pediatrics, 13*(1). https://www.semanticscholar.org/paper/fcfe4030fadd844eb95140019702093b9623a9a8 (accessed on 22 May 2025).

16. Fuleihan, R., & Etzioni, A. (2012). Primary immunodeficiency diseases: Past, present and future. *Current Opinion in Allergy and Clinical Immunology, 12*(6), 575–576. https://www.semanticscholar.org/paper/6a232551ff6ed438bfca3d4333735f5400843fae (accessed on 22 May 2025).

17. Gamal, L., Hassan, M., Mohammed, A., & Mubarak, H. (2019). Effect of nursing exercise protocol on hemodynamics and functional capacity among patients after cardiac surgery. https://core.ac.uk/download/524771840.pdf (accessed on 22 May 2025).

18. Giamello, J., Savioli, G., Longhitano, Y., Ferrari, F., D'Agnano, S., Esposito, C., Tesauro, M., *et al.* (2024). The role of acetazolamide in critical care and emergency medicine. *Journal of Geriatric Cardiology, 21*(11), 1085–1095. https://www.semanticscholar.org/paper/649155d90ac7c2336dfe2d94681f5e05c7abcff2 (accessed on 22 May 2025).

19. Glasbey, J., Bibi, S., Pata, F., Özkan, B. B., van Straten, S. V., Hodson, J., Chapman, S., *et al.* (2021). P131: Transferring critically ill COVID-19 patients in ITU—A multidisciplinary training exercise. *BJS Open, 5*(1). https://www.semanticscholar.org/paper/129b1add1cb076ba8595b5c6fa6bd2f695db0de4 (accessed on 22 May 2025).

20. Hadzic, N. (2012). Review: Medical management of 'failing' Kasai portoenterostomy. https://core.ac.uk/download/478307962.pdf (accessed on 22 May 2025).

21. Härgestam, M., Jacobsson, M., Bååthe, F., & Brulin, E. (2023). Challenges in preserving the "good doctor" norm: Physicians' discourses on changes to the medical logic during the initial wave of the COVID-19 pandemic. *Frontiers in Psychology, 14*. https://www.semanticscholar.org/paper/90d091b697ff6bd6be495ae2beecb8e0e93b6ab4 (accessed on 22 May 2025).

22. Hosie, A., Siddiqi, N., Featherstone, I., Johnson, M. J., Lawlor, P., Bush, S., Amgarth-Duff, I., *et al.* (2019). Inclusion, characteristics and outcomes of people requiring palliative care in studies of non-pharmacological interventions for delirium: A systematic review. *Palliative*

Medicine, 33(8), 878–899. https://www.semanticscholar.org/paper/032e7651eabab2c81dc51f01c50cf8155c937cb3 (accessed on 22 May 2025).

23. Johnson, M., Butts, I. R., Ashworth, R., Smith, J., Marik, P., Davies, W., & Rothschild, C. (2025). Navigating critical moments: The importance of spiritual and psychosocial collaboration in addressing coping in the pediatric ICU. *Clinical Practice in Pediatric Psychology*. https://www.semanticscholar.org/paper/42f23a1829fd12677ae5168cb0b3977ebf0f6206 (accessed on 22 May 2025).
24. Kassutto, S., & Baston, C. (2023). Entrusting the process: Assessment of critical care ultrasound skills in fellowship trainees. *ATS Scholar, 4*, 8–11. https://www.semanticscholar.org/paper/ba2d29c9b384635e5754d0cf5cff6843c22ce9ab (accessed on 22 May 2025).
25. Kim, J. H., Goo, B., & Nam, S. S. (2022). A spadework for integrative medicine-based critical pathways for facial palsy: Web-based survey from traditional Korean medicine doctors. *Medicine, 101*. https://www.semanticscholar.org/paper/4146cbefa47b2aa41dcdd7646cd7b9c7988a42b9 (accessed on 22 May 2025).
26. Kochanek, P. M., Tasker, R. C., Carney, N., Totten, A. M., Adelson, P. D., Selden, N. R., Davis-O'Reilly, C., *et al.* (2019). Guidelines for the management of pediatric severe traumatic brain injury, third edition: Update of the Brain Trauma Foundation Guidelines. *Pediatric Critical Care Medicine, 20*(Suppl 1), S1–S82. https://doi.org/10.1097/pcc.0000000000001735.
27. Kruk, M. E., Gage, A., Arsenault, C., Jordan, K., Leslie, H. H., Roder-DeWan, S., Adeyi, O., *et al.* (2018). High-quality health systems in the Sustainable Development Goals era: Time for a revolution. *The Lancet Global Health, 6*, e1196–e1252. https://doi.org/10.1016/s2214-109x(18)30386-3.
28. McGain, F. (2018). The Washington Manual of Critical Care (3rd ed.). *Anesthesia & Analgesia*. https://www.semanticscholar.org/paper/e9c7f0e5d86fd23c34a1b9f60fe68987de2f2a5f (accessed on 22 May 2025).
29. Medetalibeyoğlu, H., Velichko, Y., Hart, E. M., & Bagci, U. (2024). Foundational artificial intelligence models and modern medical practice. *BJR Artificial Intelligence, 2*(1). https://www.semanticscholar.org/paper/eb08ca9f819f54fe8eb3110a4a9feb22fad35ca1 (accessed on 22 May 2025).
30. Meloy, P. G., Rutz, D. R., & Bhambri, A. (2022). 3rd-degree atrioventricular block. *Journal of Education & Teaching in Emergency Medicine, 7*, O1–O28. https://www.semanticscholar.org/paper/173a12b75f9b972652f4835633cce64cef81a460 (accessed on 22 May 2025).
31. Misseri, G., Piattoli, M., Cuttone, G., Gregoretti, C., & Bignami, E. (2024). Artificial intelligence for mechanical ventilation: A transformative shift in critical care. *Therapeutic Advances in Pulmonary and Critical Care Medicine, 19*(1). https://www.semanticscholar.org/paper/b3be8979647c7302fd325411dc302e4a58e2209d (accessed on 22 May 2025).
32. Mojtabaee, M., Mohsenzadeh, M., & Sadegh Beigee, F. (2017). Deceased organ donation from pediatric donors: Does the literature really help us? (Implication for more powerful guidelines). *Transplantation, 101*(Suppl 1), S31. https://www.semanticscholar.org/paper/62a0b848333e22d585ff22cd2d59eba806533b98 (accessed on 22 May 2025).
33. Nowak-Węgrzyn, A., Chehade, M., Groetch, M., Spergel, J. M., Wood, R. J. K., Allen, K. J., Atkins, D., *et al.* (2017). International consensus guidelines for the diagnosis and management of food protein–induced enterocolitis syndrome: Executive summary—Workgroup Report of the

Adverse Reactions to Foods Committee, American Academy of Allergy, Asthma & Immunology. *Journal of Allergy and Clinical Immunology, 139*(4), 1111–1126.e4. https://doi.org/10.1016/j.jaci.2016.12.966.

34. Parrish, R., Ciarkowski, S. L., Aguero, D., Benavides, S., Bohannon, D. Z., Guharoy, R., & On Behalf of the United States Pharmacopeia Compounding Expert Panel. (2022). Creating data standards to support the electronic transmission of compounded nonsterile preparations (CNSPs): Perspectives of a United States Pharmacopeia expert panel. *Children, 9*. https://www.semanticscholar.org/paper/d2062c23024a81c72f9248a4688ff297decd2f49 (accessed on 22 May 2025).

35. Penkala-Gawęcka, D., & Rajtar, M. (2016). Introduction to the special issue 'medical pluralism and beyond'. *Anthropology & Medicine, 23*(2), 129–134. https://www.semanticscholar.org/paper/9966eba7ae2ad1906ee12d2b3901088b984064b1 (accessed on 22 May 2025).

36. Ranjan, V., Shankar, S., Kumar, N., & Singh, A. (2024). Outcome assessment of patients of non-CF bronchiectasis admitted with ARF and managed with NIV as a primary mode of ventilatory support: An analytical observational study. *Indian Journal of Critical Care Medicine, 28*(Suppl 1), S56–S57. https://www.semanticscholar.org/paper/a9c97416c1c659de96b6320b83840a48e4c39fb3 (accessed on 22 May 2025).

37. Reddy, K., Calfee, C., & McAuley, D. (2021). Acute respiratory distress syndrome subphenotypes beyond the syndrome: A step toward treatable traits? *American Journal of Respiratory and Critical Care Medicine, 203*, 1449–1451. https://www.semanticscholar.org/paper/c27fe7214dca50c22acf178298c8ae7d66d95aa5 (accessed on 22 May 2025).

38. Ring, A., Sieber, W. A., Studt, J., Schuepbach, R., Ganter, C., Manz, M., Müller, A., *et al.* (2023). Indications and outcomes of patients receiving therapeutic plasma exchange under critical care conditions: A retrospective eleven-year single-center study at a tertiary care center. *Journal of Clinical Medicine, 12*(1). https://www.semanticscholar.org/paper/c66b33ae1849ed9958172b5efffbc22c9a0e791 (accessed on 22 May 2025).

39. Salinas, M., Flores, E., López-Garrigós, M., Pomares, F., Carbonell, R., *et al.* (2020). Potential serum magnesium under request in primary care: Laboratory interventions to identify patients with hypomagnesemia. *Clinical Chemistry and Laboratory Medicine (CCLM), 58*, e221–e223. https://www.semanticscholar.org/paper/1d2c1c24a25aaa3954c6f844c75b3b5db8c5291d (accessed on 22 May 2025).

40. Saqib, M., Iftikhar, M., Neha, F., Karishma, F., & Mumtaz, H. (2023). Artificial intelligence in critical illness and its impact on patient care: A comprehensive review. *Frontiers in Medicine, 10*. https://www.semanticscholar.org/paper/aea977986b62eb2bdef87cfbdeed20394449abf2 (accessed on 22 May 2025).

41. Slater, A., Rousseau, A. F., Lambe, C., Young, D., Health, D. O., Rogers, E. J., Gentles, E., *et al.* (2014). *An Evaluation of Enteral Nutrition Practices and Nutritional Provision in Children During the Entire Length of Stay in Critical Care*. https://core.ac.uk/download/20480255.pdf (accessed on 22 May 2025).

42. Smith, K. (2019). Facing history for the future of nursing. *Journal of Clinical Nursing, 29*, 1429–1431. https://doi.org/10.1111/jocn.15065.

43. Srivastava, A., Santagostino, E., Dougall, A., Kitchen, S., Sutherland, M. L., Pipe, S. W., Carção, M., *et al.* (2020). WFH guidelines for the management of hemophilia (3rd ed.). *Hemophilia, 26*(S6), 1–158. https://doi.org/10.1111/hae.14046.

44. Taggarsi, D., & Sampath, S. (2024). Acute gastrointestinal injury in critically ill patients in a South Indian intensive care unit: A prospective, observational, preliminary study. *Cureus, 16*(1). https://www.semanticscholar.org/paper/dccdb0eef2d0308e2cf171ae12afbcb73838fd03 (accessed on 22 May 2025).

45. Ullah, A., Kumar, M., Sayyar, M., Sapna, F., John, C., Memon, S., Qureshi, K., *et al.* (2023). Revolutionizing cardiac care: A comprehensive narrative review of cardiac rehabilitation and the evolution of cardiovascular medicine. *Cureus, 15*(1). https://www.semanticscholar.org/paper/e6fbe50b5ebecc63c251d02552cd7f53cceed02d (accessed on 22 May 2025).

46. Utami, R. S. (2012). The challenges and strategies to improve family-centered round: A literature review. https://media.neliti.com/media/publications/154611-EN-the-challenges-and-strategies-to-improve.pdf (accessed on 22 May 2025).

47. Wang, R., Liu, J., Ma, K., Wu, Z., Lu, J. R., Li, L., Ma, S., *et al.* (2022). Expert statement on the construction criteria of critical care department in municipal and district designated hospitals under the pandemic prevention and control. *Zhonghua Wei Zhong Bing Ji Jiu Yi Xue, 34*(6), 561–570. https://www.semanticscholar.org/paper/e0daa85b3ea072ef10ccefd69cf49dd5f5fcdc9a (accessed on 22 May 2025).

48. Wani, S. J., Ganaie, B., Jalal, A., Shah, S., Hafiz, U., Qadri, S. M., & Qadri, U. (2025). Prognostic significance of the HALP index in predicting mortality in COVID-19 hospitalisations: A retrospective cohort study from a tertiary care hospital in Northern India. *National Journal of Laboratory Medicine*. https://www.semanticscholar.org/paper/6783857acf30499d97e3c6a654b4b73bb920b507 (accessed on 22 May 2025).

49. Webb, T., Boyer, T. J., Mitchell, S., & Eddy, C. S. (2020). Intraoperative sepsis: A simulation case for anesthesiology residents. *MedEdPORTAL, 16*. https://www.semanticscholar.org/paper/7b6c9b79267b60c3521b1f6dfdd91c2e411ff9b2 (accessed on 22 May 2025).

50. Zhao, L., Xie, Y. X., & Wang, C. (2020). Recommendations for respiratory rehabilitation in adults with coronavirus disease 2019. *Chinese Medical Journal, 133*, 1595–1602. https://doi.org/10.1097/cm9.0000000000000848.

ASSESSMENT AND DIAGNOSIS IN CRITICAL CARE

2

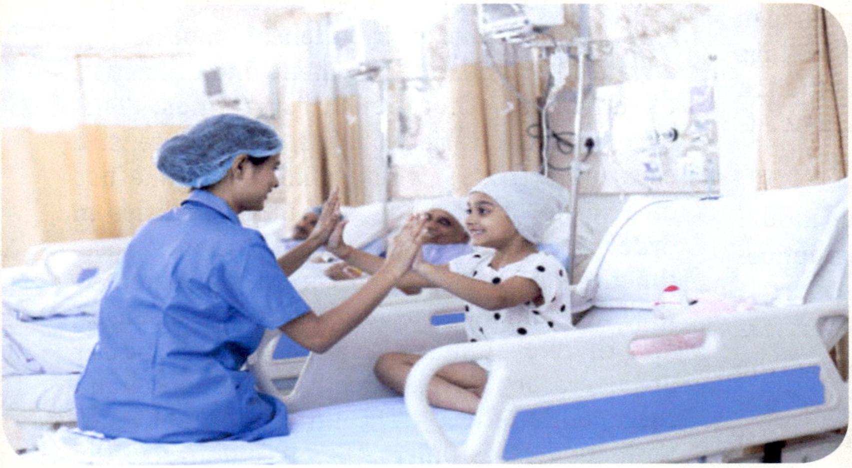

LEARNING OBJECTIVES

After studying this chapter, you will be able to:

1. Describe the role of assessment in critical care.
2. Define diagnostic tools and techniques.
3. Explain the clinical judgment in diagnosis.
4. Discuss multidisciplinary approach to assessment.
5. Understand the challenges in assessment and diagnosis.

Introduction

Diagnosis and patient status determination are critical foundations in critical care on which evidence-based practice interventions are designed. Clinicians, particularly nurses, must utilize systematically the nursing process, a critical thinking model for optimal patient outcomes. Through the use of broad knowledge and tried-and-true frameworks, clinicians are better able to navigate complicated patient presentations so that all phases of the process—assessment, diagnosis, planning, implementation, and evaluation—are carried out with precision and commitment. Despite this, various research studies have documented glaring differences in the application of this process, particularly where resources are scarce and the health workforce is not adequately trained, as measured by outcomes that demonstrate a high level of poor knowledge of the nursing process among healthcare providers (Abdullah *et al.*, 2025). This further goes to underscore the urgent requirement for training programs designed to improve clinical competence in critical care environments. Surmounting the impediments to practical assessment and diagnosis in critical care is central to improving patient outcomes. Various factors will counteract healthcare professionals in the task, among them poor time, poor education, and poor collaboration among career stakeholders. Research shows that nursing shortages and excessive workload often prevent nurses from undertaking thorough assessments, thus compromising the quality of care being offered (Abdullah *et al.*, 2025). Apart from that, the absence of coordinated support from the health administration can further worsen the issues to lead to feelings of overburden among nurses and insufficient preparedness to address the sophisticated needs of critical care.

This implies that a structured model of planning the nursing process, evidence-based practice, and administrative support is required to overcome such systemic barriers towards improved patient care. Moreover, the study of chronic illnesses like heart failure proves the essential application of synthesis of assessment and diagnosis in integrated patient management. Under palliative care, for instance, the establishment of effective communication frameworks and application of nursing care plans grounded in Basic Human Needs Theory has the remarkable effect of actually enhancing patients' quality of life in dealing with end-stage disease.

With the utilization of standardized tools like the Barthel Index and the Edmonton Symptom Scale, nurses can identify the needs of the patients and implement uniform individualized care plans for addressing complex symptomology. With this integrated clinical effort, evidence-based practice is not only being advanced, but teamwork culture is also being improved among health professionals, thereby increasing the overall integrity of critical care diagnosis and assessment. Hence, critically examining these areas is critical to the continued enhancement of patient care within the evolving health care environment.

Definition of Critical Care

Critical care needs to be defined in terms of diagnosis and assessment because it deals with specialized medical treatment for patients with potentially life-threatening conditions or injuries. It is based on the notion that instant and proper treatment has a tremendous potential to change patient outcomes. Critical care is characterized by intensive monitoring, advanced diagnostic equipment, and utilization of advanced therapeutic strategies. This encompasses a variety of sites, such as intensive care units (ICUs), where clinicians make use of a variety of technologies and modalities in order to augment and maintain patients' basic functions. Such advanced care is mandated by the uncertainty and severity of critical diseases, and therefore, multidisciplinary interventions are necessary for enhanced patient safety and therapeutic efficacy. The intricacy that comes with such cases only serves to emphasize the need for systematic assessment and diagnosis to ensure thorough coverage of the short- and long-term care needs of the patients. Secondly, the dynamic nature of definitions of critical care requires ongoing reevaluation of the factors considered when making decisions on eligibility for intensive care. Evolution of protocols, such as the advent of high-flow nasal oxygen and updated diagnostic criteria, is a reflection of the dynamism in this specialty (Lim *et al.*, 2024). It is these innovations that are bequeathed by both patient safety requirements and clinical creativity. Clarity in the definition of critical care enables inter-provider communication, process flows within the emergency setting, and determines the patient management approach. Furthermore, the use of patient preference in decision-making is also one of the most vital aspects in effective treatment planning. Emphasizing collaborative decision-making values the unique circumstances and beliefs of the patients, significantly increasing their autonomy in the face of severe health conditions (Lim *et al.*, 2024). A more layered approach not only delineates the steps in intensive care but also thoroughly revises how care is considered and delivered. The consequence of a clear definition of critical care extends to clinical practice and research, emphasizing the necessity of consensus regarding the criteria for diagnosis. Their clarification can lead to improved patient outcomes and improved utilization of healthcare resources. The need for a widely accepted definition is also increased by the increasing complexity of patient presentations and diverse settings wherein care is provided, including low-resource environments (Matthay *et al.*, 2023). By revisiting and revising the definitions of critical care, health systems are well-positioned to predict the challenges posed by acute illness, ensuring that evaluation and diagnosis remain relevant, effective, and practical. Lastly, a correct comprehension of critical care facilitates an easier provision of in-depth assessment and interventions, which form the basis of high-standard patient-led practice in critical environments. This ongoing debate, thus, is important since it summarizes the evolving process of care based on re-surging evidence and patients' needs.

Importance of Assessment and Diagnosis

The importance of assessment and diagnosis in critical care cannot be overstated because they directly influence patient outcomes and the effectiveness of interventions. Appropriate assessments lead to the identification of some health issues and the formulation of corresponding treatment plans. In the high-risk environment of a critical care unit, rapid and precise evaluations are important for addressing the sophisticated needs of the patients. For instance, hospital length of stay (LOS) data-driven insights help caregivers better comprehend the complexity of patient care to inform decisions that enhance the recovery experience while minimizing complications of extended hospital stays. Methods such as propensity scoring can render these assessments distinctive, enabling clinicians to tailor interventions and optimize the utilization of resources, thus facilitating a more compassionate care setting as exemplified through our findings on the association between LOS and patient outcomes (Allam, 2024) (Figure 2.1).

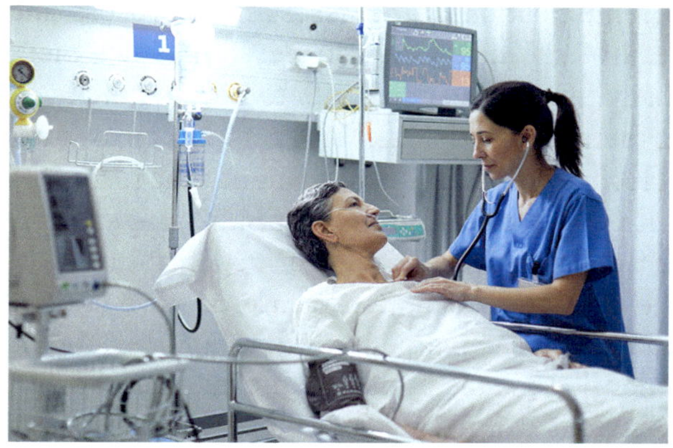

Figure 2.1. Assessment and diagnosis in critical care.

Source: https://www.monash.edu/__data/assets/image/0004/2769025/Clinical-patient-on-ward.jpg.

In addition, the introduction of new-age technologies such as machine learning serves to further establish the revolutionary nature of critical care diagnosis and evaluation. Through algorithms being utilized for handling large volumes of data, healthcare practitioners are better able to achieve diagnostic precision, which is paramount for effective treatment of acute illnesses. Use of advanced analytical solutions, such as the XGBoost algorithm to study cardiovascular disease, is a prime example of how data analysis influences clinical decisions and enhances patient treatment in general (Aditi *et al.*, 2024). Such technologies not only enhance diagnostic precision but also help us understand the trends and nature of diseases in order to make timely and knowledge-based decisions regarding patient needs. This marriage of technology and evaluation practice serves to emphasize the importance of continued assessment in the generation of new therapeutic processes and the best patient care. Lastly, the need to develop a patient-centered model of diagnosis and assessment in critical care settings is highest in advancing patient autonomy and satisfaction. By placing explicit communication of the assessment process and result first, healthcare professionals are more likely to empower patients to become included in their care decisions. It is an approach towards prioritizing patient involvement that resonates with new care models emphasizing single-patient pathways, as described in studies of the dynamics of patient-centered care (Allam, 2024). By closing gaps in data and leveraging emerging means of health information sharing, clinicians can form a more integrated image of patients' situations and potential interventions. In the end, an excessive focus on diagnosis and assessment, in addition to enhancing health outcomes, has the effect of creating the emotional and psychological stability of the patients, which enhances their role as active agents in the cure.

2.1. The Role of Assessment in Critical Care

Learning Outcome

1. Discuss the types of assessments used in critical care
2. Explain the importance of timely assessments
3. Identify the impact of assessment on patient outcomes

Assessment within critical care settings plays an important role in guiding the direction of treatment and patient outcomes. Systematic and detailed assessments by health care workers establish the severity level of a patient's condition, an issue that is particularly important with acute critical illnesses under consideration. Rapid assessment with vital signs, laboratory, and imaging provides essential information that informs decision-making. In the case of interstitial lung diseases (ILD), for instance, pre-transplant evaluation is a critical factor in determining transplant suitability, based on the combination of pulmonary function tests imaging studies. These assessments not only help identify the stage of the disease but also help to plan interventions that are necessary because it is essential to identify patients' health status in order to obtain optimal outcomes of lung transplantation and solve associated complications in intensive care units (Georgakopoulou, 2025). The use of advanced diagnostic equipment optimizes the accuracy of assessments in intensive care units. Techniques such as magnetic resonance imaging (MRI) and other new imaging techniques have transformed the practice of evaluation. MRI is indeed unique with its ability to produce high-contrast images of soft tissues and is a gold standard for malignancy staging and diagnosis. It is of tremendous importance in critical care, where early and accurate diagnosis can dramatically alter treatment protocols. Moreover, in very serious diseases where interventions are needed, like in ILD, the ability to ascertain the lung involvement from imaging accurately equips clinicians with negotiating power to plan integrated management plans with pre- and post-transplant in consideration. Continuous innovation in these technologies makes assessment increasingly accurate, and ultimately, improved and smarter decisions lead to better patient outcomes (AlHarbi *et al.*, 2024). Second, critical care assessment is not dependent on technology; it also needs to incorporate an integrated process of assessing patients. It entails the evaluation of psychosocial needs, nutrition, and comorbidities that affect care outcomes. There, therefore, needs to be interdisciplinary collaboration in order to gain holistic information from varied viewpoints of healthcare providers. Interdisciplinary collaboration ensures that patient evaluations are comprehensive and include all the determinants that shape recovery. Strategic assessment then extends beyond individual patient care, influencing protocols and pathways for care that enhance overall clinical effectiveness. Through the application of systems-based assessment, critical care teams can maximize diagnostic accuracy and direct interventions toward addressing the multi-dimensional needs of critically ill patients, thus improving the quality of care in such high-stakes environments.

2.1.1. Types of Assessments Used in Critical Care

In critical care settings, various types of assessment are employed to facilitate adequate patient evaluation and management. Measurement of vital signs, such as heart rate, blood pressure, respiratory rate, and temperature, is one of these types of assessment. These values are extremely crucial markers of a patient's hemodynamic stability and can signal impending complications like shock or infection. Furthermore, laboratory investigations such as imaging and blood tests enable the diagnosis of underlying pathologies that require early intervention (Figure 2.2).

The proper utilization of these tests allows clinicians to make evidence-based treatment and intervention, and hence supports the importance of sequential assessment in critically ill patients. Another critical assessment tool is the assessment of organ function, particularly for acute kidney injury (AKI), which occurs frequently in critically ill patients. Utilization of the standardized criteria, such as Kidney Disease: Improving Global Outcomes (KDIGO) guidelines, assists doctors in the detection of AKI that is not clinically evident. Underdiagnosis of ICU patients with AKI were highlighted in a recent study by the observation that a large percentage of cases were unidentified by physicians even after fulfilling criteria (Assante *et al.*, 2025).

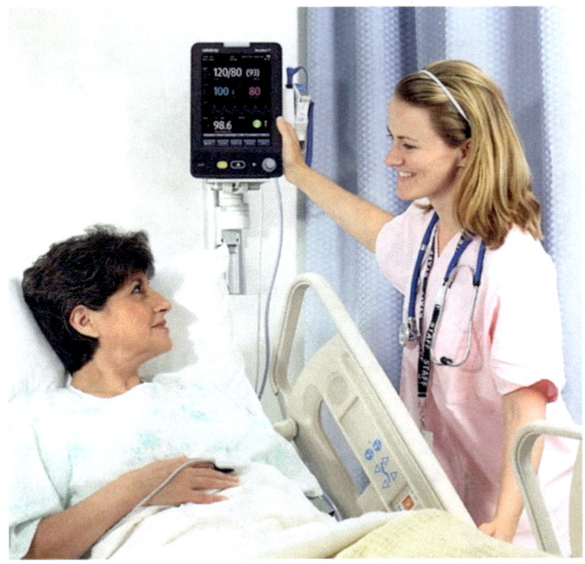

Figure 2.2. Vital signs monitor.

Source: https://mindray.scene7.com/is/image/mindray/3_.pic_hd?$news-kv-894x566$.

Not only does this injurious diagnostic gap delay ICU and hospital stay but also heightens the risk of mortality, stressing the importance of improved surveillance and early identification of such disease to yield optimal patient outcomes. In addition to traditional evaluation modalities, new technologies are increasingly being integrated into critical care assessment. For example, infrared thermography (IRT) is a quick and non-invasive method of temperature change monitoring, which can be an effective diagnostic technique. Application of IRT in animal science has proven its effectiveness in the identification of health disorders, such as mastitis in dairy ruminants (Korelidou *et al.*, 2024). Though employed mainly in veterinary medicine, future applications of IRT for the identification of physiological abnormalities in human patients are rather impressive. Ongoing exploration for newer technologies and evaluation of the functional challenges of such could pave the way for broader applications in critical care and ultimately enhance diagnostic sensitivity and patient safety (Figure 2.3).

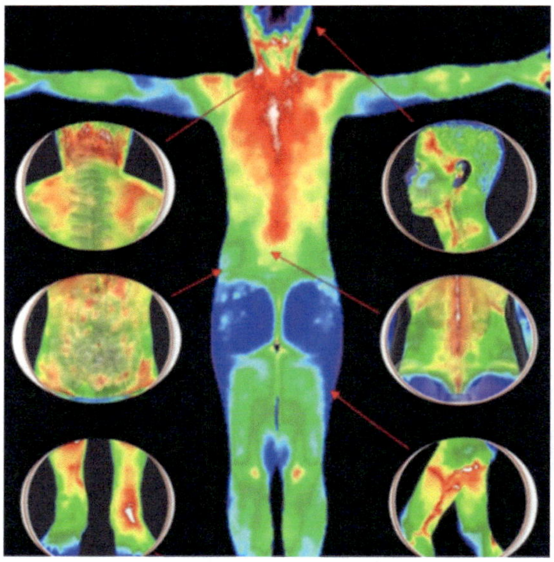

Figure 2.3. Infrared thermography (IRT).

Source: https://i.pinimg.com/originals/24/83/26/24832650896ab91351d007d74293a0a3.jpg.

2.1.2. Importance of Timely Assessments

Premature assessment is key to the attainment of optimal patient outcomes in critical care. Early identification of patient condition makes it possible to prevent complications that will further complicate existing health issues, and even trigger severe morbidity or mortality. The urgency involved dictates the necessity for standardized assessment processes that permit rapid determination of life-sustaining cues and presentation. Early diagnosis not only lays the ground for improved resource utilization but also improves treatment planning. For example, in Morquio A syndrome, orthopedic complications related to delayed evaluation can have a significant impact on the patient's quality of life, as highlighted in the guidelines for management of extremity deformities, where the importance of early diagnosis and intervention is highlighted (Bache *et al.*, 2014). The initial assessment culture of critical care units must therefore be employed to tackle multifaceted health concerns effectively. Initial assessment should also be utilized to monitor patients in the critical care units constantly. Situations in the units shift rapidly, and constant re-assessment must be undertaken to keep up with any decline promptly. The ability to monitor changes in the clinical condition of a patient facilitates corrective interventions on time that can lead to saving lives. For instance, information on patients' lifestyles and their impact on oral health, as well as the overall body, highlights the possible dangers of failing to assess such lifestyles at early stages (Berisha *et al.*, 2023). With the incorporation of the comprehensive evaluation of patient behaviors, clinicians can formulate well-focused plans that address underlying causes more effectively, hence leading to better overall outcomes of care. The multidisciplinary plan, combined with timely assessments, enhances the plans, once more highlighting the necessity of diligence in detail in following the well-being of the patients. Besides the direct facilitation of the patient outcome, timely assessments also optimize the coordination of the health practitioners in the critical care settings. Effective and coordinated care is dependent on clear communication among team members regarding the status of patients. By ongoing assessment and reporting in a timely fashion, team members can make decisions in accordance with shifting patient needs. This organized system of care proves particularly beneficial for complex conditions involving multi-specialties, such as in Morquio A syndrome management, where pediatric, genetic, and orthopedic concerns must converge (Bache *et al.*, 2014). Cultivating a culture of providing early diagnosis works not just for the individual patient but the whole health provision system, sowing seeds towards better outcomes through collaborative watchfulness and intervention strategies.

2.1.3. Impact of Assessment on Patient Outcomes

The impact of critical care nursing assessment on patient outcomes is immense, and it is generally the basis on which the right treatment plans are developed. During assessment, healthcare practitioners take into account several factors of a patient's health, including nursing complexity and health literacy, which are important predictors of clinical outcomes. It has been reported that high nursing complexity is strongly linked to adverse patient outcomes, including increased mortality. Specifically, high nursing complexity and low health literacy patients were most vulnerable to death, identifying where these two forces intersect in generating patient death rates. Thus, complete assessments not only inform clinical decision-making but also facilitate early identification of vulnerable patients thereby informing prompt intervention that can improve overall patient outcomes and the quality of critical care provided (Cocchieri *et al.*, 2025). Other than nursing expertise, no part of diagnostic testing, including point-of-care ultrasound (POCUS), can be overstressed when it comes to maximizing patient outcomes in intensive care. POCUS has been a clinician's goldmine where they can visualize illnesses such as pericardial effusions in real time, which, had they gone unnoticed, would lead to complications. Its ability to measure and demarcate pericardial effusion has a direct impact on clinical decision-making in the sense that it allows clinicians to differentiate critical information about a patient's hemodynamic status and underlying pathology. By detecting cardiac tamponade or other life-threatening pathology with a rapid diagnosis, POCUS provides clinicians with the information required to respond promptly, thereby enhancing patient outcomes. The integration of POCUS as part of standard assessment reinforces the importance of timely and precise assessments in stabilizing complex cases in critical care settings (de Azevedo *et al.*, 2024). Additionally, the coordinated impact of thorough assessments in critical care is to maximize systemic healthcare outcomes beyond the isolated patient. By way of structured processes to nursing complexity and engagement with advanced diagnostic equipment like POCUS, healthcare institutions can build an environment of anticipatory patient management. This is important, especially with the potential for wide variation in health outcomes that is caused by bad assessment. As has been proven with evidence, those individuals who have high nursing complexity and low health literacy are at increased risk for mortality and hospital readmission, showing why clear communication and education interventions, as well as clinical assessment, are necessary. Thus, the process of optimization of the evaluation process and resulting interventions not only enhances the outcome of patients but also optimizes the efficacy of care overall in critical care models (Cocchieri *et al.*, 2025; de Azevedo *et al.*, 2024) (Figure 2.4).

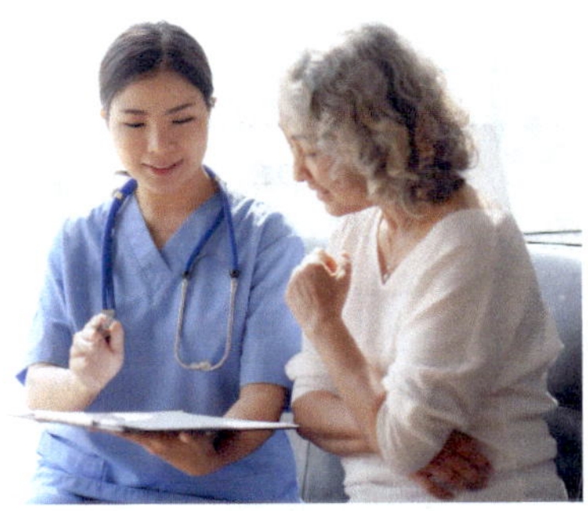

Figure 2.4. The impact of critical care nursing assessment on patient outcomes.

Source: https://www.oecd.org/adobe/dynamicmedia/deliver/dm-aid--757adc79-d680-43f0-96df-c9231a5318c2/shutterstock-2261501289.jpg?preferwebp=true&quality=80.

Test Your Knowledge

1. What types of assessments are commonly used in critical care settings?
2. Why is timely assessment crucial in managing critically ill patients?

2.2. Diagnostic Tools and Techniques

Learning Outcome

1. Discuss the laboratory tests and their significance
2. Define imaging studies in critical care
3. Explain the monitoring technologies and their applications

Within critical care settings, the use of sophisticated diagnostic technology and techniques is crucial to successful patient monitoring and management. EEG is a prime mechanism for the observation of live brain activity, allowing medical professionals to make accurate diagnoses of seizures and other neurological disorders. Single-channel EEG information within traditional applications is insufficient in providing an accurate picture; however, developments with multi-view information fusion techniques have enhanced accuracy up to this point. These newer methods integrate spatial, temporal, and frequency data, and hence present a more integral view of cerebral dynamics. This EEG signal improvement can potentially function better within critical care by enabling improved measurement and intervention in an appropriate time, particularly in acute neurologic illness where there is a need for intense monitoring (Patir *et al.*, 2025). Employing Diagnostic and Statistical Manual of Mental Disorders (DSM-V) criteria is more evident with the prevalence of comorbidities, for instance, perioperative neurocognitive disorders (PNDs), which are very common in critical care environments. PNDs have been revealed to negatively impact on postoperative recovery, proving the need for accurate diagnostic processes. Global assessment tends to employ a combination of neuropsychological screening measures such as the Clock Drawing Test, Mini-Mental State Examination, and Montreal Cognitive Assessment. These diagnostic tests enable clinicians to gauge the probability and severity of PNDs and take into account causative factors, such as the extent of pre-existing neurocognitive impairment and chronic inflammation. Neuroimaging modalities and biochemical markers are also significant adjuncts in enhancing the sensitivity of diagnosis, emphasizing the intricate interaction of diagnostic modalities in intensive care (Lakshminarayanan *et al.*, 2024). Addressing the complexities of diagnostic challenges in critical care depends on technology and methodological adjustments, and research being continuous. Application of risk reduction strategies, particularly prior to surgery, is likely to have significant effects on outcome by reducing the incidence of postoperative complications. Emerging strategies like brain plasticity-based therapy and enhanced anesthesia regimens hold potential to decrease the neurological hazards of surgery. Furthermore, having standardized diagnostic criteria and methodology for evaluating PNDs is important in order to enhance the efficacy of interventions. With the aging population, the incidence of PNDs will certainly increase, and thus, a sophisticated, systematic method for diagnosing and intervening with PNDs using both established and new diagnostic methods is needed. Advancing these techniques not only facilitates better patient results but also improves the overall framework of assessment and diagnosis in critical care (Lakshminarayanan *et al.*, 2024) (Figure 2.5).

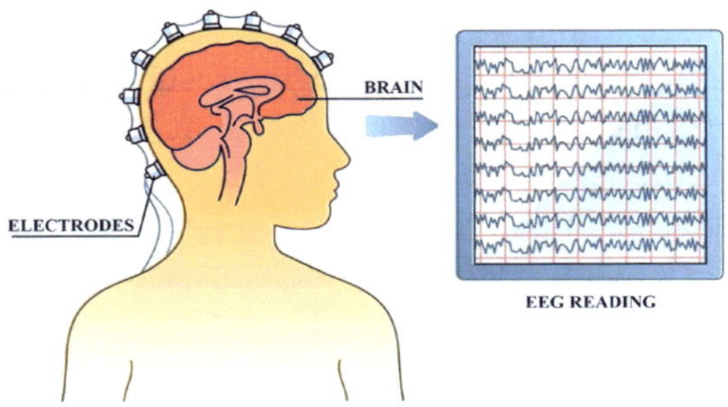

Figure 2.5. Electroencephalography (EEG).

Source: https://www.brainandentspecialist.in/wp-content/uploads/2023/12/electro.jpg.

2.2.1. Laboratory Tests and Their Significance

The role of laboratory tests in critical care cannot be overestimated, especially when it comes to the timely and accurate assessment of patients. In environments where timely decision-making is critical, these tests provide critical information regarding the patient's physiological state, guiding clinicians as to how to devise timely and effective interventions. For instance, laboratory examination can reveal important signs of systemic infections, metabolic disturbances, or hematologic abnormalities that would otherwise remain missed by physical examination. Notably, a dengue outbreak study pointed out the importance of laboratory diagnosis in identifying the clinical and hematological presentations of the patients, thereby indirectly influencing the treatment protocols and patient care (Hossain *et al.*, 2025). This indicates the potential of laboratory tests to reveal the underlying reasons behind complicated clinical presentations and emphasizes their importance in patient outcome prediction. Further, their integration into critical care unit evaluation protocols enhances the capacity for prevention and management of complications.

Tests such as a complete blood count (CBC) and some biomarker tests are used to monitor the progression of infections and the body's response to treatment. Monitoring of conditions such as thrombocytopenia and increased hematocrit levels in dengue illustrates the need for routine laboratory assessment in stress conditions with increased risk for dangerous complications (Hossain *et al.*, 2025). Such regular screening can also allow for the early detection of systemic conditions that may have an oral presentation, thereby impacting treatment planning across professions like dentistry, as seen in the utilization of lab tests for systemic health in dentistry. Such is the cross-professional application, as it is crucial to the truth behind good communication among healthcare providers.

Finally, laboratory testing helps significantly in creating a holistic view of patient health, which ultimately improves critical care clinical outcomes. As doctors rely increasingly on evidence-based practices, combining laboratory findings with patient assessments improves the quality of care. Through the adoption of an individualized approach, healthcare professionals can prevent risks associated with unknown health complexities that may complicate treatment plans. For instance, detection of underlying illnesses like diabetes or liver disease enables clinicians to tailor interventions that consider these conditions, thereby resulting in safer and more successful treatment outcomes. In conclusion, the intentional use of laboratory tests in critical care significantly enhances patient assessment and diagnosis, paving the way for life-saving clinical decisions (Figure 2.6).

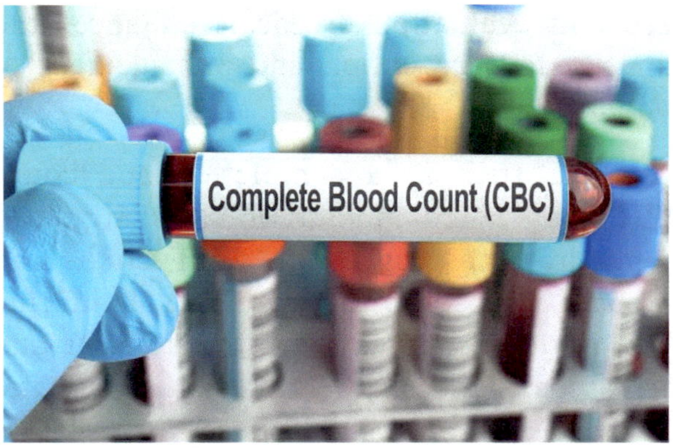

Figure 2.6. Complete blood count (CBC).

Source: https://www.metropolisindia.com/upgrade/blog/upload/25/04/cbc-test1745833156.webp.

2.2.2. Imaging Studies in Critical Care

Imaging tests are a mainstay in the diagnostic and evaluation workup of critically ill patients, providing vital information to inform clinical decision-making. Within the environment of critical care units, where rapid evaluation is often necessary, modalities such as computed tomography (CT), MRI, and ultrasound are valuable. These modalities allow early identification of potentially fatal conditions, such as subarachnoid hemorrhage (SAH), that are accompanied by high mortality if left undiagnosed. For instance, an uncontrasted CT scan can have excellent sensitivity for detecting SAH within the initial six hours since the onset of headache, which is very significant for proper handling of such emergencies. Sensitivity falls quite significantly after 24–48 hours, evoking the need for immediate imaging in acute cases where SAH could be suspected, as noted in (Rainer *et al.*, 2024). In critical illness, imaging studies are primarily used to distinguish among various pathologies. An example is acute chest syndrome in sickle cell disease patients to be diagnosed with caution by chest imaging as it may mimic other respiratory diseases. Radiographic results are crucial in the discrimination of acute chest syndrome and pneumonia or pulmonary embolism based on the similarity of the presenting symptoms, like cough, chest pain, and hypoxemia. The fact that chest X-rays can be used as a first-line imaging modality allows clinicians to determine new infiltrates and guide subsequent management strategies. Interpreting imaging results correctly, therefore, matters to emergency medicine practitioners, who have to take many differential diagnoses into account when evaluating patients experiencing respiratory distress, as outlined in (Meloy *et al.*, 2023).

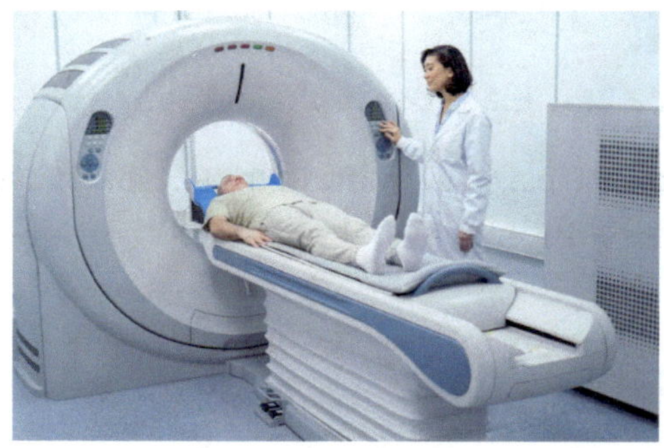

Figure 2.7. Magnetic Resonance Imaging (MRI) techniques

Source: https://www.yashodahealthcare.com/blogs/wp-content/uploads/2023/03/mri-1.jpg.

One of the key features of imaging evaluations in critical care is integrating the findings into the big picture of the clinical scenario. Imaging results do not stand in isolation; they need to be reconciled with the patient's presentation and lab work to arrive at a proper diagnosis. For instance, while a negative head CT may exclude SAH initially, the presence of certain clinical signs may necessitate further evaluation, such as lumbar puncture or CT angiogram. The crossing point between imaging results and clinical wisdom speaks to the importance of a multi-faceted patient assessment strategy in the critical care setting. Thus, imaging studies not only provide valuable diagnostic information but also enhance the entire evaluation paradigm that guides treatment plans in critically ill patients (Figure 2.7).

2.2.3. Monitoring Technologies and Their Applications

Monitoring technology has transformed critical care to the extent that medical staff can have real-time monitoring of patient states. The deployment of sophisticated monitoring systems, where multiple vital signs are reduced to comprehensible streams of data, is at the center of ensuring patient safety and efficacy of treatment. Ongoing heart monitoring, for instance, blood pressure and oxygen saturation monitoring, are now standard practice in intensive care units. These technologies allow clinicians to detect anomalies or worsening of a patient's condition in seconds, allowing timely intervention that can be life-saving. Moreover, the availability of remote monitoring capacity has increased access to intensive care, allowing healthcare practitioners to manage multiple patients simultaneously, hence maximizing resource utilization in high-demand settings. Evolution of such sophisticated systems largely relies on the importance of trustworthy monitoring in the diagnostic and assessment process of critical care units. The combination of telemedicine with mobile technologies has been proposed as a critical add-on to traditional monitoring methods in critical care. Emergent technologies have been able to use smartphones and hand-held devices not only as communication devices but also as platforms for symptom and vital sign remote monitoring. Referencing contemporary texts, mobile technologies illustrate the ability to enhance the provision of care by enabling patients to take an active role in managing their conditions. By utilizing mobile apps that have been optimized to check health monitors, patients can inform healthcare professionals in case there is a change in their condition, and hence enhance more coordinated critical care management. The ease and choice offered by these technologies also enable those based in far-flung or high-risk areas to get timely monitoring, which consequently translates into improved treatment outcomes (Susick *et al.*, 2011). The pivotal position occupied by mobile-based monitoring systems has appeal in rectifying the imperative to apply innovative solutions to the assessment of acute health challenges. The use of converged eHealth platforms is a step into the future concerning critical care monitoring. As testified by ongoing advancements in systems like the ones presented under the INTERMED project, these platforms allow for efficient interaction and information sharing between medical experts, thereby enhancing teleconsultation and telecare services (Androulidakis *et al.*, 2011).

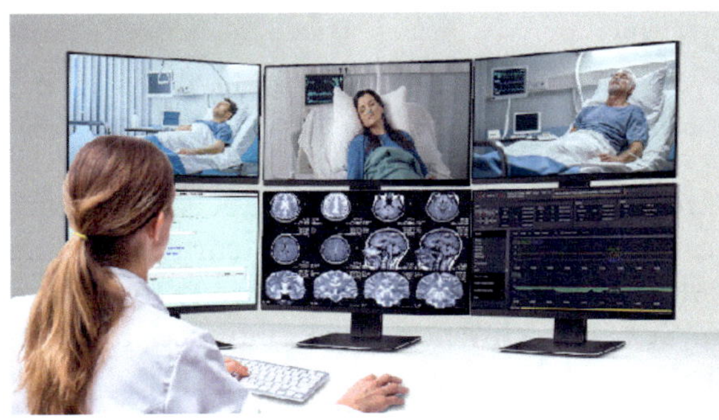

Figure 2.8. Monitoring of patient states.

Source: https://www.aver.com/AVerExpert/Tele-ICU-Transforming-Critical-Care-Delivery.

By bridging the technology divide among rural health centers, eHealth platforms leverage the advantages of telemedicine to facilitate continuous professional development among healthcare providers and enhance access to essential services for marginalized populations. This integration enables real-time analysis of patients' biosignals and imaging investigations, an element that is highly vital in areas with poor standard monitoring capacity. In addition, interoperability among diverse health technologies eliminates conflict among disparate health technologies, ushering in a harmonious approach toward patient care, building a robust framework for diagnosis and evaluation of intensive care units (Figure 2.8).

Test Your Knowledge

1. What is the significance of routine laboratory tests in critical care?
2. How are imaging studies utilized to support diagnosis in critically ill patients?

2.3. Clinical Judgment in Diagnosis

Learning Outcome

1. Describe the role of experience in clinical judgment
2. Define cognitive biases affecting diagnosis
3. Discuss the strategies to improve clinical decision-making

Clinical judgment in diagnostic decision-making is a core principle in critical care medicine, where the conditions of the patient tend to be complex and clinicians are required to make quick, sound judgments. Clinical judgment lies not merely with the presence of medical information but also with the ability to properly process diverse patient information. This intricate process is ultimately a function of nurses' and doctors' skills and experience, which determines their diagnostic accuracy to a very large extent. For instance, experts can detect patterns and irregularities in a presentation at once. New professionals may struggle to integrate information and, as a result, may misdiagnose or delay in providing care. Hence, clinical judgment needs optimization through ongoing education and mentoring to improve critical care diagnostic quality. Further, the use of systematic approaches to assess patient preference and decision models should also improve clinical judgment. As illustrated with dementia patients, shared decision-making (SDM) is crucial in such cases to honor them and their unique position despite impaired cognition. The consideration of values and preferences is crucial in this regard to make clinical decisions patient preferences and needs congruent. There is some evidence available that SDM promotes effectiveness in the SDM process, and the same can be judged by increased patient satisfaction and increased compliance with guideline recommendations. Patient-centered interventions will enable health workers to enhance clinical judgment and therefore provide enhanced and more empathetic care in high-stakes settings, as recent overviews discovered (Lim *et al.*, 2024). In the setting of critical care units, formalized nursing diagnosis serves the same primary function in enabling well-informed decision-making. Research examining the correlation between nursing diagnoses and differing levels of nursing experience has shown disparities between clinical diagnosis and the decision to judge. For instance, newly graduated nurses tend to default to simpler diagnoses, such as Activity Intolerance Risk, whereas expert clinicians prefer more complex diagnoses, like Fluid Volume Excess Risk. This divergence indicates the use of standardized nursing data systems that gather detailed patient data and diagnostic patterns. By encouraging a culture of evidence-based practice and improvement, healthcare organizations are able to enable nurses to enhance clinical judgment and support effectively in patient care planning, thus resulting in better outcomes in intensive care environments (Yang *et al.*, 2023) (Figure 2.9).

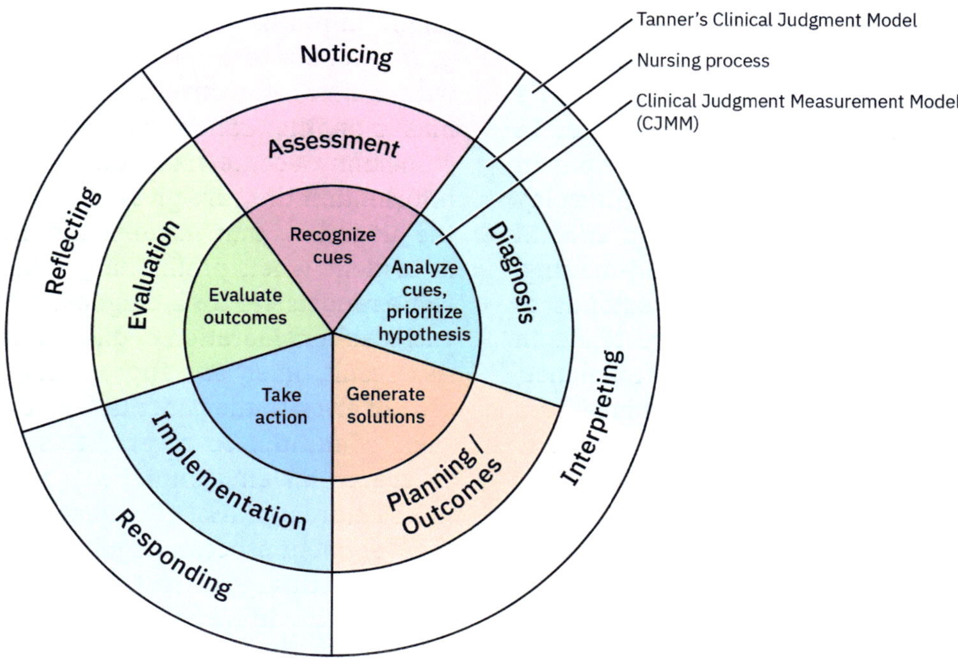

Figure 2.9. Integration of clinical judgment model and nursing process model tanner's clinical judgment model, the nursing process, and the clinical judgment measurement model work together for effective patient care.

Source: https://med.libretexts.org/Bookshelves/Nursing/Maternal-Newborn_Nursing_%28OpenStax%29/27%3A_Unfolding_Case_Study_-_Applying_Clinical_Judgment/27.02%3A_Clinical_Judgment_within_the_Nursing_Process.

2.3.1. The Role of Experience in Clinical Judgment

Experience is the major contributor to the construction of clinical judgment, particularly in critical care medicine, where there is a need for timely decision-making. Clinicians acquire a tremendous amount of experience throughout their careers, which helps them sense the subtle presentation of complex conditions. This skill is critical because clinical environments are complicated and often ambivalent, with symptoms merging across different diseases. Vetted clinicians can utilize an abundance of previous cases to search for patterns and anticipate future complications, and therefore hone their diagnostic skills. In addition, experience allows one to stratify risk, a normal aspect of patient assessment in critical care, in which physicians order interventions from most urgently to least urgently needed, according to severity of disease. As a result, seasoned clinicians are better equipped to manage high-stakes decisions, treating patients quickly and appropriately. Furthermore, combining clinical guidance with experience data lies at the core of sound clinical judgment. Clinical guidance, for example, for acute coronary syndromes (ACS), provides formalized pathways to diagnosis and treatment; yet, case complexity typically demands a tailored response. Even seasoned clinicians will look to established evidence when adapting guidelines to meet the unique needs of their patients (Chew *et al.*, 2016). Flexibility is used most precisely in intensive care, in which variability of patient response can have a highly significant impact on results. Accordingly, while guidelines ensure the consistency and reliability of clinical assessment, it is the practitioner's experience that determines best practices in how to make use of these recommendations in real time, testament to the dynamic interplay between standardized protocols and clinical acumen. Beyond individual decision-making, experience in clinical acumen also extends to team practice within the healthcare team. In critical care, where lives hang in the balance, communication and teamwork are the measures to best patient outcomes. There is generally guidance by senior clinicians, who share their knowledge with junior colleagues, supporting a culture of continuous learning. This collaboration not only improves the judgment of junior professionals but also introduces a checks and balances measure to avoid potential mistakes while evaluating patients (Page *et al.*, 2021). Synergy of experience and skill within a group of people can lead to more extensive analysis, factoring in the different angles offered to assist in reaching important decisions. Synergy between experience, clinical guidelines, and teamwork, in general, has an important impact on individual and group judgment in diagnosing and assessing patients who are critically ill.

2.3.2. Cognitive Biases Affecting Diagnosis

Cognitive bias plays a significant role in diagnosis in critical care units, as it tends to lead to misinterpretation of clinical data. One significant bias is confirmation bias, where physicians prefer evidence that favors their initial hypotheses and have a tendency to overlook contradictory evidence. Confirmation bias may lead to persistence in false diagnoses because physicians tend to base their diagnoses on early impressions or initial findings. In critical care, where timely decision-making is paramount, confirmation bias can prove disastrous. Confirmation bias needs to be eliminated; utilization of systematic diagnostic pathways might minimize its impact, allowing health professionals to approach patient evaluation with a more objective perspective. Anchoring bias is another salient cognitive bias, in which clinicians become fixed on the first piece of information they are given, unfairly preying on the judgments that ensue. In intensive care, this is evident when preliminary imaging or vital signs reports set up a diagnostic pathway that excludes consideration of differential diagnoses. As a result, timely and appropriate interventions are not given to the patients, hence deteriorating their condition. To reverse this bias, one has to create an environment in which there is incessant reappraisal of patient data throughout the treatment process. Regular interdisciplinary team meetings can foster diverse input and deconstruct entrenched assumptions, facilitating less misleading clinical judgment in assessment and diagnosis. Finally, the influence of Cognitive Dissonance cannot be eliminated from critical care diagnosis. Faced with new evidence that is incompatible with previous beliefs or diagnoses, clinicians feel uneasy mentally, a stimulus to rationalize or disavow the new evidence. This bias can hinder necessary treatment plan modifications and can block meaningful evaluation of patient progress. For instance, a clinician will refuse to change a diagnosis in light of fresh test results because of established notions. To counter this, one must establish a culture of openness and flexibility in medical practice. The encouragement of clinicians to identify and deal with cognitive dissonance can lead to improved diagnostic accuracy and ultimately better patient outcomes in critical care environments.

2.3.3. Strategies to Improve Clinical Decision-Making

Effective clinical decision-making is crucial in critical care settings, where it may be a matter of life and death for patients if done on time and properly. Multidisciplinary decision-making is one of the promising approaches to facilitate speedier decision-making. Engaging diverse clinical specialists, including physiatrists, primary care physicians, and specialists, in the process of decision-making enables improved intelligence to be gained on intricate matters, like Long COVID. Collaborative environments provide clinicians with the opportunity to integrate alternate perspectives and experiences, which can be employed to realize symptom patterns that no individual practitioner would otherwise think of. Organizational frameworks like the American Academy of Physical Medicine and Rehabilitation have encouraged this type of collaborative work by providing models and guidelines for the approach of complex health issues in an interdisciplinary environment. This approach, apart from optimizing diagnostic effectiveness, optimizes overall management approaches used for lethal diseases as it encompasses diverse views and experiences of patient treatment (Cheng *et al.*, 2025). Another crucial strategy is the implementation of evidence-based practice, whose clinical evaluations and interventions are informed by it. Standardized clinical pathway implementation can help with decision-making, streamlining, and reduction of care variation generally encountered in critical care settings. For example, leveraging current research studies and clinical trials data to guide evidence-based practice for management of specific disease state symptomology, such as Long COVID, holds promise. Through systematic use of these protocols in clinical workflows every day, clinicians can be confident that they are making evidence-based and up-to-date, research-driven decisions using the latest research and best practices. Secondly, the use of structured clinical assessments in electronic health record (EHR) systems can make it possible to document patient information on a routine basis, and thereby increase the capacity to track outcomes and optimize care pathways in the long run. This level of structuring of clinical decision-making can be highly valuable in complex cases where timely interventions are of critical importance (Campbell *et al.*, 2025). Finally, technology assists in augmenting clinical decision-making through the use of decision support systems. Such systems can display real-time data, clinical practice guidelines, and predictive analytics that warn healthcare professionals of the best action to take based on the latest patient data and current evidence.

For instance, in ICUs, monitoring algorithms tracking patient vital signs and laboratory results can prompt clinicians to potential patient status declines and thus evoke early interventions. With such technologies used, not only is the process of clinical evaluation enhanced in terms of efficiency, but also the mental workload conventionally faced by caregivers in such high-stress environments is lightened. Furthermore, creating a culture of learning and improvement with such tools can enable healthcare teams to optimize the use of technology for better patient outcomes. Taken together, all these solutions focus on improving clinical decision-making in a manner that the needs of the patient are taken care of effectively and promptly in critical care scenarios (Cheng *et al.*, 2025) (Figure 2.10).

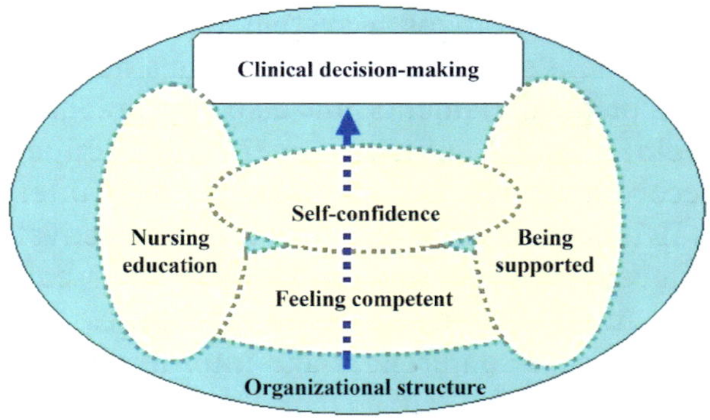

Figure 2.10. Interactive relationships between variables affecting effective clinical decision-making.

Source: https://bmcnurs.biomedcentral.com/articles/10.1186/1472-6955-3-2.

Test Your Knowledge

1. How does clinical experience influence judgment in critical care situations?
2. What are common cognitive biases that can affect diagnostic accuracy?

2.4. Multidisciplinary Approach to Assessment

Learning Outcome

1. Define collaboration among healthcare professionals
2. Identify the role of nurses in patient assessment
3. Explain the involvement of specialists in diagnosis

Multidisciplinary critical care evaluation is the solution to optimizing patient outcomes by consolidating diverse professional skills. Coordination among specialists such as critical care physicians, nurses, pharmacists, and allied health professionals in this fast-paced healthcare environment is important for accurate diagnosis and comprehensive patient care. This holistic strategy encourages a systematic analysis of the patient's condition, considering not only physiological elements but also psychological, social, and environmental influences. Accordingly, this broad understanding offers individualized interventions that are actively tailored towards the unique needs of each patient. Collaborative practice approaches, such as daily case conferences and interdisciplinary rounds, facilitate all team members' involvement in, and awareness of, all aspects of patient care, hence enhancing decision-making processes and clinical outcomes. Effective assessment in a multidisciplinary setting entails the employment of evidence-based guidelines established through collective expertise. These guidelines, such as those provided by the American Society of Hematology and other relevant organizations, guide the diagnosis of conditions such as von Willebrand disease (VWD) using a methodical process. They emphasize the importance of selected diagnostic tests, clinical findings, and prioritizing questions that impact both the clinician and patient perspectives. The multidisciplinary committee responsible for making such recommendations ensures that all aspects of patient evaluation, be it laboratory analysis, bleeding-assessment tools, are reviewed for efficacy and usability, thereby ensuring high medical standards. Such elaborate guidelines help to centralize the treatment protocols implemented in all the specialties, ultimately leading to improved consistency in critical care assessment. Additionally, the establishment of critical care assessment relies partly on the continued integration of new therapies and technology into practice. The multidisciplinary model encourages ongoing education in the latest available treatments among healthcare professionals, such as new therapeutic products and treatment modalities for bleeding disorders. Since the dawn of revolutionary therapies like gene therapy and half-life extended clotting factors, there is a dire need for coordinated education among various specialties. By creating forums for the exchange of information and team projects, healthcare professionals can become properly skilled to use the most optimal and current assessments and interventions. This is also as per guidelines given by the World Federation of Hemophilia, with the stress laid on total care being delivered by way of a well-coordinated, multidisciplinary approach (James *et al.*, 2021; Srivastava *et al.*, 2020).

2.4.1. Collaboration Among Healthcare Professionals

Effective interprofessional collaboration among healthcare providers is one of the foundations of quality care, particularly within critical care settings where patients have complex conditions that require diversified expertise. Multidisciplinary teams consisting of physicians, nurses, pharmacists, and allied health professionals in such settings provide an integrating platform for assessment and diagnosis. This collaborative strategy enhances not just the quality of care delivery but also holistic evaluations by integrating various perspectives and specialized knowledge. As illustrated by the assessment of artificial intelligence in healthcare, these collaboration practices can be enhanced by technology-supported tools that enhance diagnostic accuracy and develop personalized pathways of treatment to promote patient outcomes (Otu *et al.*, 2025). In addition, the setting of open lines of communication and shared purposes between team members is crucial in ensuring maximum effectiveness of interprofessional practice. The dynamic nature of critical care settings necessitates healthcare professionals to remain consistently flexible and attentive to shifting patient needs. With an interdisciplinary approach, ongoing learning and exchange of best practices among team members become easier. This common culture not only facilitates cross-pollination of ideas but also facilitates active participation by healthcare providers in decision-making. For instance, an interdisciplinary problem-solving approach can significantly reduce the risk of misdiagnosis, particularly in illnesses with identical clinical presentations, which also adds weight to collective assessment and discussion among specialists (Bonon, 2024). Additionally, regular interdisciplinary rounds can solidify team integration, promote professional responsibility, and create a patient-centered care culture. Lastly, collaboration training is crucial since collaborative work has immediate consequences on patient safety and quality of care. Collaboration skills training, conflict management, and shared responsibility training are crucial in readying healthcare professionals to operate in teams with ease. As healthcare settings continue to evolve, developing collaborative abilities will enhance teams' ability to handle exigencies more efficiently. Importantly, implementation of simulation-based education can provide real-life opportunities for health care providers to learn teamwork skills in real situations, preparing them for emergency conditions in critical care settings. Lastly, through embracing a philosophy of collaboration, healthcare practitioners may exceedingly well enhance their collective capacity for holistic and effective diagnoses and assessment, which is pivotal in optimizing patient outcomes in critical care environments (Figure 2.11).

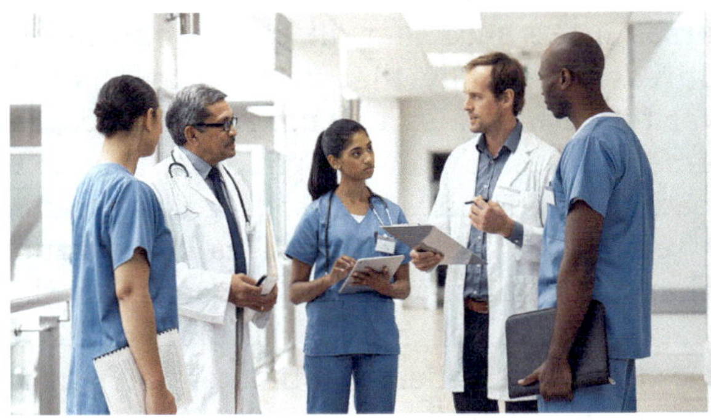

Figure 2.11. Collaboration in healthcare is key to driving better quality care.

Source: https://blog.wcei.net/wp-content/uploads/2024/06/collaborationinhealthcare.jpg.

2.4.2. Role of Nurses in Patient Assessment

The assessment role of the nurse is imperative, especially in intensive care units where fast and accurate assessments can save lives. Nurses are often the first caregivers tasked with direct contact with the patient and his/her family, so that they can gather vast clinical information. The key information from this direct source builds a whole picture of the patient's health status, such as vital signs, physical examination, and patient history. Furthermore, nurses are taught to observe small things that do not necessarily catch a doctor's eye, thus becoming critical first responders for early detection of difficulties such as deteriorating health or potential complications. Their ongoing observation plays a significant role in the establishment of individualized care plans and delivering timely interventions, which are intrinsic components in handling critically ill patients as a unit. Besides direct evaluation, nurses also play a crucial role in facilitating multidisciplinary teams to improve patient care. Their training prepares them with the necessary skills to communicate effectively among various healthcare providers like doctors, respiratory therapists, and dietitians. Being patient advocates as frontline practitioners, nurses make sure that all care problems are addressed and any that develop are handed over to the health care team. For instance, the nurse can decide how the patient responds to treatment, and this can direct drug management or requesting further tests. This coordination enhances continuity of care and ensures that treatment plans align with the evolving needs of critically ill patients, ultimately enhancing outcomes. The critical functions for nurses in treating specific conditions affirm the necessity of ongoing education and training in patient assessment techniques. Empirical research has shown that knowledge gaps can adversely affect nurses' knowledge and reaction to critical patients, particularly in areas like sepsis and diabetic foot care. For example, some studies have proven that ICU nurses have inadequate knowledge in the assessment and care of sepsis, with a high percentage having poor practice capabilities (Khan *et al.*, 2025). Similarly, a lack of adequate knowledge concerning diabetic foot care amongst nurses has been linked to poor outcomes amongst diabetes patients (Mahar *et al.*, 2024). Such findings underscore the role of advanced training programs that maximize nursing competencies in these high-stakes care fields, ultimately leading to improved assessment and diagnosis within high-stakes environments (Figure 2.12).

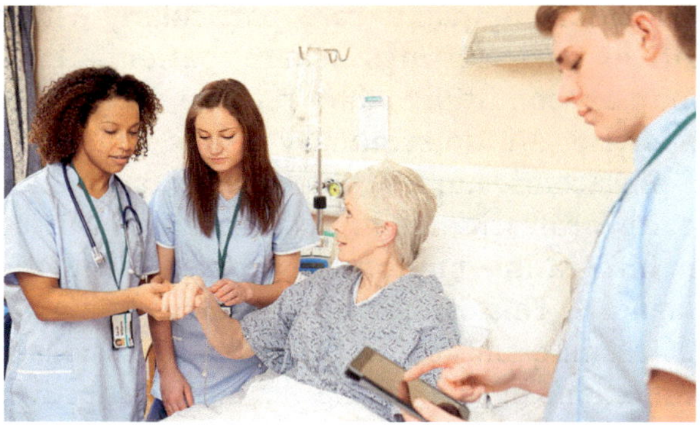

Figure 2.12. Nurses assessing a patient.

Source: https://blogs.biomedcentral.com/on-medicine/wp-content/uploads/sites/6/2023/09/nursing-assessment.jpg.

2.4.3. Involvement of Specialists in Diagnosis

The role of specialists in diagnosis is an inherent part of effective assessment and management in critical care units. In such settings, diagnosis is generally obtained through a multidisciplinary approach, involving the expertise and skills of various specialists, each contributing specialized knowledge and insights. For example, in the care of complex conditions such as pediatric cor pulmonale, it takes a team effort by pediatric cardiologists, pulmonologists, and critical care specialists to achieve proper diagnosis and subsequent management. This team effort enables comprehensive evaluation of symptoms, risk factors, and pathophysiology, thereby increasing the chances of successful intervention. Moreover, the early detection of conditions such as cor pulmonale through the utilization of sophisticated imaging and hemodynamic assessment is heavily reliant on a specialist's knowledge, thereby underscoring the significance of their involvement in critical care diagnosis (Thakur *et al.*, 2024). Specialists are not only involved in diagnosis but also have a significant role in designing personalized treatment plans based on the individual needs of patients. For instance, in neurodegenerative diseases like Parkinson's disease, timely treatment with drugs is crucial to the patient's outcome. Not only do experts provide information on the correct pharmacology of the medications, but also on the entire treatment regimen, including coordinating different care teams to follow treatment protocols. The Cambridge University Hospitals' Parkinson's disease medication management audit is an example of significant care deficits that can be filled by addressing specialty involvement, particularly to ensure timely medication administration and proper specialist evaluation (Jermola *et al.*, 2024).

This attests to the importance of a specialist's knowledge in addressing complex clinical issues that arise in critical care settings. In the practice of critical care, looking for better diagnostic practice always relies on specialist advice for optimizing patient outcomes. Specialist partnership promotes a spirit of understanding and consensus in diagnostics' decision-making, which is particularly applicable in time-sensitive conditions prevalent in critical settings. Through interprofessional rounds and case conferences, experts can provide diverse insights and evidence-based suggestions that enhance diagnostic accuracy and establish clear treatment algorithms. Moreover, producing standard protocols and promoting communication between experts can minimize risks of misdiagnosis and improve patient management , further ascertaining the importance of their presence in acute cases. The ongoing interaction of various specialists not only sustains the quality of care in such delicate situations but also promotes a platform that is conducive to both patient safety and clinical effectiveness (Thakur *et al.*, 2024).

Test Your Knowledge

1. How does collaboration among healthcare professionals benefit patient care in critical settings?
2. What is the role of nurses in the ongoing assessment of critically ill patients?

2.5. Challenges in Assessment and Diagnosis

Learning Outcome

1. Discuss the complexity of critical care patients
2. Understand the limitations of diagnostic tools
3. Define ethical considerations in diagnosis

Assessment and diagnosis within critical care settings present a multitude of challenges that can have a profound impact on patient outcomes. Arguably, one of the most trenchant challenges is the necessity to base decision-making on complex and at times ambiguous clinical indicators. Critical care patients may have multi-system dysfunction, which makes it difficult to differentiate among the etiologies of their condition. For instance, the overlapping symptoms of numerous disorders can lead to misdiagnosis or delayed treatment. Additionally, the urgent nature of critical care environments often necessitates quick decision-making that can result in hasty assessment. Such rapid assessments can exclude important details such as vital signs or laboratory testing, thereby causing harm to patients. Thus, healthcare professionals need to establish a methodical approach to assessment that minimizes the potential for omission but allows for timely intervention.

Furthermore, patient-specific factors like age, comorbidities, and communication issues also make it difficult to process the assessment and diagnosis. Patients with cognitive impairment or those who cannot communicate their symptoms, for instance, may be an extremely challenging situation in determining their health condition. Patients with dementia or severe delirium, for instance, may require other methods of assessing their needs and preferences, which will impact the shared decision-making. Traditional assessment tools are not good at capturing the nuances of an individual patient's medical issues and desires. Clinicians, therefore, need to be capable of adjusting their approach to suit different groups of patients. Patients, families, and caregivers can also be highly insightful when engaged in discussions around assessments and can facilitate a better understanding of patient's health. Multidisciplinary team participation in diagnostic work in critical care can improve assessment as it is more precise and efficient by providing a wider picture of the patient's health. Specialist collaboration, nurses, and allied health professionals through sharing specialty skills allows for combining different expertise, which is immensely valuable when dealing with unusual cases. Such collaboration is essential in the management of such challenges as in the patient with rare genetic disorders, where traditional evaluation methods cannot cope. For example, multi-disciplinary collaboration is paramount in the dental anomalies of patients with IFIH1-related disorders, where different experts collaborate to develop holistic treatment plans. Moreover, shared decision-making strategies can potentially enable patients and families to express their values and preferences in meaningful terms, bridging treatment goals with patient needs in efficient ways. In the end, it aims to moderate some of the inherent challenges in the process of assessment and diagnosis in critical care environments (Friedman *et al.*, 2025; Lim *et al.*, 2024).

2.5.1. Complexity of Critical Care Patients

The complexity of critical care patients is highlighted by the multilaterality of the medical conditions they present, which are often associated with co-occurring pathologies that need intensive and immediate intervention. Critical care patients often have complicated health problems that require a fine-tuned approach to diagnosis and assessment. The understanding of the fluctuating psychiatric diagnoses, for example, can be one of the factors that impact the management and treatment practices being used in critical care. Personalized care that responds to the distinct requirements of the patient, such as the function of support systems, is vital in seeking to enhance their wellness. Based on an understanding of the diverse profiles and requirements that come with different diagnoses, health experts can better engage with patients and their support systems, ensuring optimal overall quality of critical care interventions (Sousa *et al.*, 2024). Added to the complexity of this patient population is the high nursing workload of intensive care, which has been noted to directly influence patient outcomes. This study of nursing activity and patient care emphasizes the intensity with which critical care practitioners have to work. Exposure has shown that increased nursing workload at admission and discharge is linked to increased risks of adverse events, such as ICU readmission and medication errors. It demonstrates the importance of strategic management of workload to prevent potential complications arising from overworked healthcare personnel. Through the use of effective tools like the Nursing Activities Score (NAS), healthcare professionals can ascertain whether additional resources may be needed to avoid risks and improve patient outcomes within the critical care environment (Alhosani *et al.*, 2023). Moreover, the role of interdisciplinary communication to navigate the complexity of critical care patients cannot be overemphasized. Effective communication among healthcare staff, patients, and families is essential to effective treatment procedures. Having companions around during consultations, for example, can assist in understanding the psychological nature of a patient's condition so that physical and mental health needs are attended to. Incorporation of companions has been found to enhance communication and understanding, thereby improving treatment protocol adherence. This interprofessional approach enhances the integrative nature of critical care, emphasizing that a comprehensive approach must incorporate not only clinical evaluation but also the psychosocial elements that contribute to a patient's overall general health trajectory (Sousa *et al.*, 2024) (Figure 2.13).

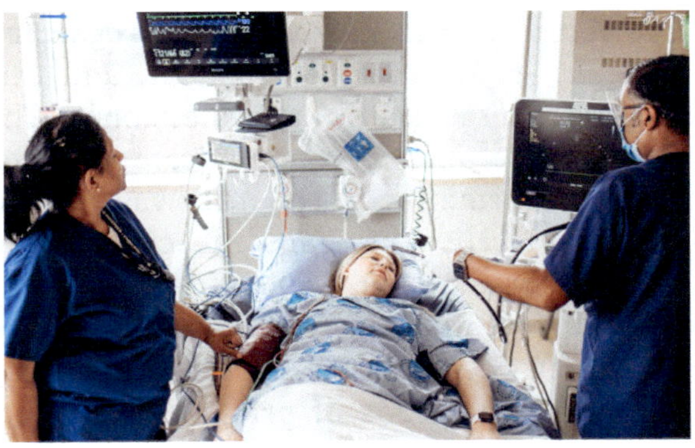

Figure 2.13. The complexity of critical care patients.

Source: https://images.squarespace-cdn.com/content/v1/5ad0e57d50a54fd13cb5d5b8/3bf62227-520b-4b98-8e53-91554a5858a8/FTFL_1000X640.png.

2.5.2. Limitations of Diagnostic Tools

Diagnostic equipment effectiveness is most critical in critical care settings, but it is never without limitations that can influence clinical judgment. A major limitation is the availability and accessibility of advanced imaging technologies like computed tomography pulmonary angiography (CTPA). Even though CTPA is the gold standard for diagnosing acute pulmonary embolism (PE), its application can be encumbered in low-resource countries and resource-limited environments, where such infrastructure does not exist (Melo *et al.*, 2025). Consequently, more rudimentary or point-of-care diagnostic systems may be entirely reliant on, which can lead to misdiagnosis or delayed treatment. The disparity in the utilization of high-quality diagnostic devices indicates the necessity of researching alternative modalities and ensuring that critical care patients receive proper utilization of accurate and timely evaluations, regardless of location. Diagnostic device accuracy and interpretation is also significant limitations that vary dramatically depending on the context of use and user expertise. For example, POCUS has emerged as an efficient and rapid replacement for traditional imaging techniques within the emergency and critical care settings. While studies have identified that POCUS demonstrates high diagnostic accuracy in conditions like PE, success relies on operator competency and experience (Melo *et al.*, 2025). Subjectivity in ultrasound interpretation causes variability in diagnostic findings, hence uncertainty in patient management. Additionally, POCUS may be limited in generating the same level of detail as usual imaging modalities, thus diagnosis may be further complicated. A guarantee of including thorough training and standardization of POCUS practice remains the panacea for mitigating these limitations and enhancing overall diagnostic test reliability in critical care. The diagnostic equipment range also encompasses their ability to be utilized in addressing the multifaceted aspects of deadly diseases. Precisely, while POCUS is a macroscopic technique of detecting gross pathological conditions, it does not possess the histopathological examination of autopsies. Furthermore, while POCUS provides immediate feedback, its inability to make specific diagnoses can lead to gaps in postmortem analysis. The POCUS controversy as a bedside autopsy raises the need for integrated solutions that combine several diagnostic modalities to offer accurate assessments. With advanced critical care environments developing further, there needs to be a common aspiration to develop synergistic diagnosis protocols that encompass new-edge imaging devices and traditional approaches. These will enhance diagnostic accuracy, enhance patient care streamlining, and ultimately yield better results in critical care environments (Figure 2.14).

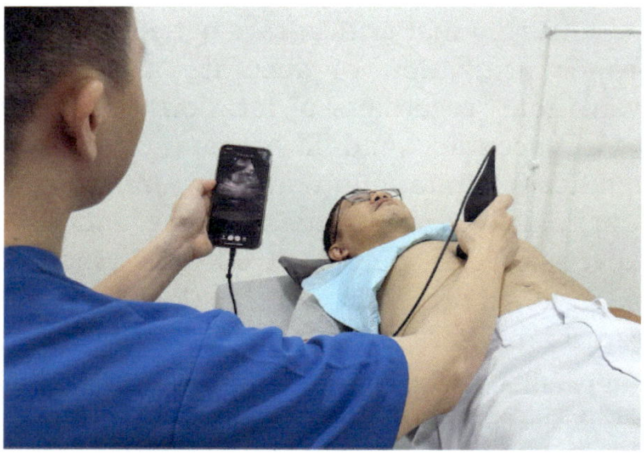

Figure 2.14. Point-of-care Ultrasound (POCUS) in critical care.

Source: https://drplus.com.sg/wp-content/uploads/2024/03/20231004_165548-scaled-e1710221798336.jpg.

2.5.3. Ethical Considerations in Diagnosis

Critical care diagnosis practice regularly leads clinicians to traverse a complex landscape of ethical dilemmas. Ethical decision-making is often required in the initial assessment of patients when their situations may not have apparent symptoms to offer. This ambiguity brings tension between requiring speed and providing treatment, and requiring precision in diagnosing. Misdiagnosis leads to incorrect treatment plans, potentially worsening the patient's situation and infringing on fundamental ethical principles such as "do no harm." Ensuring, therefore, that a thorough but rapid assessment is conducted is of cardinal importance, particularly in high-risk environments such as critical care units where every minute is precious. In addition, healthcare providers must be firm in upholding evidence-based practice for the sake of guaranteeing the integrity of their diagnostic results and respecting the patient's autonomy and informed consent throughout diagnosis (Vahanian *et al.*, 2021). Another aspect of critical care diagnosis sophistication in terms of ethics is upholding the transparency of patient and family communication. With the intricate nature of diagnostics, healthcare professionals should share open discussion on the potential risks, benefits, and unknowns of various diagnostic tests and interventions. Providing patients and their relatives with complete information empowers them to make choices regarding their care in an informed manner, and this builds trust in the healthcare professionals. The issue is to be able to communicate complex medical information straightforwardly and compassionately. This requires compassion towards the emotional well-being of families that may be subjected to sudden crises and loss of loved ones. Being transparent is not only necessary as a means of prioritizing respect for patient autonomy but also as a means of promoting mutual decision-making, in which patients and families feel heard and involved in their care process (Lambertini *et al.*, 2020). Besides, ethical considerations of diagnosis are concerned with the distribution of intensive care resources. Healthcare inequities can heighten ethical concerns, particularly when diagnostic facilities, time, and healthcare professionals are limited. Physicians will have to deal with the ethical dilemma of ranking patients according to potentially biased evaluations that, in the process, allocate favor to some groups ahead of others. Such decisions can influence the availability of treatment and may violate ethical principles of justice and equity. Therefore, the establishment of rigorous regulations on resource allocation based on evidence and equity is essential in fostering ethical practice in the diagnostic process. Critical care professionals must advocate for policies ensuring equal access to diagnostic care with ethical considerations as a core component of patient-centered care in extremely demanding medical environments (Vahanian *et al.*, 2021).

Test Your Knowledge

1. How can the limitations of diagnostic tools affect patient management in the ICU?
2. What ethical considerations must be taken into account during the diagnostic process in critical care?

SUMMARY

The evaluation and diagnosis of critical care patients are crucial for proper management and improved outcomes. Various methods, including the application of advanced technologies like AI-based language learner models (LLMs) in diagnosis, have been tried and examined in this essay. The findings indicate that LLMs possess the potential to answer multiple-choice questions as well as open-ended questions in critical care, but there exist severe restrictions on their application. Surprisingly, LLMs were found to have impairments in scenario management as well as overall clinical reasoning, which may undermine patient safety. As noted in (Chaitanya *et al.*, 2024), this phenomenon of studying LLMs in critical care highlights the importance of ongoing research to refine these tools and make them more reliable for use in clinical decision-making, thus contributing to safer care for patients. Moreover, studies of the Hindi version of the Confusion Assessment Method for the intensive care unit (CAM-ICU) provide a better example of how culture-sensitive diagnostic tools can significantly assist in delirium detection among culturally heterogeneous patient groups. Validity and reliability in Salhotra *et al.*, 2024 suggest that localized evaluation tools have to make sure healthcare workers are able to diagnose and treat life-threatening conditions effectively, thus the gap between treatment and knowledge is eliminated. The tools allow for prompt interventions, which are crucial within the high-stakes environment of critical care where an error in diagnosis may be fatal. By prioritizing inclusive diagnostic approaches, healthcare systems can enhance overall patient care in critical settings. Combining advanced diagnostic approaches and ethnically responsive test and measurement approaches becomes a critical aspect of critical care medicine practice. As the health care environment is further developing, with both technological newness and ethnic diversity included in evaluation measures, this will be an essence. Striving to bridge the gaps discovered in LLMs, and calibrating equipment like the Hindi CAM-ICU, will help in more accurate and efficient testing in critical care medicine. This continued focus on innovation and adjustment will not only improve patient outcomes, but also create the more inclusive healthcare setting, ultimately benefiting a larger population of patients at their most desperate juncture.

The critical care environment calls for patient evaluation and diagnosis to be systematized and structured to maximize the efficacy of interventions. Central to this assessment is the initial detection of life-threatening conditions, particularly respiratory and hemodynamic instability. As emphasized, the process begins with a focused history and physical examination designed to detect "must-not-miss" pathologies that can deteriorate the patient's condition. The urgency of this process is underscored by the requirement to make rapid therapeutic choices, particularly in the context of complications like elevated intracranial pressure or sudden neurovascular injury. This rapid course of assessment ends with the immediate acquisition of neuroimaging to clarify potential structural dysfunction and hence inform the subsequent stage of management schemes (Wahlster *et al.*, 2024). Also, the merging of laboratory information is crucial in making a comprehensive diagnostic picture in critically ill patients. This involves screening for systemic causes that may be masked by the acute presentations, and having the care team on high alert for developing complications like infections of the central nervous system or failure of the neuromuscular. With the final goal of saving lives, the coordination among multidisciplinary teams is important because they refer to their collective experience to resolve complex cases. Furthermore, the utilization of advanced technology such as EEG or lumbar puncture can also be strategically applied based on clinical conditions, further refining the evaluation process. Lastly, these pieces are brought together to provide a solid framework that enhances patient results through effective diagnosis and care (Marconi *et al.*, 2024). The significance of a broad framework is also underscored by the value put on the problem with critical care is also displayed in the example of a study of integrated care pathways (ICPs) for the treatment of conditions such as dementia. This shows the need for standardized approaches in offering quality care. In spite of low compliance with established guidelines reported by this study, it highlights the necessity of ongoing monitoring and calibration of assessment processes in high-stakes environments. Harmonization of ICPs against national guidelines can be employed as a benchmark for increasing care within critical settings, guaranteeing that health professionals possess the tools and information necessary to evaluate patients effectively. Lastly, the preservation of high-quality care in high-risk environments relies on constant observation and evidence-based interventions, which are paramount to the achievement of successful positive health outcomes (Wahlster *et al.*, 2024).

KEY TERMS FROM THIS CHAPTER

- Arterial blood gas (ABG)
- Assessment
- Blood pressure
- Chest X-ray
- Clinical examination
- CT scan
- Diagnosis
- Echocardiography
- Electrocardiogram (ECG)
- Electrolyte Imbalances
- Glasgow coma scale (GCS)
- Heart rate
- Hemodynamic monitoring
- MRI
- Neurological assessment
- Oxygen saturation (SpO_2)
- Pain assessment
- Pulse oximetry
- Respiratory rate
- Temperature
- Ultrasound
- Urine output monitoring
- Vital signs

CRITICAL THINKING QUESTIONS

1. **Which scoring system is commonly used to assess the severity of illness in ICU patients?**
   a. APGAR score
   b. Glasgow Coma Scale
   c. APACHE II (Acute Physiology and Chronic Health Evaluation II)
   d. Mini-Mental State Examination
2. **The Glasgow Coma Scale (GCS) is used primarily to assess which of the following?**
   a. Respiratory function
   b. Liver function
   c. Level of consciousness
   d. Renal output
3. **In critical care, which diagnostic tool is most commonly used to monitor oxygenation and ventilation status?**
   a. Chest X-ray
   b. CT scan
   c. Arterial Blood Gas (ABG) analysis
   d. ECG
4. **Which parameter is NOT included in the Sequential Organ Failure Assessment (SOFA) score?**
   a. Respiratory function
   b. Neurological status
   c. Coagulation profile
   d. Bone density
5. **What is the purpose of a central venous pressure (CVP) measurement in ICU patients?**
   a. To evaluate liver function
   b. To estimate right atrial pressure and guide fluid management
   c. To determine heart rate
   d. To assess blood glucose levels

Short Answer Questions

1. What is the primary role of assessment in critical care settings?
2. Name two commonly used diagnostic tools in critical care and briefly describe their purpose.
3. How does clinical judgment influence the diagnostic process in critically ill patients?
4. Why is a multidisciplinary approach important in patient assessment within critical care?
5. Identify one major challenge in diagnosing critically ill patients and suggest a possible solution.
6. How can continuous monitoring improve assessment outcomes in critical care environments?

Answer to Critical Thinking Questions

1. (c); 2. (c); 3. (c); 4. (d); 5. (b)

REFERENCES

1. Abdullah, R. Y., Hassan, K. H., & Yasin, M. M. (2025). Knowledge towards nursing process and barriers to implementing nursing process in health care system in Iraqi Kurdistan region. *Saudi Journal of Health Systems Research*. https://www.semanticscholar.org/paper/41f3a0395bfbfe8441e9afcd580b79ca08875f5e (accessed on 22 May 2025).
2. Aditi, A., Gupta, N. K. K., & Sharma, A. (2024). Enhanced heart disease prediction using machine learning techniques. *Journal of Intelligent Systems and Internet of Things*. https://www.semanticscholar.org/paper/de46ec7118f60613c292ada31399dafe62eea97b (accessed on 22 May 2025).
3. Albagieh, H., Aldrees, M. N., Alshamrani, A. H., Alnadhari, S. M., Almuwayni, R. M., Alotaibi, K. F., & Alayed, S. (2024). Role of laboratory tests in enhancing diagnosis and treatment planning for dentists: A review of evidence-based practices. *Cureus, 16*. https://www.semanticscholar.org/paper/088e2c5934aef9a7fd5cedf6e140408a50caae35 (accessed on 22 May 2025).
4. AlHarbi, N. M., AlHarbi, F. H., Al-Shalali, A. M. S., Alheary, W. E., Althbyani, B. M., Alaeinbawi, M. H., Alrehaili, H. A. S., *et al.* (2024). Advancing cancer care: A critical review of MRI imaging in pretherapeutic malignancy assessment. *Journal of Eco Humanism*. https://www.semanticscholar.org/paper/c9568d93158e1d4c36f812365837c018adbbe75c (accessed on 22 May 2025).
5. Alhosani, M. I., Ahmed, F., Al-Yateem, N., Mobarak, H. S., & Aburuz, M. (2023). Assessment of nursing workload and adverse events reporting among critical care nurses in the United Arab Emirates. *The Open Nursing Journal*. https://www.semanticscholar.org/paper/e4908fb8fe9353311d77054ebbf96a9045ae991f (accessed on 22 May 2025).
6. Allam, S. (2024). Advancing patient-centered care: A nationwide analysis of hospital efficiency and morbidity using innovative propensity score techniques. *Cureus, 16*. https://www.semanticscholar.org/paper/73ff6daf2b67e3d18fa74a38c99eaf117d918e2b (accessed on 22 May 2025).
7. Androulidakis, A., Bracale, U., Konnis, G., Koutsouris, G., *et al.* (2011). A feasibility study for the provision of electronic healthcare tools and services in areas of Greece, Cyprus and Italy. https://core.ac.uk/download/16664902.pdf (accessed on 22 May 2025).
8. Assante, W., Kore, S., Alavi, R., Foroshani, S., Andrabi, S., Kichloo, A., & Chugh, S. (2025). Evaluating outcomes in critically ill patients with undiagnosed acute kidney injury: A comparison of the incidence of physician-diagnosed vs KDIGO criteria-diagnosed acute kidney injury. *Proceedings, 38*(3), 266–271. https://www.semanticscholar.org/paper/5ada6cb7fb19ae05a44f20de5fd15e2442cb1467 (accessed on 22 May 2025).
9. Bache, C. E., Harmatz, P. R., Jester, A., Mackenzie, W., *et al.* (2014). Orthopedic management of the extremities in patients with Morquio A syndrome. https://core.ac.uk/download/323062594.pdf.
10. Berisha, V., Demjaha, G., Gjikolli, A., Kiseri, F., *et al.* (2023). Oral habits of patients as indicators of occlusal dysfunction: A comprehensive review. https://core.ac.uk/download/616936096.pdf (accessed on 22 May 2025).
11. Bonon, M. R. C. D. (2024). Differentiating vulgar psoriasis and tinea incognito: Challenges and implications for healthcare professionals. *Revita Systematical*. https://www.semanticscholar.org/paper/401ffcf984c2247f48b4715f4be39c9e5773a098 (accessed on 22 May 2025).

12. Bull, F., Al-Ansari, S. S., Biddle, S., Borodulin, K., Buman, M. P., Cardon, G., Carty, C., *et al.* (2020). World Health Organization 2020 guidelines on physical activity and sedentary behavior. *British Journal of Sports Medicine, 54*, 1451–1462. https://doi.org/10.1136/bjsports-2020-102955.

13. Campbell, K., Torrence-Hill, J., Whitten, K. A., Abbud, M., Querubin, J. A., Stewart, C., Dobre, M., *et al.* (2025). Abstract 987: Enhancing oncology navigation services: A mixed methods approach to developing an EHR power form to improve metrics and reporting. *Cancer Research*. https://www.semanticscholar.org/paper/b1d6d0d81f9b02a702a1ab92089af033fce82140 (accessed on 22 May 2025).

14. Chaitanya, K., Pavan, N., Reddy, K., & Gpvn, S. (2024). Chatbots in the ICU: Unveiling the accuracy and limitations of AI in critical care knowledge assessment. *Indian Journal of Critical Care Medicine, 28*, S139–S142. https://www.semanticscholar.org/paper/0f9985d397e8e2a64e9d3963b94cd1066fcc6c61 (accessed on 22 May 2025).

15. Cheng, A. L., Herman, E., Abramoff, B. A., Anderson, J., Azola, A., Baratta, J. M., Bartels, M. N., *et al.* (2025). Multidisciplinary collaborative guidance on the assessment and treatment of patients with Long COVID: A compendium statement. *PM&R: The Journal of Injury, Function, and Rehabilitation*. https://www.semanticscholar.org/paper/e9bd7c0b0cc281b0495e85211df2081086d574a5 (accessed on 22 May 2025).

16. Chew, D. P., Scott, I., Cullen, L., French, J., Briffa, T., Tideman, P., Woodruffe, S., *et al.* (2016). National Heart Foundation of Australia & Cardiac Society of Australia and New Zealand: Australian clinical guidelines for the management of acute coronary syndromes 2016. *Heart, Lung and Circulation, 25*, 895–951. https://doi.org/10.1016/j.hlc.2016.06.789.

17. Cocchieri, E., Cristofori, M., Nurchis, M. C., Nursing and Public Health Group, Damiani, G., & Cesare, M. (2025). Nursing complexity and health literacy as determinants of patient outcomes: A prospective one-year multicenter cohort study. *Nursing Reports, 15*. https://www.semanticscholar.org/paper/0f553316bf0621f51ce4310fd48111f66d0549cb (accessed on 22 May 2025).

18. De Freitas, L., Carregari, J. A., Garcia, A. C. M., Chini, L. T., Costa, A. C. B., & Fava, S. M. C. L. (2024). Nursing care plan for people with heart failure in palliative care. *Latin American Journal of Palliative Care*. https://www.semanticscholar.org/paper/99cc7bd7f839930b255fdfab834227721567c604 (accessed on 22 May 2025).

19. Friedman, C. S., Ari, T., Ünsal, G., Balci, T., Morrison, M., & Ari, N. (2025). Overlap diagnostic odyssey and full mouth rehabilitation of a juvenile patient with IFIH1-related disorder: A case of Aicardi-Goutières and Singleton Merten syndromes overlap. *Special Care in Dentistry, 45*. https://www.semanticscholar.org/paper/838d66d3eafd536f18b7060e34f0f99ffca058e1 (accessed on 22 May 2025).

20. Georgakopoulou, V. (2025). Optimizing patient outcomes in interstitial lung disease through pre- and post-transplant management strategies. *World Journal of Transplantation*. https://www.semanticscholar.org/paper/74d796ce4e10c18b673a1a8aa1a7e0fab37d130e (accessed on 22 May 2025).

21. Hossain, M. J., Das, M., Shahjahan, M., Islam, M. W., & Towhid, S. (2025). Clinical and hematological manifestation of dengue patients in 2022 outbreak: A tertiary care hospital-based cross-sectional study. *Health Science Reports, 8*. https://www.semanticscholar.org/paper/e8fd54a2b101ea7a1788f9ae1f3ddd056c7f7574 (accessed on 22 May 2025).

22. Izquierdo-Pretel, G. (2025). From cadavers to soundwaves: The evolution of autopsy in medical diagnosis and the rise of point-of-care ultrasound. *Cureus, 17*. https://www.semanticscholar.org/paper/da12499df83d7e7b1116a09a31bf0776fa82ffe5 (accessed on 22 May 2025).

23. James, P., Connell, N. T., Ameer, B., Di Paola, J., Eikenboom, J., Giraud, N., Haberichter, S. L., *et al.* (2021). ASH ISTH NHF WFH 2021 guidelines on the diagnosis of von Willebrand disease. *Blood Advances, 5*, 280–300. https://doi.org/10.1182/bloodadvances.2020003265.

24. Jermola, E., & McDonald, M. (2024). eHospitals and Parkinson's disease care: Audit insights from an EPIC-integrated hospital. *International Journal of Pharmacy Practice*. https://www.semanticscholar.org/paper/7a8b4a5c620f24e44596f393741218f6d1600117 (accessed on 22 May 2025).

25. Khan, I., Ashfaq, S., & Khushid, K. (2025). Evaluate analysis and decision-making of nurses regarding sepsis assessment and management in critically ill patients. *Biological and Clinical Sciences Research Journal*. https://www.semanticscholar.org/paper/65e433a72d72232d3bb095e10c92fc859de8ecab (accessed on 22 May 2025).

26. Korelidou, V., Simitzis, P., Massouras, T., & Gelasakis, A. (2024). Infrared thermography as a diagnostic tool for the assessment of mastitis in dairy ruminants. *Animals, 14*. https://www.semanticscholar.org/paper/ad4c86876865d90e0e75e6e2e16441a3d6c184c9 (accessed on 22 May 2025).

27. Lakshminarayanan, S., Aboobacker, M., Brar, A., Manoj, M. P., Elnimer, M. M. E. I., Marepalli, A., Shukla, K., *et al.* (2024). Advancing perioperative neurocognitive health: A critical review of predictive tools, diagnostic methods, and interventional strategies. *Cureus, 16*. https://www.semanticscholar.org/paper/0e46286a488b3a5f274c896a849891caac7c1978 (accessed on 22 May 2025).

28. Lambertini, M., Toss, A., Passaro, A., Criscitiello, C., Cremolini, C., Cardone, C., Loupakis, F., *et al.* (2020). Cancer care during the spread of coronavirus disease 2019 (COVID-19) in Italy: Young oncologists' perspective. *ESMO Open, 5*, e000759. https://doi.org/10.1136/esmoopen-2020-000759.

29. Lim, H., Choe, Y., Hwang, J., Choi, S. H., Kim, S. J., Lee, J. H., Woo, J. I., *et al.* (2024). Preference assessment in dementia care: Systematic literature review. *Alzheimer's & Dementia, 20*. https://www.semanticscholar.org/paper/3070ed954a3818b2e280a8c7f634f20e05caa4fc (accessed on 22 May 2025).

30. Mahar, S., Soomro, F., Haque, A., Zakarya, M., Jamali, I. A., Rai, Y., & Gul, S. (2024). Assessment of the knowledge levels of nurses of diabetic foot care management and to determine influencing factors. *Social Science Review Archives*. https://www.semanticscholar.org/paper/ea675ddc6099ace8755ee34068674fe5bfcf2596 (accessed on 22 May 2025).

31. Marconi, S., Pani, M., Salemme, S., Lazzeri, G., Sardu, C., Bacigalupo, I., Lorenzini, P., *et al.* (2024). Assessment of integrated care pathways for dementia in Italy according to the national guidance. *The European Journal of Public Health, 34*. https://www.semanticscholar.org/paper/4be9c1d2994f937a45a976b521bbbbefac621ebd (accessed on 22 May 2025).

32. Matthay, M., Arabi, Y., Arroliga, A., Bernard, G., Bersten, A., Brochard, L., Calfee, C., *et al.* (2023). A new global definition of acute respiratory distress syndrome. *American Journal of Respiratory and Critical Care Medicine, 209*, 37–47. https://www.semanticscholar.org/paper/a1460aa39563d339b120298e5952c0b4cf26e092 (accessed on 22 May 2025).

33. Melo, R. H., Gioli-Pereira, L., Lourenço, I. D., Passos, R. H., Bernardo, A. T., & Volpicelli, G. (2025). Diagnostic accuracy of multi-organ point-of-care ultrasound for pulmonary embolism in critically ill patients: A systematic review and meta-analysis. *Critical Care, 29*. https://www.semanticscholar.org/paper/98a195aff601a5756d05893a9fdd04d49f60f1ca (accessed on 22 May 2025).

34. Meloy, P. G., Rutz, D. R., & Bhambri, A. (2023). Acute chest syndrome. *Journal of Education & Teaching in Emergency Medicine, 8*, O1–O23. https://www.semanticscholar.org/paper/19db50ef41095c800884649893878816lf5b8c0c (accessed on 22 May 2025).

35. Moura de Azevedo, S., Duarte, R., Krowicki, J., Vázquez, D., Arroja, S. P. F., & Mariz, J. (2024). Heart in focus: Advancing pericardial effusion diagnosis with point-of-care ultrasound. *Cureus, 16*. https://www.semanticscholar.org/paper/f3ef173120964304dcb303c9131d4ff0857a31f7 (accessed on 22 May 2025).

36. Otu, W., Khan, M. U., Javed, H. T., & Sheikh, I. S. (2025). Artificial intelligence in epilepsy education. *Advanced Neurology*. https://www.semanticscholar.org/paper/0d102f137bdbbca104e81372b030e0e1a39469ec (accessed on 22 May 2025).

37. Page, M. J., Moher, D., Bossuyt, P. M., Boutron, I., Hoffmann, T., Mulrow, C. D., Shamseer, L., *et al.* (2021). PRISMA 2020 explanation and elaboration: Updated guidance and exemplars for reporting systematic reviews. *BMJ*. https://doi.org/10.1136/bmj.n160.

38. Patir, B., Jyoti, C., Kumar, P., & Hazarika, A. (2025). Multi-view information fusion for EEG signal in health care monitoring: A systematic review for modeling new strategies. *Journal of Information Systems Engineering and Management*. https://www.semanticscholar.org/paper/ec379bd93280881a21845f10fb6b216c7f068e1c (accessed on 22 May 2025).

39. Rainer, R., Reynolds, B. C., Adeli, C., & San Miguel, C. E. (2024). Subarachnoid hemorrhage causing a seizure: An assessment simulation for medical students. *Journal of Education & Teaching in Emergency Medicine*, *9*, S30–S64. https://www.semanticscholar.org/paper/dc9d21ca0eb876150c02b1c12e8dc4bbbf408e56 (accessed on 22 May 2025).

40. Salhotra, R., Bose, A., Srivastava, S., Mohta, M., Pandarinathan, K., & Rautela, R. (2024). Reliability and validity of Hindi version of the Confusion Assessment Method for Intensive Care Unit (CAM-ICU) for diagnosis of delirium: A cohort study. *Indian Journal of Critical Care Medicine, 28*, 958–962. https://www.semanticscholar.org/paper/aea985eec8aefe6ab0893d09a9c80f7d8e2fe10a (accessed on 22 May 2025).

41. Sousa, C., Correia, Z., & Ramos, J. (2024). Tell me who you're coming with, I'll tell you what you have! *European Psychiatry, 67*(Suppl), S816–S817. https://www.semanticscholar.org/paper/703eb0fd0f98b951d91816bb4641b48fe68f9a88 (accessed on 22 May 2025).

42. Srivastava, A., Santagostino, E., Dougall, A., Kitchen, S., Sutherland, M. L., Pipe, S. W., Carção, M., *et al.* (2020). WFH guidelines for the management of hemophilia (3rd ed.). *Hemophilia, 26*, 1–158. https://doi.org/10.1111/hae.14046.

43. Susick, M. (2011). *Application of Smartphone Technology in The Management and Treatment of Mental Illnesses*. https://core.ac.uk/download/12206606.pdf (accessed on 22 May 2025).

44. Thakur, Y., Meshram, R., & Taksande, A. (2024). Navigating pediatric cor pulmonale: A comprehensive review of diagnosis and management. *Cureus, 16*. https://www.semanticscholar.org/paper/0c55d708784169569baf14219459599de5d6815e (accessed on 22 May 2025).

45. Vahanian, A., Beyersdorf, F., Praz, F., Milojevic, M., Baldus, S., Bauersachs, J., Capodanno, D., *et al.* (2021). 2021 ESC/EACTS guidelines for the management of valvular heart disease. *European Heart Journal, 43*, 561–632. https://doi.org/10.1093/eurheartj/ehab395.

46. Wahlster, S., & Johnson, N. J. (2024). The neurocritical care examination and workup. *CONTINUUM: Lifelong Learning in Neurology, 30*, 556–587. https://www.semanticscholar.org/paper/703a215d87fc762b8114d9de0c59ea3260129c05 (accessed on 22 May 2025).

47. Yang, L., Xu, Y., Ji, X., Wang, Z., Cao, C., Chong, P., & Wu, Z. (2023). Analysis of intensive care unit nursing clinical judgment and selection of nursing diagnosis for cerebral hemorrhage. *CIN: Computers, Informatics, Nursing, 41*, 789–795. https://www.semanticscholar.org/paper/cad0987a1f4fa32f4c0e01d7ec4b1b5f5e774378 (accessed on 22 May 2025).

AIRWAY MANAGEMENT AND RESPIRATORY SUPPORT

3

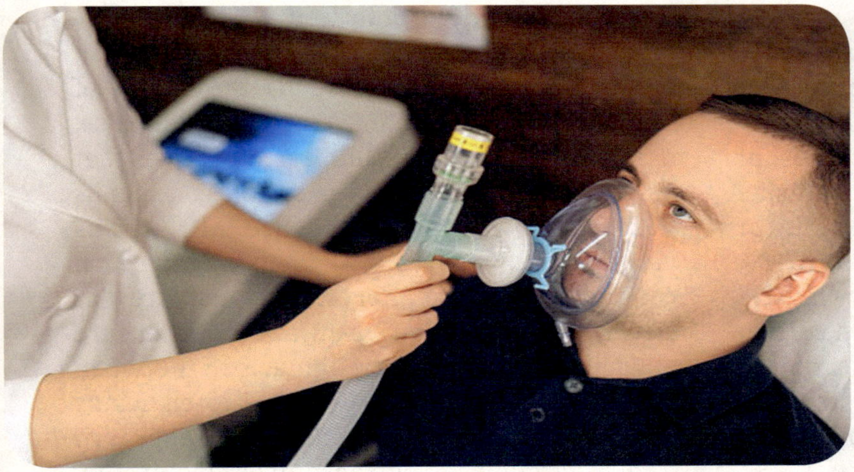

LEARNING OBJECTIVES

After studying this chapter, you will be able to:

1. Identify the anatomy of the respiratory system.
2. Discuss the assessment of airway patency.
3. Explain the techniques for airway management.
4. Define the respiratory support methods.
5. Identify potential complications of airway management.
6. Explain the current trends and innovations in airway management.

Introduction

Airway handling and respiratory care are top priorities in the practice of critical care and emergency medicine, especially when there are respiratory pathologies such as those encountered in the case of COVID-19. The complexity of airway handling begins with the recognition of respiratory distress and the early execution of the proper interventions. Good airway management not only ensures adequate oxygenation but also prevents the evolution of hypoxic injuries that can develop due to the ongoing absence of adequate ventilation. Additionally, with advancements in technology, there have also arisen advanced devices that improve patient outcomes, particularly in situations where everyday practices are not enough. Knowledge of these advances within the framework of clinical protocols is essential in training healthcare practitioners assigned to administer emergency care. The area of emergency medical services (EMS) has increasingly seen the vital importance of remaining within the set guidelines for taking care of the airway. As a backward-looking study indicates, deviations from accepted practice can lead to suboptimal treatment of patients requiring respiratory intervention. The authors of this research found that in 90% of the scenarios, EMS personnel did not initially use less invasive practices prior to using more invasive practices. This trend highlights an area of important potential for enhancement in training and adherence to guidelines in EMS environments. The consequence of such findings suggests the necessity for continued assessment of the practice of airway management to ensure that guidelines leave room to respond to the evolving nature of patient care under emergencies, particularly in the context of complications posed by illnesses like COVID-19 (Ofei-Dodoo *et al.*, 2023). More studies of specialized respiratory support mechanisms demonstrate the growing recognition of chronic respiratory morbidities of COVID-19, or long COVID. Patients with respiratory muscle weakness can significantly benefit from certain rehabilitation protocols, like the application of low-cost respiratory muscle strength training (RMST) devices. A case study demonstrated how a patient who was undergoing RMST showed considerable improvement in muscle performance, thereby facilitating an early return to normal respiratory function. The experience highlights the need for the integration of technological advancements into rehabilitation interventions as a way of enhancing respiratory support for recovering patients. Ultimately, airway management innovation must take into account both short-term acute intervention and establishing full rehabilitation protocols to treat long-term respiratory health complications (Kandel *et al.*, 2024).

Definition of Airway Management

The airway management principle is critical in both everyday practice medicine and emergency treatment, aiming to secure a patient's airway as patent and safe as possible to enable adequate ventilation. Relative to respiratory support, airway management is the group of methods and devices to maintain or restart ventilation, particularly in those at risk for respiratory compromise or threat of obstruction. Securing an airway is paramount as any compromise can lead to suboptimal oxygenation and subsequent hypoxia that can be severe and potentially life-threatening. Management of the airway entails knowledge of the physiology behind it, individual patient characteristics, and intervention techniques appropriate for the situation that range from simple positioning to complex surgical intervention where indicated. In respiratory-distressed neonates, patient outcomes can be significantly determined by the choice of methods for airway management. For instance, there have been recent comparative studies that have evaluated the efficacy of bubble continuous positive airway pressure (B-CPAP) versus ventilator CPAP (V-CPAP) in managing such conditions. The two interventions help prevent airway collapse during expiration and ensure oxygenation, thus the comparison between treatment interventions provided to clinicians (Pak *et al.*, 2023). An evidence-based approach to airway management encompasses not only the selection of devices but also patients' needs and the effectiveness assessment of selected interventions. This synthesis demonstrates that airway management is not merely technical proficiency but a comprehensive practice with clinical expertise and adaptability. Airway management complications continue after initial stabilization and require ongoing assessment and modifications of intervention strategies. Ventilation-associated pneumonia (VAP) and barotrauma are severe problems with mechanical ventilation, particularly in acute respiratory distress syndrome (ARDS), and are present with a 23% frequency rate among ventilated patients (Robinson *et al.*, 2021). Thus, the idea of airway management must incorporate awareness and prevention of such complications and ensure adequate ventilation. Lastly, effective airway management also encompasses predictive anticipation of potential complications and preventive application of measures to safeguard patient well-being, which validates the complex nature of this core clinical skill (Figure 3.1).

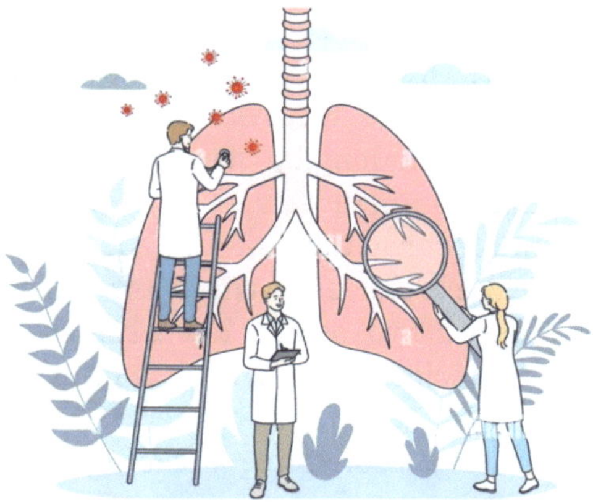

Figure 3.1. The airway management.

Source: https://media.licdn.com/dms/image/v2/D5612AQHFDsu1O4r94w/article-cover_image-shrink_720_1280/article-cover_image-shrink_720_1280/0/1726717244307?e=2147483647&v=beta&t=cNyA-dl_VSiOZn6C8KR4RF1YceBmrWcyOVDm6Sb6JEc.

Importance of Respiratory Support

The position played by respiratory support in the clinical setting cannot be emphasized enough, particularly when taking care of patients with compromised respiratory function. Appropriate airway management and ongoing respiratory support are key determinants that ensure patients are well oxygenated and ventilated and hence do not suffer from respiratory failure. This is most apparent within pediatric populations reliant on home invasive mechanical ventilation (HIMV), where the complexity of ventilator setting titration and respiratory monitoring is augmented by the necessity for individualized treatment. As expressed by recent studies, family education and support are the most important determinants of success, which enables caregivers to respond effectively to their child's condition at home, regardless of complication risk with HIMV. Through appropriate education and training, medical professionals can empower families with the requisite resources necessary to act quickly in response to respiratory complications, thus improving patient outcomes and quality of life (Tekin *et al.*, 2024). In neonatal care, the need for respiratory assistance is directly realized in conditions like neonatal respiratory distress syndrome (NRDS). Preterm infants often have disabling issues due to defective surfactant production, faulty lung function, along with issues of oxygenation. Data proves that interaction among respiratory therapy and body rehabilitation techniques enhances the treatment of NRDS and stresses the requirement for interdisciplinary management in neonatal care. Treatments such as the administration of exogenous surfactant, along with a combination of various rehabilitation techniques, are proven to enhance respiratory function and hence stabilize preterm infants. This interdisciplinary approach highlights the importance of individualized respiratory interventions that not only bring immediate respiratory relief but also improve long-term opportunities for high-risk groups (Sharath *et al.*, 2024). Further, respiratory support is important beyond emergency care, influencing long-term healthcare policy and patient recovery. Chronic respiratory patients, such as those with chronic obstructive pulmonary disease (COPD) or asthma, benefit from ongoing respiratory support to maintain optimal lung function and avoid exacerbations. Such conditions typically demand the coordinated treatment of pharmacologic therapies and respiratory support devices that are designed to ensure airway patency as well as successful gas exchange. This underscores the larger implications of respiratory care in chronic disease management, where regular monitoring and intervention can significantly enhance patients' daily existence and functional autonomy. In the end, the value of respiratory support is its capacity to accommodate the dynamic requirements of patients along the continuum of care—ranging from acute interventions to chronic care approaches—so that health is maintained in the long term and quality of life is enhanced.

3.1. Anatomy of the Respiratory System

Learning Outcome

1. Define major components of the respiratory system
2. Explain the function of the airway in respiration
3. Identify the common anatomical variations affecting airway management

The anatomy of the respiratory system is intricately organized to facilitate the crucial functions of gas exchange and control. Comprising the upper and lower respiratory tracts, the system begins in the nasal cavity, where air is warmed, humidified, and filtered. Air flows from the nasal passages into the pharynx and larynx, which are not only airways but also serve critical functions of phonation and airway guarding during the process of swallowing. Once these structures have been passed through, the trachea bifurcates into the bronchi, which further branch out into smaller bronchioles in the lungs. This complex network of branching significantly increases the surface area used for the exchange of gases, through which oxygen is absorbed into the blood and carbon dioxide is eliminated. Familiarity with this anatomy is critical to effective airway management and respiratory therapy since interventions so frequently rely on an appreciation of these structures and functions. In the acute care environment, complications related to the anatomy of the respiratory tract can significantly impair airway management interventions. Trismus or anatomical deformities can complicate intubation, making usual methods unsuitable. For instance, in the case of masseter muscle rigidity (MMR) due to succinylcholine injection, usual oro-pharyngeal intubation can be unsuccessful due to minimal jaw mobility, and other methods such as blind nasal intubation must be employed. Although it is not the first-line usual method of airway management, blind nasal intubation has proved successful in challenging scenarios. The ability to manage complex airway anatomy in such cases underscores the value of comprehensive anatomical expertise, as clinicians must shape their methods to attain the utmost patient safety and performance in crucial interventions (Chowdhury *et al.*, 2025). Further advancements in respiratory assistance measures are also driving our approach to managing patients with compromised respiratory conditions. Recent technology, for instance, the application of cloud-based long short-term memory (LSTM) networks to predictive analysis for the control of ventilation, illustrates the integration of technology and anatomy. These intricate systems evaluate data from multiple medical devices in order to tailor ventilation parameters in real-time as a function of patient-specific respiratory physiology. By modifying interventions based on individual anatomical and physiological characteristics, health care providers can optimize patient outcomes with minimal risk of complications associated with mechanical ventilation. Therefore, the integration of respiratory system anatomy with the latest technological advancements like predictive ventilation represents a significant paradigm shift in airway management practice, creating new avenues to improve respiratory care in intensive care settings (Krishnamoorthi *et al.*, 2025).

3.1.1. Major Components of the Respiratory System

The respiratory system is a complex series of structures that facilitate gas exchange between the body and the environment. Essentially, structures encompass the upper and lower airway, the lungs, and associated muscles such as the diaphragm. The upper airway consists of the nasal cavity, the pharynx, and the larynx, which condition, filter, and humidify inspired air. Outside of this, the lower respiratory tract includes the bronchi and the trachea, both of which are passageways for airflow to the lungs. The lungs, where millions of alveoli are found, are the primary gas exchange sites, trapping oxygen and removing carbon dioxide. All these components must function properly, as dysfunction will generate severe respiratory problems, impacting an individual's overall health and well-being. Airway management is critical in various medical settings and remains highly dependent on understanding the anatomy of the respiratory tract. Interventions such as intubation will need correct information on the anatomical landmarks to guarantee that the airway is viable and patent. With the connection that exists between the respiratory system and the related conditions, practical training on airway management guidelines has become unavoidable. The new guidelines encourage awareness about potential complications that are faced when intubating; awareness and prevention of these complications are vital towards ensuring patient safety. Emphasizing methods such as preoxygenation and usage of latest equipment such as video laryngoscopes can greatly improve success rates in airway procedures, thus validating the use of these components in the topic of airway management and respiratory therapy (Frerk *et al.*, 2015). Besides, environmental components play a significant role in respiratory wellbeing and may lead to acute or chronic illnesses. Air pollution, for instance, contains numerous toxic substances such as particulate matter and volatile organic compounds that can penetrate the respiratory system and exacerbate asthma and Chronic Obstructive Pulmonary Disease (COPD) (Manisalidis *et al.*, 2020). While clinical practitioners concentrate on airway management, they must also be aware of the broader public health policy and environmental policies that serve to limit exposure to such pollutants. Since there is a synergistic interaction between the respiratory system and the external world, multidisciplinary interventions that integrate clinical information with environmental health principles can maximize aggregate measures of respiratory support. Hence, the building of scientific collaboration and public enlightenment is essential in combating respiratory conditions on individual and community levels (Figure 3.2).

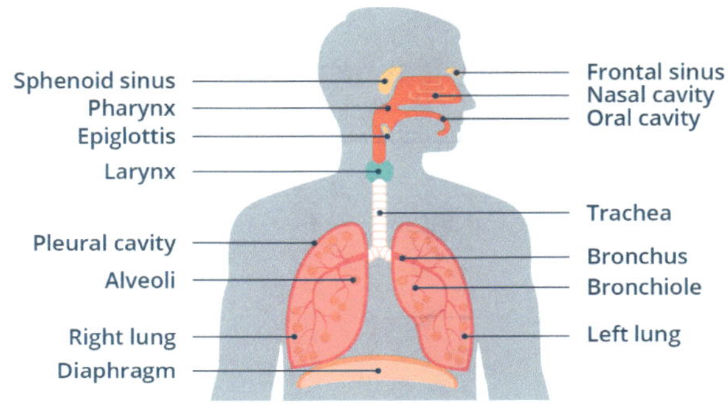

Figure 3.2. Structures of the respiratory system.

Source: https://media.healthdirect.org.au/images/inline/original/respiratory-system-bc6474.png.

3.1.2. Function of the Airway in Respiration

The airway serves a critical role in the respiratory mechanism as the pipe along which air travels into and out of the lungs. The mechanism begins in the nasal passage or the mouth, where air is filtered, warmed, and humidified prior to traveling into the trachea. The trachea branches into bronchi, which further divide into bronchioles, ultimately terminating into the alveoli-small air sacs where gas exchange occurs. Sustaining efficient airway function is important not only for the delivery of oxygen but also for the elimination of carbon dioxide. Dysfunctions of this circuit, such as airway obstruction caused by foreign bodies, inflammation, or tumors, can severely undermine respiration, leading to poor oxygenation and life-threatening states. Maintaining the integrity of the airways and knowing it is thus important in the management of respiration within clinics (Coté *et al.*, 2019) (Figure 3.3).

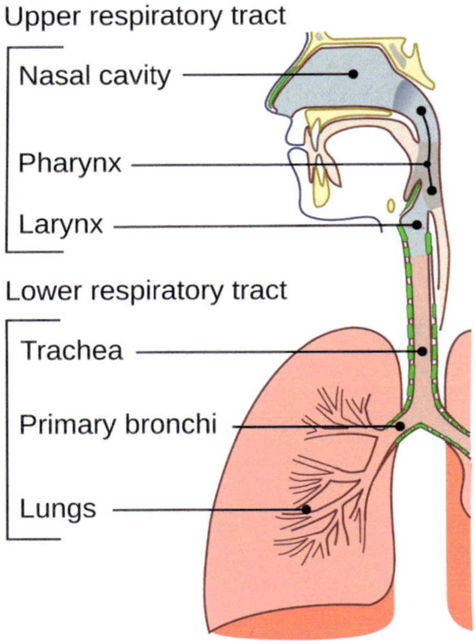

Figure 3.3. Conducting passages of the human respiratory system.

Source: https://upload.wikimedia.org/wikipedia/commons/thumb/9/9f/Illu_conducting_passages.svg/800px-Illu_conducting_passages.svg.png.

In children, the urgency of airway management cannot be overstated because an anatomical and physiological difference is evident relative to adults and can make them susceptible to more frequent airway obstruction. The small airways in children make them particularly prone to sedation or anesthesia complications, as they have a greater likelihood of apnea or compromise of the airway. A thorough and systematic airway assessment must precede procedures that require sedation. This includes assessment for conditions such as large tonsils or other factors that can predispose to increased airway obstruction risk. Proper sedation methods and the use of properly fitting age-based equipment are important in maintaining speedy and effective intervention in these cases, detailing the intricacies of pediatric airway management (Hahn *et al.*, 2013). Also, the role of the airway is not just the passage of air, but also includes defense mechanisms to shield the lungs. The epiglottis is a flap that covers the trachea while swallowing to prevent aspiration of food or liquids. Ciliated epithelium over the airway catches particles and pathogens and helps in their expulsion through mucus. This intrinsic immunological activity of the airway is essential, especially in patients with limited respiratory function or pre-existing sickness. Clinical practice to support the airway must consider both respiratory and protective airway functions to avoid hindering these vital activities through intervention, but optimize for effective ventilation and oxygenation in various clinical settings (Coté *et al.*, 2019) (Figure 3.4).

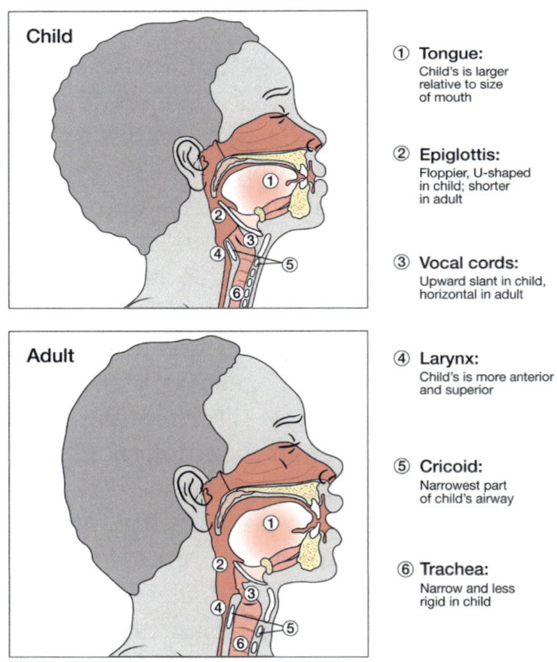

Figure 3.4. Adult and pediatric airway anatomy.

Source: https://en.wikipedia.org/wiki/Respiratory_tract#/media/File:Adult_and_pediatric_airway_anatomy.png.

3.1.3. Common Anatomical Variations Affecting Airway Management

Identification of normal anatomical variations during clinical practice that can significantly influence procedural success in airway management is essential. Protruding maxilla, hypertrophied tonsils, or a long uvula can cause narrowing of the airway and result in difficult intubation. Cervical kyphosis or lordosis can alter the position of the airway structures such that visualisation of the glottis becomes difficult. Such anatomical nuances call for careful preoperative assessment to identify the potential challenges before administering anesthesia. Therapists need to execute appropriate interventions, like an altered positioning approach or second-intention intubation equipment, to render airway administration a success in patients with some anatomical issues. Failure to take these variations into account may result in complications, which underlines the importance of customized planning in procedures of airway administration. Anatomical variations encompass more than the external structure; the internal structure is also a problem in airway management. For instance, the presence of a high-larynx, which is usually associated with congenital malformations, can complicate direct laryngoscopy and routine intubation procedures. Size and shape differences of the epiglottal structure can obstruct or facilitate entry to the glottic opening and therefore affect the choice of intubation devices. Obesity should also be considered by clinicians since it can be accountable for obesity-related effects such as more soft tissues in the airway and a greater likelihood of airway collapse when sedated. Mindfulness of such internal anatomical variations is pertinent during preparation for the most favorable airway management strategy since it is a premise for forewarning complications and selecting appropriate interventions. Advanced preoperative imaging techniques can identify these anatomical differences, thus helping ensure better patient safety and outcomes. In respiratory support scenarios as well, normal anatomical differences similarly necessitate individualized approaches to non-invasive ventilation. For example, patients with obstructive sleep apnea tend to have anatomical differences such as retrognathia or macroglossia, which render positive pressure ventilation problematic. Such anatomic difficulties may compromise the function of standard respiratory support devices, with clinicians having to look for alternative therapy, i.e., high-flow nasal cannula or BiPAP devices. Secondly, the evolving airway management scenario has brought more liberal use of preoperative noninvasive respiratory assistance in an attempt to optimize lung function, especially in patients with difficult anatomy. Guidelines now emphasize the value of thorough preoperative evaluation, considering the variation that affects airway management as well as other respiratory management, hence enabling healthcare providers to maximize the efficacy of interventions across various patient populations (Rogerson *et al.*, 2024; Vetrugno *et al.*, 2024).

Test Your Knowledge

1. What are the major components of the human respiratory system?
2. What is the primary function of the airway in the process of respiration?

3.2. Assessment of Airway Patency

Learning Outcome

1. Discuss the signs of airway obstruction
2. Explain the techniques for assessing airway patency
3. Describe the role of patient history in airway assessment

Among airway management and respiratory care competencies, airway patency evaluation is a key area of competence for health care providers. Airway patency must be maintained if successful oxygenation and ventilation are to be achieved; compromise will most likely be of critical importance to patient safety. Methods for evaluating patency of the airway include visual examination, palpation, and more advanced diagnostic procedures like fiberoptic intubation. These methods enable detection of anatomical differences, edema, or foreign bodies that would restrict respiratory function, and thus, promote the timely introduction of interventions to enhance patient outcomes. Identification of factors that affect airway patency enables the clinician to introduce interventions at the appropriate time. Continuous training coupled with the implementation of standardized assessment protocols plays a fundamental role in empowering healthcare providers to intervene appropriately in airway problems arising in critical care settings. In complex respiratory diseases, particularly in the postoperative or ICU environment, patency evaluation of the airway is more critical. The phenomenon of failed weaning from mechanical ventilation substantiates this need, where patients are unable to sustain spontaneous breathing. Failed weaning occurs in approximately 20% of ICU patients, with an increase in mortality by up to 50% (González *et al.*, 2025). To manage such risks, multifaceted approaches with clinical assessment, monitoring of patients, and technological advancements in ventilator environments are required. Such processes as utilizing a convolutional neural network (CNN) to analyze respiratory performance with spontaneous breathing trials are examples of innovative endeavors to forecast patient readiness for extubation realistically. These advances describe how the integration of technology can ease airway assessment, eventually leading to improved decision-making for patency management of the airway. In addition, the entwinement of airway patency and severe respiratory signs, such as hemoptysis, highlights the intricacy of respiratory management.

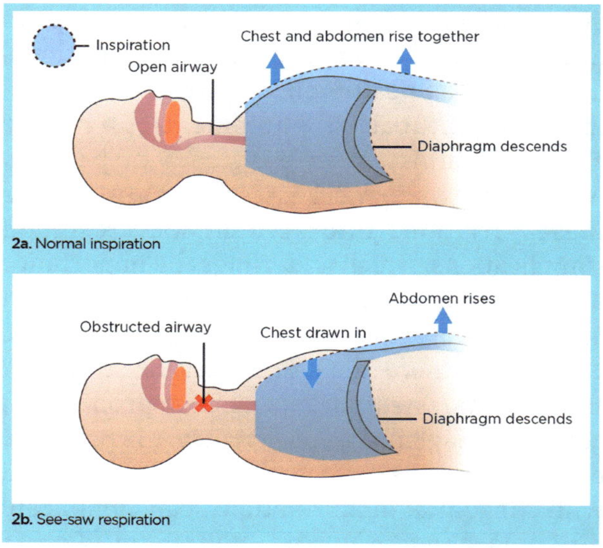

Figure 3.5. Comparison of normal and see-saw breathing.

Source: https://www.nursingtimes.net/emergency-and-critical-care/essential-critical-care-skills-4-airway-assessment-and-management-31-01-2022/.

Hemoptysis can result in the immediate compromise of airway integrity, requiring prompt interventions in order to preserve airway patency and prevent asphyxia (N/A, 2025). Management of the condition has sometimes involved other mechanisms, e.g., bronchoscopy and BAE, which have been proven to be the most efficient mechanisms for the management of hemorrhage. Standardized procedural protocols like that for the BAE are very important in enhancing clinical outcomes in patients who experience massive hemoptysis. Such protocols not only ensure timely intervention during airway emergencies but also make provisions for post-procedure care and monitoring, thereby preparing the medical caregivers adequately to maintain airway patency along the continuum of care. Through these concerted efforts, evaluation and care of airway patency can have a significant influence on overall respiratory care in high-risk environments (Figure 3.5).

3.2.1. Signs of Airway Obstruction

Recognition of airway obstruction signs is of paramount significance in the delivery of adequate airway management and respiratory treatment. Among the most exemplary of such signs is the manifestation of distressful breathing or dyspnea, which occurs in several forms, including wheezing, stridor, and even apnea. Facial expression of panic, anxiety, or distress is also critical, a sign indicating the patient is experiencing difficulty in breathing.

The patient will, in most cases, show an involuntary posture known as the tripod position, in which they will lean forward to ensure maximum airflow. Early detection of these signs will allow health professionals to distinguish between partial and total obstruction, which is essential in figuring out how pressing and what type of intervention is required. With the increasing population of vulnerable groups, including the elderly and those with neurological disability, it is crucial to recognize these signs to secure the airway in a timely and efficient way (Doppalapudi *et al.*, 2024). In addition to respiratory distress, alterations in the patient's level of communicability may suggest impending airway obstruction. Severe airflow limitation patients can become incapacitated to speak sentences, a condition known as two-to-three-word dyspnea. This sign is a critical warning sign for healthcare practitioners. Besides, cyanosis, characterized by bluish coloration of the face, lips, or extremities, is a visual presentation of inadequate oxygenation. Excessive salivation observed is also a possible indicator of difficulty in swallowing, which can accompany airway compromise due to obstruction.

Recognition of these physical and communication cues facilitates immediate action, which is critical in averting the harmful effects of airway obstruction that lasts for a long time. Inability to talk significantly heightens the need for an organized approach to airway management and patient support interventions (Szymanowski *et al.*, 2019). The integrated understanding of signs indicative of airway obstruction is not only beneficial to immediate clinical assessment but also important in predicting potential interventions. For instance, findings of acute onset choking or foreign body aspiration warrant immediate response interventions.

Effective methods of airway management must be attended to such symptoms, and clinicians must be trained in interventions such as the Heimlich maneuver or intubation based on the severity of the blockage. The use of imaging techniques, for example, fluoroscopy or bronchoscopy, could be pivotal in determining the location and the type of obstruction, particularly in complex cases. Proactive intervention in response to the recognition and acceptance of such signs can greatly reduce morbidity associated with airway obstruction, highlighting the importance of education and readiness in airway management protocols (Doppalapudi *et al.*, 2024) (Figure 3.6).

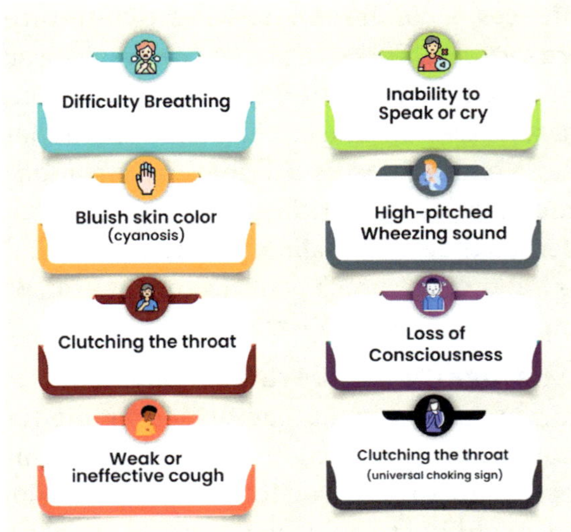
Difficulty Breathing
Inability to Speak or cry
Bluish skin color (cyanosis)
High-pitched Wheezing sound
Clutching the throat
Loss of Consciousness
Weak or ineffective cough
Clutching the throat (universal choking sign)

Figure 3.6. Sign of severe airway obstruction.

Source: https://pvpd.com/wp-content/uploads/2024/03/Signs-of-severe-airway-obstruction-including-difficulty-breathing-gasping-for-air-bluish-skin-and-inability-to-speak-or-cough-PVPD-1024x1024.png.

3.2.2. Techniques for Assessing Airway Patency

Assessment of airway patency is critical in maintaining sufficient respiratory support and management of potential complications due to airway obstruction. Various methods are employed in the assessment of airway integrity and function, with initial assessment commonly performed at the patient's bedside. Physical examination plays a crucial role in the process, whereby healthcare professionals utilize visual inspection and auscultation to determine indicators of respiratory distress or obstruction. Listening for the presence of abnormal breath sounds, such as stridor or wheezing, can alert the clinician to possible airway issues. Furthermore, success with SBTs is also a significant indicator of airway patency and calls for successful extubation procedures that challenge patient's ability to breathe successfully without mechanical aid. These initial probes provide a foundation for more invasive treatments when necessary. Where non-invasive testing is ambiguous, other diagnostic measures may be used to determine airway patency. One such measure is the cuff leak test that checks for airway edema and potential obstruction upon extubation. By measuring the air around the cuff of an endotracheal tube upon deflation, medical practitioners can obtain useful information regarding whether the airway will become patent upon extubation or not. This approach is particularly relevant in high-risk extubation failure patients since it informs the decision-making process regarding continuous respiratory support interventions (Nazir *et al.*, 2025).

Imaging studies, such as chest X-ray or CT scans, can also assist in identifying potential structural airway or lung defects that may cause obstruction and thereby inform appropriate management regimens. Health care professional care coordination is essential when one is utilizing airway patency testing. Integrating respiratory therapists, nurses, and physicians into the process ensures a multisciplinary model that guarantees patient safety and improved respiratory outcomes. Techniques such as pulmonary function tests, which measure various aspects of respiratory mechanics, can be utilized to evaluate the effectiveness of airflow and screen for obstructive or restrictive patterns. In addition, airway clearance maneuvers are critical in the care of mucus plugging and maintaining effective ventilation, especially among patients with chronic conditions such as COPD. In-depth understanding of airway obstruction mechanisms combined with effective assessment techniques is necessary for optimal airway management and facilitating timely intervention to prevent complications (Nazir *et al.*, 2025). With careful evaluation and focused methods, patient recovery and quality of life can be dramatically improved by healthcare workers in respiratory care (Figure 3.7).

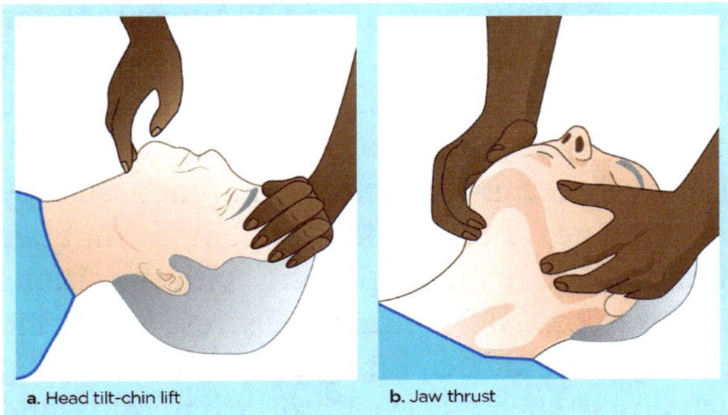

3.2.3. Role of Patient History in Airway Assessment

Understanding the role of patient history in airway assessment is key to successful airway management and respiratory treatment. A complete patient history not only reveals existing diseases that may complicate airway management—such as obstructive sleep apnea, asthma, or intubation history—but also informs clinicians about anatomical derangements that would hinder airway access. For instance, a patient with cervical spine issues may require special positioning for safety and effectiveness during airway maneuvers. Based on reviews of such historical data, clinicians can create individualized methods that account for specific patient requirements to minimize risks associated with airway interventions. As noted in emergency airway management, a thorough history of the patient is critical for effective decision-making, ultimately culminating in successful patient outcomes (Ahmed *et al.*, 2024). Patient history can also provide valuable information regarding potential respiratory complications that may arise during airway examination. Smoking history, exposure to allergens, and previous episodes of respiratory distress can be critical indicators when evaluating airway stability. These factors can contribute significantly to the patient's global risk profile, especially in the acute environment where time-sensitive interventions are called for. By systematically evaluating these variables in the context of acute respiratory failure, the clinician can better anticipate obstacles and adjust their strategy accordingly. The use of such historical results is in line with the upcoming trend of personalized medicine in airway management because it advocates for better patient safety and customized care methods (Sartini *et al.*, 2024). Apart from clinical use, patient history also facilitates proper communication between the healthcare team, enhancing airway management guidelines further. Health care professionals, such as nurses and respiratory therapists, rely on the comprehensive history to communicate effectively with each other and provide a co-ordinated response to airway emergencies. When team members are given ample historical data, they are better able to anticipate each other's requirements during the assessment and interventions, establishing greater synergy and efficacy. This commingling process points to the intrinsic dimension of interprofessional practice, according to emergency airway management literature, whereby each professional's patient history information forms a part of delivering an uninterrupted chain of care. This union of patient history and airway evaluation thus becomes a fundamental part of efficient respiratory support (Ahmed *et al.*, 2024).

Test Your Knowledge

1. What are the key signs indicating airway obstruction in a patient?
2. What techniques are commonly used to assess airway patency?

3.3. Techniques for Airway Management

Learning Outcome

1. Understand the basic airway management techniques
2. Explain the advanced airway management techniques
3. Define indications for intubation and extubation

Effective airway management is necessary in the provision of respiratory care, particularly in cases of emergency medical emergencies. The approach employed may significantly vary depending on patient condition, setting, and equipment at hand. Non-invasive ventilatory support modes, such as Continuous Positive Airway Pressure (CPAP), are typically employed first to maintain patency of the airway and allow for gas exchange. This method could be particularly beneficial in respiratory distress since it could increase oxygenation while avoiding more invasive methods. The use of such procedures is the basis for ensuring the safety of the patient and minimizing complications (Hullumani *et al.*, 2024). However, if obstructive complications arise, more advanced interventions could be needed, and a stepwise approach to airway management is therefore useful. Where earlier techniques prove to be insufficient, further developed airway management techniques, such as endotracheal intubation, may be utilized to ensure airway protection. The procedure involves threading a tube into the trachea and, in so doing, having a straight path for oxygen delivery. While intubation can significantly enhance ventilation as well as protection against aspiration, there are associated inherent risks, including trauma to the airway and adverse physiological responses (Ofei-Dodoo *et al.*, 2023). Therefore, proper training and protocol satisfaction are essential for EMS personnel and medical doctors. Clinicians' retention of proper evaluation of the requirement for invasive techniques is important in patient care since improper intubation can complicate therapy for the underlying respiratory condition. Moreover, the integration of adjunct therapy will enhance airway management techniques even more. In neonatal patients with conditions such as Neonatal Respiratory Distress Syndrome (NRDS), a multidisciplinary treatment involving techniques such as Oro Motor Stimulation and manual airway clearance maneuvers has proven to be effective (Hullumani *et al.*, 2024). These rehabilitative interventions are directed toward the enhancement of respiratory function and even neuromuscular coordination in at-risk groups. By fostering a more holistic style of management that combines traditional methods and novel therapies, medical professionals can better address the complexities of airway management. In the long run, ongoing research and mutual cooperation between medical practitioners will play an essential role in evolving these practices and ensuring all patients get the best quality of care.

3.3.1. Basic Airway Management Techniques

Successful airway management forms the basis of respiratory care, employed to provide adequate oxygenation and ventilation to critically ill patients with compromised respiratory status. Central to all maneuvers is the assessment of airway patency, in which the patient is observed for the presence of obstruction and positioned to facilitate easy breathing accordingly. The head tilt-chin lift maneuver is most commonly employed to position the airway and avoid obstruction by the tongue. Under emergency situations, uncomplicated adjuncts such as nasopharyngeal and oropharyngeal airways may be employed to achieve patency, particularly in unconscious individuals. These assist in opening up an unobstructed pathway for air, thus enhancing the effectiveness of supplemental oxygen supply systems. Proficiency in these skills and information can far surpass in making patient outcomes, with major importance on adequate oxygenation and minimizing risks of airway compromise during critical care procedures. In some cases, particularly in post-severe respiratory patients, other airway management techniques might be needed. One is the use of respiratory muscle training (RMT) devices, which may reverse the effects of respiratory muscle weakness that often affects post-acute care, such as patients with long COVID (Figure 3.8).

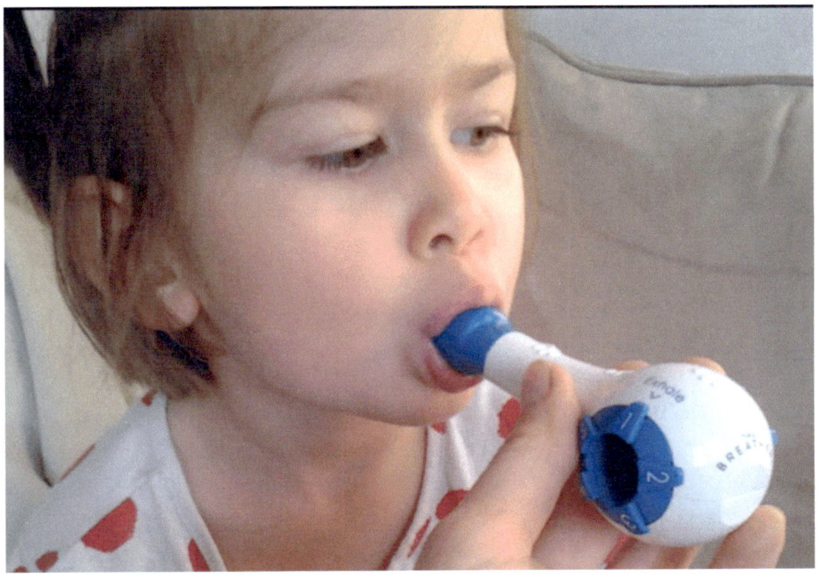

Figure 3.8. Use of respiratory muscle training (RMT) in children.

Source: https://pnmedical.com/wp-content/uploads/2018/01/rmt-kids.png.

These devices also assist in educating patients on proper breathing methods, leading to enhanced respiratory function and quality of life. Deployment of a tailor-made RMST device allowed a patient to achieve significant strides in their recuperative process, like walking for physical rehabilitation without supplemental oxygen in a limited timeframe. These advances in basic airway management indicate the need for ongoing innovation and attention during the recovery process in patients with complex respiratory conditions (Kandel *et al.*, 2024). In addition, one should point out that airway management involves not only individual interventions. There is a high demand for a multi-disciplinary approach, particularly in traumatic or acute respiratory distress syndrome. Early management following Advanced Trauma Life Support (ATLS) principles that begin with the maintenance of the airway and preservation of circulation serves as the foundation for optimal patient care. Emergency interventions such as endotracheal intubation or the implementation of chest tubes for pneumothorax drainage are vital in definitive airway management. By incorporating various medical practices like effective pain management and rehabilitation, medical professionals can treat both the physiological and psychological aspects of airway management in an integrative way. This expanded practice not only improves short-term results but also ensures long-term lung health and recovery for patients with severe challenges (Mart Símez Beleño, 2024) (Figure 3.9).

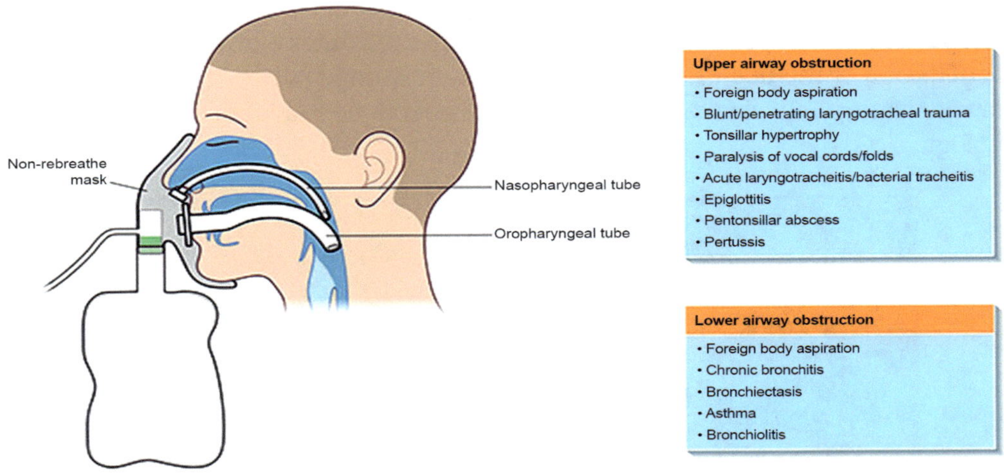

Figure 3.9. Basic airway adjuncts.

Source: https://aneskey.com/basic-airway-management-2/.

3.3.2. Advanced Airway Management Techniques

Effective airway management is a core component of respiratory care, particularly in the emergency and critical care settings. New techniques such as rapid sequence intubation (RSI) and video laryngoscopy have transformed the practice of securing the airway in acutely decompensating patients. RSI combines the use of sedative and paralytic medication to enable quick and effective intubation while minimizing the risk of aspiration and enhancing the overall success rate. Video laryngoscopy, on the other hand, is more comprehensive in airway visualization, with better visualization of vocal cords and fewer chances for complications in intubation. These measures are essential in the management of patients with severe respiratory distress or altered consciousness, enhancing safety and efficacy in managing the airway. An area of growing focus in advanced airway management is the incorporation of non-invasive methods of ventilation, including CPAP and BiPAP (Figure 3.10).

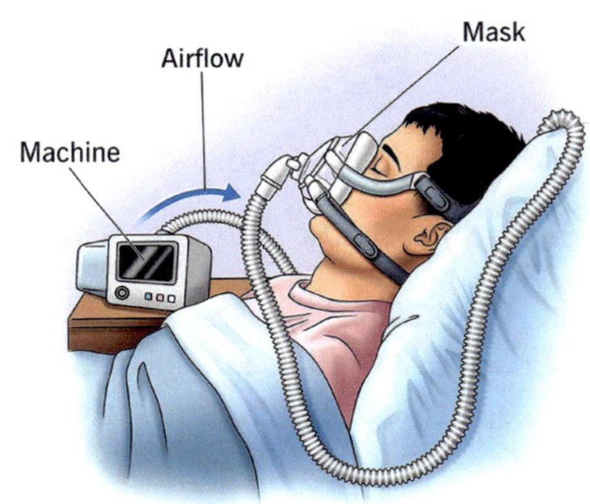

Figure 3.10. CPAP (continuous positive airway pressure) machine helps treat sleep apnea.

Source: https://my.clevelandclinic.org/-/scassets/images/org/health/articles/22043-cpap-machine.

Such techniques have proven beneficial in acute conditions such as exacerbation of COPD and acute pulmonary edema, which involve significant respiratory support without endotracheal intubation. In the management of long COVID syndromes, for instance, emerging technologies such as the tailor-made RMST device demonstrate the efficacy of employing non-invasive techniques in patients with respiratory muscle weakness. This multifaceted approach emphasizes the necessity of tailoring airway management according to the specific needs of every patient, illustrating how the advantages of technology contribute to enhanced respiratory care results. Further, the implementation of newer airway management must consider the totality of the patient's care needs, particularly in high-risk patients such as neonates. A case report examined the effect of physical rehabilitation techniques in combination with standard therapy, observing the complementary role that manual airway clearance and oro-motor stimulation can provide in improving respiratory capacity in neonates with diseases like NRDS.

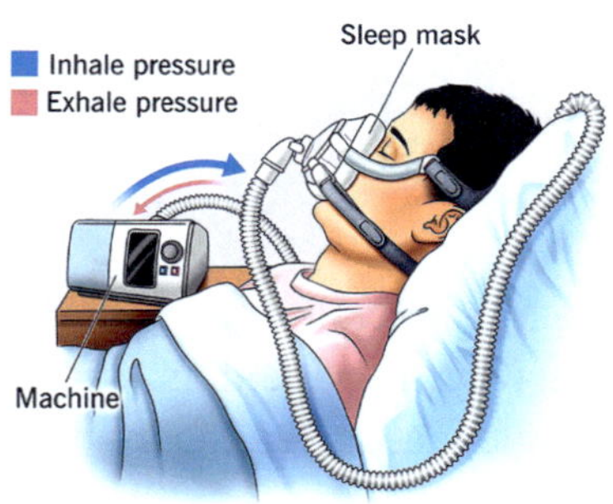

Figure 3.11. BiPAP uses a higher air pressure when you're inhaling and a lower one when you're exhaling.

Source: https://my.clevelandclinic.org/-/scassets/images/org/health/articles/24970-bipap-machine.

This interdisciplinary treatment modality suggests a shift towards more holistic treatment of airway management, and it is suggested that combining technological advancement with rehabilitative interventions can lead to enhanced clinical stability and facilitate more optimal recovery patterns. These remarks underscore the need to adopt holistic models encompassing innovative interventions and thus maximizing the overall effectiveness of airway management and respiratory support algorithms in a broad variety of clinical environments (Kandel *et al.*, 2024; Sharath *et al.*, 2024) (Figure 3.11).

3.3.3. Indications for Intubation and Extubation

In airway care and respiratory assistance, the criteria for intubation are diverse and necessary. Intubation cannot be avoided in a patient showing extreme respiratory distress or failure, an implication of which is a failure to maintain proper ventilation. This is true with the acute respiratory distress syndrome (ARDS) when there is loss of gas exchange, and mechanical ventilation becomes necessary to prevent hypoxemia and hypercapnia. Furthermore, intubation is indicated in a loss of protective airway reflexes, which can occur in patients with reduced consciousness due to trauma, overdose, or neurologic injuries. All these interventions are essential in intensive care units, where decision-making needs to be done quickly to be highly vital to patient outcomes. To provide care for such patients in an effective manner, the clinicians should have a detailed understanding of when to initiate intubation procedures and how much risk is associated with this life-supporting intervention (Phua *et al.*, 2020). In contrast, extubation or removal of the endotracheal tube must be performed following intensive evaluation of respiratory status and capacity to protect the airway of the patients. Readiness for extubation in a patient is frequently determined based on various criteria, which would include good oxygenation, stable hemodynamics, and the capability of maintaining a patent airway without any help. Notably, extubation is generally appropriate after the root cause of respiratory failure has been addressed or adequately controlled so that patients can breathe on their own. Additionally, measures for assessing readiness for extubation may include spontaneous breathing trials as well as tests of the patient's cough strength. A premature extubation will result in negative consequences in the form of airway obstruction or respiratory failure, so prudent monitoring and clinical acumen in this area of respiratory support are essential (Morris *et al.*, 2020). Evolving technologies in respiratory medicine have also immensely improved our practice of both intubation and extubation.

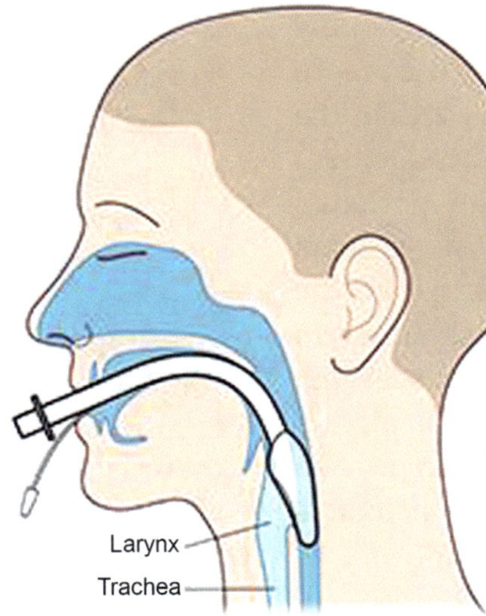

Figure 3.12. Laryngeal mask airway (SAD).

Source: https://aneskey.com/basic-airway-management-2/.

The advancements in monitoring devices and protective gear, especially in the context of the COVID-19 pandemic, have reaffirmed the need to streamline airway management practices. This includes minimizing aerosol production during treatments, which safeguards healthcare professionals and patient groups. Furthermore, weaning protocols are now widely utilized, allowing greater systematic evaluation of how ready a patient is to be weaned from mechanical ventilation to breathing spontaneously. Utilizing evidence-based guidelines and customized assessment, healthcare providers can optimize patient outcomes for airway management and respiratory support. Continuing education and training in these fields remain of paramount concern to practitioners in order to manage the complexities that come with intubation and extubation confidently, particularly in critically ill patients (Phua *et al.*, 2020) (Figure 3.12).

Test Your Knowledge

1. What are some basic techniques used in airway management?
2. What advanced techniques are employed when basic airway management is insufficient?

3.4. Respiratory Support Methods

Learning Outcome

1. Non-invasive ventilation techniques
2. Invasive ventilation methods
3. Indications for different types of respiratory support

Appropriate respiratory support methods are crucial components of airway management, particularly in patients with compromised respiratory function. Methods such as supplemental oxygenation, positive pressure ventilation, and non-invasive ventilation (NIV) are vital for enhanced patient outcomes. Supplemental oxygen is commonly given through face masks or nasal cannulas and providing relief from hypoxemia by increasing the fraction of inspired oxygen (FiO2) in the lungs of the patient. In patients with more respiratory failure or distress, positive pressure ventilation can be employed by endotracheal intubation or the application of an apparatus like CPAP. Both are employed in combination to address a spectrum of respiratory insufficiencies and provide assurance for delivering adequate oxygenation and ventilation to avert morbidity due to respiratory failure. Another important innovation in respiratory therapy is the use of the laryngeal mask airway (LMA), which has revolutionized traditional intubation techniques. The LMA offers a safer approach to the management of a patent airway that can substantially reduce the incidence of respiratory complications in anesthesia procedures. In a recent investigation, it was discovered that the LMA, when removed during deep anesthesia, had fewer respiratory complications compared to extubation under lighter anesthetics, which was a reflection of its safety in promoting airway stability (Abbasi *et al.*, 2022). Though the use of LMA minimizes risks, utmost care must be observed for potential complications such as obstruction of the airway or laryngospasm following removal. Therefore, adequately training medical staff in the correct placement and care of LMAs is essential to optimize patient safety during airway procedures. For neonates, particularly those suffering from disease states like NRDS, rehabilitation protocols have evolved into prominent adjunctive therapies beyond standard respiratory supportive interventions. The PROMPT (Physical Rehabilitation using Oro Motor Stimulation, Manual Airway Clearance Technique, Positioning, Tactile, and Kinesthetic Stimulation) protocol represents one integrated intervention with a respiratory as well as neuromuscular function approach (Hullumani *et al.*, 2024). As an integrated intervention, it is intended to optimize oxygenation and minimize ventilatory support requirements with improved neuromuscular reflexes and muscle tone. Existing clinical trials are examining the effectiveness of such treatments and have shown that applying these rehabilitative methods in combination with existing treatment may have dramatic enhancements in clinical outcomes for neonates with NRDS. As the work continues, such an outcome may revolutionize clinical practice by maximizing existing protocols and enhancing the overall care of respiratory patients.

3.4.1. Non-Invasive Ventilation Techniques

Non-invasive modalities of ventilation are a significant advance in airway management, particularly in respiratory failure cases. By delivering positive pressure support without the need for intubation, CPAP and NIV modalities achieve effective gas exchange with minimal risk of complications associated with invasive procedures. This is highly valuable in the postoperative period, as re-intubation itself can lead to increased morbidity and mortality. Studies have shown that, when used appropriately, NIV can significantly reduce the incidence of re-intubation among such groups, highlighting its role in promoting patient safety as well as rapid recovery. In addition, the studies show that NIV can decrease the occurrence of complications such as nosocomial pneumonia, highlighting its overall utility in clinical care (Pettenuzzo *et al.*, 2024) (Figure 3.13).

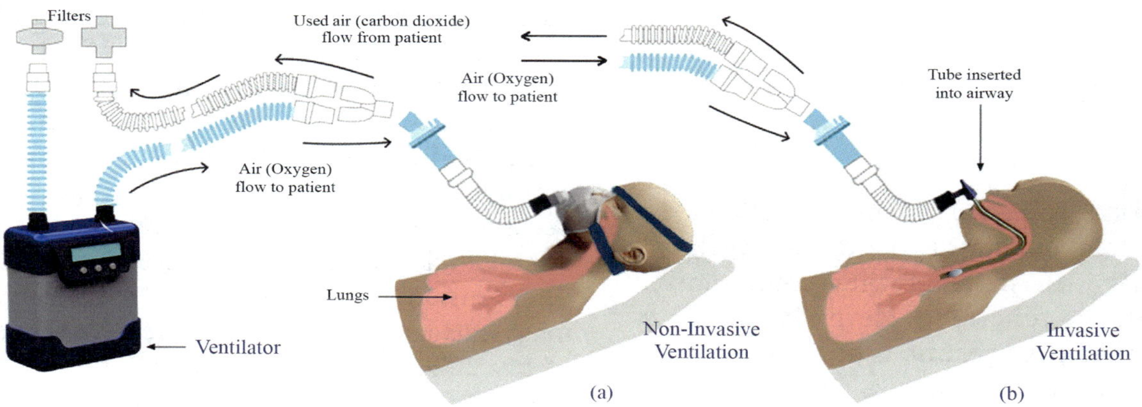

Figure 3.13. The general scheme of a) Noninvasive, and b) Invasive methods of ventilation.

Source: https://www.researchgate.net/publication/345734951/figure/fig3/AS:984193622355984@1611661453740/The-general-scheme-of-a-Noninvasive-and-b-Invasive-methods-of-ventilation.png.

The efficacy of non-invasive respiratory therapies is not only applicable to postoperative patients but has been discovered to be very beneficial to the elderly patient population, which is rapidly becoming increasingly common among the intensive care population. Elderly patients frequently present with acute respiratory failure but are too weak to tolerate invasive therapy. For such patients, non-invasive therapy may be a beneficial choice, allowing for conservative management by the caregivers and avoiding complications associated with intubation. Research indicates that the short to medium-term outcomes of NIV and other measures in elderly patients are not different from those in younger individuals if their unique comorbidities are taken into account. This adaptability makes non-invasive strategies central in the present quest to optimize respiratory care in vulnerable populations (Coppola *et al.*, 2024). Despite the advantages offered by non-invasive ventilation, patient appropriateness needs to be taken into account with care and followed up for response to treatment. Although these approaches minimize many risks, they are not complication-free, such as discomfort, interface leak, and in the worst-case scenario, failure to suppress respiratory distress. There is thus a requirement to make a proper assessment to ensure that the chosen modality accommodates patient preference and medical history. Furthermore, continuous education and updating of clinical guidelines on non-invasive ventilation are required for health professionals to ensure appropriate usage and maximize patient outcomes. With these features in place, non-invasive ventilation can serve as a cornerstone within airway management strategies, effectively handling patients in all categories of clinical settings without subjecting them to the risks of invasive procedures (Pettenuzzo *et al.*, 2024) (Figure 3.14).

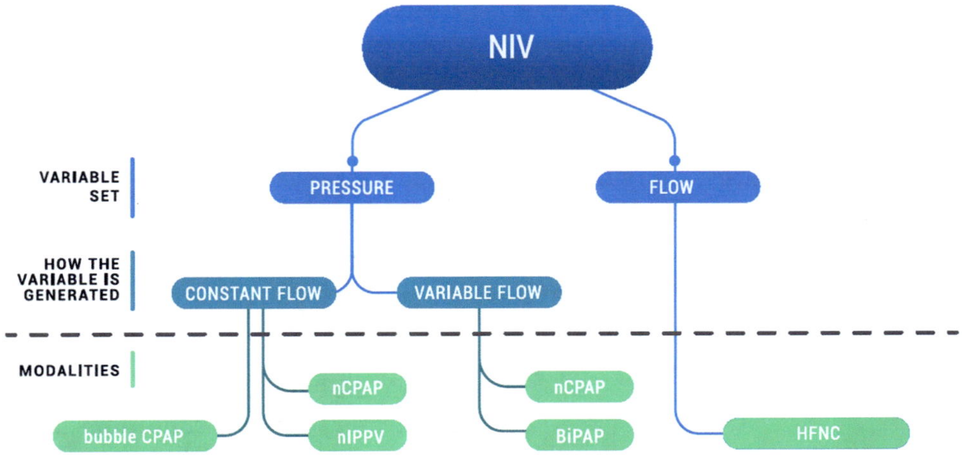

Figure 3.14. Classification of non-invasive respiratory support—according to the set parameter (pressure versus flow). Pressure-controlled modalities are classified further based on the pressure generated (constant flow versus variable flow).

Source: https://www.researchgate.net/publication/349643527/figure/fig5/AS:11431281115682128@1675051424541/Classification-of-non-invasive-respiratory-support-according-to-the-set-parameter.png

3.4.2. Invasive Ventilation Methods

Invasive ventilation modalities are integral components of airway management and respiratory therapy, particularly in a situations when non-invasive modalities are insufficient to provide sufficient ventilation and oxygenation. Among the modalities applied, endotracheal intubation and later mechanical ventilation are a routine practice employed in various clinical scenarios, mainly in patients with severe respiratory distress or failure. Ventilation strategy, including pressure-controlled or volume-controlled modes, has a significant impact on the outcome of the patient. The clinician must examine the specific needs of each patient and consider factors such as underlying diseases and degree of respiratory compromise. An understanding of the specifics of these methods is important in order to best individualize ventilatory support and minimize complications of prolonged mechanical ventilation, including ventilator-associated pneumonia and airway injury. The advent of non-invasive modalities, such as nasal continuous positive airway pressure (NCPAP) and nasal intermittent positive pressure ventilation (NIPPV), has transformed practice habits, particularly among children and patients with chronic respiratory conditions. NIPPV is found to enhance respiratory outcomes after extubation, effectively reducing the risk of respiratory failure and reintubation in preterm infants (Lemyre *et al.*, 2023). Notably, NIPPV can provide greater synchrony with the patient's respiratory effort and thus minimize discomfort and promote therapy compliance. However, these non-invasive methods are not intrinsically complication-free, a consideration that underscores the necessity for individualized patient evaluation and appropriate use of technology in airway management. Especially in certain populations, such as children with neurological disorders requiring home invasive mechanical ventilation (HIMV), the intensity of care is significantly greater (Sayar *et al.*, 2023). These patients often have paralyzed respiratory muscles and impaired ventilation due to a range of underlying diseases like spinal muscular atrophy or muscular dystrophy. Multidisciplinary treatment is required to manage them successfully, involving pediatric pulmonologists, neurologists, and specially trained nurses to deliver proper care. Major considerations involve proper ventilator mode selection, caregiver education, and airway clearance technique implementation. Maximizing ventilatory support in these at-risk populations can have a significant impact on their quality of life and health outcomes, highlighting the essential role of invasive ventilation techniques in contemporary respiratory support management (Figure 3.15).

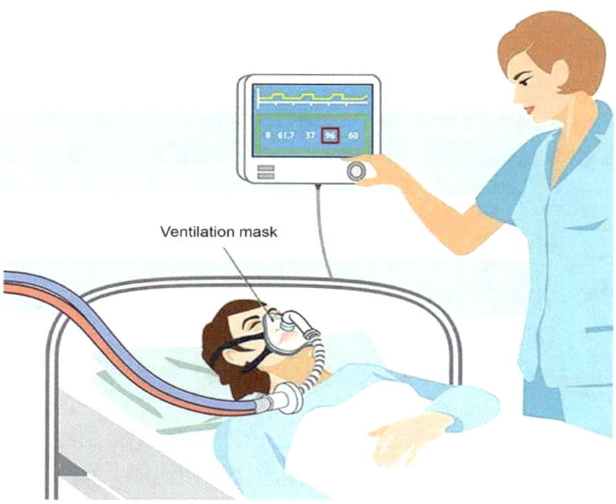

Figure 3.15. Invasive ventilation provides air through a flexible tube rather than a mask.

Source: https://www.informedhealth.org/how-does-ventilation-therapy-for-respiratory-problems-work.html.

3.4.3. Indications for Different Types of Respiratory Support

The requirement for various types of respiratory support arises due to the varied nature of respiratory diseases patients may have, particularly in critically ill patients. Patients with acute respiratory failure often require individualized interventions to provide proper oxygenation and ventilation. In such cases, NIV has proven to be useful in patients with exacerbations of COPD and cardiogenic pulmonary edema by enhancing comfort and minimizing intubation needs. In contrast, patients presenting with profound ARDS along with associated changes in level of consciousness or compromised airway reflexes will need invasive mechanical ventilation to prevent effective gas exchange and worsening respiratory distress. This personalized treatment approach enhances the importance of selecting the appropriate level of respiratory support based on each patient's presentation and underlying pathophysiologic processes (Zhao *et al.*, 2020). Under the conditions of the COVID-19 pandemic, respiratory support conditions have also evolved with better clinical knowledge of the illness. For patients with mild to moderate symptoms, supplemental oxygen may be sufficient, possibly in addition to supportive treatment alternatives emphasizing patient autonomy and comfort. As the disease progresses to more severe stages, close monitoring of respiratory parameters is mandatory, with proactive interventions to prevent compromise. There is greater popularity for high-flow nasal cannula (HFNC) oxygen therapy, which has benefits over conventional oxygen therapy in sustaining better oxygenation and reducing the work of breathing. Whereas in patients who have established respiratory failure, particularly in pneumonia or severe hypoxemia, where there is a need for intensive care unit admission, invasive ventilation is of utmost concern. Research shows early treatment helps appreciably in critically ill patients, and therefore, airway management guidelines are required (Alhazzani *et al.*, 2020). Post-discharge pulmonary rehabilitation is increasingly gaining recognition as a vital part of care for patients who have recovered from life-threatening illnesses of the respiratory tract, including those related to COVID-19. Following recovery, individuals develop residual respiratory dysfunction that can undermine their quality of life. Personalized rehabilitation programs in the form of physical training, breathing exercises, and psychological support remain key in enhancing overall recovery. Evidence indicates that personalized rehabilitation strategies have come a long way in the recovery of lung function and the alleviation of psychological distress among patients discharged. Furthermore, the integration of telemedicine has been effective in supplementing these rehabilitation processes to facilitate sustained monitoring and support by medical professionals during the course of recovery. Respiratory parameter monitoring, as well as active patient engagement within their rehabilitation schedule, identifies an effective strategy in improving recovery as well as quality of life. This integrated approach is a promising direction for the treatment of post-acute sequelae of respiratory disease (Zhao *et al.*, 2020).

Test Your Knowledge

1. What are common non-invasive ventilation techniques used in critical care?
2. When are invasive ventilation methods like mechanical ventilation required?

3.5. Complications of Airway Management

Learning Outcome

1. Define potential complications during intubation
2. Identify the risks associated with mechanical ventilation
3. Discuss the long-term effects of airway interventions

The complexity of airway management is generally added by dissimilar clinical conditions, and as a result, potential complications with profound impacts on patient outcomes of such complications, difficult intubation is foremost and typically results from anatomical distortions, obesity, or prior surgical alterations. Practitioners thus find themselves compelled to use alternative methods of providing airway safety, such as video laryngoscopy or flexible bronchoscope intubation. Moreover, failure to properly secure an airway compromises the patient's immediate safety but may also lead to hypoxia, brain injury, or death if it is not immediately resolved. Thus, understanding the risks of airway management, as well as proper assessment and training, is essential in minimizing complications and optimizing the effectiveness of respiratory support interventions, especially in the context of critical care, wherein time is of the essence. Besides the anatomical and physiological difficulties, unexpected complications arise during airway management that necessitate specialized treatment. For instance, the use of various airways, such as endotracheal tube or supraglottic airway, can lead to unintended injury to surrounding structures, forming situations as laryngeal edema or vocal cord paralysis. In addition to that, improper positioning of these devices leads to ventilation insufficiency, which further adds to respiratory distress. In such patients as pregnant ones or neonates, such complications are significant since their unique physiological demands need to be with utmost accuracy adapted by airway management techniques. Due to this fact, a multidisciplinary team, consisting of anesthesiologists, intensivists, and obstetricians, must get involved to manage such complications while ensuring both fetal and maternal safety under high-risk procedures in respiratory care (Taksinwarajarn *et al.*, 2025). Also, airway complications are controlled not just by the intervention that happens in real time but also involve careful monitoring and follow-up post-intubation. In patients with congenital conditions in the neonatal group, special attention is paid to monitoring the potential for ventilator-induced lung injury (VILI) and other respiratory complications. These patients tend to be at higher risk due to underlying anatomical challenges and the need for surgical intervention of thoracic structures (Alberti *et al.*, 2025). Therefore, the implementation of lung-protective ventilation practice becomes paramount in minimizing such risks. With increased understanding of the technical and physiological subtleties of airway management by practitioners, continuous education and rigorous compliance with evolving best practices can significantly reduce complications. Lastly, convergence of purposeful airway management with combined respiratory assistance remains key to optimizing patient outcomes in various health settings.

3.5.1. Potential Complications During Intubation

Effective management of the airway is essential but intubation is dangerous due to a multitude of possible complications that endanger patient safety. The most significant of these risks is the risk of oral or dental trauma extended attempts at intubation that can be caused by anatomical variation or unsuspected airway obstruction. These types of trauma can be lifelong and can be caused by improper use of equipment or force. It becomes important to comprehend such risks, and anesthesia providers must be fully aware of the risk of injuries due to their interventions. Such awareness assists in building proper measures for risk prevention, such as employing alternative intubation methods or using advanced imaging to help fully assess airway status, thereby enhancing patient outcomes at this delicate procedure. In the event of complex airway management, the issues that arise due to improper intubation can be extrapolated to respiratory distress or hypoxia. Intubation can potentially exacerbate existing respiratory disease in certain patients and lead to an increased incidence of postoperative pulmonary complications such as atelectasis or pneumonia. The employment of preoperative noninvasive respiratory support (NRS) has gained prominence as a way to optimize lung function before intubation, effectively reducing airway management hazards. Greater ventilatory support can fight hypoxia and expand lung volumes, providing a safer environment for intubation. Employing these advanced techniques not only addresses problems in the short term but also offers a baseline measurement of respiratory health, indicating that airway management issues must include patient-specific factors and anticipated complications to derive optimal benefits, as evidenced is found in newer findings (Vetrugno *et al.*, 2024) (Figure 3.16).

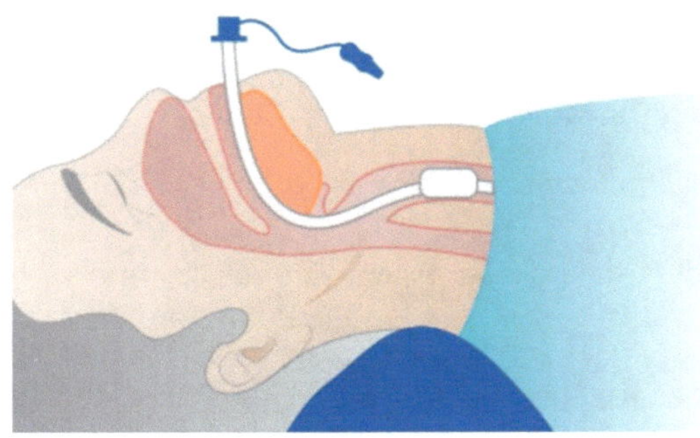

Figure 3.16. Endotracheal tube (ETT).

Source: https://www.nursingtimes.net/emergency-and-critical-care/essential-critical-care-skills-4-airway-assessment-and-management-31-01-2022/.

Beyond respiratory and dental complications, intubation techniques such as submental intubation are now second-line techniques that may even minimize some risks inherent with routine techniques. The technique, typically being discussed in facial trauma, comes with its own set of complications. Complications may arise due to incorrect placement of the tube or lack of training with the technique, leading to scarring or infection postoperatively. Nevertheless, studies indicate that the benefits of submental intubation overcome such risks with appropriate protocols. Raising awareness about the technique and its usefulness in overcoming problems related to facial trauma raises its usage in clinical practice. Cumulatively, accurate evaluation of potential intubation complications, both by method, is crucial to further advance airway management procedures on the premise of the continuous interaction between patient safety and innovative medical procedures (Mahajan *et al.*, 2024) (Figure 3.17).

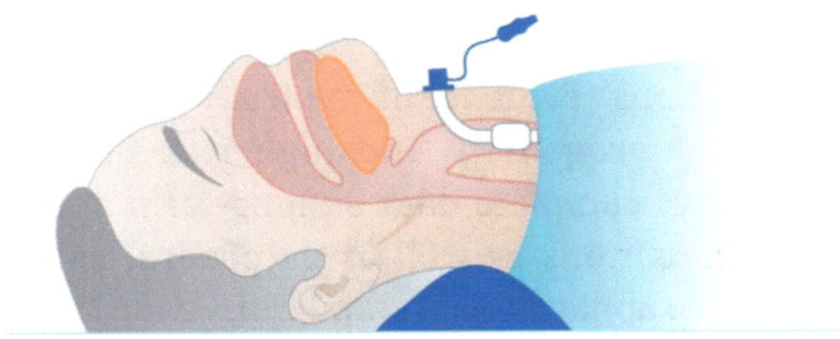

Figure 3.17. Tracheostomy tube.

Source: https://www.nursingtimes.net/emergency-and-critical-care/essential-critical-care-skills-4-airway-assessment-and-management-31-01-2022/.

3.5.2. Risks Associated with Mechanical Ventilation

Mechanical ventilation is also linked with numerous risks that can potentially impact patient outcomes in a major way. The most critical of these risks is the development of ventilator-associated pneumonia (VAP), a nosocomial infection developed as a result of the entry of bacteria into the lung via the endotracheal tube. The infection not only adds to hospital length of stay but also increases the cost of care and exacerbates the clinical course of patients who are critically ill. Moreover, mechanical ventilation may also result in barotrauma and volutrauma, which include lung tissue damage from excessive ventilator settings, pressure, or volume. These complications require close observation and adjustment of ventilation parameters to minimize possible lung injuries and to maximize airway management, thereby demonstrating the intricate balance of adequate respiratory assistance provision and prevention of related risks. Moreover, the risk of respiratory muscle deconditioning is of significant concern in patients undergoing extended mechanical ventilation. If patients are not allowed to breathe spontaneously for extended durations, then the diaphragm and other inspiratory muscles become weakened, and respiratory function is compromised. It can reduce the process of weaning from mechanical ventilation and thus prolong the duration of ventilator dependency. Such a phenomenon is particularly relevant in critically ill patients, including those with acute respiratory distress syndrome, in which lung injury is prevalent. Evolution of interventions such as early mobilization and diaphragm-specific training can prevent these effects, creating a critical consideration in the care of mechanically ventilated patients. These approaches emphasize the requirement for proactive and early care to augment recovery trajectories and mitigate the risks from prolonged mechanical ventilation. In addition, an understanding of interactions between mechanical ventilation and comorbidities is essential in the management of associated risks. For example, patients with the presence of underlying trauma or experiencing severe illness like COVID-19 face specific challenges that can add to the impact of mechanical ventilation. For trauma, such as acute respiratory distress syndrome, the risk can become compounded when conventional ventilatory strategies fail, causing conditions such as refractory hypoxemia. Newer modalities, such as airway pressure release ventilation, have been shown to provide benefits under these circumstances, suggesting an imperative for innovation in airway management in an effort to improve patient outcomes. Effective control of these risks must be achieved through an interdisciplinary approach of several specialties and individualized care plans aimed at the specific requirements of each patient, ultimately maximizing overall respiratory support and safety in critical care settings (Figure 3.18).

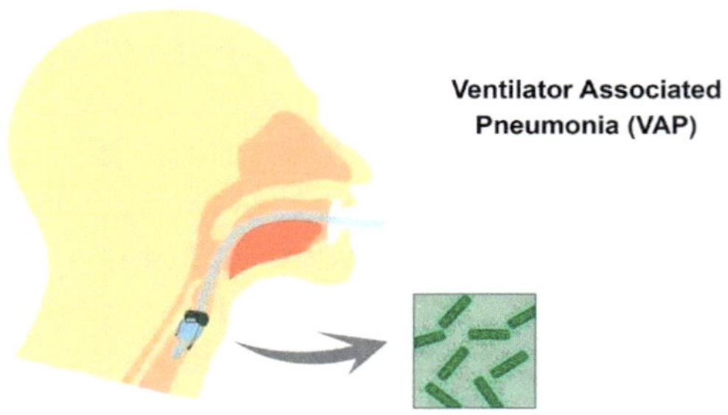

Figure 3.18. Ventilator-associated pneumonia (VAP).

Source: https://stgaccinwbsdevlrs01.blob.core.windows.net/newcorporatewbsite/blogs/June2024/2dQb3MjKXmtujgKSkoY5.webp.

3.5.3. Long-Term Effects of Airway Interventions

The long-term effects of airway interventions, particularly in the management of COPD, have drawn a lot of interest in recent research. Self-management interventions, for instance, allow patients to take care of themselves by learning some skills that help them manage their condition better. Evidence suggests these interventions have the potential to improve health-related quality of life (HRQoL) as assessed by the St. George's Respiratory Questionnaire (SGRQ), although they failed to achieve the minimally clinically important difference (MCID) standard. Interestingly, those treated with self-management had a lower rate of hospitalizations for respiratory reasons, suggesting application of these strategies may reduce healthcare utilization long-term. Yet, the strength of evidence is moderate to low because there is considerable inherent bias in most studies, primarily due to the absence of blinding in self-management interventions. This brings into focus the importance of research to demarcate these benefits further (Schrijver *et al.*, 2022). Besides self-management strategies, the use of digital interventions in managing COPD is also an area with the potential to further improve patient outcomes.

Computer-based aids, which provide self-management support, have been investigated for their ability to enhance healthier behaviors and patient activation. There is some evidence for modest improvements in quality of life and exercise capacity over the long term, although the evidence is unclear. Specifically, the confidence of such digital interventions' evidence is typically rated low due to heterogeneity and high risk of bias, and lack of complete data on long-term effects on exacerbations as well as on general health status. The application of standardized measures and generalized protocols may be capable of enhancing the robustness of subsequent research in determining the effectiveness of digital self-management in COPD treatment (Janjua *et al.*, 2021). Finally, finding the long-term impacts of airway interventions needs to be done in an integrated way that brings together traditional self-management actions and the new place of digital technologies. The interplay between these two types of intervention can produce synergistic effects, thereby improving patient compliance and activation of their treatment plans. Future research should aim to evaluate long-term outcomes in diverse patient populations and healthcare settings and emphasize behavior change methodology to promote long-term change. A more sophisticated appreciation of the long-term effects of these interventions will allow healthcare professionals to individualize strategies that meet specific patient needs, ultimately improving respiratory health and well-being for patients with chronic airway conditions (Janjua *et al.*, 2021; Schrijver *et al.*, 2022).

Test Your Knowledge

1. What are the common risks linked to prolonged mechanical ventilation?
2. What long-term effects may result from repeated or extended airway interventions?

3.6. Current Trends and Innovations

Learning Outcome

1. Explain the advances in airway management technology
2. Understand the emerging techniques in respiratory support
3. Define future directions in airway management research

In the last decade, remarkable progress in airway management and respiratory care has been observed, spurred on by an increased desire to improve patient outcomes within the critical care environment. Newer technologies, like high-flow nasal cannula systems and non-invasive positive pressure ventilation, have become par for the course, enhancing oxygenation with less distress to the respiratory system. These advances reflect a trend toward fewer invasive techniques, supporting improved tolerance and comfort of patients undergoing treatment. In addition, telemedicine's application in respiratory therapy has been more common, allowing clinicians to monitor patients remotely, making appropriate interventions whenever necessary. These trends identify the need for patient-centered approaches, which maximize individual needs and wants combined with effective respiratory management. The COVID-19 pandemic further accelerated innovations in airway management practices, specifically the safety of healthcare workers and the integrity of personal protective equipment (PPE). The necessity to safeguard front-line workers has necessitated the pursuit of different decontamination methods for reusable PPE, as traditional approaches fall short. New technologies such as vaporized hydrogen peroxide (VH2O2) and UV irradiation are being explored to find out if they can decontaminate masks and respirators without impairing their functionality. This measure not only plays an important role in stemming the ongoing health crisis but also provides a foundation for sustainable respiratory support treatment protocols. Prioritization of effective PPE management is complemented by a broader shift toward new solutions addressing underlying healthcare supply chain issues to ultimately enhance patient safety and healthcare resilience (Rowan *et al.*, 2020). Furthermore, heightened recognition of long-term respiratory diseases, such as asthma and COPD, has driven new trends in personalized medicine and prevention-oriented care strategies. Progress in analytics of data and wearable technology allows real-time monitoring of respiratory conditions in patients, encouraging proactive management of such diseases. With rising rates of chronic diseases, the inclusion of nutrition and lifestyle management is more and more highlighted, with an appreciation of their invaluable contributions to the risk reduction of disease. Recent reviews highlight the importance of individualized interventions that account for both environmental and genetic influences, to overcome barriers to effective self-management of respiratory health (Budrevi Ačiūtė *et al.*, 2020). Such an integrated prevention and chronic disease approach is a sea change in healthcare delivery, with an emphasis on the necessity of multidisciplinary therapy for improved patient outcomes in airway management and respiratory care.

3.6.1. Advances in Airway Management Technology

Advances in technology for airway management have revolutionized the critical care practice, especially for severe respiratory conditions such as ARDS. The development of Veno-venous Extracorporeal Membrane Oxygenation (VV ECMO) is a significant leap in ARDS patient management who do not respond to conventional mechanical ventilation. This technique allows greater gas exchange, thus reducing the load on the lungs, decreasing excessive airway pressures, and thus providing a therapeutic environment for lung healing. Recent studies indicate that application of VV ECMO not only decreases mortality in ARDS patients but also sustains a higher proportion of survival, as evidenced presents the observed survivor proportion of 58.6% in treated cases within intensive care units (Maqbool *et al.*, 2024). These results validate the need for continued use of ECMO technology in normal respiratory support protocols. The integration of ultrasound technology in airway management has improved the precision of invasive anesthetic and critical care procedures. Ultrasound is an effective point-of-care diagnostic instrument that enables clinicians to visualize internal anatomical structures and facilitate the proper positioning of airway devices. Lung ultrasound evolution has expanded its application, especially with the COVID-19 pandemic, when prompt assessment of pulmonary conditions was paramount. In offering instant and dynamic evaluation of lung status, this technology offers discrimination between various respiratory illnesses and adjustment of mechanical ventilation therapy according to this. The development of lung ultrasound has consequently become unavoidable as it is now recognized to not only offer a diagnosis but also to report real-time treatment effectiveness, keeping up with the evolving airway management solutions trends (Szab Mó *et al.*, 2023). Other than ultrasound technology and ECMO, further development of airway devices and adjuncts remains crucial to effective respiratory management. Supportive technologies such as video laryngoscopes and newer supraglottic airway devices exist, with enhanced visualization and success at placement during intubation. They decrease the risk of complications associated with routine intubation techniques, such as airway trauma or esophageal placement, and improve success rates in difficult airway cases. Moreover, new technology targets an easy-to-use design that meets the requirements of operators of varied skills, thereby optimizing patient outcomes across various healthcare settings. These innovations reflect the ongoing development of airway management technologies, ultimately with a view to developing respiratory support strategies and reducing patient risk during critical care interventions (Figure 3.19).

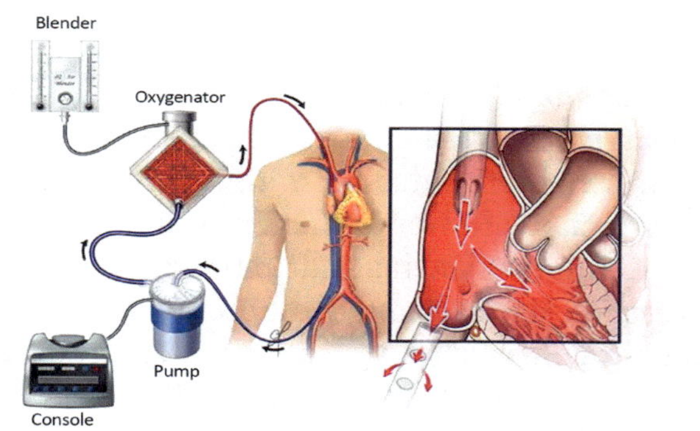

Figure 3.19. Venovenous (VV) extracorporeal membrane oxygenation (ECMO) is a temporary mechanical assistance device that allows for prolonged cardiopulmonary support.

Source: https://consultqd.clevelandclinic.org/venovenous-extracorporeal-membrane-oxygenation-for-lung-failure.

3.6.2. Emerging Techniques in Respiratory Support

Emerging techniques for respiratory support are increasingly gaining prominence in maximizing patient outcomes within various clinical settings.

As healthcare progresses, new techniques and technologies are being incorporated to maximize standard airway management methods. Advanced devices such as HFNC therapy and NIV machines are changing the trend. HFNC therapy provides warmed, humidified oxygen at higher flow rates, which reflects decreased work of breathing and improved oxygenation without the inconvenience and complications associated with invasive mechanical ventilation. The method is a significant innovation, particularly in emergency and critical care, as it facilitates caregivers in delivering effective respiratory therapy with decreased invasiveness. In addition, the inclusion of new monitoring technologies provides a significant break from respiratory management. Real-time and point-of-care ultrasonography are increasingly being applied to monitor lung function and guide therapy. These technologies enable clinicians to make informed decisions regarding patient treatment and enhance communication between multidisciplinary team members. In addition, the development of artificial intelligence (AI)-based algorithms capable of predicting respiratory distress or failure is a promising field for early intervention. By catching patterns of worsening before criticality, these techniques can do much to improve the prognosis for patients requiring respiratory support. High-risk population-specific interventions, such as neonates, are also emerging into the forefront as being key to optimizing respiratory support. NRDS, caused primarily by surfactant deficiency, necessitates both pharmacologic and supportive therapy. Recent evidence has shown that combined physical rehabilitation interventions such as oro-motor stimulation and manual airway clearance can improve respiratory outcomes in NRDS infants. These interventions, when combined with standard surfactant therapy, have been demonstrated to improve lung function and overall stability in the affected newborns, showing the merit of a multi-modal approach to the treatment of complicated respiratory disease. The integration of such newer technologies and philosophies into respiratory care programs is necessary to optimize care and improve long-term outcomes.

3.6.3. Future Directions in Airway Management Research

As airway management continues to evolve, there is a highly thrilling pipeline of future studies involving the integration of leading-edge technologies such as microfluidics and organ-on-a-chip systems. Both of these technologies allow researchers to mimic complex respiratory systems in the laboratory, providing a closer simulation of human physiology. The microengineered systems have the potential to revolutionize the way research is conducted on respiratory disease, as well as evaluate therapeutic intervention. With the innovation of microenvironments that simulate the intricate airway architecture, scientists can now explore disease mechanisms, test drug activity, and explore individualized therapies. This move away from the standard models into the sophisticated organ-on-a-chip technology is one of the major steps towards achieving outcomes that better translate to patient care and later into an improvement in the general quality of airway management and respiratory support therapy in clinics (Azizipour *et al.*, 2020). Another important area for future research is the optimization of airway management strategy in the setting of infectious disease, particularly emphasizing the COVID-19 pandemic. Highly contagious pathogens pose issues of importance that identify the necessity of successful airway interventions, which are both effective at patient outcomes and safe for healthcare workers. Future research should focus on enhancing new non-invasive ventilation practices and maximizing intubation protocols to minimize aerosol generation during procedures. Moreover, the pandemic has also brought out the need for planning for backup in the PPE supply chains. Enhanced reprocessing of PPE and new products that are easy to decontaminate are important in maintaining healthcare workers' health and ensuring continuity of care during respiratory emergencies (Rowan *et al.*, 2020). Finally, interdisciplinary collaboration will necessarily be the key to defining the future course of airway management research. Interdisciplinary bridging between fields as disparate as engineering, medicine, and public health can allow for multicomponent solutions tailored to resolving complex airway management problems. For instance, artificial intelligence can be applied in monitoring and assessment devices to enhance real-time decision-making processes, which provide clinicians with critical data that will aid interventions. In addition, community engagement in research can be utilized to gain a clearer understanding of particular issues faced within diverse populations, leading to more equitable solutions towards respiratory care. By facilitating multidisciplinary collaboration and participation of different stakeholders, the science of airway management can guarantee that its research activities cover adequately the multifaceted needs of patients and healthcare systems (Azizipour *et al.*, 2020).

Test Your Knowledge

1. What recent advances have improved airway management technology?
2. What emerging techniques are being developed for respiratory support?

SUMMARY

It has numerous critical remarks founded on the evidence of airway management and respiratory support, particularly where complications from mechanical ventilation are concerned. The unplanned extubation process is a significant challenge in intensive care settings, with incidence rates of 0.3% to 1.4% for intubated patients. This activity has severe consequences, as it is coupled with higher mechanical ventilation time, longer ICU stay, and higher morbidity, stressing the importance of better training and awareness for clinical staff. The data indicate a high need for institutions to prioritize education and standardization of protocol more in the management of endotracheal intubation and post-intubation mechanical ventilation, ultimately decreasing the rate of unplanned extubation and complications (Gulafshan *et al.*, 2021). Thus, creating an integrated plan of airway management can drastically improve the outcome of patients in the critical care setting. No less important is the judicious administration of oxygen in perioperative management, given that it plays a double role as both therapeutic and a potential cause of side effects. While oxygen is primarily utilized to prevent hypoxemia, its easy access can pose complications exemplified by oxidative stress and respiratory-related complications such as atelectasis. Evidence has advocated selective oxygen delivery with specific titration targets in individual patient requirements. Even though a proper FiO_2 is required in maintaining adequate arterial oxygenation, the latest evidence has revealed that elevated levels are responsible for undesirable cardiovascular reactions. Practitioners must thus be prudent in their use of oxygen therapy, referring to established guidelines so that they can minimize risks and achieve optimal outcomes in patients undergoing perioperative surgery (Soriano *et al.*, 2019). Effective management of airways and respiratory care is essential in maintaining optimum patient care in hospitals. The subtleties of interventions like oxygen therapy and mechanical ventilation accentuate the delicate balance that healthcare professionals must attain in order to provide effective and safe interventions. Vigilance in continuous education and rigorous compliance with evidence-based airway management protocols can significantly reduce complications like unplanned extubation. Conversely, thorough knowledge of the physiological effects of oxygen therapy will enable clinicians to utilize it judiciously, ultimately maximizing patient safety and recovery outcomes. Altogether, this synthesis of thoughts brings to the forefront the importance of an integrated approach in airway management and respiratory support and opens the door to better care for the patient in acute.

A thorough understanding of airway management and respiratory support is a priority during the perioperative period, particularly in CSR tumor patients. The tumors, most notably pituitary adenomas, possess unique complexities that warrant meticulous planning. CSR tumor patients share typical features involving water-electrolyte disturbance, cardiovascular factors, and airway accessibility issues. As seen, these issues require a multidisciplinary patient planning for surgery. Anesthesia planning must consider potential complications of postoperative respiratory disease and endocrine deficiencies that are often exaggerated by the specific surgical techniques employed, e.g., endoscopic transnasal-transsphenoidal access. The conclusions reached via a variety of literature bear out the pressing need for prudence and holistic control measures in such cases, with a focus on collaborative interventions by health practitioners involved in the patient's care (Tsentsiper *et al.*, 2024). Additionally, the neonatal airway management scenario is highly affected by the restricted application and familiarity of the LMA among HCPs. A survey revealed an acute shortage of clinical experience with the LMA, where around 79% of the surveyed population had no practical exposure.

This gap points to the hesitation of HCPs in embracing the LMA as an appropriate substitute for endotracheal intubation, and perhaps a stalemate in training models. While most indicated having received some form of training, confidence and ability in LMA insertion reported were moderately low, particularly among registered nurses and midwives. These findings provide a strong need to enhance training programs in such a manner that neonatal HCPs are competent to utilize LMAs, prioritizing safety and outcomes for airway management during neonatal resuscitation (Robin *et al.*, 2023). Incorporation of such knowledge surrounding airway management proves necessary gaps in the adult and neonatal care settings' knowledge base. The controversy surrounding CSR tumors illustrates the complexity entailed in preoperative preparation of patients for surgery, i.e., anesthetic management and postoperative monitoring. Concurrently, the outcome of the survey on neonatal practice illustrates an appalling lack of confidence and skill in dealing with laryngeal masks. Such findings not only underscore the necessity for improved training and educational programs but also reflect the necessity for ongoing research and development on approaches to managing the airway. By encouraging collaboration among healthcare professionals and prioritizing training programs, health systems can enhance the quality of respiratory care provided for patients across various populations and clinical settings, ultimately resulting in healthier outcomes.

KEY TERMS FROM THIS CHAPTER

- Airway adjuncts
- Airway patency
- Bag-valve-mask (BVM)
- Capnography
- Continuous positive airway pressure (CPAP)
- Difficult airway
- Endotracheal intubation
- Laryngeal mask airway (LMA)
- Airway management
- Apneic oxygenation
- Bi-level positive airway pressure (BiPAP)
- Confirming tube placement
- Cricothyrotomy
- Direct laryngoscopy
- End-tidal CO_2 ($EtCO_2$)
- Mechanical ventilation

CRITICAL THINKING QUESTIONS

1. **What is the primary purpose of endotracheal intubation in critical care?**
   a. To administer intravenous medications
   b. To monitor cardiac activity
   c. To maintain a secure airway and assist with ventilation
   d. To drain pleural fluid
2. **Which device delivers the highest concentration of oxygen among the following?**
   a. Nasal cannula
   b. Simple face mask
   c. Non-rebreather mask
   d. Venturi mask
3. **Which condition is most likely to require mechanical ventilation?**
   a. Mild fever
   b. Acute respiratory distress syndrome (ARDS)
   c. Controlled asthma
   d. Hypertension
4. **What is the correct position of the head and neck for optimal bag-valve-mask (BVM) ventilation in an unconscious patient?**
   a. Flexed neck and extended head
   b. Neutral position
   c. Head tilt and chin lift
   d. Chin tucked to chest
5. **Which of the following is a potential complication of prolonged mechanical ventilation?**
   a. Hypoglycemia
   b. Deep vein thrombosis
   c. Ventilator-associated pneumonia (VAP)
   d. Appendicitis

Short Answer Questions

1. What are the major anatomical structures involved in the human respiratory system?
2. How is airway patency assessed in critically ill patients?
3. Name two common techniques used for airway management and their indications.
4. What are the main methods of providing respiratory support in critical care?
5. List one potential complication of airway management and how it can be prevented.
6. What is one recent innovation in airway management, and how has it improved patient outcomes?

Answer to Critical Thinking Questions

1. (c); 2. (c); 3. (b); 4. (c); 5. (c)

REFERENCES

1. Abbasi, S., Siddiqui, K., & Qamar-ul-Hoda, M. (2022). Adverse respiratory events after removal of laryngeal mask airway in deep anesthesia versus awake state in children: A randomized trial. *Cureus, 14*. https://www.semanticscholar.org/paper/0aec8e2bc96f3d6e56eea0e88fc2594a50fb6cc6 (accessed on 22 May 2025).
2. Alberti, P., Ade-Ajayi, N., & Greenough, A. (2025). Respiratory support strategies for surgical neonates: A review. *Children, 12*. https://www.semanticscholar.org/paper/5d8231e2a5d40317de1ae6c8bd364ad1247daae1 (accessed on 22 May 2025).
3. Alhazzani, W., Møller, M. H., Arabi, Y. M., Loeb, M., Gong, M. N., Fan, E., Oczkowski, S., *et al.* (2020). Surviving Sepsis Campaign: Guidelines on the management of critically ill adults with coronavirus disease 2019 (COVID-19). *Intensive Care Medicine, 46*, 854–887. https://doi.org/10.1007/s00134-020-06022-5.
4. Alqahtani, K. S., Alshamrani, R. A., Alanazi, S. O., AlJarbou, A. S., Alharthi, F. S., Alzahrani, M. M., Alromaihi, A. J., *et al.* (2024). Guidelines for safe extubating and respiratory rehabilitation in the intensive care unit. *International Journal of Community Medicine and Public Health*. https://www.semanticscholar.org/paper/752423322dc6aa859e20aed2cf26a454aa4e6363 (accessed on 22 May 2025).
5. Azizipour, N., Avazpour, R., Rosenzweig, D. H., Sawan, M., & Ajji, A. (2020). Evolution of biochip technology: A review from lab-on-a-chip to organ-on-a-chip. *Micromachines, 11*, 599. https://doi.org/10.3390/mi11060599.
6. Budrevičiūtė, A., Damiati, S., Sabir, D. K., Önder, K., Schuller-Goetzburg, P., Plakys, G., Katileviciute, A., *et al.* (2020). Management and prevention strategies for non-communicable diseases (NCDs) and their risk factors. *Frontiers in Public Health, 8*. https://doi.org/10.3389/fpubh.2020.574111.
7. Chowdhury, R., Nair, A. K., Kamalam, D., & Jaishankar, R. (2025). Blind nasal intubation as a rescue strategy in difficult airway management. *HCA Healthcare Journal of Medicine, 6*(1), 79–81. https://www.semanticscholar.org/paper/a55137d043c803060952495782af7ebd3cbc859d (accessed on 22 May 2025).
8. Coppola, S., Radovanovic, D., Pozzi, T., Danzo, F., Rocco, C., Lazzaroni, G., Santus, P., *et al.* (2024). Non-invasive respiratory support in elderly hospitalized patients. *Expert Review of Respiratory Medicine*. https://www.semanticscholar.org/paper/ebbd49166da3258301ba12c83f99b51b7db9ab6d (accessed on 22 May 2025).
9. Coté, C. J., & Wilson, S. (2019). Guidelines for monitoring and management of pediatric patients before, during, and after sedation for diagnostic and therapeutic procedures. *Pediatrics, 143*. https://doi.org/10.1542/peds.2019-1000.
10. Doppalapudi, S., Fortuzi, K., Qasim, A., Yordanka, D. S., & Khaja, M. (2024). Glass in the airways: A bronchoscopy challenge. *Cureus, 16*. https://www.semanticscholar.org/paper/29b729467f8586a1bb1cd45b8420d5ec35fd9200 (accessed on 22 May 2025).
11. Frerk, C., Mitchell, V. S., McNarry, A. F., Mendonca, C., Bhagrath, R., Patel, A., O'Sullivan, E. P., *et al.* (2015). Difficult Airway Society 2015 guidelines for management of unanticipated difficult intubation in adults. *British Journal of Anesthesia, 115*, 827–848. https://doi.org/10.1093/bja/aev371.

12. González, H., Arizmendi, C., & Giraldo, B. F. (2025). Development of a deep learning model for the prediction of ventilator weaning. https://www.semanticscholar.org/paper/cbde1eed35fc8ce17048264f3fc5b7b37c6589a7 (accessed on 22 May 2025).

13. Gulafshan, & Umadevi, K. A. (2021). Effectiveness of teaching program on knowledge of clinical nurses regarding risk of unplanned extubating of patients with mechanical ventilation at a selected hospital, Bangalore. *6*, 452–459. https://www.semanticscholar.org/paper/f7935f8faf97020f32c9e0eade128972b97d1c82 (accessed on 22 May 2025).

14. Hahn, R. T., Abraham, T. P., Adams, M., Bruce, C. J., Glas, K. E., Lang, R. M., Reeves, S. T., *et al.* (2013). Guidelines for performing a comprehensive transesophageal echocardiographic examination. *Anesthesia & Analgesia, 118*, 21–68. https://doi.org/10.1213/ane.0000000000000016.

15. Hansel, J., Fuchs, A., Radcliffe, G., Sotiriou, A., Rivett, K., Bohnenblust, V., Grimes, R., *et al.* (2025). International consensus-based core outcome set for airway management clinical trials and observational studies: The Airway Terminology and Outcome Measures (ATOM) protocol. *BMJ Open, 15*. https://www.semanticscholar.org/paper/884bd6e01689935d178e08b0a382d2e6f193ab1b (accessed on 22 May 2025).

16. Hatem, A., Alqhtani, S., Alsalmi, K. A., Jweed, H., Almokhls, S., Alshammari, A. O., Mutlaq, S., *et al.* (2024). Emergency airway management: The critical role of nurses and respiratory therapists. *Power System Technology*. https://www.semanticscholar.org/paper/e6c04d59f823e1a903863399644c4a58abbf4dad (accessed on 22 May 2025).

17. Hullumani, S. V., Qureshi, M. I., & Raghuveer, R. (2024). Effect of physical rehabilitation using oromotor stimulation, manual airway clearance technique, positioning, tactile and kinesthetic stimulation (PROMPT) protocol on respiratory and neuromuscular function in neonatal respiratory distress syndrome (NRDS): A protocol for randomized controlled trial. *F1000Research*. https://www.semanticscholar.org/paper/4681f9e2e98ff5213b4b7fcb1a3c18db73369c59 (accessed on 22 May 2025).

18. Janjua, S., Banchoff, E., Threapleton, C. J. D., Prigmore, S., Fletcher, J., & Disler, R. T. (2021). Digital interventions for the management of chronic obstructive pulmonary disease. *The Cochrane Database of Systematic Reviews, 4*, CD013246. https://www.semanticscholar.org/paper/2a1349c1b396b8baeab499fde50fcceb16849f9e (accessed on 22 May 2025).

19. Kandel, A., Knulst, A., Riggsbee, J., Riggsbee, S. O., Tamang, S., Bhattarai, H. B., & Karn, M. (2024). Use of locally produced novel low-cost 3D printed respiratory muscle strength trainer device (RMSTD) for long COVID-rehabilitation: An innovative case report. *Case Reports in Medicine, 2024*. https://www.semanticscholar.org/paper/83d9023a1892175e79346ebd6f804193f8722a12 (accessed on 22 May 2025).

20. Krishnamoorthi, S. K., Karthi, G., Radhika, M., Rathinam, A. R., Raju, A. R., Pinjarkar, L., & Srinivasan, C. (2025). Advancing airway management for ventilation optimization in critical healthcare with cloud computing and deep learning. *Indonesian Journal of Electrical Engineering and Computer Science*. https://www.semanticscholar.org/paper/a4bab0a9b6ec2b291d1a770b26366a375ec6a811 (accessed on 22 May 2025).

21. Lemyre, B., Deguise, M., Benson, P., Kirpalani, H., De Paoli, A. D., & Davis, P. (2023). Nasal intermittent positive pressure ventilation (NIPPV) versus nasal continuous positive airway pressure (NCPAP) for preterm neonates after extubating. *The Cochrane Database of Systematic Reviews, 7*, CD003212. https://www.semanticscholar.org/paper/5e80d5fe7240190a5c736900abc20c583a309b5b (accessed on 22 May 2025).

22. Mahajan, A. D., Daithankar, S., Dholabhai, P., Singh, A. P., Shah, A. R., & Shah, N. P. (2024). Unlocking the potential of submental intubation–Redefining airway management in craniomaxillofacial trauma patients. *Craniomaxillofacial Trauma & Reconstruction*. https://www.semanticscholar.org/paper/3662b158913164fe6d285d2d04a372b705293a90 (accessed on 22 May 2025).

23. Manisalidis, I., Stavropoulou, E., Stavropoulos, A., & Bezirtzoglou, E. (2020). Environmental and health impacts of air pollution: A review. *Frontiers in Public Health, 8*. https://doi.org/10.3389/fpubh.2020.00014.

24. Maqbool, K., Dewan, S., & Chauhan, M. (2024). Short term outcome of Veno venous extracorporeal membrane oxygenation in patients of ARDS presenting at tertiary care center–An observational study. *Indian Journal of Critical Care Medicine, 28*, S106–S117. https://www.semanticscholar.org/paper/ea4337c7bb73a46a509d90da9d9937486c88bcad (accessed on 22 May 2025).

25. Martínez Beleño, S. (2024). Initial assessment and stabilization of thoracic trauma in pediatric patients: A narrative review. *Global Journal for Research Analysis*. https://www.semanticscholar.org/paper/c14fb38e0f528ab843499f48aafd6e289ca6b854 (accessed on 22 May 2025).

26. Morris, S., Fader, A. N., Milad, M. P., & Dionisi, H. (2020). Understanding the "scope" of the problem: Why laparoscopy is considered safe during the COVID-19 pandemic. *Journal of Minimally Invasive Gynecology, 27*, 789–791. https://doi.org/10.1016/j.jmig.2020.04.002.

27. Nazir, A., & Clementius, B. (2025). Airway mucus hypersecretion in chronic obstructive pulmonary disease patients: From basic pathophysiology to rehabilitation approaches. *Surabaya Physical Medicine and Rehabilitation Journal*. https://www.semanticscholar.org/paper/3f1ddb9d7b029039bdfeb30103021e96aa0bb64d (accessed on 22 May 2025).

28. Ofei-Dodoo, S., Falahat, M., Duncan, L., & Hoang, M. (2023). Emergency medical services personnel compliance with escalating airway algorithm protocol. *Annals of Family Medicine, 21*(Suppl 3). https://www.semanticscholar.org/paper/650233d699ba8d396085a6f39089aa62c1b656bf (accessed on 22 May 2025).

29. Pak, I. S., Imran, K., Sherazi, H., Riaz, S., Abbas, Y., Ali, M., *et al.* (2023). Comparison of bubble CPAP versus conventional ventilation in neonates having respiratory distress. *Annals of PIMS–Shaheed Zulfiqar Ali Bhutto Medical University*. https://www.semanticscholar.org/paper/1090a6c9281b7c37999cd5a8a48219076282f9be (accessed on 22 May 2025).

30. Pavliša, G., Gašparović, K., Puretić, H., Ljubicic, L., Nekić, A., Vukovic, V., Vukančić, K., *et al.* (2023). Noninvasive mechanical ventilation in COVID-19 related acute respiratory failure. *Acta Clinica Croatia, 62*, 125–131. https://www.semanticscholar.org/paper/824cf2d32b0097df4c8d964d3e8d40cc5ce3a361 (accessed on 22 May 2025).

31. Pettenuzzo, T., Boscolo, A., Pistollato, E., Pretto, C., Giacon, T. A., Frasson, S., Carbotti, F. M., *et al.* (2024). Effects of non-invasive respiratory support in post-operative patients: A systematic review and network meta-analysis. *Critical Care, 28*. https://www.semanticscholar.org/paper/f88802b6cf25d6d00190dfd3551382968fa40727 (accessed on 22 May 2025).

32. Phua, J., Weng, L., Ling, L., Egi, M., Lim, C. M., Divatia, J. V., Shrestha, B. R., *et al.* (2020). Intensive care management of coronavirus disease 2019 (COVID-19): Challenges and recommendations. *The Lancet Respiratory Medicine, 8*, 506–517. https://doi.org/10.1016/s2213-2600(20)30161-2.

33. Robin, B., Soghier, L., Vachharajani, A., & Moussa, A. (2023). Laryngeal mask airway clinical use and training: A survey of North American neonatal health care professionals. *American Journal of Perinatology*. https://www.semanticscholar.org/paper/5be62212778ddc86384dc35dbb4cabcc6dd751d5 (accessed on 22 May 2025).

34. Robinson, T., & Scullion, J. (2021). Acute respiratory distress syndrome (ARDS). *Oxford Handbook of Respiratory Nursing*. https://www.semanticscholar.org/paper/ed570af4907fd057aaa280362dbc751812f3b61a (accessed on 22 May 2025).

35. Rogerson, C., White, B. R., Smith, M., Hogan, A. H., Abu-Sultaneh, S., Carroll, C. L., & Shein, S. (2024). Institutional variability in respiratory support use for pediatric critical asthma: A multicenter retrospective study. *Annals of the American Thoracic Society*. https://www.semanticscholar.org/paper/e24d98cda5bb41e4f13df7cbeb18ca3968f8eeba (accessed on 22 May 2025).

36. Rovira Soriano, L., & De Andrés, J. D. (2019). ESRA19-0514 Perioperative administration of oxygen risks and benefits intraoperative hyperoxia is a valuable recommendation? *Regional Anesthesia & Pain Medicine, 44*, A36–A38. https://www.semanticscholar.org/paper/11ae5f37c864860889a38eab42b11d5232e1fabc (accessed on 22 May 2025).

37. Rowan, N. J., & Laffey, J. G. (2020). Challenges and solutions for addressing critical shortage of supply chain for personal and protective equipment (PPE) arising from coronavirus disease (COVID-19) pandemic–Case study from the Republic of Ireland. *Science of the Total Environment, 725*, 138532. https://doi.org/10.1016/j.scitotenv.2020.138532.

38. Sartini, S., Ferrari, L., Cutuli, O., Castellani, L., Bagnasco, M., Corsello, L. M., Bracco, C., *et al.* (2024). The role of POCUS in acute respiratory failure: A narrative review on airway and breathing assessment. *Journal of Clinical Medicine, 13*. https://www.semanticscholar.org/paper/a484d78b3a05dae3339043d0b75beea3c715af95 (accessed on 22 May 2025).

39. Sayar, Y., Yıldırım, M., & Teber, S. (2023). Management of neurological problems in children on home invasive mechanical ventilation. *Pediatric Pulmonology*. https://www.semanticscholar.org/paper/404989678ca42f1c7086500beee2546dd0c79225 (accessed on 22 May 2025).

40. Schrijver, J., Lenferink, A., Brusse-Keizer, M., Zwerink, M., van der Valk, P., van der Palen, J., & Effing, T. (2022). Self-management for people with chronic obstructive pulmonary disease. *The Cochrane Database of Systematic Reviews, 1*, CD002990. https://www.semanticscholar.org/paper/f3d471fd93af581bd7c7da0a1103927878979e13 (accessed on 22 May 2025).

41. Sharath, H., Qureshi, M. I., Raghuveer, R., Saklecha, A., & Nadipena, P. T. (2024). The effect of physical rehabilitation on oro-motor stimulation, manual airway clearance, positioning, and tactile stimulation (PROMPT) on neonates with respiratory distress syndrome. *Cureus, 16*. https://www.semanticscholar.org/paper/18e97e6ddb5f3d448915d11269ceff7fb31639be (accessed on 22 May 2025).

42. Su, J., Tie, X., Chen, Y., Zou, T., & Yin, W. (2024). Successful application of airway pressure release ventilation in a child with severe acute respiratory distress syndrome induced by trauma: A case report. *BMC Pulmonary Medicine, 24*. https://www.semanticscholar.org/paper/10cbb63c719608326ac8851baff359dada0b467c (accessed on 22 May 2025).

43. Szabó, M., Orosz, G., Iványi, Z., & Darvas, K. (2023). [Use of thoracic and lung ultrasound in general anesthesia]. *Orvosi Hetilap, 164*(22), 864–870. https://www.semanticscholar.org/paper/f65517309525099356bbad481827411acd35f061 (accessed on 22 May 2025).

44. Szymanowski, D., Bax, P., & Behar, P. (2019). Cervical teratoma causing airway obstruction in a premature infant. *Ear, Nose & Throat Journal, 100*, 335–336. https://www.semanticscholar.org/paper/18c150a2c9628b4692fd7b5e5e3492ebb7688800 (accessed on 22 May 2025).

45. Taksinwarajarn, T., & Petnak, T. (2025). Management of critically ill obstetric patients. *Clinical Critical Care*. https://www.semanticscholar.org/paper/6a5aaeacd0656f595d295ff1fb6a6c8779f96c60 (accessed on 22 May 2025).

46. Tekin, M., & Çobanoğlu, N. (2024). Management of respiratory problems in children on home invasive mechanical ventilation. *Pediatric Pulmonology*. https://www.semanticscholar.org/paper/9e10c6ca19642876b573e9d6413b98df55471b52 (accessed on 22 May 2025).

47. Tsentsiper, L. M., Petrova, A. O., Terekhov, I. S., Leyderman, I., Gulyaev, D. A., Ulitin, A., Samochernykh, K., *et al.* (2024). Some features of the perioperative management of patients with a tumor of the chiasmal cellaria region: A review. *Annals of Critical Care*. https://www.semanticscholar.org/paper/e50b516ba7f338ebbecfdd48dccc39aeaffcc319 (accessed on 22 May 2025).

48. Vetrugno, L., Deana, C., Colaianni-Alfonso, N., Tritapepe, F., Fierro, C., & Maggiore, S. M. (2024). Noninvasive respiratory support in the perioperative setting: A narrative review. *Frontiers in Medicine, 11*. https://www.semanticscholar.org/paper/a66696ab9dbeefb45f484c36d3cdd0253e7e2a48 (accessed on 22 May 2025).

49. Zhao, L., Xie, Y. X., & Wang, C. (2020). Recommendations for respiratory rehabilitation in adults with coronavirus disease 2019. *Chinese Medical Journal, 133*, 1595–1602. https://doi.org/10.1097/cm9.0000000000000848.

HEMODYNAMIC MONITORING AND MANAGEMENT

4

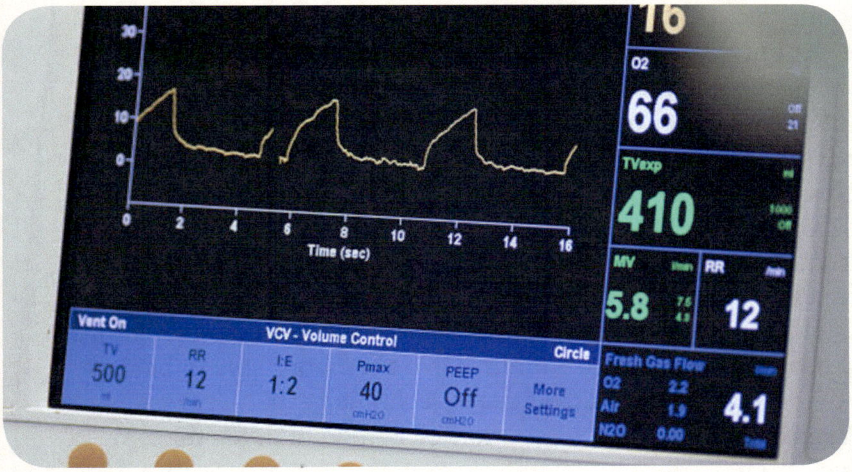

LEARNING OBJECTIVES

After studying this chapter, you will be able to:

1. Describe the principles of hemodynamics.
2. Identify the techniques of hemodynamic monitoring.
3. Define indications for hemodynamic monitoring.
4. Discuss the interpretation of hemodynamic data.
5. Explain the hemodynamic management strategies.
6. Understand the challenges in hemodynamic monitoring.

Introduction

Hemodynamic monitoring is a crucial aspect of patient care, especially for patients with diseases such as sepsis and septic shock. These diseases are characterized by potentially fatal organ dysfunction resulting from an exaggerated host response to infection that can have a profound effect on mortality. Effective hemodynamic monitoring provides early detection of abnormalities in circulation, which triggers clinical interventions toward normalizing tissue perfusion and oxygenation. Various techniques, including direct arterial pressure monitoring and less invasive measurement, provide clinicians with the information they need so that educated decisions can be made. The necessity of precise monitoring is extremely important in sepsis, where rapid therapeutic interventions significantly increase survival chances, underlining the importance of hemodynamic intelligence in critical care settings (Evans *et al.*, 2021). Sepsis essentially alters hemodynamic stability, typically resulting in hypotension and compromised organ perfusion. Sepsis management in septic shock entails aggressive fluid resuscitation and drug administration, primarily through vasopressors to maintain cardiac output and provide mean arterial pressure. Current guidelines recommend a goal mean arterial pressure of at least 65 mm Hg, illustrating the delicate balance between fluid overload and hypoperfusion states that create difficulty in patient outcomes (Wild *et al.*, 2020). An understanding of the fundamental physiological hemodynamic mechanisms of stroke volume and vascular resistance plays an important role in tailoring interventions that address both the immediate and continuing needs of the patient. Such critical insight underlies guidelines such as fluid resuscitation protocols, once more emphasizing the use of dynamic monitoring towards improved therapeutic results. The use of advanced hemodynamic monitoring technology has revolutionized patient care in critical care. Data recording and processing systems provide clinicians with an overall image of a patients hemodynamic function and provide consequent increased responsiveness to states of abrupt change. The application of parameters such as blood lactate levels as a resuscitation aid assists health professionals in deciding on timely interventions in treatment planning. Additionally, improvements in monitoring trends have assisted in the increase of evidence-based practice, and consequently, adherence to entrenched protocols that optimize outcomes for patients experiencing severe hemodynamic compromise. In summary, the significance of successful hemodynamic monitoring in septic management is a reflection of its pivotal role as a survival rate determinant and evidence-based practice driving future critical care management intervention developments (Evans *et al.*, 2021).

Definition of Hemodynamic Monitoring

Hemodynamic monitoring forms an essential component of the management of the patient, particularly in perioperative and critical care settings. Hemodynamic monitoring is the ongoing assessment of cardiovascular function as quantified using the parameters of blood pressure, heart rate, and cardiac output. The overall purpose of hemodynamic monitoring is to gain accurate, contemporaneous information pertaining to a patient's cardiovascular status that can potentially affect clinical decision-making and direct timely intervention. As it provides information about the hemodynamic stability of the patient, it assumes a vital role in directing therapy and minimizing the risk of carrying out varied surgical and medical procedures. As a dynamic specialty, the development of hemodynamic monitoring equipment reflects technological innovation, and shifting toward increasingly noninvasive methods, which can enhance patient comfort and safety during emergent interventions (Bilotta, 2017). During the recent past, the focus of hemodynamic monitoring shifted from purely invasive techniques to the inclusion of more forms of noninvasive methods. This is because of the advances in technology that have enabled better separation of hemodynamic status with precise measurement without subjecting patients to harm from invasive procedures. Noninvasive monitoring methods, such as ultrasound-based technologies and modern-day optical devices, are becoming more crucial in clinical practice. These not only enhance patient satisfaction but also enable monitoring across a wider group of patients, even those with less acute illness. Integration of these technologies allows for a better understanding of the cardiovascular dynamics of a patient, and hence, healthcare practitioners introduce goal-directed therapies to optimize hemodynamic management (Karakitsos *et al.*, 2014). The integration of hemodynamic monitoring into clinical practice also emphasizes its applicability towards minimizing perioperative complications, as well as improving patient outcomes. Systematic hemodynamic assessment makes possible the early detection of potential complications and thus enables immediate medical intervention with the potential to radically alter patient trajectories. With an era in which surgical procedures are becoming increasingly complex and patient populations increasingly heterogeneous, the capacity to monitor hemodynamic status in real time is increasingly important to health care providers. As ongoing research and clinical trials evaluate the validity of these emerging monitoring tools, their findings will undoubtedly influence best practice and future directions in hemodynamic care, solidifying the role of monitoring systems as a central component of quality patient care across healthcare environments (Bilotta, 2017) (Figure 4.1).

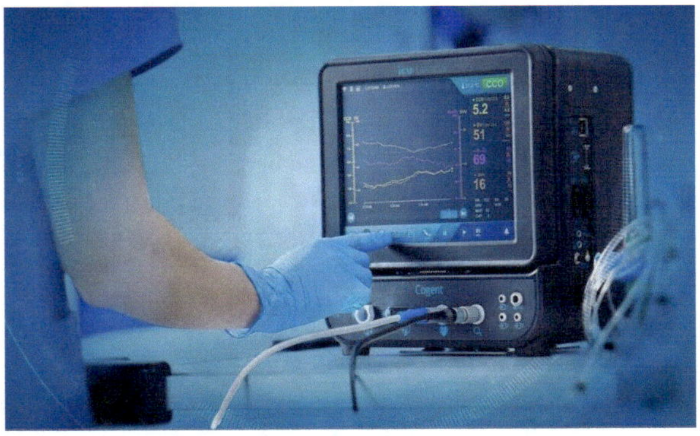

Figure 4.1. Hemodynamic monitoring.

Source: https://www.dicardiology.com/sites/default/files/field/image/Hemodynamic-Monitoring-Market-Website-New-e1659953386571.jpeg.

Importance in Clinical Settings

The utility of hemodynamic monitoring in clinical practice cannot be stressed enough, particularly in surgical procedures where precise regulation of fluid status and hemodynamic function is of utmost concern. Monitoring of parameters such as mean arterial pressure, cardiac output, and systemic vascular resistance directs anesthetic management and ensures adequate organ perfusion. Emerging methods, like the Hypotension Probability Indicator (HPI), are designed to forecast reductions in mean arterial pressure in particular, reflecting a shift away from traditional fluid therapy strategies. Instead of questioning during stationary moments, adaptive strategies emphasizing information in real-time can lead to improved patient outcomes and fewer complications. This change of strategy is necessary due to the danger associated with flap hypo-perfusion in reconstructive surgery, which would have a direct relation with healing and success of surgery as a whole (Lauretta *et al.*, 2018). The incorporation of state-of-the-art monitoring technologies, such as transpulmonary thermodilution (TPTD), makes way for enhanced efficacy in hemodynamic management in clinical practice. TPTD is a necessary tool in the estimation of pulmonary edema, facilitating clinicians to quantitatively observe water accumulation in the lungs. Quantification is not only crucial in terms of fluid therapy optimization but also in the discrimination between various types of pulmonary edema, which assists in appropriate and early interventions. With clinical practices targeting the prevention of potentially damaging fluid accumulation through fluid administration minimization, TPTD assists in monitoring and handling these parameters optimally. Such precise hemodynamic monitoring allows for more tailored therapeutic strategies in critically ill perioperative patients, emphasizing the pivotal role of advanced monitoring techniques in contemporary surgical care (Assaad *et al.*, 2017). Ultimately, optimization of hemodynamic monitoring protocols results in improved patient protection and surgical outcomes. Real-time hemodynamic parameter assessment and fluid management ensure that clinical professionals have improved diagnostic and predictive tools. An integrated monitoring strategy incorporating both conventional and novel modalities facilitates improved decision-making by multidisciplinary groups. This collaborative practice is particularly valuable in settings where effective anesthesiologist-surgeon-nurse communication is desirable. The comingling of aggressive hemodynamic management strategies underscores the need for ongoing practice improvement and research to enhance clinical outcomes and the quality of care provided to critically ill patients (Assaad *et al.*, 2017; Lauretta *et al.*, 2018).

4.1. Principles of Hemodynamics

Learning Outcome

1. Key concepts in hemodynamics
2. Factors affecting blood flow and pressure
3. Role of the cardiovascular system

It is essential to comprehend the principles of hemodynamics in order to perform hemodynamic monitoring and management optimally, especially in critically ill patients. Hemodynamics is defined as the dynamics of the circulation of blood within the circulatory system and involves the study of heart function, blood pressure, volume, and resistance. The most important factors influencing hemodynamics are cardiac output, systemic vascular resistance, and preload and afterload dynamics. Cardiac output, the volume of blood discharged by the heart each minute, is a critical measure of cardiac function and can be regulated by stroke volume and heart rate. Monitoring these measurements, clinicians can assess the level of perfusion of vital organs to intervene timely in order to attain the best patient outcomes (Evans *et al.*, 2021). Besides, more advanced hemodynamic techniques enable a comprehensive evaluation of cardiovascular health, eventually facilitating the treatment of conditions like shock and sepsis. Ohm's Law also describes blood flow versus resistance dynamics, in hemodynamics formulated as flow (Q) equals pressure (ΔP) over resistance (R). This fundamental principle illustrates that for blood to circulate effectively, sufficient pressure must be present to balance vascular resistance. Vascular resistance changes will have considerable implications on hemodynamic variables, particularly in the event of shock episodes, whereby vasodilation will decrease systemic vascular resistance. Thus, grasping pressure and flow interaction justifies why achieving the best mean arterial pressure (MAP) is imperative in critically ill patients, most notably septic shock (Evans *et al.*, 2021). Practically, the maintenance of a MAP of 65 mm Hg or higher is typically recommended because it is correlated with improved organ perfusion and decreased mortality.

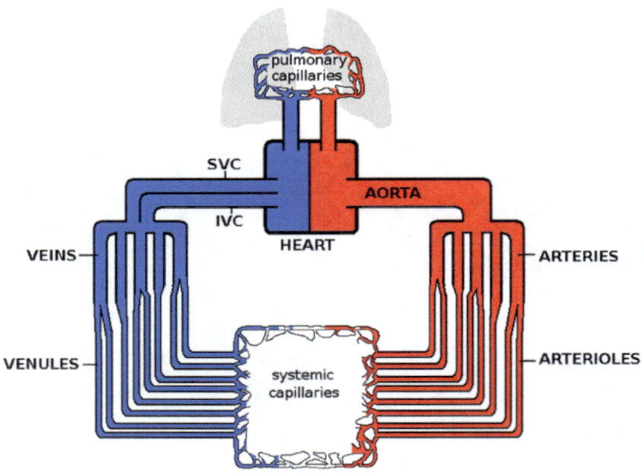

Figure 4.2. Diagram of the circulatory system.

Source: https://en.wikipedia.org/wiki/Hemodynamics#/media/File:Diagram_of_human_circulatory_system.gif.

Optimal hemodynamic care depends on precise measurement and interpretation of hemodynamic indicators, typically supported by advanced monitoring techniques. Invasive procedures such as CVP and pulmonary artery catheterization allow clinicians to gain direct pressure and flow measurements inside the heart and large vascular bed. Invasive procedures supplement non-invasive procedures such as echocardiography and impedance cardiography and provide a better grasp of cardiac function and fluid balance. The integration of innovative technologies, like the monitoring of dynamic cardiac output, is promising to provide precise fluid management and adjustment of vasopressor therapy in patients with sepsis or septic shock. Monitoring technologies not only verify the effectiveness of interventions but also help clinicians to predict the evolution of a patient's hemodynamic status, making possible a proactive model of critical care management (Figure 4.2).

4.1.1. Key Concepts in Hemodynamics

It is important to understand hemodynamics in order to optimize patient outcomes in a wide variety of other kinds of medical settings, most significantly surgery and intensive care. The cardinal axiom of hemodynamics is that of cardiac output, or that quantity of blood pumped per minute by the heart. This figure is priceless to calculate overall tissue perfusion, particularly in shock or fluid-resuscitated patients. Both invasive and non-invasive hemodynamic monitoring gives the clinician instant information regarding cardiovascular function. Accurate measurement of parameters like blood pressure, heart rate, and stroke volume can direct therapy and influence interventions such as fluid infusion or pharmacologic intervention. Newer technology improves the accuracy of such measurements, as recently documented in the literature. Thus, detailed knowledge of hemodynamic concepts improves the clinician's ability to optimally tackle complex cases of patients. Fluid management plays a key role in hemodynamic monitoring, particularly in the setting of enhanced recovery after surgery (ERAS) protocols. Goal-directed fluid therapy (GDT) is a core tenet of these protocols, the objective being to optimise fluid status and prevent under- and over-hydration-related complications. GDT consists of careful observation of several physiological parameters, such as cardiac output, heart rate, and blood pressure, to enable early fluid adjustment. Moreover, it requires individually adapted fluid management guidelines according to the specific physiological response of every patient (Rola *et al.*, 2020). Since the use of GDT has led to improved patient outcomes, i.e., fewer postoperative complications and shorter hospital stay, it is now part of modern surgical practice. By adopting a logical concept of fluid therapy, health professionals can optimize the performance of perioperative care and minimize risks due to fluid imbalance. The hemodynamics behavior at the physiological level is a reflection of the complexity of the human system and must be carefully observed. For instance, interaction among preload, afterload, and contractility is key to understanding the function of the heart and response to some of the hemodynamic stresses. Preload is the initial deformation of cardiac muscle fibers due to direct association with venous return, and afterload is the resistance against which the heart must eject the blood. Hemodynamic monitoring practices, like invasive measures like pulmonary artery catheters and non-invasive monitoring in the form of echocardiography, enable us to comprehend these parameters in a better way. Also, acute respiratory distress syndrome (ARDS) is a case of convergence of hemodynamic principles and respiratory therapy aimed at providing proper ventilation and perfusion in critical care cases (Rola *et al.*, 2020). By thorough investigation and continuous monitoring of hemodynamic parameters, healthcare professionals can provide targeted interventions, hence minimizing patient morbidity and mortality rates.

4.1.2. Factors Affecting Blood Flow and Pressure

The physiology of flow and blood pressure is regulated by a series of physiological parameters that need a thorough study in hemodynamic monitoring and management. The vascular resistance is one of the prime determinants and is functionally dependent almost entirely on the size of the blood vessel. The resistance in the smaller vessels is greater because there is more frictional force on the moving blood. Consequently, a change in the diameter of a vessel, either through vasodilation or vasoconstriction, may cause drastic changes in the blood pressure and speed of blood flow. Other properties of blood, like viscosity, which is very sensitive to the concentration of hematocrit, also have a vital role to play. Increased viscosity may cause heightened resistance and, therefore, an increase in blood pressure. It is required for the forecasting of cardiovascular responses under various pathological conditions and in guiding appropriate management strategies, as its deviation from normal hemodynamics may lead to serious complications and require clinical intervention.

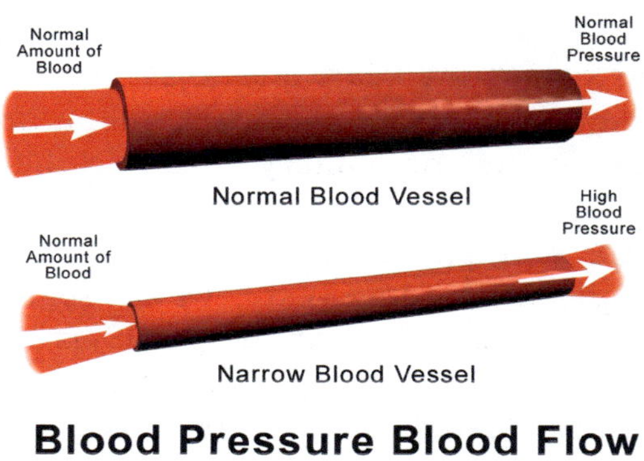

Figure 4.3. Illustration demonstrating how vessel narrowing, or vasoconstriction, increases blood pressure.

Source: https://upload.wikimedia.org/wikipedia/commons/thumb/0/0c/Blausen_0092_BloodPressureFlow.png/500px-Blausen_0092_BloodPressureFlow.png.

The dynamic relationship between stroke volume and heart rate, which collectively determine cardiac output, is another important determinant of blood pressure and flow. Cardiac output is required for sufficient tissue perfusion and normal blood pressure. In conditions of exercise or stress, the heart raises its heart rate and stroke volume to meet elevated metabolic demands. However, heart failure conditions lower stroke volume, necessitating compensation in the form of a raised heart rate. Dynamic interaction between these parameters underscores the importance of hemodynamic monitoring in the clinical setup in which patients may exhibit compromised cardiac function. Advanced monitoring techniques such as multimodal physiological modeling can provide valuable information about cardiovascular status and aid in designing interventions accordingly, thereby promoting enhanced patient outcomes through effective management of blood flow and pressure dynamics (Xiang *et al.*, 2024) (Figure 4.3).

Finally, conditions outside the cardiovascular system, including environmental temperature and lifestyle components, heavily influence blood pressure and circulation. To illustrate, long-term exposure to cold will lead to vasoconstriction and elevated blood pressure, and excess heat leads to vasodilation, reducing peripheral resistance and blood pressure. Lifestyle components, including diet, exercise, and stress reduction, also have vital roles in determining total cardiovascular function. For example, excessive sodium intake is linked to fluid overload and hypertension, whereas regular physical activity leads to maintained optimal values of blood pressure. The application of wearable technologies to measure blood pressure is a unique chance to examine such determinants in real time to facilitate the management of hypertension with regard to physiological as well as lifestyle determinants of cardiovascular dynamics. As we continue to build our knowledge of these variables, we enhance our capacity to monitor and sustain hemodynamic health in an ideal manner (Butter *et al.*, 2024).

4.1.3. Role of the Cardiovascular System

Cardiovascular system plays a crucial role in hemodynamic homeostasis of the body. It facilitates the transport of blood, which delivers oxygen and nutrients to tissue and removes metabolic end products. In addition to being essential for cell function, normal circulation is equally important for regulation of tissue perfusion with varying physiological requirements, e.g., exercise or stress. In hemodynamic monitoring, it is equally important to study the dynamics of blood pressure, cardiac output, and systemic vascular resistance. Proper maintenance of these parameters can prevent conditions such as hypovolemia and cardiac failure, which can undermine the safety and recovery of a patient, especially in high-risk surgeries.

A combination of measurement of cardiac function and vascular response allows clinicians to make intelligent choices regarding fluid resuscitation and vasopressor therapy and to maximize patient outcomes. The intricacy of cardiovascular physiology makes the use of precise hemodynamic monitoring modalities a necessity. Both invasive and non-invasive modalities have proliferated to provide dynamic assessment of cardiovascular status. Ongoing monitoring of the variables like cardiac output, blood pressure variation, and systemic vascular resistance can allow intervention on time. For example, echocardiography has been an invasive yet effective tool of real-time hemodynamic evaluation of cardiac function and volume status, exemplified by recent data. New technologies augment the clinician's ability of early shock states detection and optimization of interventions thereto. Such hemodynamic monitoring is dynamic rather than static but, more importantly, needs to be interpreted and revised constantly, especially in the case of critical care situations where a patient could have more than one comorbid illness simultaneously. As such, the incorporation of novel monitoring metrics into practice is part of enhancing perioperative care and outcomes for patients who undergo surgery. In high-risk surgical candidates, the cardiovascular system's capacity to sustain tissue perfusion determines perioperative outcome. Inadequate vascular reserve usually comes with poor tissue oxygenation and risk for complications such as organ failure or longer recovery time. These complications are further confounded by inadequate fluid management, cardiac dysfunction, and hypovolemia, thus further justifying hemodynamic monitoring. Clinical opinion concurs that proper hemodynamics monitoring allows for early detection of instability, which informs appropriate intervention to provide sufficient permissive pressures. It takes joint effort from medical personnel in conjunction with technical progress to detect high-risk patients and optimize treatment. Continuous observing and clinical evaluation in a cycle ensures constant attention to patient safety and effective management of the cardiovascular system, leading to better results in surgery and general health of patients (Aseni *et al.*, 2019; Flythe *et al.*, 2020) (Figure 4.4).

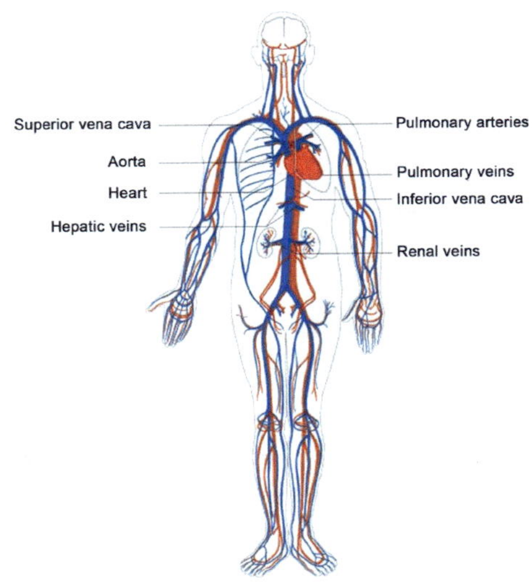

Figure 4.4. Cardiovascular system.

Source: https://www.cardiosecur.com/fileadmin/content/Fachartikel/Cardiovascular_system_EN_2.jpg.

Test Your Knowledge

1. What are the key concepts involved in understanding hemodynamics?
2. What factors influence blood flow and blood pressure in the body?

4.2. Techniques of Hemodynamic Monitoring

Learning Outcome

1. Discuss the invasive monitoring methods
2. Understand the non-invasive monitoring methods
3. Define the comparison of monitoring techniques

Hemodynamic monitoring is the basis for management of the patient's cardiovascular instability due to the fact that hemodynamic monitoring gives an indication of heart function and circulatory well-being of the body. Hemodynamic monitoring methods are broadly divided into non-invasive and invasive modalities that inherently have merits and demerits. Invasive methods such as arterial catheterization and central venous pressure deliver direct blood pressure, cardiac output, and systemic vascular resistance measurement. These methods are particularly valuable in critically ill individuals where precise titration of medication and fluid is required to attain hemodynamic stability. The high accuracy coupled with the immediate feedback that these procedures are capable of delivering in emergency conditions renders them invaluable in operating room and intensive care environments, as seen from case series of challenging surgeries like radical cystectomy with ileal conduit diversion (Gohad *et al.*, 2025). Lower-risk non-invasive methods can remain a significant part to play in hemodynamic monitoring. Impedance cardiography and echocardiography are methods through which cardiac function and hemodynamic status can be ascertained by clinicians without recourse to invasive techniques. Transthoracic echocardiography, for example, can provide immediate data regarding cardiac chamber size, global blood flow dynamics, and function. These approaches are particularly indicated in patients who may be able to withstand the risks of invasive monitoring, such as patients in compromised circulatory status or with bleeding disorders. There has been technological progress that has raised the accuracy and worth of these non-invasive techniques and made them a viable option to continuous monitoring in stable patients, and preoperative and postoperative management where hemodynamic evolution must be monitored at all times (Howsmon *et al.*, 2024). The addition of newer monitoring devices has also improved hemodynamic assessment. For instance, statistical process monitoring (SPM) techniques, originally identified in manufacturing processes, have lately been employed as a novel tool for high-frequency vital sign and hemodynamic data monitoring. This is because the capability to create multivariate trajectory maps makes it easier to monitor trends and interactions among various hemodynamic variables over time. This monitoring can also improve identification of anticipated parameter abnormalities in post-operative states, and early intervention can be facilitated in patients with congenital heart disease or recovery from complicated surgery (Howsmon *et al.*, 2024). Enhanced hemodynamic monitoring will allow the implementation of a blend of invasive and non-invasive technologies, supported by newer analytical methods to data, to provide improved patient outcomes based on more accurate and tailored management methods (Figure 4.5).

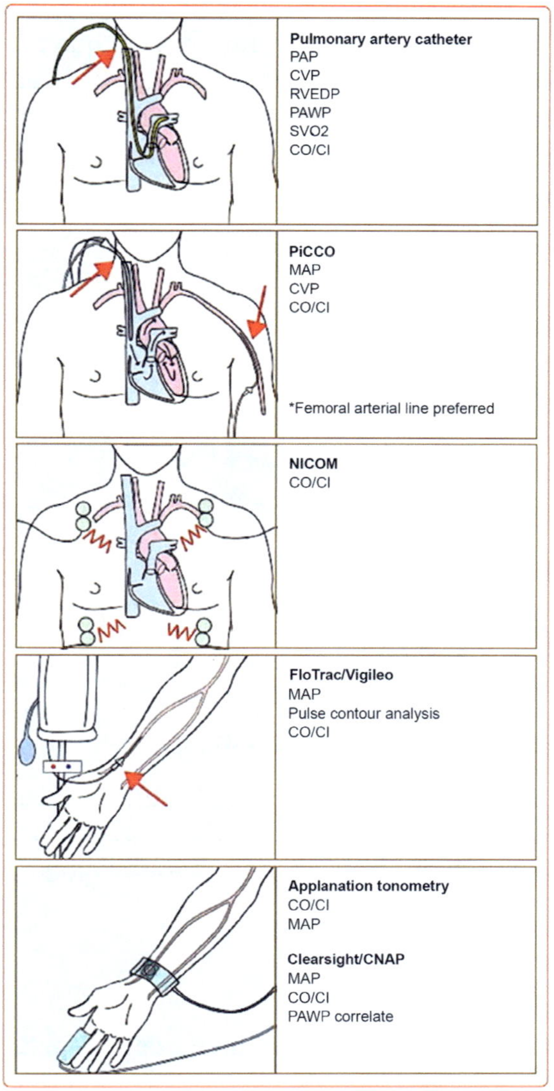

Figure 4.5. Hemodynamic Monitoring Devices and Associated Measured Indices.

Source: https://www.uscjournal.com/articles/contemporary-review-hemodynamic-monitoring-critical-care-setting.

4.2.1. Invasive Monitoring Methods

In hemodynamic monitoring, invasive methods are essential instruments in the measurement of cardiovascular performance in critically ill patients with critical medical illnesses. Certain such interventions, e.g., pulmonary artery catheterization and transpulmonary thermodilution, allow direct measurement of central venous pressure, cardiac output, and pulmonary artery pressures. Such measurements form the basis for guiding therapeutic intervention, particularly in critically ill patients and patients with significant surgery.

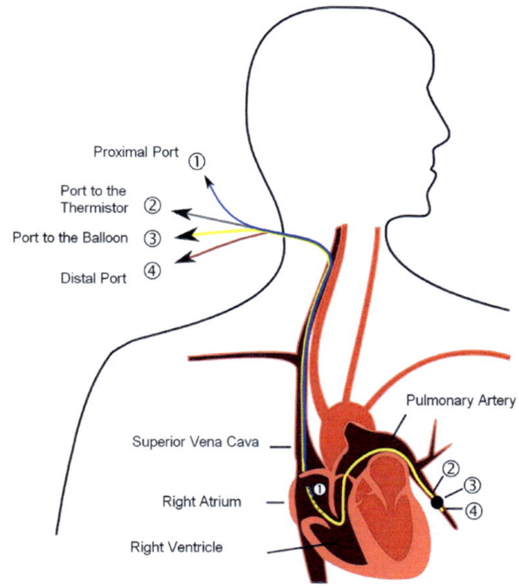

Figure 4.6. Diagram of pulmonary artery catheter.

Source: https://en.wikipedia.org/wiki/Pulmonary_artery_catheter#/media/File:Pulmonary_artery_catheter_english.JPG.

While older monitoring modalities are constrained in dynamic situations, invasive modalities provide real-time, continuous measurement that enables more informed clinical decision-making. This advantage enables practitioners to tailor fluid resuscitation and vasoactive therapy to individual patient needs. Therefore, the application of invasive monitoring methods in hemodynamic management programs can significantly improve patient outcomes, particularly where there is a necessity for quick and accurate determination to be done expediently, as outlined in existing literature (Bosso *et al.*, 2025). Invasive monitoring methods are differentiated from the rest by the fact that they can generate detailed reports regarding a patient's hemodynamic status. For instance, use of the Pulmonary Artery Catheter (PAC) is possible to determine left atrial pressure and to estimate cardiac output by using thermodilution techniques. This is a very valuable way of establishing a number of circulatory states, i.e., cardiogenic shock or hypovolemia, that are hard to attain with non-invasive devices (Figure 4.6).

Furthermore, the ability to monitor parameters like stroke volume and systemic vascular resistance at all times provides a comprehensive view of cardiovascular dynamics. High-tech equipment, including the pulse index contour continuous cardiac output (PiCCO), is invasive and non-invasive in its method of obtaining critical parameters in such a way as to ensure safety and comfort in the patient. Thus, technically more sophisticated and resource- and training-dependent invasive monitoring modalities have benefits which can significantly enhance patient management (Andrei *et al.*, 2024). However, use of invasive monitoring modalities is also related to important challenges and implications. Complication risk in the form of infection, bleeding, or thrombosis necessitates consideration of scrupulous patient selection and surveillance protocols. Furthermore, the cost of disposable equipment and the specialized training personnel needed to implement and interpret the data are significant disincentives to their widespread use. Despite as much as these barriers exist, the accuracy and immediate feedback provided by the invasive methods often justify the cost within the critical care environment. Technology advances and research ensue with decreasing complications, further simplifying the invasive methods. Also, as practitioners become more expert at applying invasive monitoring systems, the likelihood of more positive patient outcomes due to tailored therapy increases with each passing day, highlighting the benefit of adding such techniques into existing hemodynamic management regimens (Bosso *et al.*, 2025) (Figure 4.7).

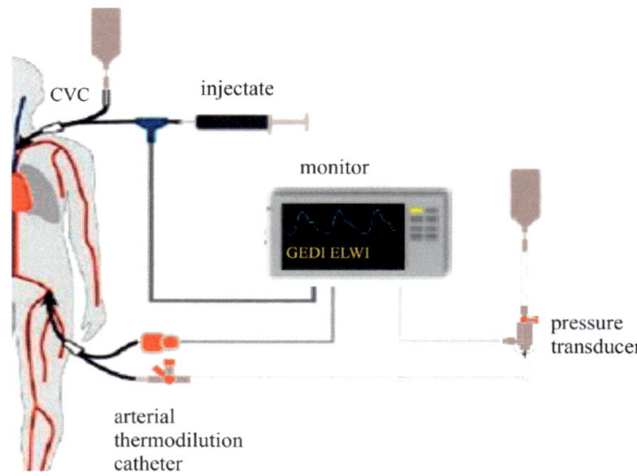

Figure 4.7. PiCCO technique.

Source: https://www.mdpi.com/medicina/medicina-60-01884/article_deploy/html/images/medicina-60-01884-g002-550.jpg.

4.2.2. Non-Invasive Monitoring Methods

Non-invasive monitoring methods are part of hemodynamic management as they guarantee that actual physiological information is received without the dangers associated with invasive techniques. They employ technologies such as bioimpedance, Doppler ultrasonography, and sphygmomanometry advancements to estimate parameters such as cardiac output, stroke volume, and blood pressure. With these modalities, the clinician is capable of ascertaining information about a patient's hemodynamic status without the threat of complications from traditional invasive monitoring. For instance, the reliability of non-invasive technologies makes them a safe option for use on a continuous basis to monitor in dynamic clinical situations, e.g., during surgery or in critically ill individuals. The ongoing development and innovation of such technologies render them a vital component of modern practice since they offer clinicians the tools required to make informed decisions in patient care and bring an added dimension of safety measures in high-risk environments. The introduction of non-invasive monitoring methods into modern clinical practice yet again solidifies their potential to diagnose and treat disorders such as circulatory shock. Evidence shows that such approaches are a pound of gold in fluid responsiveness assessment, a crucial element of prescriptive therapeutic intervention. of perhaps even greater significance, though, is the ability of non-invasive approaches to track preload status and guide fluid therapy, thus precluding over-reliance on empirical formulae that fail to accurately represent an individual patient's specific situation. The implications are as far-reaching as to allow clinicians to individualize fluid therapy with dynamic data, which can potentially maximize patient outcomes during high-risk surgery. Recent consensus statements suggest that the incorporation of dynamic non-invasive monitoring technologies has the potential to increase awareness and understanding of a patient's hemodynamic status, leading finally to enhanced clinical decision-making in the intensive care unit (Babaev *et al.*, 2014). Practical application of non-invasive monitoring methods has also been described in intraoperative fluid infusion, where precision and sensitivity are most critically vital. The move towards dynamic monitoring is a shift in paradigms paradigm in fluid management, because new non-invasive equipment is able to assess hemodynamic alterations quickly and precisely. The innovation is put into perspective by case studies that show effective results with the use of non-invasive techniques, disseminating a wide benefit over traditional invasive techniques, especially for risky surgery (Gutierrez *et al.*, 2013). Also, combined with the evolving healthcare landscape, cost-effectiveness and patient-friendliness of non-invasive monitoring render it increasingly popular in various clinical settings. Responding, safe, and effective monitoring delivery has helped to supplement improved patient outcomes and safety, increasing the value and credibility of such approaches in contemporary hemodynamic care (Figure 4.8).

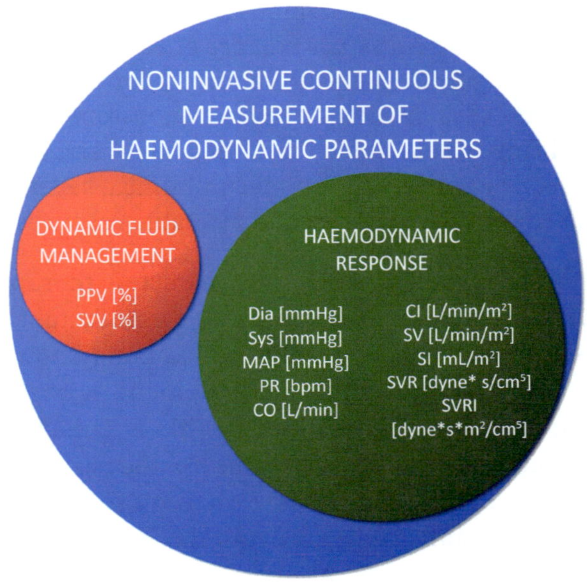

Figure 4.8. Haemodynamic parameters measured with non-invasive methods and their units.

Source: https://www.mdpi.com/jcm/jcm-10-04929/article_deploy/html/images/jcm-10-04929-g002-550.jpg.

4.2.3. Comparison of Monitoring Techniques

In hemodynamic monitoring, a variety of methods have been employed, each with advantages and disadvantages. Invasive methods, such as pulmonary artery catheterization, allow for careful assessment of cardiac output and proper heart function. They provide instant feedback that is indispensable in the management of critically ill patients with complicated cardiovascular diseases. They are, nevertheless, linked with possible complications like infection and thrombosis, which undermine patient safety. On the other hand, non-invasive techniques such as echocardiography and bioimpedance monitoring provide safer options at a lower expense without sacrificing valuable hemodynamic information. While less precise than invasive measures, technology has brought them to be as precise and dependable as necessary in the hemodynamic critical care environment. An astute balance of each's reward and danger is thereby required for optimal patient care in hemodynamic monitoring. In addition, the choice of monitoring strategy must be appropriate for specific clinical settings based on patient status and available resources.

For instance, early goal-directed therapy with a focus on expedited hemodynamic assessment and intervention has been shown to result in substantial improvement in septic patients (Evans *et al.*, 2021). This is guideline recommended by interventions like the Surviving Sepsis Campaign, which encourages rapid identification of hemodynamic abnormality to direct therapy appropriately (Evans *et al.*, 2021). In such instances, the use of non-invasive monitoring, like that with ultrasound or continuous blood pressure monitoring always has the advantage of instant regulation without exposing patients to risks associated with invasive monitoring. Moreover, as more focus by healthcare organizations is placed on the safety of the patient and cost containment, use of advanced monitoring technologies offers a possible route towards successful hemodynamic management. Finally, the optimal strategy would be a combined synergistic inclusion of strategies in coping with evolving critically ill patients' needs. Finally, integration of the monitoring techniques within an integrated management strategy remains the mainstay for maximizing overall patient outcomes. Continuing education in the latest hemodynamic monitoring modalities and proper use in clinical practice remains a need.

Multidisciplinary protocols that include invasive and non-invasive monitoring strategies have been found to enhance compliance with clinical practice guidelines and patient outcomes (Evans *et al.*, 2021). In addition, as the practice of medicine has become increasingly personalized in the care of patients, the ability to interpret and integrate information from multiple modes of monitoring is increasingly critical. By promoting cooperation among healthcare teams and adopting advances in monitoring technology, clinicians can achieve a more accurate hemodynamic status and directly influence therapy with bearing upon ultimate patient recovery in intensive care units.

Test Your Knowledge

1. What are common invasive methods used for hemodynamic monitoring?
2. Which non-invasive techniques are frequently used to assess patient status?

4.3. Indications for Hemodynamic Monitoring

Learning Outcome

1. Discuss the critical care scenarios
2. Define surgical settings
3. Explain the management of chronic conditions

The indications for hemodynamic monitoring have expanded significantly with the nature of growing patient complexity in various clinical settings. Hemodynamic monitoring is significant in the treatment of patients who come in with shock, heart failure, and sepsis, in which precise measurement of cardiovascular parameters is paramount in shaping treatment maneuvers. For instance, patients with acute myocardial infarction should be closely monitored so their cardiac function can be assessed and hemodynamic compromise appreciated early. Proper hemodynamic assessment will trigger timely intervention that can enhance outcomes in patients, reduce complications, and shorten hospital stays. Besides this, risky patients such as patients undergoing high-risk procedures, i.e., cardiac and major vascular surgery, also need close hemodynamic monitoring to observe intra- and post-operatively occurring changes. Another important application of hemodynamic monitoring is observed in the treatment of critically ill patients who are admitted to intensive care units (ICUs). These patients typically present with multi-organ impairment with deranged normal physiological compensation, for which sensitive monitoring techniques are required. In particular, CVP monitoring can provide valuable information regarding a patient's intravascular volume and right ventricular function and guide fluid resuscitation and pharmacologic maneuvers. In addition, having an arterial line in place allows for continuous monitoring of blood pressure and frequent blood withdrawal, enhancing the ability of the clinicians to make immediate adjustments to the treatment regimen. Again highlighted in the recent investigation, a lack of monitoring has adverse consequences, reiterated the importance of hemodynamic watchfulness in such highly lucrative environments (Choi *et al.*, 2021). The inclusion of hemodynamic information in the clinical bedside assessment is an easy step toward maximizing patient care during these critical periods. Lastly, hemodynamic monitoring is the challenge of developing individualized therapeutic plans for chronic disease patients, such as pulmonary hypertension or end-stage heart failure, that can adapt over time with progressive hemodynamics. Values trends such as cardiac output and pulmonary artery pressure are not only helpful for acute management but also for the individualization of longer-term treatment regimens. This makes personalized medicine possible, where physicians can make use of advanced therapies such as circulatory support or inotrope infusion, where necessary. In addition, the presence of newer technology, including non-invasive hemodynamic monitoring devices, makes it more convenient and accessible to detect early hemodynamic changes on an outpatient basis. Therefore, knowledge of the hemodynamic monitoring markers is necessary in order to enhance the patient outcome of those receiving medical or surgical therapy, especially those who are considered to be high-risk categories (Scanavacca *et al.*, 2016).

4.3.1. Critical Care Scenarios

In intensive care areas, effective hemodynamic monitoring is paramount for diagnosing and managing patients' acute illness. The ICUs are the initial centers where high-interventional procedures are performed, particularly for those having severe cardiovascular disease. Admission protocols of cardiovascular intensive care units (CICUs) are different, and therefore, there is a need for regulatory standards to direct the improvement of patient outcomes. According to a multicenter trial, admission behavior and application of scarce critical care therapies

(CCRx) differ significantly between institutions, impacting the worldwide critical care of critically ill patients. Surprisingly, patients with higher CCRx presented higher rates of comorbid conditions and adverse outcomes, which proved the need for tailored hemodynamic monitoring practices consistent with patient acuity and institutional capacity (Donnelly *et al.*, 2024). Volume management is a foundation of critical care hemodynamic monitoring. Fluid overload, a ubiquitous process in heart failure and critical illness, is risky and complex in multiple organ systems. The clinician's dilemma is accurate volume status determination since traditional methods fall short of their potential. Current best practice at the cutting edge is advocating a multiparameter approach that integrates various diagnostic modalities—such as clinical assessment, biomarkers, and point-of-care ultrasonography—to assess fluid balance in patients more precisely . With the holistic assessment, clinicians can create an evidence-based method of therapy that achieves adequate tissue perfusion to prevent tissue hypoxia without increasing the risk of fluid overload, morbidity, and mortality (Koratala *et al.*, 2022). Optimization of fluid therapy, in turn, remains an anchor of hemodynamic management in such high-risk settings. Stratification of patients in critical illness scenarios based on their hemodynamic status also has important implications for treatment and outcome. The onset of states like shock mandates urgent assessment of hemodynamics to direct therapeutic intervention. Fluid resuscitation, vasopressors, and mechanical circulatory support may be needed to resuscitate the patient. The comprehension of how these interventions talk across to each other and affect organ system perfusion is of crucial significance to CICU clinicians managing complex patients. More CCRx use patients admitted to CICUs have variable mortality, emphasizing the balance of the severity of the patient and institutional influences on affecting clinical practice. Thus, ongoing research and clinical audit become the need of the hour to maximize hemodynamic monitoring techniques and verify intervention protocols for the best patient outcomes in severe cases of care (Donnelly *et al.*, 2024) (Figure 4.9).

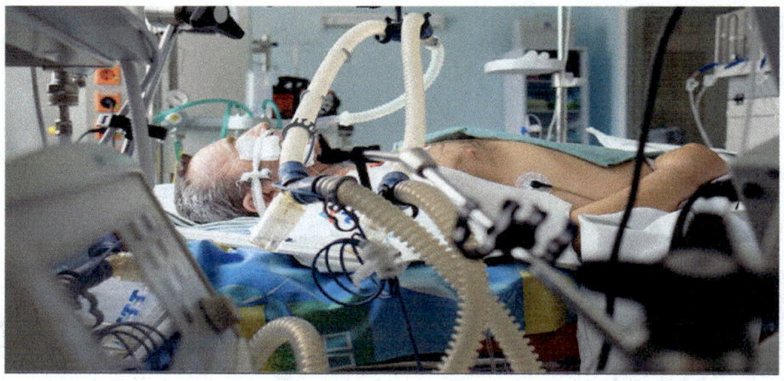

Figure 4.9. Cardiac intensive care units face an ever more complex patient population.

Source: https://d14d5nk8lue86f.cloudfront.net/s3fs-public/2017-04/4.28.17.care_.unit_.header.jpg.

4.3.2. Surgical Settings

Operating rooms are essential rooms where hemodynamic monitoring and management are essential determinants of patient outcomes. The anesthesiologist and surgeon have to coordinate efforts to maintain stable hemodynamics so that complications during procedures can be avoided. Choice of the anesthetic drugs and fluids significantly influences patients' physiological status, making it essential to have continuous vigilance and close observation. Patients with myoclonic epilepsy with ragged red fibers and other multifactorial disorders have emphasized the need for individualized anesthetic care to correct the special susceptibility of neuromuscular function and energy metabolism. Such patients require the application of continuous hemodynamic monitoring and proper fine-tuning of anesthetic management to prevent such complications as respiratory depression and lactic acidosis due to anesthetic intervention (Lee *et al.*, 2024). In addition, the presence of co-morbid psychiatric illness, e.g., self-inflicted stab injuries to the abdomen, complicates attaining hemodynamic stability during surgery. These patients, who also come with schizophrenia or drug abuse, pose special challenges that are more than just one mode of treatment. The surgeons have to deal with not only the physical trauma but also psychological management, which has a significant influence on the hemodynamic parameters. In-depth evaluation and care strategies are seen to be necessary in such a situation, thus the intervention of psychiatric evaluation and postoperative care. This kind of dual model of care is conducive to recovery and avoids possible complications related to hemodynamic instability (Adhikari, 2024) (Figure 4.10).

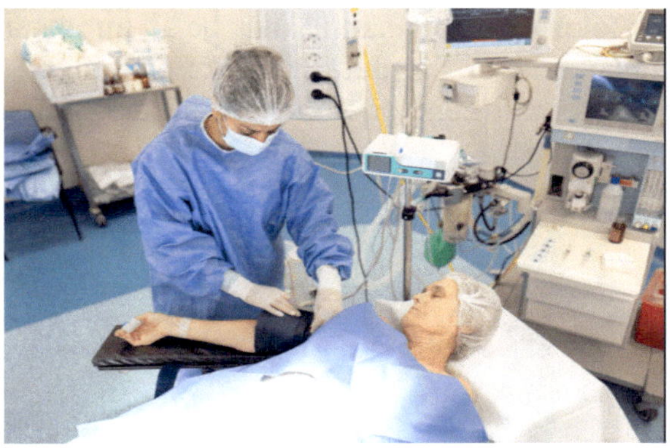

Figure 4.10. Operating room settings.

Source: https://hospitalprocedures.org/wp-content/uploads/2024/03/Hemodynamic-Monitoring.png.

In addition to considering physiological and psychological factors, operating rooms also need to focus on aggressive perioperative monitoring for perfect hemodynamic control. Continuous monitoring of key vital signs, including blood pressure, heart rate, and oxygen saturation, enables the delivery of information critical to timely intervention. Utilization of advanced technologies like invasive arterial blood pressure monitoring supports the precision of hemodynamic measurement, enabling clinicians to detect early departures from expected parameters. Moreover, educational courses for operating personnel on the hemodynamic effects of various anesthetic drugs are valuable. Training for correct utilization of tailored treatment protocols ensures proper utilization, ultimately leading to improved surgical outcomes and safety for the patient (Adhikari, 2024; Lee *et al.*, 2024).

4.3.3. Management of Chronic Conditions

Treatment of chronic illness has increasingly become an essential aspect of healthcare, most notably hemodynamic monitoring. Diabetes, hypertension, and cardiovascular illness are all chronic illnesses that must be intervened and monitored repeatedly, as well as separately. Pharmacologic management is only one aspect of successful management, and lifestyle modification, patient education, and follow-up also play a crucial part. For example, diabetic patients are liable to develop complications that influence their hemodynamic status to a considerable extent and require stringent management of blood glucose as well as blood pressure, and cardiovascular function. Appreciating the interconnection between these factors can enable clinicians to make evidence-based decisions leading to improved outcomes. Each patient comes with a unique set of conditions that dictate the particular management approach, validating the importance of personalized care for chronic disease management, particularly among comorbid patients. The effect of chronic disease on patient vulnerability during medical emergencies, such as the COVID-19 pandemic, has been far-reaching and varied. Research has also proven that patients with severe or comorbid diseases have augmented fears of getting into contact with infectious diseases, and these are also driving forces for vaccine hesitancy. Vaccination acceptance among patients with chronic disease was greatly influenced due to fear concerning the impact of COVID-19 vaccines on disease control among patients with chronic disease in a study of chronic disease patients' acceptance of vaccines. This hesitation is caused by subjective susceptibility to unwanted effects of the disease, and thus it becomes difficult to decide on being vaccinated. Excess information on vaccines can also cause patients to be empowered and influenced accordingly by health-seeking behavior. Hence, intervention of such issues through improved communication and patient-centered care can reduce anxiety and increase adherence to preventive measures, thus improving health outcomes among people with chronic disease (Choi *et al.*, 2023). Apart from psychological management, the use of systematic tools in evaluation can enhance chronic pain management, particularly in musculoskeletal disorders prevalent in patients with chronic diseases. The use of validated instruments to measure pain within primary care allows practitioners to assess pain more effectively and tailor interventions in response. Results from a single randomized controlled trial identified that the introduction of pain assessment had a statistically significant reduction in writing prescriptions for higher-level analgesics, which showed overall improvements in standards of pain management. The results did note, though, that this did not always equate to greater pain relief compared to conventional practice. This raises important questions about the appropriateness of standardized test instruments, suggesting that their use should be determined by context and patient-specific needs. Generally, consideration of the nuances of managing chronic illness, particularly hemodynamic, may be an important determinant of the determinants of quality of life and treatment outcome in patients (Huas *et al.*, 2006).

Test Your Knowledge

1. What are common hemodynamic challenges in critical care scenarios?
2. How is hemodynamic monitoring utilized in surgical settings?

4.4. Interpretation of Hemodynamic Data

Learning Outcome

1. Understanding key parameters
2. Discuss the clinical significance of data interpretation
3. Identify the common pitfalls in data analysis

Hemodynamic reading interpretation is critical in clinical decision-making and management of most medical conditions, particularly surgical and intensive care. Hemodynamic monitoring enables clinicians to measure performance of the cardiovascular system so that they can assess such factors as cardiac output, pressure, and fluid status. Accurate interpretation of the data is necessary because it guides treatment direction, particularly in shock management and fluid resuscitation. Subtleties of interpretation of hemodynamic data can directly influence patient outcomes, as a specific type of shock can be established with proper analysis of hemodynamic parameters. Proper interpretation is not followed, so that inappropriate intervention may occur, and the patient's condition can further deteriorate, making management pathways complex, with special emphasis on gaining a firm understanding of data interpretation procedures in hemodynamic monitoring. New technology has significantly enhanced hemodynamic monitoring equipment on hand, but the problem of proper interpretation of data remains the largest problem. The technology of transcranial Doppler (TCD) has started to evolve in its applications, particularly with the advent of neurointerventional therapy. TCD offers bedside real-time monitoring, not just concerning cardiac function but also cerebral hemodynamics. It is useful as it complements artificial intelligence systems that can process gigantic data sets rapidly and efficiently. For instance, TCD capability for cerebral autoregulation and collateral assessment is important in deciding to evaluate clinical outcomes following interventions such as endovascular thrombectomy. Thus, a proper understanding of these elaborate data is capable of enhancing patient selection based on criteria and effectiveness of interventions in general, and thus, it is an irreplaceable member of the current hemodynamic monitoring bench (Baik, 2024).

Hemodynamic data interpretation management also addresses issues of fluid resuscitation complexity, particularly in shock conditions. Fluid therapy is not only essential in hypovolemic or distributive shock patients but also hampers recovery in patients and results in further complications like organ failure. Its excess or improper use results in further complications. It is hence extremely important to make appropriate hemodynamic measurements to guide fluid management algorithms. Some monitoring techniques provide extremely valuable information about a patient's fluid responsiveness and tolerance, and intensivists use them to refine volume status. But excessive reliance on forceful misinterpretation of data will inadvertently accelerate mortality and morbidity rates. Therefore, forceful training in the hemodynamic data interpretation and understanding its role in fluid management has to be given utmost priority in bedside practice (Kashani *et al.*, 2022) (Figure 4.11).

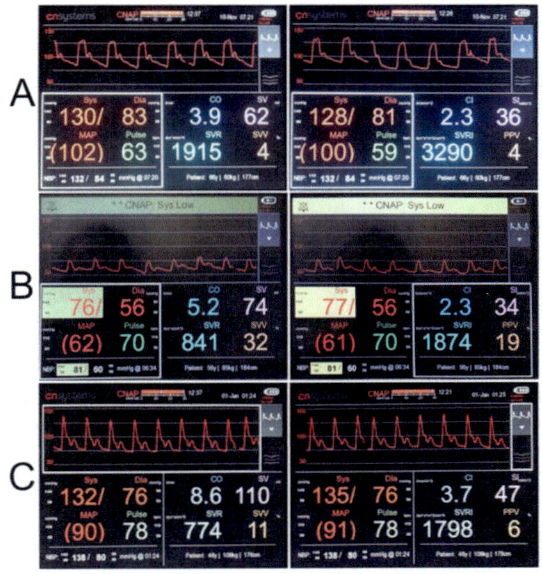

Figure 4.11. Record of measured haemodynamic parameters in patients.

Source: https://www.mdpi.com/jcm/jcm-10-04929/article_deploy/html/images/jcm-10-04929-g003-550.jpg.

4.4.1. Understanding Key Parameters

To manage critically ill patients, information about some of the key parameters is crucial in hemodynamic monitoring. Important parameters like cardiac output, blood pressure, and systemic vascular resistance are indicators of cardiovascular performance and play an important role in decision-making in treatment. Advanced techniques, such as cardiac ultrasound and transpulmonary thermodilution, allow for precise real-time measurement of these parameters by clinicians to allow for individualized clinical management to optimize patient benefit. Their adoption is not just sporty accuracy; they allow clinicians to make many diagnoses of forms of shock and other terminal complications so that therapeutic maneuvers can be appropriately instituted. Since the consensus guidelines outline, these methods are groundbreaking in translating intricate hemodynamic information to meaningful leads to direct care in critically ill patients (Andrei *et al.*, 2024). To better appreciate the vital role monitoring plays in hemodynamic therapy, one should recall that advancing technologies offer uninterrupted monitoring. Wearable device technology, or the flexible adaptive sensing tonometry (FAST) system, has been one of the most important breakthroughs in hemodynamic assessment capability. The novel device functions by using flexible iontronic sensing to facilitate a complete understanding of important parameters like blood pressure and heart rate in real-time. This technology not only makes the measurement process easier but also offers prompt medical intervention, thus decreasing the cardiovascular event risks. In this regard, real-time hemodynamic monitoring can be a potential area for anticipatory care management and patient safety, considering how accurate FAST is in ensuring medical-grade level precision for all parameters (Deng *et al.*, 2024). Moreover, hemodynamic parameter evaluation extends far beyond data acquisition in the raw sense; instead, it involves interpretation of such measurements within a clinical setting to optimize patient outcomes. For instance, understanding of the interplay between systemic vascular resistance and cardiac output is paramount to the determination of states of shock and management of attempts at fluid resuscitation. Explanation of such hemodynamic parameters by proper knowledge is evidence for decision-making of the administration of vasoactive agents to finally stabilize critically ill patients. In addition, other advanced analytic methods and parameters at the patient level need to be considered during this evaluation process in order to facilitate an integrative treatment for a patient's hemodynamic profile. As illustrated in recent research, syncretism between conventional practice and the latest technology can effectively complement clinical decision-making, which will support improved intensive care management practices (Andrei *et al.*, 2024; Deng *et al.*, 2024).

4.4.2. Clinical Significance of Data Interpretation

Under hemodynamic monitoring, clinical relevance in interpreting information cannot be overstressed. Appropriate interpretation of values for hemodynamic monitors such as cardiac output and peripheral resistance is a crucial determinant of critical care patient management. With the advent of non-invasive monitor instruments such as the NICaS monitor, critical hemodynamic information to direct clinical decision making has been streamlined. For instance, decreased cardiac output and increased total peripheral resistance have been linked to increased in-hospital mortality among patients with COVID-19, highlighting the importance of early treatment based on such justifications. Clinicians with proven evidence can better adjust fluid resuscitation and pharmacologic interventions, ultimately leading to improved outcomes for patients in intensive care settings. Accuracy in hemodynamic data interpretation thereby rises directly with clinical practice patterns and patient safety. In addition, medical staff education and training define the effect of data interpretation in hemodynamic monitoring to a great extent. Recent studies show that many nurses operating advanced hemodynamic monitoring machinery are still ill-educated regarding their use, and that this may lead to inappropriate interpretation of severe warning signs. This information deficiency can cause inefficient or late hemodynamic status adaptation to patients, eventually compromising patient safety. As an example, it has been established that improvements in hemodynamic monitoring care accuracy have been realized with a significant improvement in staff competence. With the incorporation of education, training, and access to operation manuals, nurses experienced a significant improvement in hemodynamic monitoring accuracy. These interventions led to the immediate reporting to physicians in instances where there were abnormalities, thereby enabling clinical intervention and indicating the necessity of ongoing training in clinical practice (Huang *et al.*, 2024). Finally, the extent of implications of accurate data interpretation goes beyond immediate clinical decisions to include overall general health care outcomes as well. Proper hemodynamic monitoring and interpretation can potentially lead to more efficient use of resources in intensive care units. For instance, identification of trends among hemodynamic variables enables preventive use of management strategies that are aimed at decreasing the need for invasive therapy, keeping patient risk in check, and decreasing the cost of treatment. Furthermore, as highlighted in previous studies, the correlation between hemodynamic monitoring data and patient outcomes is evidence of optimizing treatment protocols in healthcare systems. The NICaS device, for example, through its non-invasive hemodynamic status estimation, offers real-time monitoring with the potential to guide fluid management and optimize overall care (Zabeeda *et al.*, 2024). Thus, a thoughtful use of hemodynamic monitoring data can significantly enhance patient care and hospital productivity in intensive care.

4.4.3. Common Pitfalls in Data Analysis

Data analysis is among the chief instruments in the art of hemodynamic management and monitoring by which valuable information is extracted from patient information. While analyses are most frequently derailed by typical problems, fewer now than ever before. One of the most frequent mistakes made is the failure to incorporate data quality, which can generate spurious conclusions and result in clinical errors. Lack of source verification not only confirms the authenticity of results but also their applicability in real clinical scenarios. For example, without strict controls, differences in the collection methods will skew results in volatile environments such as intensive care units. This points to the critical role of healthcare professionals, through stringent data governance processes, to ensure that decision-making information accurately reflects patient condition and treatment response. The second trap, namely the major one, is the abuse or misuse of statistical methods employed in data analysis to the detriment of inference drawn from hemodynamic studies. Statistical tests can be misused inadvertently by analysts due to ignorance or a lack of sensitivity towards assumptions of such methods. They can result in misleading conclusions, such as reporting spurious correlation or differences when there are none. With newer technology, the use of sophisticated analytical techniques requires technical expertise and tactical wisdom. Doctors must possess complete control over statistical thinking so that they can manage these complexities successfully. By spending on training healthcare staff, organizations can enhance the validity and relevance of data analysis, thereby facilitating patient management strategies and outcomes. Lastly, failure to notice the importance of longitudinal observation and iterative analysis can thwart the potential of hemodynamic data analysis. Health practitioners will tend to evaluate data in isolation without any thought of real-time observation and longitudinal monitoring. This myopia diminishes the scope for the acquisition of trends and changes in patient status, critical to evoke adequate interventions on time. As emphasized in certain studies, with emphasis on effective cloud cost management methods in startup environments, multi-dimensional approaches yield stronger outcomes (Khan, 2024). Similarly, embracing continuous feedback loops in hemodynamic monitoring can offer sophisticated data and enhance decision-making strategies. By actively avoiding such data analysis errors, medical practitioners can optimize hemodynamic management guidelines and achieve improved outcomes in the care of patients (Herrera *et al.*, 2022).

Test Your Knowledge

1. Why is accurate interpretation of clinical data essential for patient management?
2. What are common pitfalls to avoid when analyzing patient monitoring data?

4.5. Hemodynamic Management Strategies

Learning Outcome

1. Define pharmacological interventions
2. Understand the fluid management techniques
3. Discuss the use of advanced technologies in hemodynamic monitoring

Proper hemodynamic management strategies are essential to maximize patient outcomes, particularly in surgical and critical care settings. Continuous hemodynamic parameter monitoring, such as blood pressure, heart rate, cardiac output, and central venous pressure, is an essential strategy. Through the application of sophisticated technologies such as arterial catheters and non-invasive monitoring devices, practitioners can derive real-time data regarding a patient's hemodynamic status. This ongoing assessment permits early interventions to prevent complications like hypotension and shock, hence ensuring hemodynamic stability. When examples like severe pulmonary hypertension present, careful planning and vigilant monitoring are highlighted, as in the case of an 86-year-old patient with emergent orthopedic surgery. This case demonstrated the tight inter-professional teamwork between the surgical and anesthesiology team and careful fluid management go a long way in achieving a good outcome when managing challenging hemodynamic problems (Khan *et al.*, 2024). Incorporating pharmacologic strategies along with close monitoring significantly enhances hemodynamic management. Inotropes and vasopressors are frequently utilized to enhance the cardiac output and maintain adequate blood pressure in critically ill patients. In addition, magnesium sulfate infusion has also proven to be a potential agent for reversal of hemodynamic instability during procedures such as laryngoscopy and tracheal intubation. Its vasodilating and antiarrhythmic effects make it a perfect way of stabilizing patients during perioperative care, particularly in post-ENT surgeries, where hemodynamic changes are the norm. Critical literature review of magnesium sulfate reveals potential benefits and safety issues, prompting clinicians to consider criteria for patient selection and optimal dosing regimen best practices (Sawant *et al.*, 2024). The upcoming evidence favors the need to personalize therapy according to a patient's specific hemodynamic needs. Multidisciplinary coordination takes precedence to effectively implement hemodynamic management regimens. This comprehensive management ensures multi-aspect care that encompasses preoperative optimization, intraoperative monitoring, and postoperative recovery. Optimal communication among surgical, anesthetic, and nursing teams facilitates immediate adjustment of management algorithms based on real-time hemodynamic data. The synergy among pharmacologic and non-pharmacologic therapies offers a holistic model to address the complexity of hemodynamic instability. For instance, approaches may include cautious fluid resuscitation optimized with diuretics for overload management with specific surgical requirements in mind. The overall concept is to remain focused on preserving maximal hemodynamic stability along the patient's care continuum and thereby reducing risk for complications as well as improving perioperative results overall. This synergistic set of guidelines underscores the dynamic nature of hemodynamic monitoring and management in today's clinical settings (Figure 4.12).

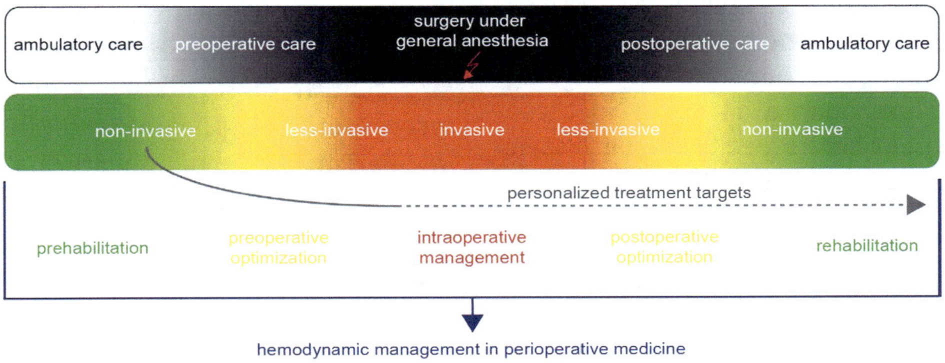

Figure 4.12. Non-invasive hemodynamic monitoring for hemodynamic management in perioperative medicine.

Source: https://www.researchgate.net/publication/321247448/figure/fig1/AS:11431281153661216@1682521505225/Non-invasive-hemodynamic-monitoring-for-hemodynamic-management-in-perioperative-medicine.tif.

4.5.1. Pharmacological Interventions

Pharmacological therapy is an essential component of hemodynamic instability management, especially in the case of ARDS patients. In these clinical situations, vasopressor and inotrope administration ensures sustained perfusion pressure and cardiac output. Norepinephrine and dobutamine are drugs that are frequently used to respond to decreased systemic vascular resistance and enhanced myocardial contractility. Research has established that application of these agents, along with modern hemodynamic monitoring, can calibrate hemodynamic measurements and ultimately enhance patient outcomes. Standardized protocols to include appropriate pharmacologic intervention and total monitoring significantly enhance the quality of care provided to critically ill patients (Gupta *et al.*, 2025). It is an integrative approach that is needed to address the polyfactorial contribution of factors to hemodynamic instability. Further, the efficacy of various pharmacologic agents must be retested over and over in practice to ensure that they are being used at their optimal capacity. Personalized medicine is the focus of ongoing research, where protocols for treatment are optimized according to patient response, comorbidity, and prior pharmacological history. For instance, use of newer medications, including GLP-1 receptor agonists and SGLT2 inhibitors, has been found to offer pronounced benefits in managing cardiovascular and renal outcomes while concurrently offering glycemic control in diabetic patients (Upadhye *et al.*, 2025). The gains speak volumes about the significance of pharmacologic interventions that, besides stabilizing hemodynamics, treat pathophysiologic processes, hence offering a more integrated response to patient management. Continuing education and research on pharmacologic effects will optimize the efficacy of these interventions in hemodynamic monitoring. Clinical practice, considering the evolving pharmacological intervention dynamics, will need to be kept abreast and incorporate new information that influences treatment modalities. The creation of combination drugs like dual GLP-1/GIP receptor agonists is proof of the promising potential of new pharmacologic strategies to achieve maximal glycemic and hemodynamic control (Upadhye *et al.*, 2025). Furthermore, ongoing investigations into long-term safety in these newer medications are needed to establish their role in prolonged clinical use.

These considerations highlight the need for health care providers to remain current with new evidence regarding pharmacologic management. Consequently, the integration of the newest hemodynamic monitoring with personalized pharmacologic regimens will eventually lead to improved clinical outcomes, reducing cardiovascular and metabolic disorder-related complications among critically ill patients (Gupta *et al.*, 2025).

4.5.2. Fluid Management Techniques

Successful fluid management is crucial in the environment of hemodynamic monitoring and management, particularly with complex procedures such as radical cystectomy with ileal conduit diversion. In patients with comorbidities such as hypertension and renal insufficiency, dehydration has to be handled with utmost care to maintain hemodynamic stability. As an example, invasive monitoring through modalities such as CVP monitoring enables clinicians to make informed decisions regarding fluid resuscitation. With continuous hemodynamic parameter monitoring, clinicians can fine-tune cardiovascular performance and sustain renal perfusion in a way that minimizes the risks of postoperative processes. Such holistic care requires fluid management plans suited to patient-specific factors and monitoring to facilitate the best outcomes in high-risk operative patients (Gohad *et al.*, 2025).

Moreover, recent advances in fluid management techniques, particularly in organ transplantation, accentuate the need for multi-directional homeostatic management. Evidence has shown that the use of machine perfusion and greater intraoperative monitoring are central to regulating fluid balance and preventing complications of fluid overload or deficit. Regional anesthesia techniques, alongside judicious fluid administration, aid in postoperative pain relief without precipitating hemodynamic instability.

As identified in recent literature, understanding of cardiovascular risk assessment is central in this context, allowing clinicians to personalize fluid therapy that precludes adverse effects on the heart and kidneys. This statistical backing bolsters the argument that understanding fluid dynamics in hemodynamic management can significantly enhance patient outcomes (Katayama *et al.*, 2025). Integration of advanced fluid management techniques into the art of hemodynamic monitoring has become increasingly sophisticated, bearing witness to enhanced understanding of surgical patient care.

Clinicians must remain vigilant not only during surgery but also during the postoperative recovery process in order to successfully monitor fluid status. Early mobilization, anti-complication prevention, and multimodal analgesia application are further priorities that reinforce the strategy for hemodynamic management. This holistic strategy recognizes that fluid management is not simply the issue of ensuring adequate circulatory volume, but also in maximizing global patient well-being. Achieving effective surgical outcomes involves the fluid management regimens always being evaluated in conjunction with real-time monitoring and a global view of each patient's unique physiological states (Gohad *et al.*, 2025; Katayama *et al.*, 2025) (Figure 4.13).

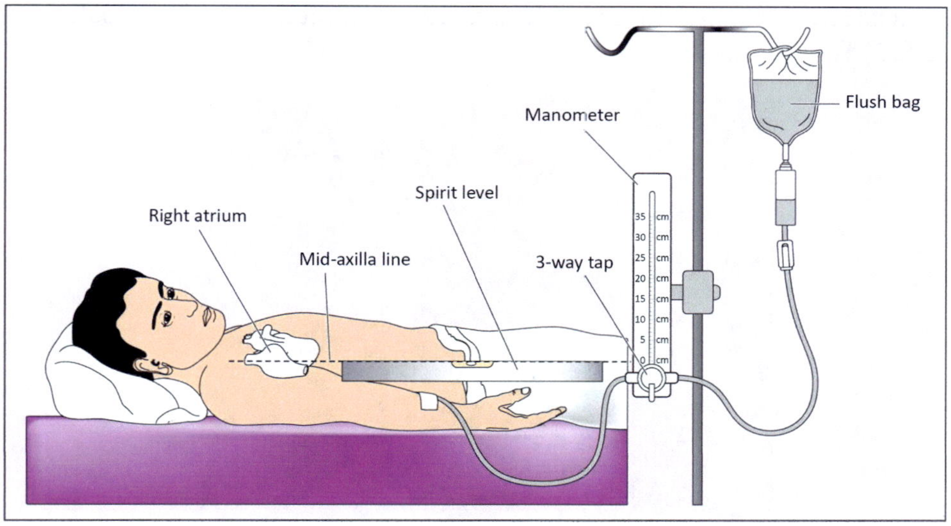

Figure 4.13. Central venous pressure (CVP).

Source: https://activelifemed.com/wp-content/uploads/2024/07/Central-Venous-Pressure-CVP-Line.jpg.

4.5.3. Use of Advanced Technologies

Blending state-of-the-art technologies in hemodynamic monitoring is revolutionizing patient management and outcomes, particularly in critical care settings. The traditional methods, although simple, are limited by their invasive nature and potentially misleading information, particularly in very dynamic situations, like trauma. Recent innovations consist of non-invasive arterial pressure monitoring and impedance cardiography, which significantly enhance real-time cardiovascular assessment. In addition to reducing the risks of invasive interventions, these technologies promote more accurate and unbroken monitoring of data. Current evidence suggests that these devices have been very promising in refining perioperative management guidelines, ultimately translating to better patient outcomes and fewer complications for polytraumatized patients placed under anesthesia (Bosso *et al.*, 2025). Besides, the utilization of advanced hemodynamic monitoring techniques plays an important role in goal-directed therapy to maximize fluid management and enhance patient stability with interventions. Dynamic parameters such as stroke volume variation and pulse pressure variation serve with greater predictive value to assess fluid responsiveness compared with static variables, thus permitting timely decisions by the clinician. The potential to tailor fluid resuscitation protocols with real-time feedback ensures personalized care, critical in high-risk environments. With healthcare moving towards precision medicine, such technologies are fast becoming standards of best practice in hemodynamic care (Bosso *et al.*, 2025). Despite perceived gains provided by such technologies, numerous stumbling blocks must be addressed for their widespread deployment. Financial constraints and the high cost of advanced monitoring systems can limit availability, particularly in resource-deprived environments. Additionally, introducing such technologies into common clinical use requires huge training efforts and expertise on the part of clinicians. Bridging these challenges with systematic training programs and clearer cost-benefit analyses is critical to enabling more general clinical use. Future research should aim to advance these monitoring technologies, render them more precise, and enhance their utility for application in other healthcare environments in order to provide maximum benefit to patient management (Bosso *et al.*, 2025) (Figure 4.14).

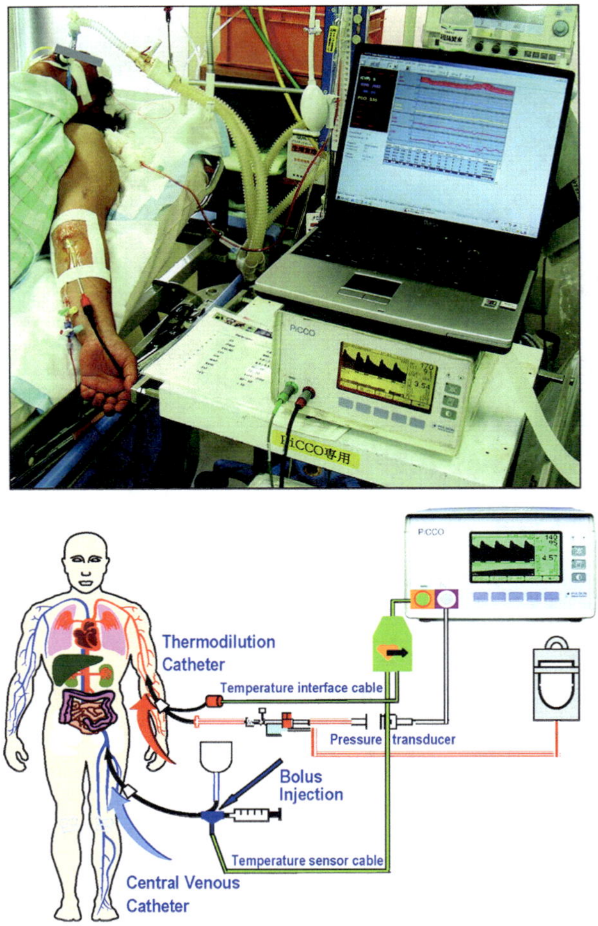

Figure 4.14. Single-indicator transpulmonary thermodilution system. Schematic illustration of the transpulmonary thermodilution system (PiCCO) was modified with permission from Pulsion medical systems.

Source: https://www.ahajournals.org/doi/10.1161/strokeaha.107.484634.

Test Your Knowledge

1. What techniques are used to manage fluids in critically ill patients?
2. How are advanced technologies utilized in modern hemodynamic management?

4.6. Challenges in Hemodynamic Monitoring

Learning Outcome

1. Explain the limitations of current monitoring techniques.
2. Discuss the patient variability and its impact.
3. Define ethical considerations in monitoring.

The intricacies of hemodynamic monitoring have numerous challenges that can impact patient outcomes significantly, especially in the critically ill patient. Early and precise assessment of hemodynamic status is essential for effective management, especially in critically ill patients with hemodynamic disorders such as cardiogenic shock and sepsis. Hemodynamic instability tends to necessitate invasive monitoring techniques, and these have associated risks like infection and vascular-related complications. Moreover, their findings can be misled by variability amongst individual patients, inherent comorbidities, and the co-existence of multiple organ dysfunction syndromes. Physicians need to make the dismal job of distinguishing between physiological and pathophysiological responses, and a good understanding of complex monitoring systems and their limitations is therefore necessary. This makes it crucial that there is continuous education and training for healthcare providers to maximize their skills in hemodynamic interpretation and management methods, which finally translates to enhanced patient care in critical areas. Another big challenge when monitoring hemodynamics is the integration and standardization of all modalities of monitoring. The physicians utilize a blend of invasive and non-invasive techniques to gain information about a patient's circulatory status. However, discrepancies between information obtained through various modalities may lead to confusion and potential mismanagement. For instance, while pulmonary artery catheters provide reliable readings of pulmonary pressure and cardiac output, they may be associated with high complications, discouraging their use. Alternatively, non-invasive methods such as echocardiography or impedance cardiography might be less accurate but carry lower risks. The challenge, therefore, is to develop an interdisciplinary strategy that synthesizes the information from these disparate methods, enhancing clinical decision-making without compromising safety for the patient. Emphasis on the principles of evidence-based practice can guarantee this synthesis, enabling a more integrative approach to hemodynamic stability in critically ill patients. In addition, the evolving landscape of technology in hemodynamic monitoring poses opportunities and challenges. The technological innovation in continuous monitoring devices and analytics has the potential to enhance patient assessment significantly but will also pose an issue of data overload and interpretation. Clinicians will find it difficult to cull relevant information from the sheer volume of data generated and, consequently, experience decision fatigue or delayed intervention. As highlighted in the clinical setting, particularly in sepsis management, prompt intervention will be essential to minimizing morbidity and mortality rates. Therefore, it is important to develop effective monitoring systems with an emphasis on important data, as well as training modules that can equip healthcare professionals with the ability to comprehend and utilize real-time data. Through these challenges, the medical fraternity can improve the management of hemodynamic instability and ensure improved outcomes for critically ill patients, as evidenced by recent clinical protocols and guidelines within this field (Blumer *et al.*, 2025; Sirohi *et al.*, 2025).

4.6.1. Limitations of Current Monitoring Techniques

Limitations of available hemodynamic monitoring techniques have a profound impact on patient management in intensive care settings. Traditional methods, while providing essential measurements like cardiac output and blood pressure, typically do not accommodate the complex physiological alterations of critically ill patients. For instance, traditional invasive techniques like central venous pressure monitoring may not accurately reflect actual hemodynamic status due to factors like intrathoracic pressure fluctuation and body position. Additionally, single-point measurement can lead to incorrect diagnosis of a patient's cardiovascular condition, particularly in dynamic or unstable conditions. More complex techniques, such as transpulmonary thermodilution, give more comprehensive data but are not universally available and add extra risks, limiting their utility in the majority of healthcare centers (Andrei *et al.*, 2024). Hence, it is necessary to critically review the current monitoring tools for their enhancement in terms of reliability and for enabling enhanced patient outcomes. The introduction of newer technologies such as cardiac ultrasound and noninvasive continuous blood pressure monitoring reflects an added sophistication on the limitations of current hemodynamic monitoring techniques. While these technologies offer more accurate and contemporaneous information, they remain beset with concerns of operator dependency and training requirements. Cardiac ultrasound, for instance, needs a skilled operator, and therefore, the quality of assessment could be greatly impacted by the practitioner's experience. Further, the habitus of the body might impact ultrasound measurement accuracy. Similarly, monitoring equipment continuously may be susceptible to noise and motion artifacts, leading to invalid information (Andrei *et al.*, 2024). Hence, despite advancement, these factors constrain the total effectiveness of modern monitoring techniques, invoking reconsideration of their use in clinical practice. Lastly, even new measures like transdermal glucose monitoring sensors illustrate ongoing challenges to continuous and accurate hemodynamic assessment. Whereas these biosensors provide hope for minimally invasive techniques for real-time monitoring, they also have their constraints. Issues of calibration, sensitivity, and physiological response restrict the utility of such devices in a dynamic environment. Furthermore, skin irritation and constant sensor replacement might exclude patient compliance and hence the utility of the resulting data. This highlights an essential limitation: while technology might exist for the reporting of continuous data, practical constraints often diminish its utility in high-stakes applications, affirming the need for ongoing research and development to enhance the accuracy and reliability of such monitoring systems in hemodynamic care.

4.6.2. Patient Variability and Its Impact

Patient heterogeneity is a major issue in hemodynamic monitoring and treatment since variability among patients can have a powerful effect on the interpretation of data as well as on subsequent clinical actions. Age, comorbidities, and genetics cause variability in BP and heart rate responses across patients. For instance, patients with stroke exhibit variable post-stroke blood pressure variability (BPV) on a wide range, as has been determined in studies that explore the relationship between sampling rate and BP pattern. Such heterogeneity necessitates patient-specific monitoring approaches, and hence the necessity of individual patient profiling to provide maximum effectiveness of treatment and better health outcomes. Personalized approaches in hemodynamic management are expected to result in improved complication prediction and comprehensive care pathways. Furthermore, the application of remote patient monitoring (RPM) technology has played a critical role in the management of patient heterogeneity. RPM enables continuous data accumulation for improving the estimation of hemodynamic parameters with time. This is particularly important for the case of chronic conditions, where abrupt changes in a patient's state can lead to serious adverse events. A clinical example of a patient with heart failure showed RPM's power in detecting and reacting to health state variability. While RPM initially did not result in alerts, remote viewing of the patient's baseline parameters through the clinical telehealth nurse interface achieved huge reductions in management, excluding costly interventions. Therefore, not only can RPM account for individual heterogeneity but also improves the timeliness of clinical interventions. Patient heterogeneity also identifies the need for ongoing research in the optimal design and operation of hemodynamic monitoring equipment.

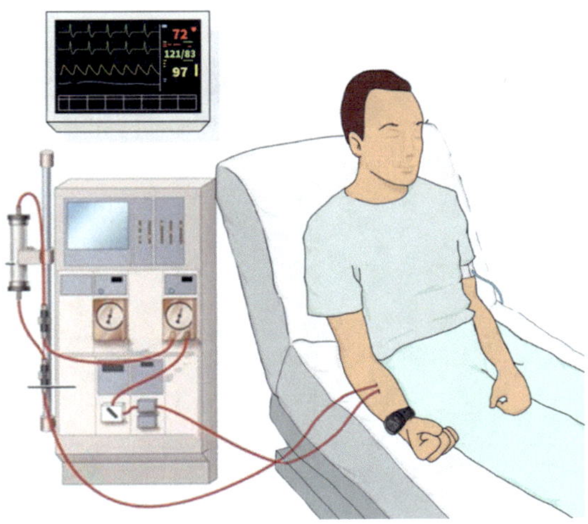

Figure 4.15. Patient heterogeneity.

Source: https://www.mdpi.com/biomedicines/biomedicines-12-01177/article_deploy/html/images/biomedicines-12-01177-g001.png.

The latest evidence on BP sampling intervals demonstrates that the accuracy of detection of change in sensing by BP deteriorates with a rise in sampling intervals and impacts clinical reliability. In settings like acute ischemic stroke, where real-time sensing of blood pressure variability is crucial, the relationship between sampling interval and detection accuracy becomes critical. The findings indicate that while the BPV could have consistent levels for some BPs, more extended sample periods will produce vast misperceptions about patient status. Therefore, future technology in RPM must address the consequences of patient heterogeneity so that patient monitor equipment is accurate and responsive and ultimately aid in improved patient outcomes in hemodynamic management (Ball *et al.*, 2024; Creton *et al.*, 2024) (Figure 4.15).

4.6.3. Ethical Considerations in Monitoring

The fast rate of hemodynamic monitoring technology raises deep ethical issues regarding patient autonomy and informed consent. As clinical advancements, particularly in critical care, enhance patients' conditions, monitoring devices have grown more intricate, possibly concealing information from patients regarding their conditions and treatment regimens. Medical personnel must see to it that patients—or their representatives—are well-informed regarding risks and benefits of various monitoring techniques, invasive or non-invasive. The ethical principle of autonomy supports patients' rights to informed choices concerning their treatment, such as being informed about how being constantly monitored impacts their quality of life and privacy. Failure to discuss the above factors leads to distress and feelings of loss of control among patients, destroying their confidence in the health care system and the monitoring measures applied to guarantee their health. Another significant ethical issue is the application of data collected using hemodynamic monitoring systems. Technology has enabled the collection of extensive patient data that proves useful in identifying personal and population health trends. The application raises issues about patient data privacy and abuse of sensitive information. Ethical stewardship also calls for healthcare providers to not only ensure the validity of the information but also the safe storage and transmission of the same while keeping the confidentiality intact. Moreover, the recent controversy in AI also points towards the ethical guidelines in using it for monitoring patients. Since clinicians employ AI for diagnostic and care-optimization purposes, ethical considerations related to data ownership, consent with respect to data use, and algorithmic bias on the quality of care and fairness among different patient populations must be addressed (Vincent *et al.*, 2020). Furthermore, it is incumbent on the nursing profession to address ethical concerns surrounding hemodynamic monitoring, particularly with critically ill patients who require aggressive interdisciplinary interventions. RNs must balance the technical needs of the monitoring against their professional mandate to act in their patients' best interest. These comprise not only intimate scrutiny of patients' physiological status and potential complications but also communication with patients regarding implications for invasive monitoring approaches that are not in line with patients' values or preferences. Ethical dilemmas of need extend to the end-of-life care situations, whereby monitoring prolongs suffering rather than improving quality of life. In making such agonizing decisions, RNs ought to incorporate an ethical framework in practice for improved patient and family care to ensure that their care is patient-centered and aligns with standard ethical guidelines, especially for high-acuity patients (Botsch *et al.*, 2019).

Test Your Knowledge

1. What are the main limitations of current hemodynamic monitoring techniques?
2. How does patient variability affect the accuracy of monitoring data?

SUMMARY

The significance of hemodynamic monitoring and control cannot be overemphasized, particularly under critical care, where patient outcome largely depends on the stability of the cardiovascular system. Suggestions forwarded for monitoring MAP are made to provide insight into the best way to manage patients with acute traumatic SCI. The guidelines suggest monitoring MAP targets between 75–80 mmHg as a lower target, and the prevention of crossing an upper target of 90–95 mmHg for the sake of maximizing spinal cord perfusion. The new guidelines are an expression of greater sensitivity to the dictates of greater subtlety in control of blood pressure and acceptance of gaps in current knowledge as it presents itself in the literature on hemodynamic interventions (Kwon *et al.*, 2024). Furthermore, modifications of current practice, founded on newer data, will be needed to carry on the clinical practices in the pediatric groups as well. For instance, neonatal hypotension is a case with singular challenges that are far different from the adult critical care situation. Uniformity in diagnostic criteria among clinicians underlines the need for standardized guidelines to guide interventions such as volume expansion and inotropes. Greater reliance on technologies such as echocardiography can potentially yield vital information about neonatal hemodynamic status, and this would eventually result in enhanced management regimens within the NICU (Das *et al.*, 2024). This brings us to a pressing need for harmonization among providers for hypotension treatment in vulnerable populations. Lastly, the dynamic evolving context of hemodynamic management accentuates the importance of continuous education and guideline dissemination among physicians. As a means of practice and knowledge bridging, the integration of evidence-based guidelines can foster consistency in the management of patients, particularly when considering the diversity in clinical presentations. The recognition of the low level of evidence for MAP management reiterates the importance of continuous research to confirm the implications of the guidelines. Finally, with the practice of these enhanced procedures now adopted by clinicians, the potential of revolutionary improvement in the outcomes of acute and chronic hemodynamic instability is within reach, setting an example for the direction of future development in the practice (Kwon *et al.*, 2024).

Effective hemodynamic monitoring plays an important role in the clinical management of the patient, particularly during invasive procedures. The conventional measurement of fluid has been routine on static values of central venous pressure and urine output. These, however, are increasingly being seen with limitations in well representing the intravascular volume status of a patient. The development of dynamic monitoring methods has given clinicians more accurate tools to direct fluid therapy, especially in the critically ill surgical setting. Minimally invasive steps advance practice to several benefits, such as fewer patient morbidities and enhanced postoperative recovery. During surgery, like resuscitative abdominal procedures, dynamic monitoring facilitates real-time adjustment of fluid administration, maximizing care to the patient and reducing volume overload or under-resuscitation morbidity (Gutierrez *et al.*, 2013). The application of advanced hemodynamic monitoring can transform therapy for cardiovascular disease patients. The current evidence has demonstrated the dual effect of particular diabetes and cardiovascular risk management pharmacologic drugs. For instance, drugs such as empagliflozin, a sodium-glucose cotransporter two inhibitor, have been reported to dramatically reduce CV mortality and hospitalization due to HF. The pathways for these actions are believed to be through hemodynamic and metabolic actions, thus introducing a new intersection of treatment in diabetes and cardiovascular disease

(Januzzi *et al.*, 2017). This two-dimensional strategy serves to meet the need for an integrated methodology of hemodynamic monitoring, which takes into account both the physiologic dynamics of fluid infusion as well as the pharmacologic impact of therapy regimens on cardiovascular stability. Beyond this, hemodynamic parameter evaluation must likewise not be solely preoccupied with immediate operative outcomes but also with the patient's long-term prognosis. Adoption of guidelines that utilize advanced monitoring systems introduces improved decision-making and successful interventions. For instance, it is possible to monitor cardiac index and stroke volume variation in real time, enabling clinicians to tailor fluid resuscitation protocols according to physiological response in real time. This active management minimizes complications, facilitates faster recovery, and ultimately lowers mortality rates among critical care patients. With ongoing developments in hemodynamic monitoring, the multidisciplinary approach of synthesizing viewpoints from surgery, cardiology, and drug therapy will be critical to achieving optimal management and facilitating maximal patient outcomes. This integration emphasizes the central importance of combined hemodynamic management to contemporary medical practice.

KEY TERMS FROM THIS CHAPTER

- Arterial line
- Blood pressure (BP)
- Cardiac index (CI)
- Cardiac output (CO)
- Central venous catheter
- Central venous pressure (CVP)
- Dynamic parameters
- Echocardiography
- Fluid responsiveness
- Heart rate (HR)
- Hemodynamic monitoring
- Invasive monitoring
- Mean arterial pressure (MAP)
- Mixed venous oxygen Ssaturation (SvO_2)
- Passive leg raise (PLR) test
- Point-of-care ultrasound (POCUS)

CRITICAL THINKING QUESTIONS

1. **Which of the following is commonly monitored in hemodynamic assessments to evaluate the heart's pumping ability?**
   a. Central venous pressure (CVP)
   b. Arterial blood pressure (ABP)
   c. Cardiac output (CO)
   d. Oxygen saturation (SpO_2)
2. **What is the primary purpose of measuring central venous pressure (CVP) in critically ill patients?**
   a. To evaluate left ventricular function
   b. To estimate the volume status and right ventricular function
   c. To assess oxygenation levels
   d. To monitor electrolyte imbalance
3. **Invasive arterial pressure monitoring is typically used for which of the following reasons?**
   a. To measure cardiac output
   b. To assess mean arterial pressure (MAP) and blood volume
   c. To monitor urine output
   d. To estimate liver function
4. **Which of the following drugs is commonly used to increase blood pressure in patients with shock?**
   a. Furosemide
   b. Epinephrine
   c. Metformin
   d. Amlodipine
5. **The use of a pulmonary artery catheter is indicated for which of the following purposes in critically ill patients?**
   a. To monitor blood glucose levels
   b. To assess cardiac output, pulmonary artery pressure, and mixed venous oxygen saturation
   c. To provide mechanical ventilation
   d. To measure intracranial pressure

Short Answer Questions

1. What are the basic principles of hemodynamics, and how do they apply to critical care?
2. What are two commonly used techniques for hemodynamic monitoring, and how do they work?
3. When are hemodynamic monitoring techniques typically indicated in a clinical setting?
4. How is hemodynamic data interpreted to assess a patient's cardiovascular status?
5. What are two key strategies for managing hemodynamics in critically ill patients?
6. What are some of the challenges encountered during hemodynamic monitoring in critically ill patients?

Answer to Critical Thinking Questions

1. (c); 2. (b); 3. (b); 4. (b); 5. (b)

REFERENCES

1. Adhikari, P. (2024). Integrated psychiatric and surgical care in managing self-inflicted abdominal trauma: A case report in a resource-limited setting. *Annals of Medicine and Surgery, 86*, 6810–6813. https://www.semanticscholar.org/paper/f2f73dc256d3335a5f553a2b1e2c19cec9840fd0 (accessed on 22 May 2025).

2. Andrei, M., Drăgoescu, N., Stănculescu, A., Chiuțu, L., Drăgoescu, O., & Istrătoaie, O. (2024). PiCCO or cardiac ultrasound? Which is better for hemodynamic monitoring in ICU? *Medicina, 60*. https://www.semanticscholar.org/paper/648d76b342bb454a1e4a73cc326bbd8fffa79c1e (accessed on 22 May 2025).

3. Aseni, P., Orsenigo, S., Storti, E., Pulici, M., & Arlati, S. (2019). Current concepts of perioperative monitoring in high-risk surgical patients: A review. *Patient Safety in Surgery, 13*. https://doi.org/10.1186/s13037-019-0213-5.

4. Assaad, S., Perrino, A., & Shelley, B. (2017). *Transpulmonary Thermodilution: Its Role in Assessment of Lung Water and Pulmonary Edema*. https://core.ac.uk/download/82958547.pdf.

5. Babaev, A., Bourgoin, A., Combes, A., Dubin, A., Geppert, A., van Gestel, A., Perel, A., *et al.* (2014). Consensus on circulatory shock and hemodynamic monitoring. *Task Force of the European Society of Intensive Care Medicine*. https://core.ac.uk/download/29469500.pdf (accessed on 22 May 2025).

6. Baik, M. (2024). Transcranial Doppler in neurointerventional: Applications in endovascular thrombectomy and carotid artery stenting. *Journal of Neurosonology and Neuroimaging*. https://www.semanticscholar.org/paper/558589c85a677d7d74590eb47e37baf74aabcff3 (accessed on 22 May 2025).

7. Ball, J. D., Panerai, R., Henstock, T., & Minhas, J. (2024). Arterial blood pressure monitoring in stroke cohorts: The impact of reduced sampling rates to optimise remote patient monitoring. *Blood Pressure Monitoring*. https://www.semanticscholar.org/paper/9bad16dad45001e1095d838c5aeef0a7e32b9158 (accessed on 22 May 2025).

8. Bilotta, F. (2017). Neuroanesthesiology: The ineludible path toward super-specialty. *Current Opinion in Anesthesiology, 30*(5), 525–526. https://www.semanticscholar.org/paper/bc63eb7493a24a1748f9160bf7034c0ec43c3b46 (accessed on 22 May 2025).

9. Blumer, V., Hanff, T. C., Gage, A., Schrage, B., & Kanwar, M. K. (2025). Cardiogenic shock teams: Past, present, and future directions. *Circulation: Heart Failure*. https://www.semanticscholar.org/paper/26da0697a94e9adedc8b9043dbed15f3bc5176f0 (accessed on 22 May 2025).

10. Bosso, H., Augusto, T. A., Maluf, E. S., Mateus, M., *et al.* (2025). Advanced hemodynamic monitoring in polytraumatized patients: A comprehensive review. *Journal of Medical Science and Evidences*. https://www.semanticscholar.org/paper/ea32219474a2324856917957bcb001a1b041766e (accessed on 22 May 2025).

11. Botsch, E., Protain, E., Smith, A. R., & Szilagyi, R. (2019). Nursing implications in the ECMO patient. In *Advances in Extracorporeal Membrane Oxygenation* (Vol. 3). https://www.semanticscholar.org/paper/67e6711826ca17030832911b49b3febe79b6a4ac (accessed on 22 May 2025).

12. Butter, J. K., Miller, A. P., & Obonin, S. S. (2024). Impact of thermal and hemodynamic factors on blood flow in magnetized arteries: A mathematical perspective. *International Journal of*

Mathematics and Statistics Studies. https://www.semanticscholar.org/paper/39f4f69995b22f0ec6a04aaccdbbc0f2eda9e70f (accessed on 22 May 2025).

13. Castellano, A., Bailo, M., Cicone, F., Carideo, L., Quartuccio, N., Mortini, P., Falini, A., *et al.* (2021). Advanced imaging techniques for radiotherapy planning of gliomas. *Cancers, 13*, 1063. https://doi.org/10.3390/cancers13051063.
14. Choi, J. H., Lee, J., Park, E., Bae, S., Kim, D., Kim, Y. H., & Choi, I. (2021). Nutrition and metabolism research abstracts. *JPEN. Journal of Parenteral and Enteral Nutrition, 45*(S1), 7–240. https://www.semanticscholar.org/paper/02cbd73c3bb6faeac33e59cc28bf6d9f1085eba0 (accessed on 22 May 2025).
15. Choi, T., Chan, B., Grech, L., Kwok, A., Webber, K., Wong, J., Nguyen, M., *et al.* (2023). Factors influencing COVID-19 vaccine hesitancy among patients with serious chronic illnesses during the initial Australian vaccine rollout: A multi-centre qualitative analysis using the Health Belief Model. *Vaccines, 11*. https://www.semanticscholar.org/paper/e2c9992ab160a8b7f25c447cb9cdbfaeb4a5619b (accessed on 22 May 2025).
16. Creton, S., Saadi, M., Monfort, H., Yaghobian, S., Pages, N., Nisse-Durgeat, S., & Diebold, B. (2024). The clinical impact and good practices of remote patient monitoring for chronic heart failure: A French case report. *Patient Preference and Adherence, 18*, 131–135. https://www.semanticscholar.org/paper/77fdfbc000e297fd6537def1163c1a8b74f43ed0 (accessed on 22 May 2025).
17. Das, R., Nagpal, R., Deshpande, S., Kumar, G., Singh, A., Kallimath, A., & Suryawanshi, P. (2024). A survey on management practices of hypotension in preterm neonates: An Indian perspective. *Frontiers in Pediatrics, 12*. https://www.semanticscholar.org/paper/afd4990eaa4f13f960c3579e39b5b6e04613fd5e (accessed on 22 May 2025).
18. Deng, M., Du, C., Fang, J., Xu, C., Guo, C., Huang, J., Li, K., *et al.* (2024). Flexible adaptive sensing tonometry for medical-grade multi-parametric hemodynamic monitoring. *npj Flexible Electronics*. https://www.semanticscholar.org/paper/0fcfc56cbd1e9428f2dfd1350f2b3997ce8baaf5 (accessed on 22 May 2025).
19. Donnelly, S., Barnett, C. F., Bohula, E., Chaudhry, S., Chonde, M. D., Cooper, H., Daniels, L. B., *et al.* (2024). Interhospital variation in admissions managed with critical care therapies or invasive hemodynamic monitoring in tertiary cardiac intensive care units: An analysis from the Critical Care Cardiology Trials Network Registry. *Circulation: Cardiovascular Quality and Outcomes, 17*, e010092. https://www.semanticscholar.org/paper/c4db4021a81e4b5f70232dd109fd18ec4727fe4b (accessed on 22 May 2025).
20. Dua, A., Debnath, A., Kumar, K., Mazumder, R., Mazumder, A., Singh, R., Mangal, S., *et al.* (2024). Advancements of glucose monitoring biosensor: Current state, generations of technological progress, and innovation dynamics. *Current Pharmaceutical Biotechnology*. https://www.semanticscholar.org/paper/9c143c9e8110173dcde2b4e7f1fad98e3b6d3580 (accessed on 22 May 2025).
21. Evans, L., Rhodes, A., Alhazzani, W., Antonelli, M., Coopersmith, C. M., French, C., Machado, F. R., *et al.* (2021). Surviving Sepsis Campaign: International guidelines for management of sepsis and septic shock 2021. *Critical Care Medicine, 49*, e1063–e1143. https://doi.org/10.1097/ccm.0000000000005337.

22. Flythe, J. E., Chang, T. I., Gallagher, M., Lindley, E., Madero, M., Sarafidis, P., Unruh, M. L., *et al.* (2020). Blood pressure and volume management in dialysis: Conclusions from a Kidney Disease: Improving Global Outcomes (KDIGO) Controversies Conference. *Kidney International, 97*, 861–876. https://doi.org/10.1016/j.kint.2020.01.046.
23. Gohad, R., Jain, S., & Paul, A. (2025). Anesthetic management and perioperative care in a high-risk patient with bladder cancer, hypertension, and chronic kidney disease undergoing radical cystectomy with ileal conduit urinary diversion: A case report. *Multidisciplinary Science Journal*. https://www.semanticscholar.org/paper/2190998a0e7eeeb0d4d61b58aa1124625e3d6c80 (accessed on 22 May 2025).
24. Gupta, S. K., Krishnatray, D., & Kanani, R. (2025). Anesthesia management in patients with acute respiratory distress syndrome (ARDS). *Journal of Neonatal Surgery*. https://www.semanticscholar.org/paper/8354d5ecd7ac6d42a07d35f0bd334305f4b260ca (accessed on 22 May 2025).
25. Gutierrez, M. C., Liu, H., & Moore, P. G. (2013). *Goal-Directed Therapy in Intraoperative Fluid and Hemodynamic Management*. https://core.ac.uk/download/323069925.pdf.
26. Herrera, P., Marazuela, M. A., Formentin, G., & Hofmann, T. (2022). Towards an effective application of parameter estimation and uncertainty analysis to mathematical groundwater models. *SN Applied Sciences, 4*. https://www.semanticscholar.org/paper/b6fc855c4511bc0bc41e660f6490089d5a844222 (accessed on 22 May 2025).
27. Howsmon, D., Mikulski, M., Kabra, N., Northrup, J., Stromberg, D., Fraser, C. D., Mery, C., *et al.* (2024). Statistical process monitoring creates a hemodynamic trajectory map after pediatric cardiac surgery: A case study of the arterial switch operation. *Bioengineering & Translational Medicine, 9*. https://www.semanticscholar.org/paper/129f477b7982c66f1fb6d5c51d2bf8d1bf3bd731 (accessed on 22 May 2025).
28. Huang, J. J., Yu, C. C., & Lo, H. Y. (2024). Using multiple strategies to improve the accuracy of hemodynamic monitoring. *Hu Li Za Zhi: The Journal of Nursing, 71*(1), 72–80. https://www.semanticscholar.org/paper/a6b9bf099cd2df27dca0a4648a8ec991d8634509 (accessed on 22 May 2025).
29. Huas, D., Pouchain, B., Gay, B., Avouac, B., Bouvenot, G., & The French College of Teachers in General Practice. (2006). Assessing chronic pain in general practice: Are guidelines relevant? A cluster randomized controlled trial. *The European Journal of General Practice, 12*, 52–57. https://www.semanticscholar.org/paper/c79618f664d73fc814f1a362fa9b29b6c35b238a (accessed on 22 May 2025).
30. Januzzi Jr., J. L., Petrie, M. C., Sattar, N., Zinman, B., *et al.* (2017). Novel diabetes drugs and the cardiovascular specialist. https://core.ac.uk/download/82893969.pdf (accessed on 22 May 2025).
31. Karakitsos, D., El Barbary, M., Gillman, L., Papalois, A., & Shiloh, A. (2014). Critical care and perioperative monitoring. *The Scientific World Journal, 2014*. https://www.semanticscholar.org/paper/5d1bf6b3597952064d302be7ef8ebdd129cd985a (accessed on 22 May 2025).
32. Kashani, K., Omer, T., & Shaw, A. (2022). The intensivist's perspective of shock, volume management, and hemodynamic monitoring. *Clinical Journal of the American Society of Nephrology (CJASN)*. https://www.semanticscholar.org/paper/80fdc167a8a9cf9fc9a41a6588e4e6c6b3ec391a (accessed on 22 May 2025).

33. Katayama, A., Patel, P., Pianelli, A., Wang, R., & Sakai, T. (2025). Abdominal organ transplantation: Noteworthy literature in 2024. *Seminars in Cardiothoracic and Vascular Anesthesia.* https://www.semanticscholar.org/paper/8680976651fa90b9d9f96cbf613ebec753f4e83c (accessed on 22 May 2025).

34. Kendrick, J. B., Kaye, A., Tong, Y., Belani, K., Urman, R., Hoffman, C., & Liu, H. (2019). Goal-directed fluid therapy in the perioperative setting. *Journal of Anesthesiology, Clinical Pharmacology, 35,* S29–S34. https://www.semanticscholar.org/paper/a3808a214399614cc3166392b6b50634b5860148 (accessed on 22 May 2025).

35. Khan, E., Nawaz, S., Inam, K., Alali, M., & Waqas, M. (2024). Anesthesia strategies for the perioperative management of severe pulmonary hypertension in emergency orthopedic surgery: A case report. *Cureus, 16.* https://www.semanticscholar.org/paper/7c0934772b96d744f663152a56bd3588767bb084 (accessed on 22 May 2025).

36. Khan, S. (2024). Cloud cost management for startups: Strategies for success. *International Journal of Scientific Research in Computer Science, Engineering and Information Technology.* https://www.semanticscholar.org/paper/3de281df98fb17aceee2657197879419e3b93962 (accessed on 22 May 2025).

37. Koratala, A., Ronco, C., & Kazory, A. (2022). Diagnosis of fluid overload: From conventional to contemporary concepts. *Cardiorenal Medicine, 12,* 141–154. https://www.semanticscholar.org/paper/4b6d3857d183d5a77126dd53fd6295df4c62a54e (accessed on 22 May 2025).

38. Kwon, B. K., Tetreault, L. A., Martin, A. R., Arnold, P. M., Marco, R., Newcombe, V. F. J., Zipser, C., *et al.* (2024). A clinical practice guideline for the management of patients with acute spinal cord injury: Recommendations on hemodynamic management. *Global Spine Journal, 14,* 187S–211S. https://www.semanticscholar.org/paper/7493e0c2f859604e5dd6f44d288bb5977ea790f5 (accessed on 22 May 2025).

39. Lauretta, M. P., Caporali, L., Manera, S., Prucher, G. M., & Melotti, R. M. (2018). *Anesthetic Challenging in Microsurgical Flap Reconstruction: A Systematic Review.* https://core.ac.uk/download/188826841.pdf (accessed on 22 May 2025).

40. Lee, E., Kim, J., & Lee, G. (2024). Advanced anesthetic management strategies in patients with myoclonic epilepsy with ragged red fibers (MERRF). *Asian Journal of Multidisciplinary Research & Review.* https://www.semanticscholar.org/paper/13e07ef117f0b250ca12b965b26dbe1f328879e6 (accessed on 22 May 2025).

41. Pazouki, S., Jamshidi, M. B., Jalali, M., & Tafreshi, A. (2025). The integration of big data in FinTech: Review of enhancing financial services through advanced technologies. *World Journal of Advanced Research and Reviews.* https://www.semanticscholar.org/paper/025d71b5036675b8e66cc4b8e6ad36108b5bbb66 (accessed on 22 May 2025).

42. Rola, P., Farkas, J. D., Spiegel, R. J., Kyle-Sidell, C., Weingart, S., Duggan, L., Garrone, M., *et al.* (2020). Rethinking the early intubation paradigm of COVID-19: Time to change gears? *Clinical and Experimental Emergency Medicine, 7,* 78–80. https://www.semanticscholar.org/paper/bb5650269c903d1c1331bf0356f25c792b6873aa (accessed on 22 May 2025).

43. Sawant, U., & Sen, J. (2024). A comprehensive review of magnesium sulfate infusion: Unveiling the impact on hemodynamic stability during laryngoscopy and tracheal intubation in ear, nose, and throat surgeries. *Cureus, 16.* https://www.semanticscholar.org/paper/0ff4b63a7b01c19ab1478783743038ffa1e91302 (accessed on 22 May 2025).

44. Scanavacca, M., & Darrieux, F. (2016). Factors in deciding between novel and traditional oral anticoagulants to prevent embolism in atrial fibrillation patients. *Arquivos Brasileiros de Cardiologia, 106*, 1–3. https://www.semanticscholar.org/paper/e55a8e67f2bd93417e12789e7a90d0a354e345ea (accessed on 22 May 2025).

45. Sirohi, D., Kumar, D., & Choudhary, R. (2025). Anesthetic considerations for critically ill patients with sepsis. *International Journal of Current Pharmaceutical Research*. https://www.semanticscholar.org/paper/3d412220070ea0aedc6acedc3b63ca8a59a405f5 (accessed on 22 May 2025).

46. Upadhye, K. S., Patidar, H., Bamnia, N., & Yadav, N. (2025). HbA1c reduction strategies: An overview of pharmacological interventions. *National Journal of Pharmacology and Therapeutics*. https://www.semanticscholar.org/paper/88e96b4b3443eca4cdfe869da64761eaac78f182 (accessed on 22 May 2025).

47. Vincent, J., & Artigas, A. (2020). Challenges in critical care. *Seminars in Respiratory and Critical Care Medicine, 42*, 001. https://www.semanticscholar.org/paper/3d8a197a321fa05243722a375a4b3a0d23b09b12 (accessed on 22 May 2025).

48. Wild, K. T., Rintoul, N. E., Kattan, J., & Gray, B. W. (2020). Extracorporeal Life Support Organization (ELSO): Guidelines for neonatal respiratory failure. *ASAIO Journal, 66*, 463–470. https://doi.org/10.1097/mat.0000000000001153.

49. Xiang, T., Zhang, Y., & Zhang, Y. (2024). A novel multimodal physiological model for the noninvasive and continuous measurements of arterial blood pressure. In *2024 46th Annual International Conference of the IEEE Engineering in Medicine and Biology Society (EMBC)*. https://www.semanticscholar.org/paper/3f2a251d0dcf2e2d73d34d22438b809a22bb8d1a (accessed on 22 May 2025).

50. Zabeeda, W., Cohen, J. B., Reiner Benaim, A., Zarour, S., Lichter, Y., Matot, I., & Goren, O. (2024). Utility of NICaS non-invasive hemodynamic monitoring in critically ill patients with COVID-19. *Journal of Clinical Medicine, 13*. https://www.semanticscholar.org/paper/ba9ac0a415e5c7db80a97bed9363d1c22d21a757 (accessed on 22 May 2025).

SHOCK MANAGEMENT

5

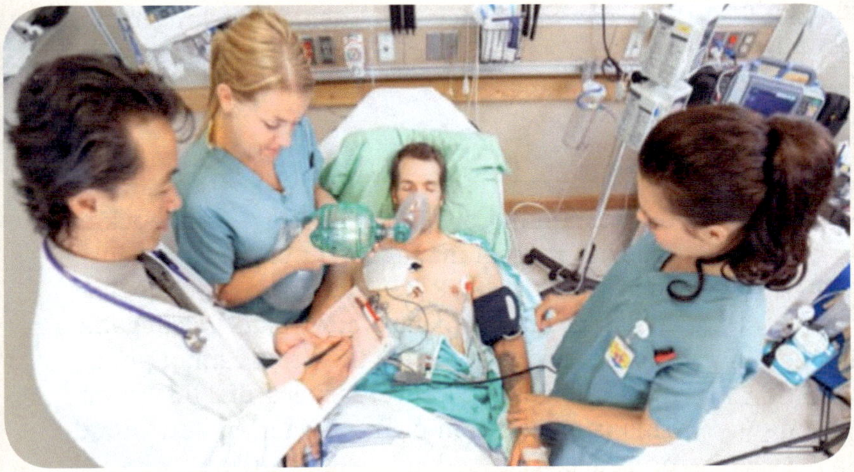

LEARNING OBJECTIVES

After studying this chapter, you will be able to:

1. List the types of shock.
2. Explain physiological responses to shock.
3. Describe the shock management techniques.
4. Elaborate psychological aspects of shock.

Introduction

In examining the complexities of shock management, it is important to give a background explanation of this life-threatening medical condition and it's role in patient care. Shock, by definition, as an insufficiency of function in the circulatory system to provide adequate blood flow to body tissues, can lead to severe dysfunction of the organs and death if not addressed at once. Numerous etiologies have been associated with shock development, including traumatic injury, severe infections, and obstetric complications. Particularly, the Non-Pneumatic Anti-Shock Garment has been a lifesaving intervention in obstetric hemorrhage and has been shown to be effective in stabilizing patients with life-threatening conditions (Adebisi *et al.*, 2025). Nevertheless, with its potential, the fact that the intervention is not being used to its full extent due to such restrictions as inadequate access and absence of training indicates an urgent need for enhanced solutions aimed at enhancing its utilization and eventually reducing maternal mortality and morbidity (Adebisi *et al.*, 2025). In essence, total shock management thus requires an interprofessional strategy with both immediate clinical maneuvers and system reform.

Definition of Shock

Shock is a critical medical condition whose definition is founded on the body's failure to maintain adequate blood perfusion and thereby insufficient oxygen delivery to tissues. This physiological state can be caused by various factors with hemorrhagic, cardiogenic, distributive, and obstructive etiologies, all of which would cause significant impairments of organ function unless addressed immediately.

It is essential to appreciate the definition of shock because it forms the foundation of successful management regimens used to restore hemodynamic stability. The European Society of Cardiology points out that clinicians are required to consider a broad range of factors, including patient history as well as clinical presentation, in diagnosing and managing shock to obtain a proper response (Pelliccia *et al.*, 2020). Also, the complexity of shock is further supported by the potential psychological effect it has, which manifests in the form of diseases like post-traumatic stress disorder, complicating patient recovery and highlighting the importance of comprehensive shock management (Bryant, 2019).

Importance of Shock Management

In determining the importance of managing shock, it is evident that organizations must respond well to sudden disruptions in a bid to maintain their operational sustainability intact. As Meyer et al. (1990) observe, extreme disruptions can have the ability to fundamentally shift industry trends and overwhelm the strongest organizations. The pandemic of coronavirus disease 19 is a contemporary icon of such shocks, compelling firms to adapt quickly to new external conditions, e.g., a shift towards home working and altered consumer behavior (Hitt *et al.*, 2020). The stakes are high; organisations with high shock management capability not only survive crises but can even emerge stronger by leveraging new opportunities. Moreover, as per the organisational and work psychology review, the pandemic has heightened stress and joblessness, and efficient shock management practice becomes necessary to insulate against these impacts (Kniffin *et al.*, 2020). Hence, an ability to implement effective shock management measures is crucial for achieving long-term, sustainable success in an evolving business environment.

Types of Shock

Understanding of the various types of shock is crucial for ideal management of shock because each type of shock has a unique physiological challenge and its management plan. Cardiogenic shock is produced when the heart cannot pump, most often due to a severe myocardial infarction. This is a condition characterized by low blood pressure, reduced urine output, and altered mental status that necessitates interventions such as venoarterial extracorporeal membrane oxygenation (VA ECMO) to achieve circulation and oxygenation in severe cases (Lorusso *et al.*, 2021).

Septic shock, on the contrary, occurs as a result of widespread infection that leads to vasodilation and multi-organ failure, where early identification and aggressive fluid resuscitation are indicated. Additionally, hypovolemic shock due to massive blood loss or dehydration requires rapid fluid replacement to restore circulatory volume to normal. Treatment of every shock type differs significantly, bringing to the fore the necessity of differentiated approaches in emergency medical treatment. Shock management hinges on the recognition of such differences to prevent morbidity and mortality in patients.

Overview of Physiological Responses

Physiological responses to shock are complex and involve a variety of systems that work towards maintaining homeostasis despite compromised circulation and cellular perfusion. Primarily regulated by neuroendocrine responses, these responses include sympathetic nervous system stimulation, which results in increased heart rate and constriction of blood vessels to produce perfusion to vital organs. Meanwhile, hormonal responses such as catecholamine release and stimulation of the renin-angiotensin-aldosterone system promote water retention and further vasoconstriction. While these adaptive responses may stabilize the person in the short term, they potentially exacerbate injury inadvertently via mechanisms such as ischemia-reperfusion injury, leading to local inflammation and possible systemic effects (Ali *et al.*, 2020). Hence, determining the interaction of these physiological reactions is important for managing shock to avert undesirable effects and institute effective therapeutic interventions that can maintain recovery without bringing about further harm (Intergovernmental Panel on Climate Change, 2023). In the development of complete treatment regimens within clinical environments, this matters.

Psychological Impact of Shock

The psychological impact of shock, particularly in situations of high tension such as pandemics and natural disasters, can be deep-rooted and long-lasting. Trauma survivors may experience a range of psychological reactions including acute stress disorder, anxiety, and post-traumatic stress disorder (PTSD). Significantly, the COVID-19 pandemic has amplified these effects, upsetting clinicians' sense of order and control, thus increasing their susceptibility to burnout and emotional exhaustion (Dewey *et al.*, 2020). The psychological distress of watching suffering and death without being able to intervene can lead to moral injury among health practitioners, hence complicating recovery and coping. To combat these psychological effects, mindfulness interventions became a successful approach, increasing moment-to-moment awareness and overall favorable mental health results (Creswell, 2016). The provision of supportive interventions and mental health interventions is essential in combating the psychological sequelae of shock and protecting the well-being of the victims.

Historical Context of Shock Management

From the past to the present, shock management has evolved significantly, all courtesy of cultural practices and scientific research. Early conceptualization of shock was primarily focused on external physical symptoms, and in doing so, it could easily fail to capture psychological elements that accompany traumatic experiences. As scholars embarked on exploring community reactions to tragedies, it was evident that stories constructed by cultural contexts are essential for constructing effective shock management. Societies use narrative, painting, and music to contextualize experience and thereby convert trauma into social memory, underpinning resilience and preparedness (Starosta, 2024). At the same time, integration of trauma life support practices in the health care environment maximized shock management, emphasizing prompt intervention and goal-directed fluid resuscitation (Mamalchi *et al.*, 2024). Through the integration of historical insights with contemporary practices, healthcare professionals are in a better place to address the advanced needs of shock patients in a way that deals with both physical and psychological care.

5.1. Types of Shock

Learning Outcome

1. Define hypovolemic shock, cardiogenic shock, and distributive shock
2. Explain the obstructive shock, neurogenic shock, and septic shock
3. Discuss the anaphylactic shock, traumatic shock, and psychogenic shock

Understanding the various forms of shock is key to managing this potentially life-threatening condition. Shock can be generally categorized into five primary types: hypovolemic, cardiogenic, distributive, obstructive, and neurogenic shock, each with its distinct physiological issues. Hypovolemic shock, which is often caused by severe blood volume loss, needs to be treated immediately by fluid resuscitation to restore the circulation. Conversely, cardiogenic shock results from underperformance of the heart, usually due to myocardial infarction, where treatment involves vigorous measures like veno-arterial extracorporeal membrane oxygenation (ECMO) to augment cardiac output and perfusion (Zhang *et al.*, 2024). Distributive shock, including septic shock, is defined by vasodilation and reduced distribution of blood pressure, which requires careful attention to infection control and fluid resuscitation. Additionally, obstructive shock, as in cases of pulmonary embolism, can significantly limit the passage of blood; hence the need for immediate discovery and correction of the obstructing factor. All types of shock necessitate a tailored form of treatment to effectively manage recovery.

5.1.1. Hypovolemic Shock

Hypovolemic shock is an acute condition brought about by direct fluid loss, leading to reduced blood volume and, in turn, insufficient perfusion of the tissues. Hypovolemic shock may be brought about by various causes, including traumatic hemorrhage, dehydration, or bleeding in the internal organs, including spontaneous retroperitoneal hematoma and rectus sheath hematoma. For instance, in anticoagulant therapy, the patient may present with the sudden onset of signs such as abdominal pain, hypotension, and tachycardia, with impending shock as in (Chen *et al.*, 2025; Kırkan *et al.*, 2022). Early identification and treatment are essential to treat hypovolemic shock effectively. Treatment is typically with aggressive fluid resuscitation and the institution of the cause of blood loss. In extreme situations, interventions like angiographic embolization can be performed to manage the hemodynamic condition of the patient. Hypovolemic shock management, particularly in susceptible populations, highlights the importance of watchfulness and early intervention to provide an improved prognosis for patients (Figure 5.1).

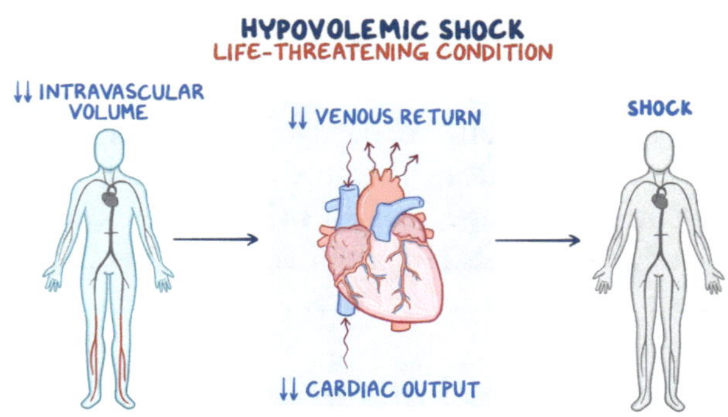

Figure 5.1. Hypovolemic shock.

Source: https://osmose-it.s3.amazonaws.com/Jtzz0RSNQguKnyeem-xpP_SpSKSribfD/_.jpg.

5.1.2. Cardiogenic Shock

Cardiogenic shock is a foreboding clinical syndrome with failure of the heart to produce sufficiency circulation with systemic hypoperfusion and tissue-deprived critical oxygenation. It is usually caused in the acute myocardial infarct setting when the heart muscle is severely damaged, and thus there is decreased cardiac output. Despite advancing treatment practices, cardiogenic shock is a difficult condition with in-hospital mortality being aggressively high at 40%–50% in these patients (Crispino *et al.*, 2025). Management of this disorder demands a delicate compromise between pharmacological interventions and the application of mechanical circulatory assistive devices, both necessary to stabilize hemodynamics and address the underlying pathology. Also, present approaches emphasize the significance of timely diagnosis and personalized treatment regimens, particularly in non-ischaemic diseases, as these have been proven to greatly improve patient results and survival (Mahajna *et al.*, 2025) (Figure 5.2).

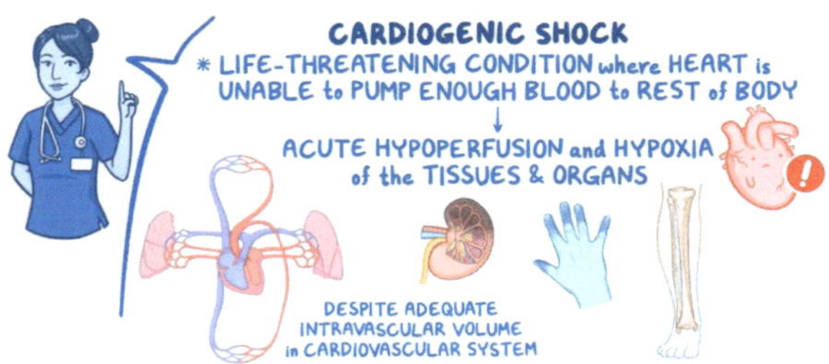

Figure 5.2. Cardiogenic shock.

Source: https://www.osmosis.org/_next/image?url=https%3A%2F%2Fd16qt3wv6xm098.cloudfront.net%2FXsSa6RCURk6wH3yYPhBlPNkPT8m0A5J_%2F_.jpg&w=3840&q=75.

5.1.3. Distributive Shock

Distributive shock is a critical condition with the overall dilation of blood vessels, causing reduced perfusion despite adequate blood volume. It is most commonly due to severe infections, such as septic shock, where inflammatory mediators lead to a drop in vascular resistance, with a resultant inadequate flow to vital organs. It is important to monitor the physiological parameters in distributive shock; e.g., research identifies a significant reduction in mean arterial blood pressure and lactate concentrations, reflecting tissue hypoxia and metabolic stress, necessitating intervention (Obonyo *et al.*, 2024). Early identification and timely therapeutic measures in the form of fluid loading and vasoactive medications are essential to reverse the effects of distributive shock and improve outcomes (Williams, 2025). Proper management not only alleviates the acute crisis but also avoids long-term sequelae of this potentially fatal disease, emphasizing the need for comprehensive shock management practices (Figure 5.3).

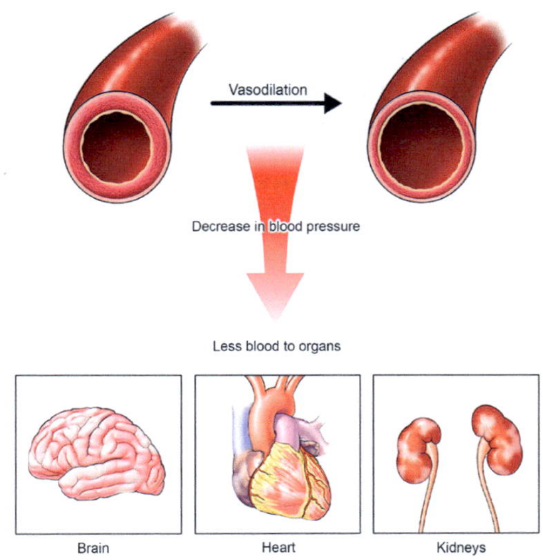

Figure 5.3. Excessively relaxed blood vessels in distributive shock are unable to deliver enough blood.

Source: https://my.clevelandclinic.org/-/scassets/images/org/health/articles/22762-distributive-shock.

5.1.4. Obstructive Shock

Obstructive shock is a sinister condition where there is interference with the circulation of blood, thereby preventing adequate circulation and oxygenation of tissues, thus compromising cellular metabolism. Obstructive shock can be caused by a variety of etiologies, among them pulmonary embolism, tension pneumothorax, or cardiac tamponade, all of which result in decreased venous return and subsequent cardiac output. There is an early need to identify obstructive shock since the underlying etiologies would require specific interventions such as relief of pressure in pneumothorax or drainage of fluid in tamponade conditions. Effective treatment modalities are crucial; these involve pharmacologic and mechanical interventions aimed at restoring hemodynamic stability. Early detection and therapy can improve patient outcomes considerably, emphasizing the need for appreciation not only of obstructive shock pathophysiology but also of the need for specific strategies in managing shock, as described in veterinary and clinical practice literature (Mahajna *et al.*, 2025; Williams, 2025) (Figure 5.4).

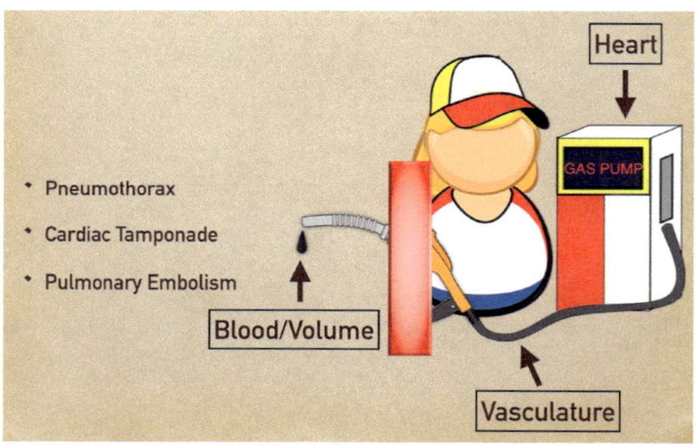

Figure 5.4. Obstructive shock.

Source: https://images.squarespace-cdn.com/content/v1/5e48489da899cd0942494 3db/1582229877751-EATHIPB7OMEW7L2INWSB/obstructive+shock.

5.1.5. Neurogenic Shock

Neurogenic shock, commonly associated with spinal injuries, leads to extreme cardiovascular instability by interrupting sympathetic nervous pathways. The syndrome is characterized by bradycardia and hypotension as a consequence of vasodilation and decreased vascular resistance, thereby impairing the ability of the body to maintain blood pressure and perfusion of vital organs. While in the treatment of shock, an early intervention is essential; resuscitation of blood pressure and heart rate with fluid resuscitation and appropriate use of vasopressors may be a savior. Finally, an understanding of the underlying pathophysiology, e.g., the role of the autonomic nervous system, is required to maximize outcomes in the patient with neurogenic shock. This in consideration aligns with the recent literature that highlights early intervention and specialized care in spinal cord injury, which can play an impactful role in long-term recovery as well as quality of life (Hachem *et al.*, 2017). Additionally, the intricate interaction between neurogenic shock and physiological systems warrants the implementation of total management strategies (Gheblawi *et al.*, 2020) (Figure 5.5).

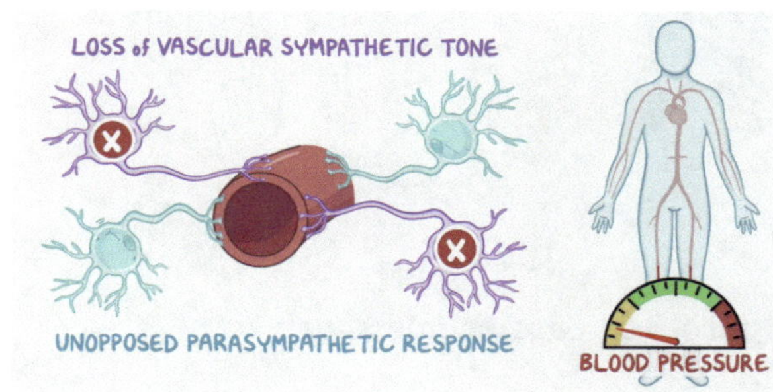

Figure 5.5. Neurogenic shock.

Source: https://d16qt3wv6xm098.cloudfront.net/VQ7eQpeNQVCkmRf1-wh110ahTQCke6Ix/_.jpg.

5.1.6. Septic Shock

Septic shock is a severe form of sepsis that includes sustained hypotension despite adequate fluid resuscitation, leading to inadequate blood flow and tissue perfusion. Septic shock should be immediately identified and treated, where timely treatment is vital in reducing morbidity and mortality rates. A multicenter observational study identified the diagnostic subtleties of septic shock, particularly with infective endocarditis, and highlighted the utility of echocardiography and blood cultures in establishing accurate diagnoses and initiating timely treatment (Lnu *et al.*, 2025). Furthermore, special populations, such as pregnant women, are faced with difficulties associated with physiological changes that conceal the diagnosis of sepsis, thereby posing challenges for early interventions (Islamy *et al.*, 2025). Aggressive fluid resuscitation, early administration of broad-spectrum antibiotics, and vasopressor therapy are effective treatments that target stabilizing hemodynamics and optimizing organ function. Treatment for septic shock is thus comprehensive to improve patient outcomes (Figure 5.6).

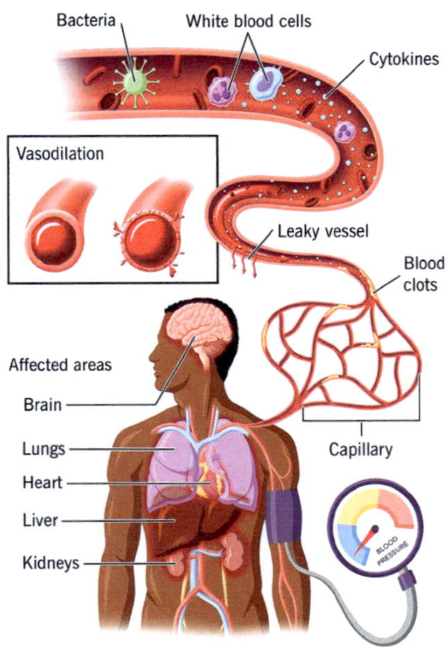

Figure 5.6. Septic shock.

Source: https://my.clevelandclinic.org/-/scassets/images/org/health/articles/23255-septic-shock.

5.1.7. Anaphylactic Shock

Anaphylactic shock is a fatal, severe disorder brought about by an out-of-proportion allergic response to specific stimuli, including certain foods, drugs, or insect stings. This acute presentation results in the subsequent rapid onset of symptoms: airway obstruction, profound drops in blood pressure, and cardiovascular collapse, which renders the immediate necessity for shock control so critical. The immediate administration of epinephrine is the primary management of anaphylaxis, which reverses the physiological process of the reaction. Even though epinephrine is available, access to it is not consistent across the world, and over 65% of countries lack sufficient supplies of auto-injectable adrenaline, thus preventing appropriate control of anaphylactic attacks (Tanno *et al.*, 2018). Also, the understanding of the various clinical presentations because of food allergies and their relation with anaphylactic shock is essential in regard to developing preventive measures along with enhancing response mechanisms in cases of emergencies (Pleşca *et al.*, 2017). It relies on timely intervention and improved accessibility of drugs needed (Figure 5.7).

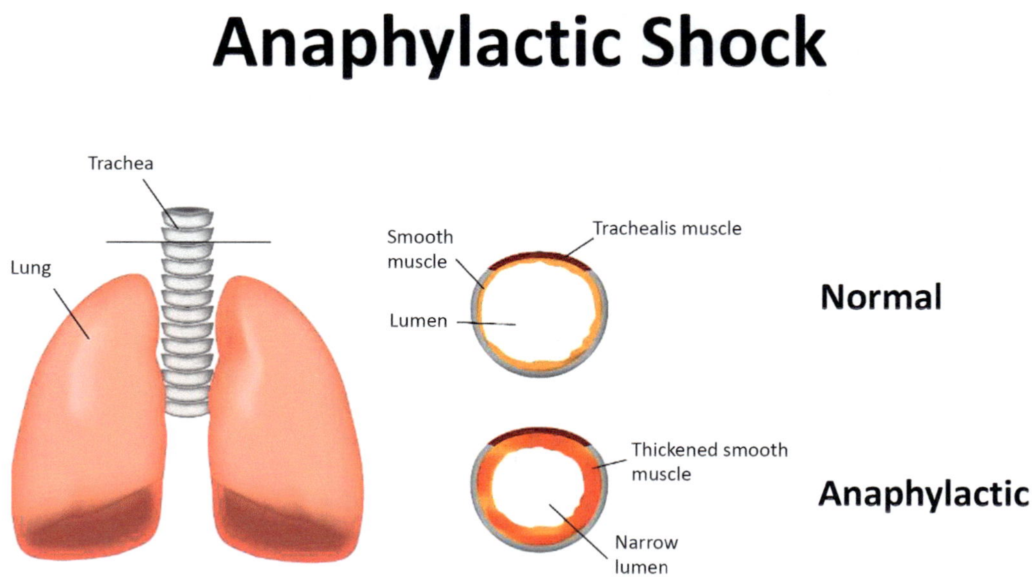

Figure 5.7. Anaphylactic shock.

Source: https://external-content.duckduckgo.com/iu/?u=https%3A%2F%2Fwww.firstaidshow.com%2Fwp-content%2Fuploads%2F2020%2F12%2FIdiopathic-Anaphylaxis.jpg&f=1&nofb=1&ipt=41e7445d23e7ad9862fa0b88e1861856a8795fc336ed5c88037ff10e32ab6c3d.

5.1.8. Traumatic Shock

Traumatic shock is an emergent condition that occurs following severe physical trauma, with decreased rate of circulation and consequent physiological dysfunctions. Management must be achieved in a state of urgency to avoid progression into complications such as organ failure. A tailored protocol could include aggressive fluid resuscitation and cautious administration of vasopressors.

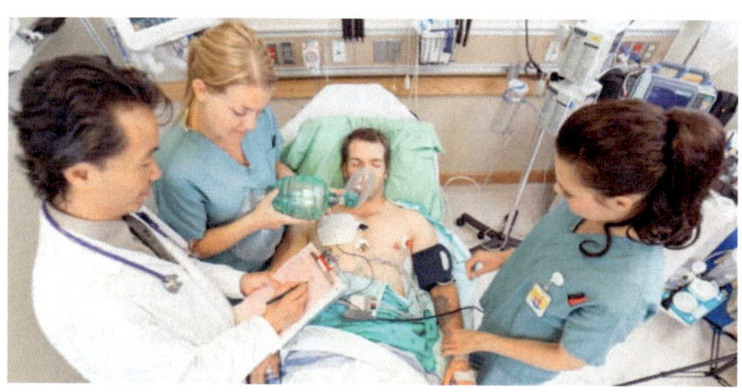

Figure 5.8. Traumatic shock can manifest itself in various forms, depending on the nature and extent of the injury.

Source: https://lh7-rt.googleusercontent.com/docsz/AD_4nXe8p-2NFYBKzkY5CMyKlVoHqu1xjOs5jyLssVXORfCJvorqhHVy2FrZnyxvVtoMVFUlrdaZyIkoB1YkjdjxJbeSULOUhstq52fWia4zIotiSc_KnkwPPwHXquis6KPw2FEL4gDwFQ?key=8AsP1VLh912vQwuzMJoT-W3g.

For instance, as highlighted in the recent study, initiation of noradrenaline is of utmost importance in the management of septic shock, an unfortunate complication of trauma patients, to restore hemodynamic stability (Kotani *et al.*, 2025). In addition, the use of adjunct therapies, such as valproic acid in combination with fresh frozen plasma, has also been hopeful in preventing neurological impairments in traumatic brain injury cases, thus promising recovery outcomes (Bhatti *et al.*, 2024). Appreciation of the complex characteristics of traumatic shock is important for clinicians to maximize patient management at times of crisis (Figure 5.8).

5.1.9. Psychogenic Shock

Psychogenic shock, a reversible condition typically caused by intense emotional stress or trauma, is a model to conventional paradigms of shock management that are primarily related to physiological causes. Unlike cardiogenic or hypovolemic shock, where systemic hypoperfusion results from biological causes, psychogenic shock is due to psychological stimuli and has symptoms such as fainting or palpitations without a recognizable organic cause. Management of this type of shock requires a multi-disciplinary approach depending on the mental status of the patient. Early identification of symptoms, accompanied by reassurance and supportive psychological management, lies at the heart of recovery, as evidenced by the effective triage regimens used in emergency scenes of mixed severity, such as those reported with mass casualty events (Pan *et al.*, 2025). Further, identifying the interplay between physical and emotional health can increase clinicians' ability to implement evidence-based treatments, ultimately leading to improved patient outcomes for psychogenic shock (Mahajna *et al.*, 2025).

Test Your Knowledge

1. How do hypovolemic, cardiogenic, and distributive shock differ in their underlying causes?

- What are the key features that distinguish obstructive, neurogenic, and septic shock?

5.2. Physiological Responses to Shock

Learning Outcome

1. Discuss the body's initial response
2. Identify the role of the autonomic nervous system
3. Explain the hormonal changes during shock
4. Define the impact on cardiovascular system
5. Understand the effects on respiratory function
6. Define metabolic changes
7. Discuss neurological implications
8. Explain the long-term physiological consequences

The physiological responses to shock are a complex interaction of adaptive processes attempting to restore homeostasis in the face of an acute stressor. Following exposure of a creature to shock, the creature deploys a sequence of hormonal responses with the obligatory activation of the hypothalamic-pituitary-adrenal axis, culminating in catecholamine release, which mediates tachycardia and augmented cardiac output in order to generate augmented blood flow to vital organs. Moreover, metabolic alterations occur with elevated levels of enzymes such as aspartate aminotransferase and alanine aminotransferase, reflecting oxidative stress and cellular damage. of special interest, organisms, such as freshwater drum, have been observed to possess significant biochemical resistance to shifting salinities, exhibiting tolerance under stress (Amankwah *et al.*, 2025). Furthermore, species like Ceratitis capitata have heightened antioxidant enzyme activity when subjected to heat stress, an indication of the importance of these physiological responses in formulating effective policies for the management of shock (Fouda *et al.*, 2025).

5.2.1. Body's Initial Response

The primary response of the body to shock plays a key role in determining the follow-up management strategy employed to reverse the physiological derangements created by traumatic insult. When exposed to shock, the body uses compensatory mechanisms such as tachycardia and vasoconstriction to maintain perfusion of important organs. This immediate response depends on the extent and type of shock, whether hemorrhagic, cardiogenic, or septic. With hemorrhagic shock, urgent recognition and hemostasis come into play, placing emphasis on the need for immediate physiological interventions in restoring circulation and oxygenation (Bonanno, 2022). Furthermore, the triggering of stress response mechanisms, including the release of heat shock proteins, is an adaptation mechanism targeted at inducing cellular tolerance (Hunter-Manseau *et al.*, 2024). Appreciation of these initial responses not only assists with timely intervention but also reveals the intricate interplay of physiologic events that have profound effects on the outcome in the treatment of shock.

5.2.2. Role of the Autonomic Nervous System (ANS)

The ANS is critical in the management of shock primarily through its effect on cardiovascular hemodynamics and homeostasis.

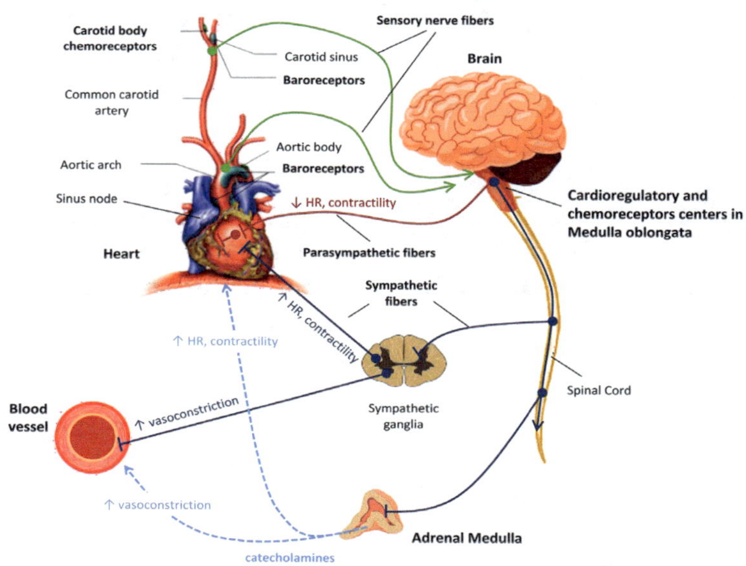

Figure 5.9. Illustration of the short-term autonomic nervous system (ANS) regulatory mechanisms of the cardiovascular system.

Source: https://annalsofintensivecare.springeropen.com/articles/10.1186/s13613-021-00869-7.

Made up of the parasympathetic and sympathetic branches, the ANS regulates heart rate, vascular tone, and gastrointestinal function, all of which are important to maintaining perfusion in shock conditions. Upon stress in the body, the sympathetic nervous system is activated with the release of catecholamines that raise cardiac output and peripheral vasoconstriction, and therefore divert blood supply to vital organs. The parasympathetic system, whose overall action is inhibitory, reverses stress by restoring equilibrium. This equilibrium is essential to clinical care for shocky patients, where imbalance will exacerbate or lead to multiple organ dysfunction. Effective management of shock depends on the application of this understanding of the ANS in order to reduce injury and promote therapeutic interventions towards improved patient outcomes, particularly for critically ill patients. (McClave *et al.*, 2016; Zeppenfeld *et al.*, 2022) (Figure 5.9).

5.2.3. Hormonal Changes During Shock

The physiological reaction to shock is characterized by dramatic hormonal alterations with the goal of restoring homeostasis and protecting vital organ function. In reaction to shock, the body engages the hypothalamic-pituitary-adrenal (HPA) axis, leading to elevated release of cortisol and other stress hormones. This response is important because cortisol increases glucose availability for energy, inhibits inflammatory responses, and regulates the immune response, thus seeking to avoid further injury to tissues. Hormonal changes also affect the sympathetic nervous system, stimulating the release of catecholamines such as adrenaline and noradrenaline, which accelerate heart rate and vascular resistance to counteract hypotension. In children, these endocrine adjustments are particularly important due to their distinct metabolic requirements during trauma, as noted in the evidence regarding pediatric burn care, highlighting the explanation of hormonal alteration to inform successful therapies (Pelizzo *et al.*, 2025). Also, the interaction of hormone levels and disease states, such as in psoriasis, is indicative of the delicate balance required for recuperation at its optimum during periods of shock (Cassalia *et al.*, 2025) (Figure 5.10).

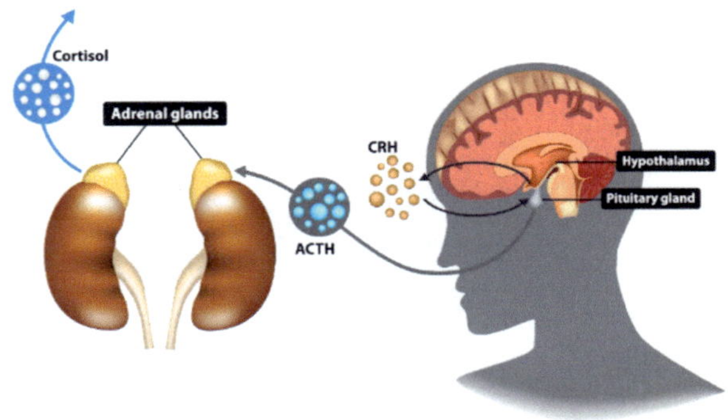

Figure 5.10. Hypothalamic-pituitary-adrenal (HPA) axis.

Source: https://www.simplypsychology.org/wp-content/uploads/hpa_axis.jpg.

5.2.4. Impact on Cardiovascular System

The impact of shock on the cardiovascular system is profound and intricate, and it plays a significant role in contributing to morbidity and mortality rates among the victims. In the state of shock, either hypovolemic, cardiogenic, or septic, the body experiences a cascade of hemodynamic changes that lead to a reduction in cardiac output and compromised tissue perfusion. This state not only raises the heart rate in an attempt to maintain blood circulation but also triggers compensatory mechanisms that can ultimately be detrimental, such as systemic vasodilation of septic shock, which potentially results in severe hypotension and organ damage. Evidence has shown that conditions like COVID-19 worsen shock states, leading to complications such as venous thromboembolism that further impair cardiovascular function and lead to increased mortality (Wichmann, 2020). Erectile dysfunction has also been established as a risk marker for underlying cardiovascular disease (Burnett *et al.*, 2018), showing ubiquitous relationships between shock states and cardiovascular status (Figure 5.11).

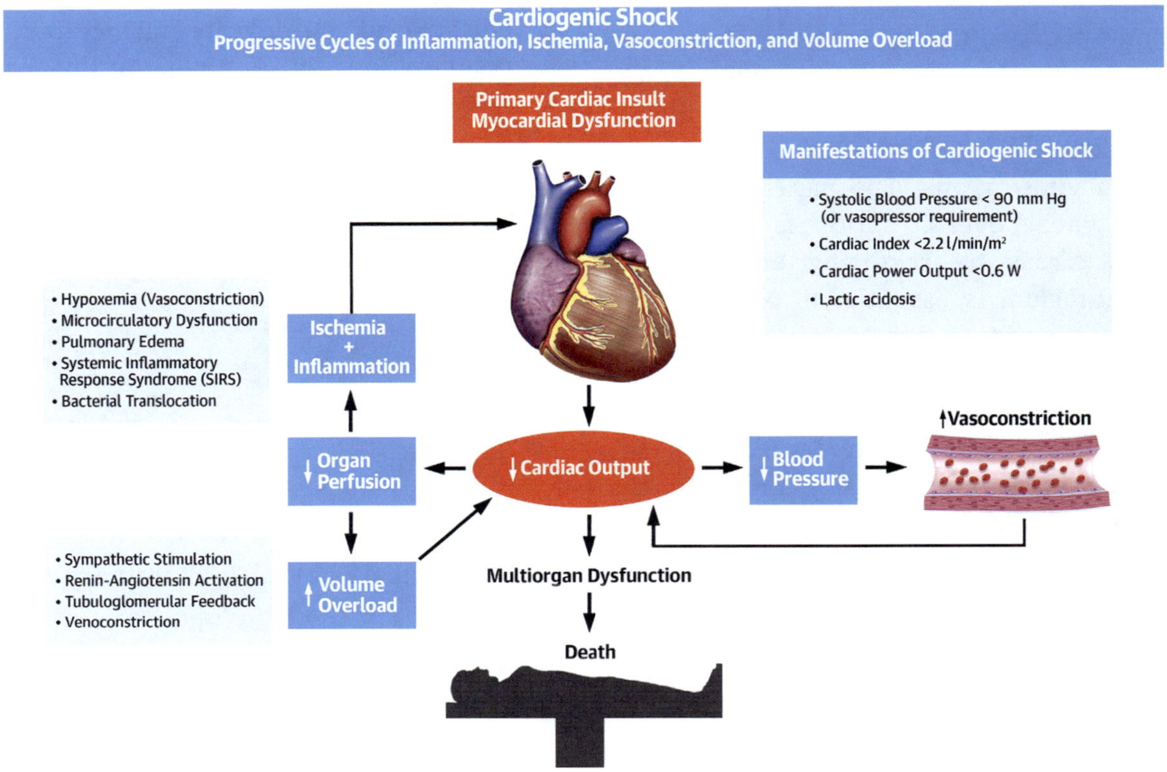

Figure 5.11. Pathophysiology of cardiogenic shock.

Source: https://ars.els-cdn.com/content/image/1-s2.0-S2213177920305138-gr1.jpg.

5.2.5. Effects on Respiratory Function

In shock management, effects on respiratory function are multifaceted and critically significant. Cardiogenic shock patients may have widely differing levels of respiratory distress and need variable treatment with direct consequences for outcome. Accrual evidence indicates disparate modalities of respiratory assistance with different consequences for patient survival, especially in intensive care settings. It has been observed that non-invasive ventilation (NIV) is linked with improved survival in well-weighed patients in comparison to invasive mechanical ventilation (IMV) which, on the other hand, is often linked with poorer mortality (Tavecchia *et al.*, 2024). ECMO is increasingly used for severe respiratory failure, but long-term pulmonary function following ECMO treatment is not markedly superior to in conventionally treated patients (Wang *et al.*, 2024). Therefore, optimization and understanding of the respiratory support strategy are essential to effective shock management and patient prognoses (Figure 5.12).

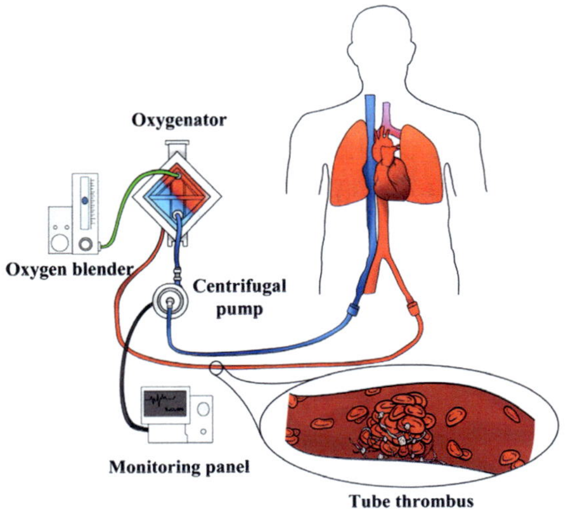

Figure 5.12. Extracorporeal membrane oxygenation (ECMO).

Source: https://www.researchgate.net/profile/Wei-Tong-16/publication/372196708/figure/fig1/AS:11431281175616740@1689836926458/Extracorporeal-Membrane-Oxygenation-ECMO-is-composed-of-five-parts-a-centrifugal-pump.png.

5.2.6. Metabolic Changes

During shock management, understanding the related metabolic changes is significant in treatment and patient outcomes. During shock, the body responds to perfusion deficiency by initiating a chain of metabolic responses to support the function of vital organs. This is best seen in burn patients, wherein the stress of injury induces hypermetabolism characterized by increased oxygen consumption and raised caloric needs, and requires strict observation of fluid resuscitation and nutrition therapy (Alwahbi *et al.*, 2024). Further, disturbances of the metabolic pathways also manifest in various forms, such as increased catecholamine release and disturbances in glucose metabolism, making the clinical presentation complex. Insects, being poikilotherms, are a fascinating analogue, as their metabolic rates adjust with environmental temperature, with the inference that metabolic plasticity is a widespread biological theme in different species under stress (Kumar *et al.*, 2024). Understanding these metabolic adjustments is crucial for effectively designing shock management interventions.

5.2.7. Neurological Implications

The neurologic effects of shock are ominous, as the brain is very vulnerable to the changes in systemic flow and oxygenation that characterize the condition. During shock bursts, particularly hemorrhagic or septic shock, cerebral perfusion may become compromised, leading to a cascade of cell injury by an inadequate delivery of oxygen and nutrients.

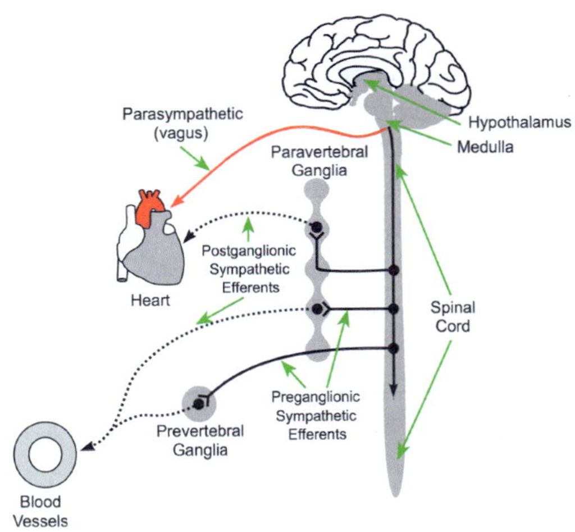

Figure 5.13. Neurological implications of shock.

Source: https://media.springernature.com/lw685/springer-static/image/prt%3A978-3-642-00418-6%2F14/MediaObjects/978-3-642-00418-6_14_Part_Fig1-480_HTML.gif.

Such a deficit may result in cognitive dysfunction, loss of consciousness, and even permanent neurological sequelae. Recent data show the importance of early intervention in patients with severe shock states, where recognition and correction of coagulopathy are crucial in the preservation of neurological function. For instance, the Surviving Sepsis Campaign identifies that immediate hemodynamic support may decrease risk of brain injury (Alhazzani *et al.*, 2020). Furthermore, traumatic injury management guidelines of major bleeding consider that early, individualized treatment strategies are needed to optimize neurological outcomes (Spahn *et al.*, 2019). As such, neurological considerations must be included in shock management guidelines (Figure 5.13).

5.2.8. Long-Term Physiological Consequences

The long-term physiological consequences of shock are profoundly embedded, spanning across various organ systems and overall well-being. During shock, particularly hypovolemic or septic shock, the resultant acute stress has been found to trigger a cascade of cellular function-altering metabolic pathways and inhibiting recovery (Galluzzi *et al.*, 2018). Such interruption manifests in the form of prolonged inflammatory processes and potential long-term organ dysfunction, significantly increasing morbidity in trauma patients. Research has established that the relationship between effective shock control and prevention of such long-term outcomes is vital; therefore, ongoing preoccupation with bleeding and coagulopathy management in trauma patients has become a priority (Rossaint *et al.*, 2016). Understanding these consequences underscores the imperative to focus not only on short-term survival of patients but also on recovery patterns, identifying that shock management is the key to preventing future long-term illness. Thus, the implications of shock go much beyond initial treatment, infusing a value on comprehensive care plans.

5.2.9. Recovery Processes

When it comes to the management of shock, how the processes of recovery are done is of utmost importance, particularly in vulnerable populations such as the elderly. Recovery from severe conditions such as sepsis is not only immediate medical treatment but also understanding the long-term implications for such patients. As mentioned earlier, elderly patients are liable to sudden deterioration in the functions of major organs, necessitating intensive treatments and intensive analysis of their physiological problems (Karcioglu *et al.*, 2022). The healing processes should also involve organizational interventions that consider environmental shocks impacting care delivery. For instance, public agencies must distinguish between anticipated and unanticipated shocks, employing proactive recovery measures that fuel performance and resilience in a time of crisis (Hawes *et al.*, 2020). An equal focus on patient recovery at the individual level and organizational preparedness at the system level is thus essential to good shock management, rendering care immediate as well as enduring.

Test Your Knowledge

1. How does the autonomic nervous system contribute to the shock response?
2. What hormonal changes occur during shock, and how do they affect the cardiovascular system?

5.3. Shock Management Techniques

Learning Outcome

1. Define immediate first aid measures
2. Understand the fluid resuscitation strategies
3. Discuss medications used in shock management
4. Explain the surgical interventions
5. Understand the monitoring vital signs
6. Analyze the psychological support for patients
7. Describe the role of emergency services
8. Identify the importance of training and preparedness

Effective shock management approaches are necessary to mitigate the adverse effects of various types of shocks, such as socio-economic crises, natural disasters, and health emergencies. For instance, in the context of food security, the COVID-19 pandemic has exposed local food systems' vulnerabilities, particularly for low and middle-income countries. Evidence shows that lockdown measures drastically eroded income and purchasing power, raising food insecurity in the vulnerable populations (Béné, 2020). Resilience can be strengthened by a strategic framework focusing on collaborative action. Using collective objectives and cross-sector partnerships, stakeholders can address the complexities of global issues more effectively (George *et al.*, 2016). Also, encouraging the adoption of specific interventions can empower communities and policy-makers so that they can withstand subsequent shocks even as they encourage sustainable behavior in local systems. Thus, integrating these techniques not only solves immediate problems but also enhances the overall resilience of impacted sectors.

5.3.1. Immediate First Aid Measures

Within the context of shock treatment, initial first aid is the key to stabilizing the patient and avoiding further compounding of the illness. Successful interventions start with maintaining an open airway and positioning the patient so as to be comfortable, usually lying down with the legs raised to facilitate circulation to the vital organs. The supply of oxygen can ease the symptoms of hypoxia and is especially useful in the case of shock caused by respiratory distress. According to Fišer *et al.* (2024), identification of the shock category is important for tailored first aid because it informs subsequent steps, such as the administration of bronchodilators in asthma or stopping lethal bleeding in traumatic accidents. Further, public education on first aid interventions is needed, particularly for scenarios of accidents due to products like aluminum phosphide, where timely intervention lessens dire outcomes to health (Nada *et al.*, 2024). All these steps form the foundation of effective shock control in cases of emergencies.

5.3.2. Fluid Resuscitation Strategies

Fluid resuscitation methods are of prime importance in effective shock management, particularly in hemorrhagic shock when rapid action is of utmost necessity. Restoration of hemodynamic stability is the primary focus through immediate correction of blood loss and optimal enhancement of cardiac output. Methods such as titrated hypotensive resuscitation and damage control surgery acknowledge the importance of assessing the patient's response to fluid administration because careful observation is most likely to prevent aggravation of ischemia and subsequent multiorgan failure. The point is that until bleeding has been controlled, the rest of the resuscitative measures may be futile; thus, fluid replacement must be accomplished with caution. Studies also highlight gaining knowledge on the physiological classification of shock, as this guides practitioners to tailor treatment to individual cases, making prospects for good outcomes in critically ill patients with the potentially fatal disease (Bonanno, 2022; World Health Organization, 2020) (Figure 5.14).

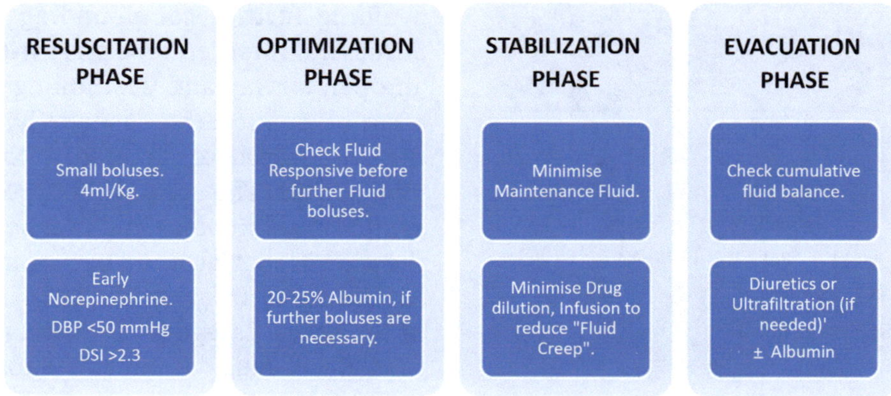

Figure 5.14. Fluid management in septic shock.

Source: https://media.springernature.com/lw685/springer-static/image/chp%3A10.1007%2F978-3-031-42205-8_14/MediaObjects/475156_1_En_14_Fig2_HTML.png.

5.3.3. Medications Used in Shock Management

Shock management involves the nuanced administration of drugs depending on the nature and etiology of shock, either septic, cardiogenic, hypovolemic, or anaphylactic. Fluid resuscitation is performed as a first treatment to restore circulation and perfusion. Subsequently, vasopressors like norepinephrine are applied in order to raise blood pressure by causing vasoconstriction of vessels, something that is necessary in septic shock, where there is excessive vascular dilation. In cardiogenic shock, inotropic therapy such as dobutamine may augment the cardiac output and thereby enhance perfusion at the end-organ level. Glucocorticoids may also be employed in septic shock to reverse adrenal insufficiency and promote hemodynamic stability. The choice of drug must be individualized to the patient based on consideration of drug-drug interactions and the pathophysiology of the illness, as illustrated in revised clinical guidelines emphasizing a stepwise approach to medication in the management of shock (Burnett *et al.*, 2018).

5.3.4. Surgical Interventions

Surgical interventions are categorically necessary in the treatment of all forms of shock, particularly where medical intervention is not sufficient. In cases of increased intracranial pressure (ICP), availing neurosurgical interventions such as decompressive craniectomy depends on the failure of medical treatment, perhaps at the expense of substantial risks such as hypotension and cardiovascular complications (Lin *et al.*, 2025). Current studies highlight the fine type of strategy to be followed in such situations where prompt surgical intervention can lead to improved results, particularly in traumatic brain injury and other neurosurgical disorders. Even with abdominal echinococcosis, laparoscopic surgery is a useful procedure, lowering postoperative morbidity but needing a judicious technique to prevent such complications as cyst rupture and subsequent anaphylactic shock (Slavu *et al.*, 2024). Thus, the strategic application of surgical interventions in the management of shock accentuates the need for personalized care planning that takes both short-term needs and long-term patient health into account.

5.3.5. Monitoring Vital Signs

Vital signs monitoring is vital in shock management since it provides instant feedback regarding a patient's physiological status and guides the direction of therapy. Criterions such as heart rate, blood pressure, respiratory rate, and oxygen saturation are essential indicators of hemodynamic stability and can represent the trajectory or resolution of shock. For instance, the early decline in blood pressure may be a predictor of septic shock development, to which fluid resuscitation and possible vasopressor treatment would need to be initiated immediately (Medeiros *et al.*, 2017). Furthermore, constant monitoring of these parameters allows medical professionals to initiate timely interventions, enhancing patient outcomes during critical conditions. Educational simulations also confirm the requirement for early identification of essential signs in emergencies via demonstration of short-term impacts of early interventions upon survival rates under such conditions as hemorrhagic shock (Tarver *et al.*, 2021). Thus, systematic and vigilant monitoring of vital signs becomes a natural component of effective shock management methods (Figure 5.15).

Sign	What It Means
Increased Pulse	Body increasing cardiac output
Pale, Cool, Moist Skin	Increased vascular tone; blood moved away from skin to vital organs
Nausea	Reduced blood to the gut
Increased Respirations	Maximizing oxygenation, reducing acidosis
Altered Mental Status	Brain feeling the affects of hypoxia/reduced circulation

Figure 5.15. Identify the shock.

Source: https://limmereducation.com/article/vital-sign-trends-in-shock.

5.3.6. Psychological Support for Patients

Psychological treatment of shock patients forms an important aspect of integral shock management. As the patient undergoes the psychological stress associated with sudden medical crises, physical and mental well-being should also be treated with equal concern by healthcare providers. Anxiety, fear, and confusion can aggravate the physical symptoms of shock and hence, disrupt recovery. Evidence shows that specifically tailored psychological interventions could go some way toward mitigating such affective burdens, maintaining resilience, and reinforcing coping mechanisms (Zeppenfeld *et al.*, 2022). Furthermore, during global health emergencies such as the COVID-19 outbreak, patients' psychological stress has been exacerbated, and there is a great necessity for a healthy support system within the healthcare setting to counteract these problems (Chen *et al.*, 2020). By integrating psychological support into shock management procedures, doctors not only maximize the overall treatment of their patients but also establish a friendly atmosphere that facilitates body recovery while emphasizing the body-mind connection in the recovery process

5.3.7. Role of Emergency Services

Emergency services are tasked with the job of effectively treating shock, a potentially life-threatening condition in need of immediate care. The ability of emergency medical technicians (EMTs) and paramedics to rapidly evaluate and respond is crucial, particularly in stressful situations where seconds count. Through the implementation of interventions such as the "proximity response" principle, emergency services are able to position equipment closer to areas where demand is greatest, thus reducing response times significantly (Teng *et al.*, 2024). Moreover, during behavioral health emergencies, EMS ought to possess clearly established protocols for effective and safe care. The total initiatives set forth, such as process maps that detail the response from a 9–1–1 call through hospital transport, emphasize the need for increased integration and standardization of emergency protocols (Cheung *et al.*, 2024). Lastly, the enhancement of emergency services not only optimizes the management of shock but also fosters a more effective health system capable of responding adaptively to diverse exigent health needs.

5.3.8. Importance of Training and Preparedness

Integrated management of shock calls for effective readiness and training mechanisms that are vital in minimizing risks during an emergency. Hazardous environments, such as offshore oil platforms, are model cases for constant training aimed at guaranteeing robust safety protocols, as mentioned in Aderamo *et al.* (2024). Training that involves virtual reality simulations of crisis scenarios equips staff with the skills to respond as needed in the event of an emergency, thereby reducing human error and enhancing decision-making processes. In addition, integration of new technologies such as real-time data analysis and surveillance systems can enhance response efficacy, as argued in Soyege *et al.* (2024). By encouraging a culture of preparedness and collaboration among stakeholders, organizations can not only maximize their response capacities on a day-to-day level but also build resilience to address future crises. Ultimately, spending on training and preparedness remains paramount to safeguarding lives and minimizing environmental and economic effects during important incidents.

Test Your Knowledge

1. What are the key strategies for fluid resuscitation in shock patients?
2. Which medications are commonly used in the treatment of various types of shock?

5.4. Psychological Aspects of Shock

Learning Outcome

1. Discuss the emotional responses to shock
2. Understand the coping mechanisms
3. Identify the impact on mental health
4. Describe the role of support systems
5. Analyze the long-term psychological effects
6. Explain the importance of counseling
7. Discuss the strategies for mental resilience
8. Identify the community support initiatives
9. Discuss the research on psychological recovery

Psychological conditions of shock are of relevance to our knowledge of how individuals react to traumatic experiences and cope with the consequent emotional responses. Shock may disrupt mental functioning, inducing states of confusion, apprehension, and even states of indifference to emotions, which, unless properly addressed, may act as obstacles to recovery. Research findings show that such emotional responses typically emanate from the stresses inherent in traumatic experiences, augmented by workplace pressures or interpersonal conflicts, where emotional intelligence is vital in managing responses to these experiences (Gomathi *et al.*, 2024). Furthermore, the interactive dynamics that come into play are able to create complexity layers, especially when in environments where there are generational differences, such that shock perceptions and affective outcomes are different (Оксана Сєдашова *et al.*, 2025). Accordingly, it is necessary that the manager implements measures to create psychological resilience among the team, resulting in the build-up of a support network to enhance shock recovery and management in general.

5.4.1. Emotional Responses to Shock

The shock experience can lead to the most intense emotional responses, which significantly impact the ability of an individual to respond resiliently to the situation. Individuals respond initially in disbelief, numbness, or denial as a manifestation of the psychological defense against the traumatic nature of the shock experienced. As the truth becomes apparent, feelings of anxiety, fear, and anger may arise, making the emotional scenario more complicated and leading to potential long-term psychological effects such as post-traumatic stress disorder (PTSD). The emotional effect may also rely on individual differences, demographics, and prior experience, as suggested in current work and organizational psychology literature (Kniffin *et al.*, 2020). It is imperative to appreciate these emotional responses in shock management, as resilient, supportive interventions can provide resilience and hasten recovery. In addition, the appreciation of the potential for varied emotional experience enables health professionals to tailor their approach to meet the varied needs of the affected (McClave *et al.*, 2016) (Figure 5.16).

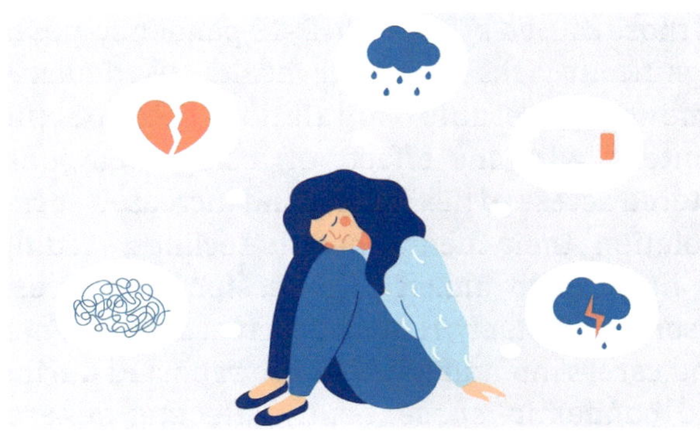

Figure 5.16. Post-traumatic stress disorder.

Source: https://www.teachermagazine.com/assets/images/teacher/Understanding-PTSD.jpg.

5.4.2. Coping Mechanisms

Coping styles form a critical component of shock management to enable individuals to adjust to unforeseen and generally disruptive incidents. Various coping strategies emerge as crucial to ensure psychological hardiness; among these are self-empowering coping styles, social support, and emotional trigger identification. Research indicates that personal coping mechanisms such as mindfulness and time management can effectively minimize stress reactions to shocking events. Further, social connectedness encourages the sense of belongingness and support that can cushion feelings typically associated with trauma (Shalini, 2024). The increasing mental health conversation on social media like TikTok illustrates how people share different coping mechanisms and validate one another's experiences, hence further legitimizing common issues with shock and anxiety (Balcıoğlu, 2024). Thus, education and promoting effective coping strategies not only enhance personal well-being but also form community resilience during times of crisis, emphasizing their pivotal role in effective shock management.

5.4.3. Impact on Mental Health

The impact of economic and social shocks, such as those caused by the COVID-19 pandemic, poses significant risks to mental health, particularly among vulnerable populations. As people contend with the effects of losing their jobs, altered access to healthcare, and increased social isolation, their mental health declines, leading to heightened anxiety, depression, and stress disorders. Notably, reported increases in parents' and carers' mental illness were reported during the pandemic, subsequently affecting general emotional family environments and negative effect on children's developmental outcomes (Yoshikawa *et al.*, 2020). The incorporation of robust human resource management approaches that encourage employee psychological well-being has been shown to enhance job satisfaction and productivity (Azizi *et al.*, 2021). Therefore, addressing the psychological effects of such shocks is imperative not just for individuals' recovery but also in creating healthy communities that could emerge and thrive after the crisis (Figure 5.17).

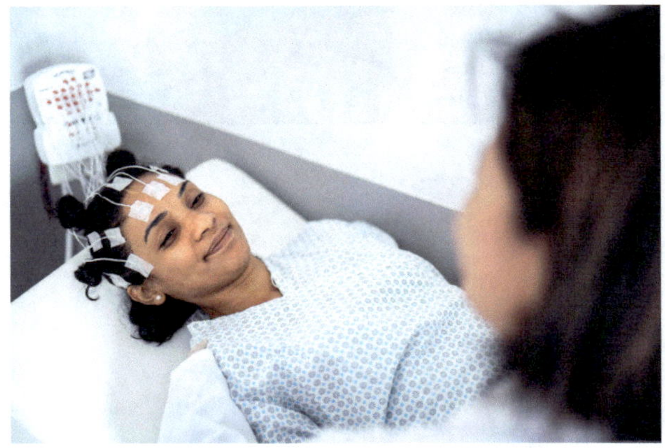

Figure 5.17. Impact on Mental Health

Source: https://www.health.com/thmb/GeTzCPEayBN5xGT4JffdLWvrctw=/6000x0/filters:no_upscale():max_bytes(150000):strip_icc()/health-GettyImages-1361394500-82a94788291447dca5744bf7a0479d18.jpg.

5.4.4. Role of Support Systems

In shock management, support systems play a very significant role in recovery and resilience. Support systems range from informal networks of relatives and friends to institutionalized agencies that provide emotional and psychological support. The necessity for a support system becomes even more paramount in high-stress scenarios, like the responses of healthcare workers during crisis like the COVID-19 pandemic. Evidence shows that supportive peers assist healthcare workers in managing the emotional pressures of their role, reducing the likelihood of burnout and improving patient care quality (Dewey *et al.*, 2020). Broad support networks may also include resources for adaptive coping capabilities, which are essential shock management elements (Intergovernmental Panel on Climate Change, 2023). By combining many forms of support, individuals are able to reconcile with the complexity in shock, and a successful response to adversity becomes possible along with long-term psychological health.

5.4.5. Long-Term Psychological Effects

The enduring psychological impact of trauma plays a significant role in the management of shock because these aspects have a crucial influence on the patterns of recovery. Traumatized patients develop chronic psychological dysregulation in the form of anxiety, depression, and PTSD. These conditions can be exacerbated by the poorly managed distress of the acute phase, and therefore, proper shock management interventions are critical. Methods such as multimodal pain control that incorporate psychological support as well as physical intervention can thwart the possibility of chronic psychological disease developing after trauma (Kim, 2025). In addition, patient education and psychological preparation before operative procedures are increasingly recognized as key to enhancing outcomes and reducing later distress (Choudhury, 2025). These integrative therapies not only allow enhanced physical outcomes but also address the psychological and emotional well-being of patients, demonstrating that holistic shock management needs to deal with both long-term and short-term mental health impacts.

5.4.6. Importance of Counseling

Counselling is also very crucial in the treatment of shock since it is a priceless resource for individuals experiencing the emotional burden of traumatic experiences. The counselling process provides a setting where the victims feel safe to express their emotions and thoughts, which provides a sense of recognition and understanding that they might desperately require. Furthermore, the counseling worked-out therapeutic relationship can enable resilience and coping so that people can more effectively handle their lives. Identity discovery and the intertwining of both offline and online identities, as given in arguments surrounding contemporary social values, are a case in point regarding the demand for counseling in today's complex world of digital technology (Zeppenfeld *et al.*, 2022). Because continued advancements in new technologies like the Metaverse are evolving, counseling access may become even more important in order to address the socio-emotional needs that will continue to arise, continuing to enhance the recovery process for survivors of shock (Park *et al.*, 2022) (Figure 5.18).

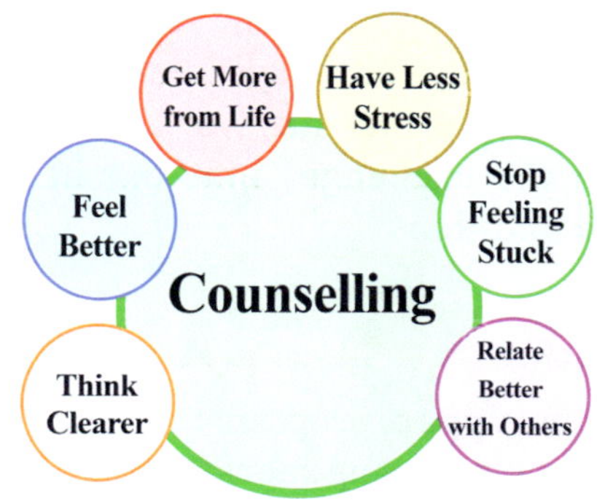
Get More from Life
Have Less Stress
Feel Better
Stop Feeling Stuck
Counselling
Think Clearer
Relate Better with Others

Figure 5.18. Benefits of psychological counseling stock.

Source: https://external-content.duckduckgo.com/iu/?u=https%3A%2F%2Fthumbs.dreamstime.com%2Fz%2Fsix-benefits-psychological-counseling-207731525.jpg&f=1&nofb=1&ipt=60f7f49e69b0f09af68be7c4fa9cc60859fe3cf0cdaf199b8175fe7d95012235.

5.4.7. Strategies for Mental Resilience

Building psychological resilience is essential in effective shock management, particularly in situations of stress. As research indicates, task-oriented coping strategies, which provide for favorable behavioral reactions to stress, are a significant element in building resilience among people exposed to occupational hazards (Koval *et al.*, 2025). Furthermore, incorporating technology-based interventions, such as mobile phone-based resilience training, has been seen to play a vital role in augmenting significant resilience in stress regulation, as evident from research demonstrating enhanced stress management in participants receiving such interventions (Lenger *et al.*, 2025). All these approaches collectively amount to an active process of self-regulation and emotional self-control needed to manage the complexities of stressful problems. Besides, organizations have to lead in creating a psychologically safe workplace through extended support structures and strength training. Although this action helps individuals adapt to current sources of stress, it also builds long-term psychological resilience and flexibility so that the workers are able to deal with the challenges inherent in stressful working conditions.

5.4.8. Community Support Initiatives

Community support programs are also the most important for managing shocks. Under conditions of economic uncertainty and social openness, these programs offer basic resources and services that enhance capacities for resilience towards all types of shocks, such as economic crises or natural disasters. Programs to empower ultra-micro debtors demonstrate the efficacy of the same as they focus on entrepreneurial skill building, financial capability, and access to technology, which ultimately sustain local economic resilience (Kurniawati *et al.*, 2025). Additionally, an integrated approach consisting of the mobilization of financial resources and adaptive governance can significantly promote household stability during adverse times. The strategy guarantees that projects remain flexible and adaptive to changing needs, optimizing the utilization of resources as well as enhancing community contribution to monitoring and evaluation (Karyeija *et al.*, 2025). Collectively, all these interventions impose a critical focus on community-led solutions as an aspect for curtailing shocks' effects as well as guaranteeing long-term socio-economic resilience.

5.4.9. Research on Psychological Recovery

The role of psychological recovery in managing shock cannot be overstated as it is a core element of integrated rehabilitation for patients who have been subjected to traumatic trauma. Research has established that patients who are recovering from severe psychological stressors such as medical emergencies or natural disasters present similar symptoms of anxiety, depression, and posttraumatic stress disorder, which require targeted intervention to recover and become resilient. Effective psychological recovery strategies include cognitive-behavioral therapy, mindfulness, and structured peer support systems, which are shown to decrease emotional distress and support adaptive coping styles. Besides, in the present pandemic, the psychological impacts of the COVID-19 tragedy have further emphasized the need for immediate psychological services in terms of psychological state recovery, as with more vulnerability due to seclusion and fear of the disease, individuals require effective psychological recovery measures in comprehensive shock management approaches (Zeppenfeld *et al.*, 2022; Zhao *et al.*, 2020).

Test Your Knowledge

1. What emotional responses are commonly observed in patients who experience shock?
2. How do coping mechanisms and support systems influence recovery from shock?

SUMMARY

In general, effective shock management calls for a comprehensive understanding of the pathophysiology underlying it and the use of evidence-based practice. With the increasing prevalence of disabling illness from shock, as highlighted by the increasing years lived with disease for the said major depressive disorder and iron-deficiency anemia (Vos *et al.*, 2017), the healthcare system must act to meet the increasing demand for skills. Furthermore, fresh definitions of sepsis and septic shock call for an emphasis on early identification and treatment, and ultimately aim to reduce mortality caused by these life-threatening syndromes (Singer *et al.*, 2016). In incorporating interprofessional approaches and tapping into developments in diagnostic criteria, patient outcomes can be radically improved. Thus, the focus will have to continue being placed on research, education, and optimization of clinical practice guidelines in order to improve the treatment of shock and complications thereof within diverse clinical settings.

Successful management of shock entails various strategies in restoring hemodynamic stability and enhancing patient outcomes. Central to such management is fluid and vasopressor therapy, particularly in septic shock, where inappropriately administered fluid resuscitation has been known to precipitate further complications. Dynamic measurements, such as the stroke volume response to passive leg raise, have been shown to have significant advantages over conventional fluid management protocols. Research confirms that application of these dynamic measures results in decreased net fluid balance, decreased renal replacement therapy rates, and decreased mechanical ventilation rates, ultimately improving chances of survival in shock patients (Douglas *et al.*, 2020). More specifically, guidelines encourage personalized fluid resuscitation care to be adjusted to fit the specific demands of each patient for greater therapeutic effectiveness (Ponikowski *et al.*, 2016). Therefore, incorporating sophisticated monitoring methods and customized fluid management can significantly affect the clinical outcome in shock care.

KEY TERMS FROM THIS CHAPTER

Anaphylactic shock	Blood products	Cardiogenic shock
Colloids	Crystalloids	Distributive shock
Dobutamine	Dopamine	Epinephrine
Fluid resuscitation	Hypovolemic shock	Inotropes
Lactic acidosis	Neurogenic shock	Norepinephrine
Obstructive shock	Perfusion	Phenylephrine

CRITICAL THINKING QUESTIONS

1. Which of the following is the first-line treatment for hypovolemic shock?

a. Vasopressors
b. Blood transfusion only
c. Rapid administration of intravenous crystalloids
d. High-dose corticosteroids

2. In septic shock, which vasopressor is considered the first-line agent to restore adequate perfusion?

a. Dopamine
b. Epinephrine
c. Vasopressin
d. Norepinephrine

3. What is the most reliable clinical sign of shock?

a. Bradycardia
b. Low urine output
c. Cyanosis
d. Warm extremities

4. Which type of shock is characterized by elevated central venous pressure (CVP) and jugular venous distension (JVD)?

a. Hypovolemic shock
b. Cardiogenic shock
c. Neurogenic shock
d. Septic shock

5. In the management of anaphylactic shock, the drug of choice is:

a. Diphenhydramine
b. Hydrocortisone
c. Epinephrine
d. Salbutamol

Short Answer Questions

1. What are the four main types of shock, and how do they differ in pathophysiology?
2. What are the classic signs and symptoms of shock across all types, and how can they help with early diagnosis?
3. How does cellular hypoperfusion contribute to lactic acidosis in shock states?
4. What is the role of serum lactate in diagnosing and monitoring shock, and what are the limitations of this marker?
5. Why is early recognition and treatment critical in shock management?

Answer to Critical Thinking Questions

1. (c); 2. (d); 3. (b); 4. (b); 5. (c)

REFERENCES

1. Adebisi, O., Afolabi, O. B., Adekanye, E. A., Aderukuola, B., Lawal, F., Akinyoade, A. R., & Odiegwu, T. I. (2025). A critical review of non-pneumatic anti-shock garment utilization in Nigerian healthcare space: Challenges, strategies and prospects to scale-*up uptake. International Journal of Clinical Obstetrics and* Gynecology. https://www.semanticscholar.org/paper/9d24d5171980e66b592fe8ac17872a9246bde7da (accessed on 22 May 2025).

2. Aderamo, A. T., Chukwuemeka, H., Olisakwe, Y. A., Adebayo, Y. A., & Esiri, A. E. (2024). Conceptualizing emergency preparedness in offshore operations: A sustainable model for crisis m*anagement. Engineering Science & Technol*ogy Journal. https://www.semanticscholar.org/paper/c29e1a6abfdeeb78c7fe4a7e61709dc1eb77b4c4 (accessed on 22 May 2025).

3. Alhazzani, W., Møller, M. H., Arabi, Y. M., Loeb, M., Gong, M. N., Fan, E., Oczk*owski,* S., et al. (2020). Surviving Sepsis Campaign: Guidelines on the management of critically ill adults with Coronavirus Disease 2019 (*COVID-19). Intensive Care M*edicine, 46(5), 854–887. https://doi.org/10.1007/s00134-020-06022-5.

4. Ali, M., Pham, A., Wang, X., Wolfram, J., & Pham, S. M. (2020). Extracellular vesicles for treatment of solid organ ischemia–reperfusi*on injury. American Journal of Transpla*ntation, 20(11), 3294–3307. https://doi.org/10.1111/ajt.16164.

5. Alwahbi, K. N., Alharbi, N. L. S., Almutairi, F. M. M., Alshammari, M., Alharbi, W. S., Aldhafeeri, M. M. M., Alharbi, *Y. F.* F., et al. (2024). Anesthesia for patients with burns: An updated review for anesthesiologists an*d nursing. Journal of E*co Humanism. https://www.semanticscholar.org/paper/c43bbec0139914157dbe4b1de2818ccbafc65deb (accessed on 22 May 2025).

6. Amankwah, J. F., Jin, W., Ma, X., Xu, P., Wen, H., Amuneke, K. E., Mungan*ga, B.* P., et al. (2025). Salinity tolerance in freshw*ater drum (Aplodinotu*s grunniens): Investigating biochemical, antioxidant, digestive enzyme, and gene expression responses to acute salini*ty stress.* Animals, 15. https://www.semanticscholar.org/paper/1cbbff233000307ba75d0afecc79913319da6c01 (accessed on 22 May 2025).

7. Azizi, M. R., Atlasi, R., Ziapour, A., Abbas, J., & Naemi, R. (2021). Innovative human resource management strategies during the COVID-19 pandemic: A systematic narrative review *approach.* Heliyon, 7, e07233. https://doi.org/10.1016/j.heliyon.2021.e07233.

8. Balcıoğlu, Y. S. (2024). Anxiety management strategies on TikTok: A discourse analysis of collective coping m*echanisms. Journal of Me*ntal Health. https://www.semanticscholar.org/paper/8ba093dbe38f256b17e12bd196f2c65834a57e25 (accessed on 22 May 2025).

9. Bhatti, U. F., Dawood, Z., Shang, Z., Jin, G., Liggett, M. R., Chtraklin, K., Liu, B., et al. (2024). Testing neuroprotective strategies in prolong*ed field care mod*el of traumatic brain injury and hemorrhagic shock. Journal of the American College of Surgeons. https://www.semanticscholar.org/paper/b4361b*45f82*47ba90e048edb4c9c1034d4254110 (accessed on 22 May 2025).

10. Bonanno, F. (2022). Management of hemorrhagic shock: Physiology appr*oach, timing and strategies. Journal of Cli*nical Medicine, 12, 260. https://www.semanticscholar.org/paper/83cbe4eca67af17e195b8fed5ed8e606ea752be6 (accessed on 22 May 2025).

11. Bryant, R. A. (2019). Post-traumatic stress disorder: A state-of-the-art r*eview of evidence and challenges.* World Psychiatry, 18(3), 259–269. https://doi.org/10.1002/wps.20656.

12. Burnett, A. L., Nehra, A., Breau, R. H., Culkin, D. J., Faraday, M. M., Hakim, L., Heidelbaugh, J. J., et al. (2018). Erectile dysfunction: AUA guideli*ne. The Journal of* Urology, 200, 633–641. https://doi.org/10.1016/j.juro.2018.05.004.

13. Béné, C. (2020). Resilience of local food systems and links to food security–A review *of so*me important concepts in the context of COVID-*19 and other shocks. Food S*ecurity, 12, 805–822. https://doi.org/10.1007/s12571-020-01076-1.

14. Cassalia, A., Lunardon, G., Frattin, G., Danese, A., Caroppo, F., & Fortina, A. B. (2025). How hormonal balance changes lives in women with *psoriasis. Journal of Clinical M*edicine, 14. https://www.semanticscholar.org/paper/4a4bfb0e8ef3874e0b8a27138e6b3c376513d16a (accessed on 22 May 2025).

15. Chaussy, C., Rassweiler, J. J., Renner, C., Th*üroff,* S., et al. (2001). Treatment of renal stones by extracorporeal shockwave lithotripsy–An update. https://core.ac.uk/download/16432642.pdf (accessed on 22 May 2025).

16. Chen, S. C., Lai, Y. H., & Tsay, S. L. (2020). Nursing perspectives on the impacts of *COVID-19. Journal of Nursing R*esearch, 28(3), e85. https://doi.org/10.1097/jnr.0000000000000389.

17. Chen, X., Li, Z., Zou, L., Lan, Y., Wu, X., & Wang, H. (2025). Spontaneous retroperitoneal hematoma after COVID-19 infection: A ca*se report. Me*dicine, 104(1). https://www.semanticscholar.org/paper/3438635c03859da3085f52ca5ef6a3ac2dc79e21 (accessed on 22 May 2025).

18. Cheung, E. H., Whitfield, D., Kipust, A., Tadeo, R., & Gausche-Hill, M. (2024). Advancing emergency medical services' (EMS) response capability for behavioral health emergencies: Los Angeles County's performance improvement i*nitiative. Prehospital Eme*rgency Care. https://www.semanticscholar.org/paper/544fb61620674004f918e712b27b113ff32d9b1f (accessed on 22 May 2025).

19. Choudhury, R. D. (2025). The role of the LCHF diet in weight management: Mechanisms and long-term susta*inability. Asian Journal of Basic Science* & Research. https://www.semanticscholar.org/paper/2d2d4bf1c7adb3fcaf5e4d73c53399449734539f (accessed on 22 May 2025).

20. Creswell, D. (2016). Mindfulness inte*rventions. Annual Review of Psy*chology, 68, 491–516. https://doi.org/10.1146/annurev-psych-042716-051139.

21. Crispino, S. P., Segreti, A., Nafisio, V., Ciancio, M., Cavallari, I., Giannone, S., *Melfi,* R., et al. (2025). Tailoring pharmacological treatment in cardiogenic shock: A narrati*ve review. Discovery M*edicine, 37(193), 222–243. https://www.semanticscholar.org/paper/2ce29d39cb53f20ccfe2146d1b2676a8030e4227 (accessed on 22 May 2025).

22. Dewey, C. M., Hingle, S., Goelz, E., & Linzer, M. (2020). Supporting clinicians during the COVID-19 *pandemic. Annals of Internal Me*dicine, 172, 752–753. https://doi.org/10.7326/m20-1033.

23. Douglas, I. S., Alapat, P., Corl, K., Exline, M. C., Forni, L. G., Holder, A. L., Kaufm*an, D.* A., et al. (2020). Fluid response evaluation in sepsis hypotension *and shock.* Chest, 158, 1431–1445. https://doi.org/10.1016/j.chest.2020.04.025.

24. Fišer, Z., & Bokan, D. (2024). Guidelines 2021: Changes in guidelines for first aid *measures. Journal Resuscitati*o Balcanica. https://www.semanticscholar.org/paper/1ded085e59a4ce781e9a80f73606bca7f24aeba3 (accessed on 22 May 2025).

25. Fouda, M., Negm, A., Germoush, M., & Mahmoud, S. (2025). Temperature and Spinosad-induced modulation of antioxidant enzyme activity and gene expression of adaptive stress-relate*d genes in Ceratit*is *capitata. Open Veterinary* Journal, 15, 108–117. https://www.semanticscholar.org/paper/0a824424863aaabc7da7551f7f6793c873e2128b (accessed on 22 May 2025).

26. Fox, R. A., Rotatori, A. F., & Switzky, H. (1981). Behavioral treatment approaches to obesity: Successes with the nonretarded and retarded. https://core.ac.uk/download/213083518.pdf (accessed on 22 May 2025).

27. Galluzzi, L., Vitale, I., Aaronson, S. A., Abrams, J., Adam, D., Agostinis, P., Alnem*ri, E.* S., et al. (2018). Molecular mechanisms of cell death: Recommendations of the Nomenclature Committee on Cell D*eath 2018. Cell Death and Differen*tiation, 25, 486–541. https://doi.org/10.1038/s41418-017-0012-4.

28. George, G., Howard-Grenville, J., Joshi, A., & Tihanyi, L. (2016). Understanding and tackling societal grand challenges through management *research. Academy of Management* Journal, 59, 1880–1895. https://doi.org/10.5465/amj.2016.4007.

29. Gheblawi, M., Wang, K., Viveiros, A., Nguyen, Q., Zhong, J. C., Turner, A. J., Raiza*da, M.* K., et al. (2020). Angiotensin-converting enzyme 2: SARS-CoV-2 receptor and regulator of the renin-angiotens*in system. Circulation Re*search, 126, 1456–1474. https://doi.org/10.1161/circresaha.120.317015.

30. Gomathi, S., & Rajeswari, A. (2024). Stress management and psychological aspects of workforces–Causes, consequences and management *strategies. GLS KALP: Journal of Multidisciplin*ary Studies. https://www.semanticscholar.org/paper/d80e4995066d5b7cc05f0a66e96f96c9a7a8fffa (accessed on 22 May 2025).

31. Hachem, L. D., Ahuja, C. S., & Fehlings, M. G. (2017). Assessment and management of acute spinal cord injury: From point of injury to rehab*ilitation. Journal of Spinal Cord M*edicine, 40, 665–675. https://doi.org/10.1080/10790268.2017.1329076.

32. Hawes, D. P., & Testa, J. R. (2020). Shocking performance: The effects of anticipated and unanticipated shocks on organizational pe*rformance. Public Administration Qu*arterly, 44, 433–461. https://www.semanticscholar.org/paper/c8e587af62a8b9ba187673c45e5b95c64acbb388 (accessed on 22 May 2025).

33. Hitt, M. A., Arregle, J. L., & Holmes, R. M. (2020). Strategic management theory in a post-pandemic and non-ergo*dic world. Journal of Management* Studies, 58(1), 259–264. https://doi.org/10.1111/joms.12646.

34. Hunter-Manseau, F., Cormier, J., & Pichaud, N. (2024). From molecular to physiological responses: Improved stress tolerance and lo*ngevity in Drosophila m*elanogaster under fluctuating therma*l regimes. The Journal of Experimen*tal Biology. https://www.semanticscholar.org/paper/ca071ec7064b64fb87e51a9cbe0eb3fa579d8b8f (accessed on 22 May 2025).

35. Intergovernmental Panel on Climate Chang*e. (2023). Climate Change 2022–Impacts, Adaptation and Vu*lnerability. https://doi.org/10.1017/9781009325844.

36. Islamy, N., Aziz, M. A., Yonata, A., Lumentut, A. M., Maelissa, M., Khaerunnisa, M., Wi*rawan,* W., et al. (2025). Sepsis and septic shock in *pregnancy. Journal La Me*dihealtico. https://www.semanticscholar.org/paper/7ddc87f0ae9cfbf062b5bd4b727252f6fb66100a (accessed on 22 May 2025).

37. Karcioglu, S., Yılmaz, S., Kılıç, M., Suzer, N. E., Ozbay, S., Tatlıparmak, A. C., & Ayan, M. (2022). Geriatric sepsis in the COVID-19 era: Challenges in diagnosis and m*anagement. International Journal of Pharmaceutical Research and Allie*d Sciences. https://www.semanticscholar.org/paper/f88e5cb00431dc812367c030479fe2937659239f (accessed on 22 May 2025).

38. Karyeija, J., Nyamboga, T. O., & Nyasimi, M. M. (2025). Eradicating household poverty in emerging economies through government change management *strategies. Asian Journal of Economics, Business and* Accounting. https://www.semanticscholar.org/paper/5988a4bc9dff8ee078d836fe4dce21f236430715 (accessed on 22 May 2025).

39. Kim, J. (2023). Current trends and practice patterns for difficult bile duct stones *in Korea. Gut an*d Liver, 17, 349–350. https://www.semanticscholar.org/paper/1ebe27b312040a47ad6e44592f926bfffa20ab0a (accessed on 22 May 2025).

40. Kim, Y. D. (2025). Association between postoperative pain management and long-term patient *outcomes. Journal of the Korean Medical* Association. https://www.semanticscholar.org/paper/bb46f1c64120a483ad1dcee92e42e1a36acdd0fe (accessed on 22 May 2025).

41. Kniffin, K. M., Narayanan, J., Anseel, F., Antonakis, J., Ashford, S. J., Bakker, A. B., Bamberger, P., et al. (2020). COVID-19 and the workplace: Implications, issues, and insights for fut*ure resear*ch and action. American Psychologist, 76, 63–77. https://doi.org/10.1037/amp0000716.

42. Kotani, Y., Ryan, N., Udy, A., & Fujii, T. (2025). Hemodynamic management of septic shock. Burns & Trauma, 13. https://www.se*mantic*scholar.org/paper/4fcd68cca88a41c4cc3b2beb21d587a4c48c4999 (accessed on 22 May 2025).

43. Koval, V., & Pidlu*zhna, S. (2025). Mental r*esilience of employees in hazardous work conditions: Psychoemotional challenges and support strategies. Public Administration and Law Revi*ew. https://www.se*manticscholar.org/paper/f77bdce542a1d50a14c0506ddfb4563b3c23db43 (accessed on 22 May 2025).

44. Kumar, H., Sagar, D., Verma, S., Rajarushi, C., R. J. S., Madhuri, E. V., Godavari, et al. (2024). Heat stress and thermoregulation in insects: Unveiling molecular *and physiological responses in ligh*t of climate change. Journal of Advances in Biology & Biotechnology. https://www.semanticscholar.org/paper/e6d6a0de9bb1c3455d07a17f6838346ffaec0b45 (accessed on 22 May 2025).

45. Kurniawati, A. D.*, Febr*ianti, P., Suryani, S., Rizky, I., & Dewi, N. G. (2025). Empowerment and literacy initiatives to enhance ultra micro debtor classe*s: Strategies for sustainable regional economi*c growth. Jurnal Akuntansi dan Bisnis. https://www.semanticscholar.org/paper/183c42f2b0fed0b727e7f57ee60a2fd058f7ce98 (accessed on 22 May 2025).

46. Kırkan, F., Ulgur, H. S., Comert, S., Erol, C., Yıldırak, M. K., & Ozkan, O. (2022). Management of spontaneous major rectus sheath hematoma in a COVID-19 patient: A case re*port and literature review.* Cureus, 14. https://www.semanticscholar.org/paper/e02273795bfda530aacce3c8e40dbc3bf75b2b68 (accessed on 22 May 2025).

47. Lenger, E., Schönthaler, A., Hantke, A., Dalkner, N., Guggemos, S., Pszeida, M., Mosbach*er, J.* A., et al. (2025). Impact of an app-based resilience training on enhancing stress regulation and menta*l health. Neurops*ychobiology. https://www.semanticscholar.org/paper/955f7e5791c5b8f1e08fd8ce47125c4c506224e3 (accessed on 22 May 2025).

48. Lin, V., Hutchinson, P. J. A., Kolias, A., Robba, C., & Wahlster, S. (2025). Timing of neurosurgical interventions for intracranial hypertension: The intensivists' and neurosurge*ons' view. Current*

*Opinion in Cr*itical Care. https://www.semanticscholar.org/paper/61dc0b0db5515b770505223606341efa82162920 (accessed on 22 May 2025).

49. Lorusso, R., Shekar, K., MacLaren, G., Schmidt, M., Pellegrino, V., Meyns, B., Ha*ft, J.* W., et al. (2021). ELSO interim guidelines for Veno arterial extracorporeal membrane oxygenation in adult cardiac *patients. ASAIO* Journal, 67(8), 827–844. https://doi.org/10.1097/mat.0000000000001510.

50. Mahajna, A., Bolotin, G., & Lorusso, R. (2025). Managing the acute cardiac functional crisis: A comprehensive review of cardiogenic shock management s*trategies. European Heart Journal Supp*lements, 27, iv4–iv11. https://www.semanticscholar.org/paper/2dc79add472c3e50500f6cd07483b113e3d6c869 (accessed on 22 May 2025).

51. Mamalchi, S. A., Matar, M., & Bass, G. A. (2024). Peri-operative strategy in resuscitation of unstable injured surgical patients: *A primer. Postgraduate Medic*al Journal. https://www.semanticscholar.org/paper/a78ffde36579052badf33d4c54742ff2b095a2f2 (accessed on 22 May 2025).

52. McClave, S. A., Taylor, B., Martindale, R. G., Warren, M., Johnson, D. R., Braunschweig, C., McCart*hy, M.* S., et al. (2016). Guidelines for the provision and assessment of nutrition support therapy in the adult critically il*l patient. Journal of Parenteral and Enteral Nu*trition, 40(2), 159–211. https://doi.org/10.1177/0148607115621863.

53. Medeiros, D., Pizarro, C. F., Cardoso, M. P., Ogawa Shibata, A. R., & Troster, E. (2017). Quality: A bridge from guidelines to *practice. Critical Ca*re Medicine. https://www.semanticscholar.org/paper/1aedb5c23eac9ffd682a21b67472b0302817acdb (accessed on 22 May 2025).

54. Nada, M. A. A. A., Elfeky, A. K. E. E., Darweesh, H., Mohamed, F. K. I., Sharif, L., Kandil, F., Elsob*ky, F.* A., et al. (2024). The effect of educational programs on parents' knowledge, behavior, and practices regarding aluminum phosphide poisoning and its first-aid *measures. BMC Ped*iatrics, 24. https://www.semanticscholar.org/paper/0574247ecfabbdc4262cdefc00382d0f710a2103 (accessed on 22 May 2025).

55. Obonyo, N., Raman, S., Suen, J. Y., Peters, K. M., Phan, M., Passmore, M., Bo*uquet,* M., et al. (2024). An ovine septic shock model of live bacterial *infusion. Intensive Care Medicine Expe*rimental, 12. https://www.semanticscholar.org/paper/cf657c027632ead7387e5a69b74f475b5baf207e (accessed on 22 May 2025).

56. Pan, T. C., Chen, Y., & He, B. (2025). Emergency treatment and management strategies for 79 patients involved in a school mass bee sting *incident. ASP Loro Journal of Biomedical and Clinical C*ase Reports. https://www.semanticscholar.org/paper/9a5f37935b707c493f9fb5df4054f290fd085839 (accessed on 22 May 2025).

57. Panagiotakis, I., Strompoula, E., & Dermatas, D. (2025). Review of national contaminated land management frameworks in front of the new EU soil monitoring law era–The case study *of Greece. Integrated Environmental Assessment and Man*agement, 21(1), 152–160. https://www.semanticscholar.org/paper/4af8b3cb4b54993d069e7254d8f9fbbc7e5e4e5e (accessed on 22 May 2025).

58. Park, S., & Kim, Y. G. (2022). A metaverse: Taxonomy, components, applications, and open c*hallenges. IEEE* Access, 10, 4209–4251. https://doi.org/10.1109/access.2021.3140175.

59. Pelizzo, V., Calcaterra, V., Marinaro, M., Baldassarre, P., Canonica, C. P. M., & Zuccotti, G. (2025). Metabolic and hormonal changes in pediatric burn patients: Mechanisms, evidence,

and care *strategies. European Burn* Journal, 6. https://www.semanticscholar.org/paper/bacfd1b3304531bc86c27fdae8bfd4ba2b1ebbdc (accessed on 22 May 2025).

60. Pelliccia, A., Sharma, S., Gati, S., Bäck, M., Börjesson, M., Caselli, S., Coll*et, J.* P., et al. (2020). 2020 ESC Guidelines on sports cardiology and exercise in patients with cardiovascular *disease. European Heart* Journal, 42, 17–96. https://doi.org/10.1093/eurheartj/ehaa605.

61. Pleșca, D., Spătariu, L., Bordei, L., Vlad, P., & Hurduc, V. (2017). OC-54 The role of prevention in food *allergies. Archives of Disease in Chi*ldhood, 102, A20–A21. https://www.semanticscholar.org/paper/ca18e9ce38925a2d07c43c1d248f0a627ec7fa9b (accessed on 22 May 2025).

62. Ponikowski, P., Voors, A. A., Anker, S. D., Bueno, H., Cleland, J. G. F., Coats, A. J. S., *Falk,* V., et al. (2016). 2016 ESC guidelines for the diagnosis and treatment of acute and chronic hear*t failure. European Heart* Journal, 37(27), 2129–2200. https://doi.org/10.1093/eurheartj/ehw128.

63. Rossaint, R., Bouillon, B., Černý, V., Coats, T., Duranteau, J., Fernández-Mondejar, E., Fili*pescu,* D., et al. (2016). The European guideline on management of major bleeding and coagulopathy following trauma: Fourt*h edition. Criti*cal Care, 20. https://doi.org/10.1186/s13054-016-1265-x.

64. Saad, L., Jamal, A., Raza, M. A., Umar, Z., Ahmad, S., Alvi, W., Khatt*ak, L.* Z., et al. (2025). Infective endocarditis in septic shock: Results from an observational multicen*ter study.* Cureus, 17. https://www.semanticscholar.org/paper/bfc7218ccc2b350ed2203bc31f92884b87bd2536 (accessed on 22 May 2025).

65. Shalini, O. (2024). Exploring coping mechanisms: A study on stress management techniques for work*ing women. International Journal of Scientific Research in Engineering and* Management. https://www.semanticscholar.org/paper/9bd8062128eba81ba471b429b6008c130e3b2b5d (accessed on 22 May 2025).

66. Singer, M., Deutschman, C. S., Seymour, C. W., Shankar-Hari, M., Annane, D., Bauer, M., Be*llomo,* R., et al. (2016). The Third International Consensus Definitions for Sepsis and Septic Shock (*Sepsis-3).* JAMA, 315(8), 801–810. https://doi.org/10.1001/jama.2016.0287.

67. Slavu, O., Munteanu, O., Gheorghiță, V., Filipoiu, F., Ursuț, B. M., Tulin, R., *Dima,* I., et al. (2024). Laparoscopic management of abdominal echinococcosis: A technical report on surgical techniques and *outcomes.* Cureus, 16. https://www.semanticscholar.org/paper/2ed7c1a379637783f8aea553fad148e0bd8c333b (accessed on 22 May 2025).

68. Soyege, O. S., Nwokedi, C. N., Tomoh, B. O., Mustapha, A. Y., Mbata, A. O., Balogun, O. D., Fork*uo, A.* Y., et al. (2024). Public health crisis management and emergency preparedness: Strengthening healthcare infrastructure against pandemics and bioterroris*m threats. Journal of Frontiers in Multidisciplinar*y Research. https://www.semanticscholar.org/paper/0c4f2d034945172fd83e46347c17418bccdc4271 (accessed on 22 May 2025).

69. Spahn, D. R., Bouillon, B., Černý, V., Duranteau, J., Filipescu, D., Hunt, B. J., Kom*adina,* R., et al. (2019). The European guideline on management of major bleeding and coagulopathy following trauma: Fift*h edition. Criti*cal Care, 23. https://doi.org/10.1186/s13054-019-2347-3.

70. Starosta, D. (2024). Raised under bad stars: Negotiating a culture of disaster pre*paredness. International Journal of Disaster Risk* Management. https://www.semanticscholar.org/paper/9a2bd1fdd083a6720da89d2c8e76e922e42a4a91 (accessed on 22 May 2025).

71. Tanno, P., & Demoly, P. (2018). How can the World Health Organization's International Classification of Diseases (ICD)-11 change the clinical management of ana*phylaxis? Expert*

*Review of Clinical Imm*unology, 14, 783–786. https://www.semanticscholar.org/paper/d361173785c024f6d23c70cf09bcb07d4b59e088 (accessed on 22 May 2025).

72. Tarver, E., Lerant, A., Orledge, J., Stevens, B., & Jefferson, G. (2021). Tracheoinnominate artery *fistula. Journal of Education & Teaching in Emergency* Medicine, 6, S62–S86. https://www.semanticscholar.org/paper/01985d940f4359d6e19687c01863a2544af672da (accessed on 22 May 2025).

73. Tavecchia, S., Frea, S., De Ferrari, G., Sorini Dini, C., Briani, M., Viola, G., Ber*taina,* M., et al. (2024). Respiratory support modalities in cardiogenic shock: Insights from a prospective multicenter *registry. European Heart Journal: Acute Cardiova*scular Care. https://www.semanticscholar.org/paper/8508881eac085b3452daa1cde899401091d22eb0 (accessed on 22 May 2025).

74. Teng, C., Yu, P., & Liu, L. (2024). A cooperative optimization model and enhanced algorithm for guided strategies in emergency mobile f*acilities. Humanities and Social Sciences Communi*cations, 11, 1–11. https://www.semanticscholar.org/paper/182412bf4f29a5975ce5b42834e7ceb1a2245fdf (accessed on 22 May 2025).

75. Vos, T., Abajobir, A. A., Abate, K. H., Abbafati, C., Abbas, K., Abd-Allah, F., Abdulkad*er, R.* S., et al. (2017). Global, regional, and national incidence, prevalence, and years lived with disability for 328 diseases and injuries for 195 countries, 1990–2016: A systematic analysis for the Global Burden of Disease *Study 2016. The* Lancet, 390(10100), 1211–1259. https://doi.org/10.1016/S0140-6736(17)32154-2.

76. Wang, B., & Ye, X. (2024). Long-term lung function recovery after ECMO versus non-ECMO management in acute respiratory failure: A systematic review and meta-*analysis. BMC Pulmonary M*edicine, 24. https://www.semanticscholar.org/paper/3385eb0aaff86dd00c759ce0b117c5b63392212f (accessed on 22 May 2025).

77. Wei, P. F. (2020). Diagnosis and treatment protocol for novel coronavirus pneumonia (trial v*ersion 7). Chinese Medical J*ournal, 133(9), 1087–1095. https://doi.org/10.1097/cm9.0000000000000819.

78. Wichmann, D. (2020). Autopsy findings and venous thromboembolism in patients with *COVID-19. Annals of Internal Me*dicine, 173, 1030. https://doi.org/10.7326/l20-1206.

79. Williams, N. (2025). Shock: What is it and how is i*t managed? The Veteri*nary Nurse. https://www.semanticscholar.org/paper/632436f014a8a5cb263b2ccdc1fb978fb217d0e8 (accessed on 22 May 2025).

80. World Health Organization. (2020). Clinical management of severe acute respiratory infection (SARI) when COVID-19 disease is suspected: Interim *guidance. Pediatria i Medycyna R*odzinna, 16(1), 9–26. https://doi.org/10.15557/pimr.2020.0003.

81. Yoshikawa, H., Wuermli, A. J., Britto, P. R., Dreyer, B. P., Leckman, J. F., Lye, S. J., Pongu*ta, L.* A., et al. (2020). Effects of the global coronavirus disease-2019 pandemic on early childhood development: Short- and long-term risks and mitigating program and polic*y actions. The Journal of Pedi*atrics, 223, 188–193. https://doi.org/10.1016/j.jpeds.2020.05.020.

82. Zeppenfeld, K., Tfelt-Hansen, J., Riva, M., Winkel, B. G., Behr, E. R., Blom, N. A., Ch*arron,* P., et al. (2022). 2022 ESC guidelines for the management of patients with ventricular arrhythmias and the prevention of sudden card*iac death. European Heart* Journal, 43, 3997–4126. https://doi.org/10.1093/eurheartj/ehac262.

83. Zhang, H., Yu, Y., Chen, D., & Shang, Y. (2024). [Annual review of clinical research on extracorporeal life support *in 2023]. Zhonghua Wei Zhong Bing Ji Jiu* Yi Xue, 36(2), 118–123. https://www.semanticscholar.org/paper/deab27798469e27c5284208c747758ddbb156d6f (accessed on 22 May 2025).

84. Zhao, L., Xie, Y. X., & Wang, C. (2020). Recommendations for respiratory rehabilitation in adults with coronavirus dis*ease 2019. Chinese Medical J*ournal, 133, 1595–1602. https://doi.org/10.1097/cm9.0000000000000848.

SEPSIS AND MULTI-ORGAN DYSFUNCTION

6

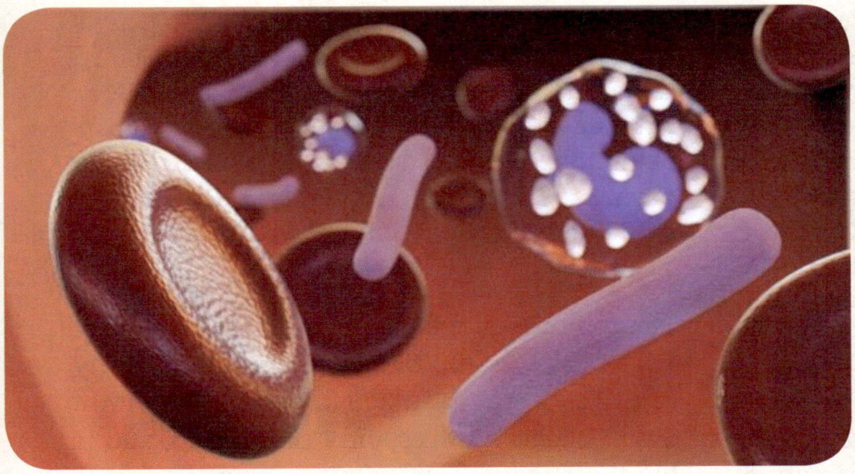

LEARNING OBJECTIVES

After studying this chapter, you will be able to:

1. Discuss about the pathophysiology of sepsis.
2. List the risk factors for sepsis.
3. Explore clinical manifestations of sepsis.
4. Understand the diagnosis of sepsis.
5. Explain the treatment strategies for sepsis.

Introduction

Sepsis is a critical medical condition that consists of a dysregulated host response to infection leading to multi-organ dysfunction. It is a complex condition arising from an infection that triggers a cascade of inflammatory reactions in the body. While most individuals possess a healthy immune system that can manage infection effectively, sepsis results when this immune response spirals out of control and causes generalized inflammation. The clinical importance of sepsis is gigantic, considering it can lead to morbidity and mortality, making early diagnosis and intervention necessary. Such a background underscores the need for ongoing research into the mechanisms by which sepsis evolves and progresses, particularly in high-risk populations such as children who may develop multi-system inflammatory syndrome due to other infecting pathogens such as COVID-19 (Jiang *et al.*, 2020). A key region of sepsis is its connection to multi-organ dysfunction syndrome (MODS), an additive failure of two or more organ systems to complicate sepsis. Pathophysiology of MODS is multifaceted, involving diminished blood supply, apoptosis, and dysregulation of cellular metabolism. As sepsis develops, its associated inflammatory response can overburden homeostatic mechanisms, leading to tissue hypoperfusion and anoxic damage to critical organs. Besides, the likelihood of acute organ failure development within a short period presents extreme challenges to clinical management. Understanding interlinkages among sepsis, immune response, and MODS will guide the creation of therapeutic interventions. Evolving evidence on biological markers, specific therapies, and the action of hormones, such as angiotensin-converting enzyme 2 (ACE2), is important for demystifying organ dysfunction pathogenesis in septic individuals (Bourgonje *et al.*, 2020). In the battle posed by the interrelated illnesses of sepsis and MODS, the medical profession concurs that prevention, early detection, and treatment must be done in an integrated manner. Advances in medical science have emphasized detecting early signs of sepsis and adopting timely treatment methods to stabilize organ function and curb inflammation. Establishing connections between sepsis, co-morbidities, and environmental determinants only serves to increase the complexity of the disease, and so a multidisciplinary approach with both clinical and public health interventions is now warranted. Additional research into the potential of treatment strategies like antibiotics, immunotherapies, and vaccines will undoubtedly shape sepsis treatment's future. As research continues to advance, it becomes increasingly necessary to make findings relevant to clinical practice guidelines in the hope of improving outcomes for sepsis and its concomitant multi-organ injury.

Definition of Sepsis

Sepsis, which is a lethal condition induced by the body's response to infection, is characterized by an uncontrolled inflammatory response that results in systemic inflammation and potential multi-organ dysfunction. On infection occurring, the body's immune response typically responds to eliminate the pathogens. In sepsis, this response is hyperactive, resulting in widespread inflammation and vascular malfunction. Clinical presentation is variable from mild to severe, with presentation most commonly fever, tachycardia, and altered mental status. Such variability in presentation is proof of the nature of sepsis in the sense that there can be variable pathophysiological responses depending on the causes of infection. The sooner that sepsis is identified and treated, the better the results, as sepsis can rapidly resolve into septic shock with enormously increased mortality. Sepsis definition has evolved across decades, reflecting progress in understanding of the disease's pathophysiology and clinical presentation.

The current definitions, developed by the Third International Consensus Definitions for Sepsis and Septic Shock (Sepsis-3), classify sepsis as organ dysfunction associated with a dysregulated host response to infection and is life-threatening. This definition emphasizes the importance of both the causative agent and the host reaction to the agent. The most widely used measure of organ dysfunction is the Sequential Organ Failure Assessment (SOFA) score, which allows clinicians to quantify the degree of organ impairment and act in a timely manner. The specificity of this definition facilitates critical communication among healthcare professionals and directs standardized treatment algorithms for suspected sepsis.

Additionally, in recent years, increasing emphasis has been laid on the association of sepsis with antimicrobial resistance (AMR), which further complicates the clinical presentation. Although sepsis itself is due to infection, the development of drug-resistant microorganisms has added to the complexity of effective management. As documented in more recent literature, the economic burden of AMR is attributed to sepsis-induced increased morbidity and mortality, especially when conventional antibiotics fail to eliminate resistant microorganisms (Murray *et al.*, 2022). Furthermore, the connection between serious infections, such as those induced by COVID-19, and MODS provides the incentive for further research into the pathophysiologic processes responsible for these syndromes (Jiang *et al.*, 2020). Understanding these interacting factors will guide more effective management practices and enhance prevention and early intervention strategies, thus ultimately preventing the bleak consequences of sepsis and its complications.

Importance of Understanding Multi-Organ Dysfunction

Knowledge about multi-organ dysfunction is significant in sepsis because it is an escalation of physiological stability to the extent that it affects patient outcomes adversely. Sepsis, infection-induced and life-threatening, can lead to an avalanche of failure of the multiple organ systems, with morbidity and mortality following this condition. Knowledge of the underlying mechanisms of multi-organ dysfunction allows clinical practitioners to identify those at increased risk, institute early interventions, and modify treatment strategies according to the needs of the individual patient.

Immune mechanisms have been investigated increasingly in recent years for the explanation of the pathologies of diseases with multi-organ dysfunction, such as severe fever with thrombocytopenia syndrome (SFTS), emphasizing the need to learn about the immune response present in such complex pathologies (Niu *et al.*, 2024). This data is important in the design of targeted therapy to reverse sepsis-induced multi-organ dysfunctions' life-threatening impact and thus improve patient care and survival. Further, the use of technology in medicine with an emphasis on machine learning is central to enhancing the understanding of multi-organ dysfunction. As noted in Post-COVID-19 Syndrome studies, the application of artificial intelligence techniques can facilitate early detection and treatment of sepsis and other multi-organ dysfunction disorders (Castro *et al.*, 2023). Machine learning algorithms can identify patterns and correlations within vast data sets that tend to evade clinicians' perception and assist in locating those at risk and facilitate timely treatment interventions.

This technological advancement is a critical milestone towards personalized medicine, where patient data customized at the individual level can be used to create personalized treatment protocols for preventing or reducing multi-organ dysfunction. Application of technology in the management of multi-organ dysfunction not only advances research but also allows clinicians to successfully improve patient outcomes. In general, the significance of understanding multi-organ dysfunction cannot be overemphasized, particularly in sepsis.

While the scientific community grapples with the varied implications of multi-organ dysfunction, enhanced research needs to be channeled toward explaining the intricate interplay between pathogen responses, immune processes, and organ systems. Insight gained from diseases like SFTS and long-COVID bridges the narrative of multi-organ dysfunction with therapeutic opportunities. Such studies will provide the basis for new ways to manage sepsis-triggered organ failures. As the healthcare landscape increasingly becomes more complex, embracing an integrated understanding of multi-organ dysfunction is the key to greater clinical performance and eventually transforming the treatment of such disorders in the future.

6.1. Pathophysiology of Sepsis

Learning Outcome

1. Understand the mechanisms of infection leading to sepsis.
2. Define immune response and inflammation.
3. Describe the role of cytokines and mediators.

Sepsis pathophysiology is directly interrelated with an abnormal immune response that initiates an excessive systemic inflammatory state. It is usually triggered by infection, and the immune system of the body overcompensates and releases pro-inflammatory cytokines and other mediators into the body. The hyper-inflammatory response not only attempts to kill the pathogen but also inadvertently injures host tissues and organs. This type of injury is amplified by the engagement of a broad range of immune cells, including neutrophils and macrophages, that drive inflammation and lead to multi-organ dysfunction. The role of extracellular vesicles (EVs), namely those exosomes shed from activated immune cells, has been of some interest in recent literature. These vesicles enable intercellular communication and significantly influence the inflammatory environment, ultimately resulting in the metabolic disturbance observed in sepsis (Gebeyehu *et al.*, 2024). As sepsis progresses, cellular energy metabolism and inflammation becomes critically important in understanding multi-organ dysfunction .

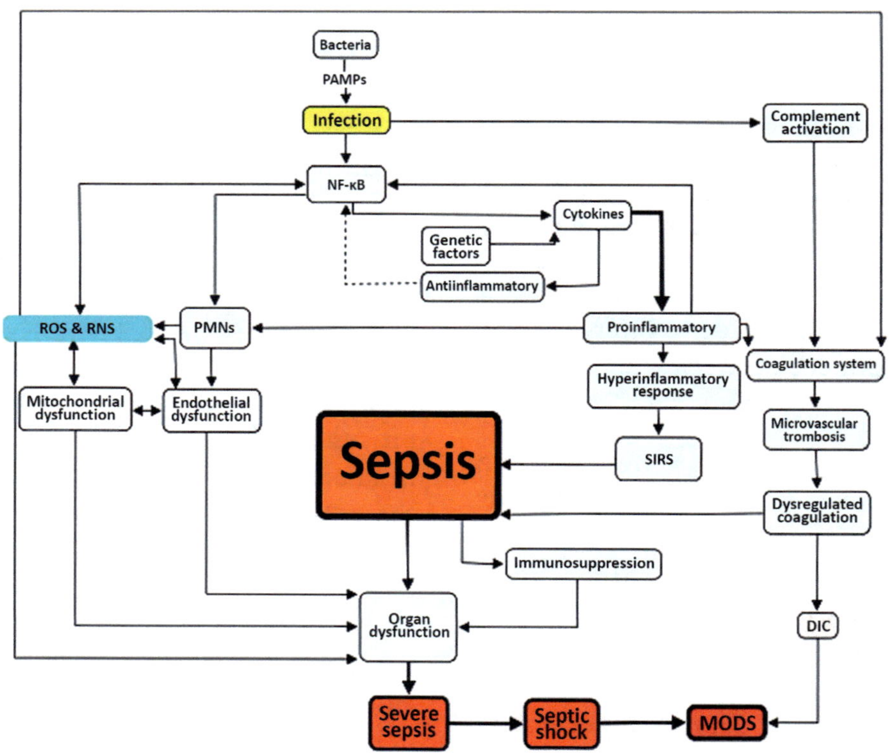

Figure 6.1. Pathophysiology of sepsis.

Source: https://www.researchgate.net/figure/Pathophysiology-of-sepsis-Several-elements-are-crucial-in-the-progression-of-the_fig1_277024240.

Cellular energy failure, due to mitochondrial dysfunction and impaired oxidative phosphorylation, typically leads to inadequate production of adenosine triphosphate (ATP). The resultant energy deficit compromises normal cellular function, organ function, and even drives cellular apoptosis. In addition, oxidative stress exacerbates the process by causing cellular macromolecule damage, including lipids, proteins, and DNA. This cascade of events demonstrates how sepsis not only alters immune homeostasis but also the very energetic demands of tissues. The comprehension of sepsis metabolic derangements will inform future therapeutic interventions to restore cellular function and enhance patient outcomes, particularly as researchers aim at alternative pathways that reverse cellular damage and promote recovery (Srdic *et al.*, 2024).

The intricate sepsis pathophysiology results in multi-organ dysfunction, a syndrome characterized by the failure of two or more organ systems. Viscera such as the liver, lungs, heart, and kidneys are particularly vulnerable to insult during septic attacks due to their midline roles in metabolism, gas exchange, and waste removal. Steatosis and derangement of drug metabolism by the liver, while acute lung injury due to inflammatory breakdown of alveolar-capillary membranes, is a common occurrence. Cardiac compromise usually manifests as myocardial depression that has the potential to drastically compromise hemodynamics. Simultaneously, renal dysfunction occurs as a secondary consequence of ischemia and inflammation, endangering fluid and electrolyte equilibrium. Awareness of such organ-specific pathways is crucial for the development of specific interventions. Recent insights into the role of gut microbiota and other emerging possible novel treatments, such as melatonin and metformin, provide new therapeutic strategies in the management of sepsis-induced multi-organ dysfunction and are expected to improve clinical outcomes (Srdic *et al.*, 2024) (Figure 6.1).

6.1.1. Mechanisms of Infection Leading to Sepsis

The etiology of sepsis as a significant public health concern is directly related to a variety of infection mechanisms that undermine the host's immune response. Sepsis occurs when pathogens, primarily bacteria, but also fungi and viruses, enter the bloodstream with a resultant hyper-inflammatory response characterized by severe tissue damage. The systemic inflammatory response is not only a result of the initial infection but is perpetuated by the host's immune dysregulation. Abnormal immune responses are capable of triggering microcirculatory alterations and mitochondrial injury in organ systems, resulting in cell death and organ dysfunction. Recent studies suggest that ferroptosis, a new form of oxidative stress and iron metabolism-related cell death, may play a significant part in the pathogenesis of sepsis by increasing inflammatory responses and promoting multi-organ failure, as explained in the cellular mechanisms review of sepsis (Huang *et al.*, 2023). When inflammation from sepsis increases, the pathogen-immune cell interaction becomes more intricate, underlining the importance of unraveling the causes of this lethal condition. Antimicrobial resistance (AMR) significantly increases the challenges brought by sepsis because infections from resistant pathogens lead to increased morbidity and mortality. It was calculated in 2019 that there were 4.95 million deaths due to bacterial AMR, demonstrating the widespread effects of resistant infection on worldwide health data (Murray *et al.*, 2022). Pairs of pathogen and drug, such as meticillin-resistant *Staphylococcus aureus*, demonstrate the widening problem of AMR since the infections tend to resist conventional treatments and are prime causes of sepsis severity (Murray *et al.*, 2022). Thus, the harmony of heightened inflammatory responses and AMR demands novel strategies for therapy and intervention in sepsis management. Understanding complex mechanisms of sepsis and infection is pivotal to therapeutic interventions. Inflammatory mediators released during infection can potentially induce a chain reaction of organ dysfunction and tissue injury, as seen in sepsis. Further, some research indicates that some pathogens can induce several immune response chains, and these can also influence the extent of sepsis that arises afterwards. Because ferroptosis has been identified as a potential key player in this action, ongoing research is looking at its specific role in the inflammatory condition and cell death in sepsis. Research into these cell processes can form the basis for new therapeutic opportunities, enhancing our ability to minimize organ dysfunction and promote survival in septic patients (Huang *et al.*, 2023). There must still be a priority to continue research into dissecting out pathways linking infection to multi-organ dysfunction to direct clinical practice in treating sepsis (Figure 6.2).

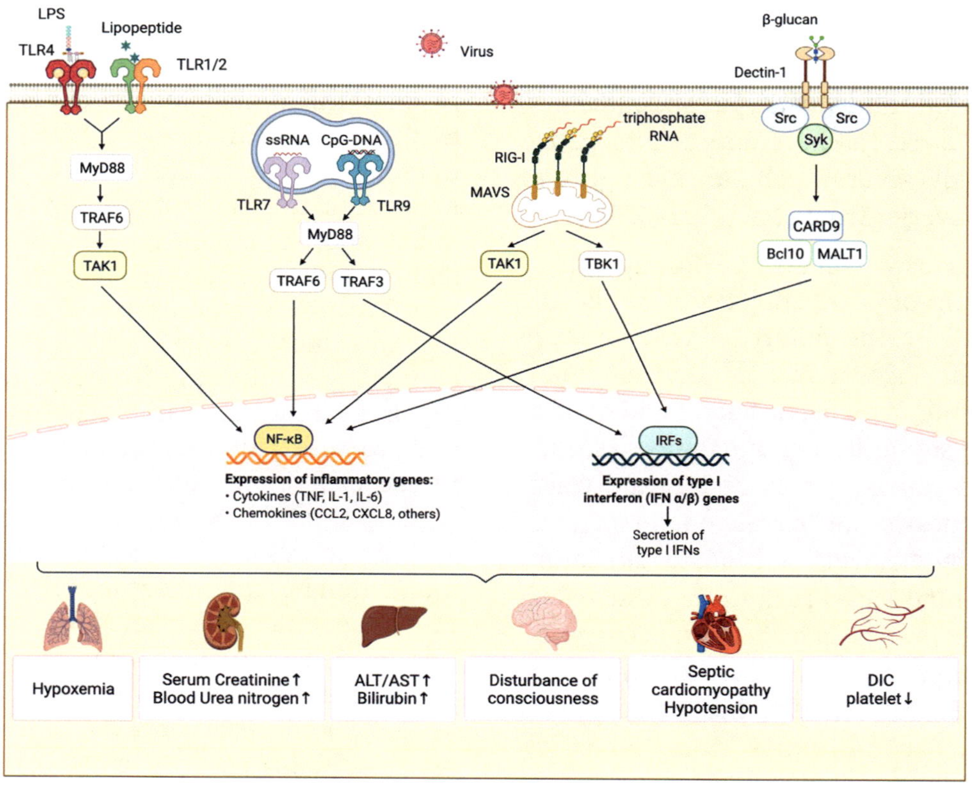

Figure 6.2. Immunity mechanism of sepsis induced by different pathogens. The predominant pathogens that cause sepsis are bacteria, fungi, and viruses. The lipopolysaccharide (LPS) in the outer membrane of Gram-negative bacteria can be recognized by TLR4, while the lipoprotein in the cell wall of Gram-positive bacteria can be bound to TLR2/TLR1.

Source: https://www.frontiersin.org/files/Articles/718089/fphar-12-718089-HTML/image_m/fphar-12-718089-g002.jpg.

6.1.2. Immune Response and Inflammation

Immune response in sepsis is a complex dance of cellular communication and inflammatory signaling, which, when disturbed, leads to multi-organ dysfunction. One of the characteristic features of septic response is the abrupt release of proinflammatory cytokines, including IL-6, TNF-α, and IL-1β. These mediators serve as alarm signals that activate immune cells to migrate into infected tissue in an attempt to contain the infection and repair damage. However, unregulated cytokine release culminates in a hyperinflammatory state—the hallmark of sepsis with widespread tissue damage and organ failure. Angiogenesis, coagulation cascade, and immunosuppression follow in general and complicate the clinical course and promote morbidity (Copaescu *et al.*, 2020). The ability to balance proinflammatory and anti-inflammatory reactions is essential for the recovery process, underpinning the significance of an exhaustive comprehension of these processes for the construction of successful treatments in septic patients. Inflammation and immune response are related in more than common terms within the framework of sepsis, in which body's defense results in systemically expressed manifestations.

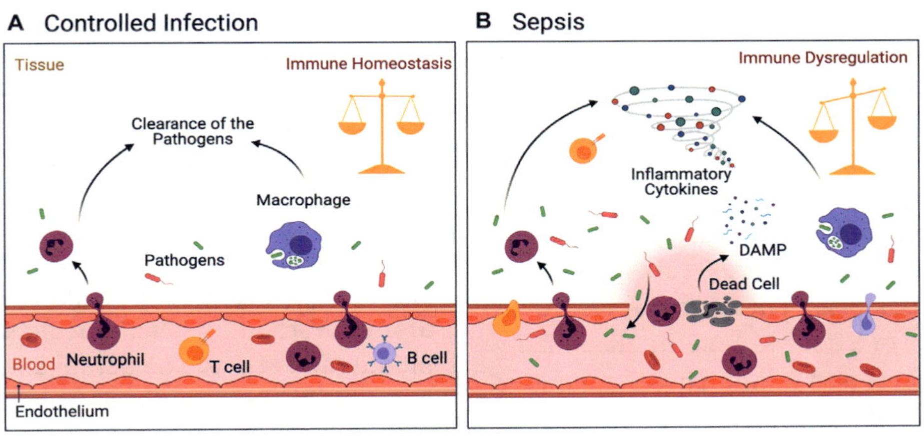

Figure 6.3. Immune response following pathogen infection. (A): Pathogen invasion induces local inflammatory response in tissues. The activated innate immune and adaptive immune cells migrate locally to tissues, inhibit microbe duplication and systematic dissemination, and finally clear the pathogen. Inflammation is controlled and immune balance of the body is achieved. (B): Heavy load infection accompanied by local damage activated innate and adaptive immune cells are in a hyperinflammatory state under the dual effects of pathogens and DAMPs. The cytokine storm generated by these cells inhibits the pathogens to a certain extent, but also leads to further tissue damage.

Source: https://www.frontiersin.org/files/Articles/718089/fphar-12-718089-HTML/image_m/fphar-12-718089-g001.jpg.

When the immune system detects a pathogen, it mounts an innate response by releasing cytokines and chemokines to recruit additional immune cells. This initial response, as much as is needed for the eradication of the pathogen, tends to spiral out of control and leads to an exaggerated inflammatory response. This dysregulation manifests as a cytokine storm, a term used to signify high circulating levels of cytokines that lead to heightened systemic inflammation

(Copaescu *et al.*, 2020). This overstimulation can ultimately lead to capillary leak syndrome, with edema of the tissues and compromised perfusion of vital organs. It is thus important to unravel the immunopathologic mechanisms governing this cascade to develop new therapies to guard against the sequelae of sepsis and enhance patient outcomes. Recent advances in therapeutic strategies aim to manipulate the immune response of septic patients by blocking major inflammatory mediators. Very notable amongst such strategies is decoy nanozyme application, which mimics macrophages to neutralize hyperinflammatory signals and oxidative stress. The clearance of reactive oxygen species by such engineered nanoparticles is effective, and cytokine release is also blocked, thereby preventing systemic hyperinflammation and reducing organ damage (Du *et al.*, 2022). Furthermore, research points out the therapeutic role of biologic agents, i.e., monoclonal antibodies targeting specific cytokines like IL-6, towards re-establishing immune homeostasis. These therapies could have the bonus of a double benefit: maximizing pathogen removal and minimizing the dangers of an unrestrained inflammatory response. With our improved understanding of sepsis immune dysregulation, the introduction of these novel therapies into practice has the potential to reframe sepsis and its associated complications management (Figure 6.3).

6.1.3. Role of Cytokines and Mediators

Appreciation of cytokine and mediator function in sepsis is essential to the understanding of the multi-organ dysfunction syndrome. Cytokines are major signaling molecules in the immune response and can be pathological as well as protective in sepsis. Pro-inflammatory cytokines such as tumor necrosis factor-alpha (TNF-α) and interleukin-1 beta (IL-1β) are released during the onset of the infection. But an unrestrained discharge of these mediators triggers systemic inflammation, resulting in organ dysfunction. So the delicate equilibrium between pro-inflammatory and anti-inflammatory reactions is essential; a predominance of pro-inflammatory cytokines is deleterious, increasing the risk of organ failure and obscuring the clinical presentation of sepsis (Shahid *et al.*, 2024). The mediators employed in sepsis are not only tasked with triggering the immune response but also orchestrating the crosstalk between different systems of the body. As much as cytokines like IL-6 and IL-10 exhibit both pro- and anti-inflammatory activities, they illustrate the multifaceted nature of the inflammatory response during sepsis. Disruption of the gut barrier is one of the significant characteristics, involving inflammatory mediators that lead to increased intestinal permeability, hence, facilitating the translocation of endotoxins and bacteria into the circulation. The condition is accountable for amplifying organ dysfunction and systemic inflammatory responses. Studies are now laying greater emphasis on the role of understanding such mechanisms, as the modulation of cytokine derangements may offer potentially therapeutic strategies to improve patient survival in sepsis (Shahid *et al.*, 2024). The action of inflammatory mediators also extends beyond immune control to modulate hemostasis and vascular integrity, adding further complexity to the pathophysiology of sepsis. Systemic circulation is predisposed to being overwhelmed by cytokines that disrupt microcirculatory hemodynamics, encouraging thrombotic activity and decreased tissue perfusion. This condition of hyper-inflammation can precipitate disseminated intravascular coagulation (DIC), a critical complication characterized by generalized clotting followed by massive bleeding due to consumption of clotting factors. The dominance of tissue-destabilizing cytokine effects therefore, necessitates ongoing investigation into potential biomarkers and targeted therapies capable of modifying such inflammatory events. Finally, the understanding of cytokines and mediator roles illuminates not only our comprehension of sepsis but also gives us an indication of how to develop improved diagnostic and therapeutic approaches in order to reduce multi-organ dysfunction (Osikov *et al.*, 2024) (Figure 6.4).

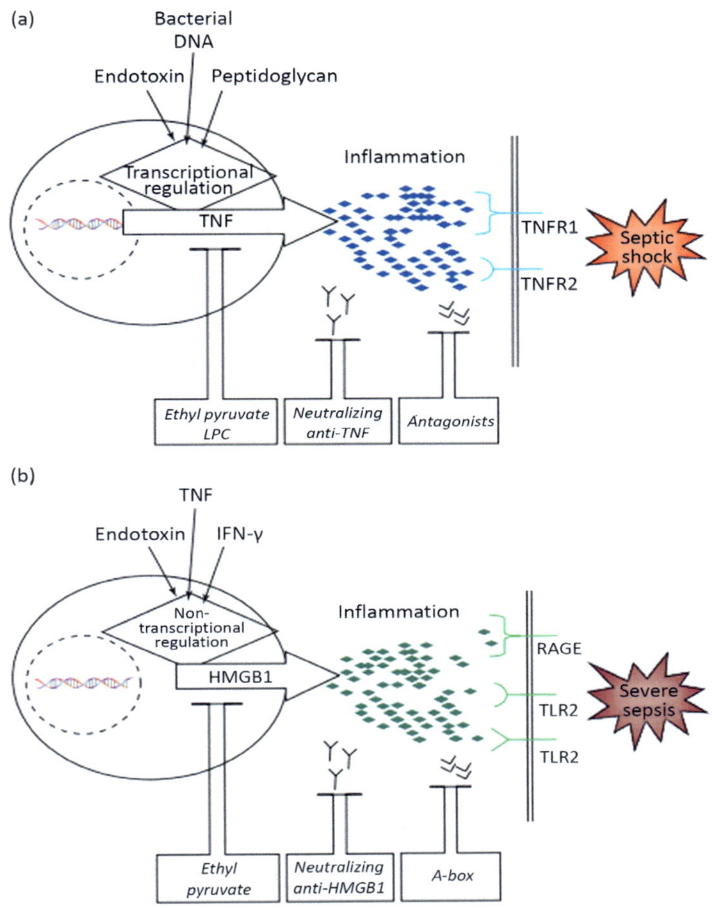

Figure 6.4. (a) TNF in septic shock; (b) HMGB1 in severe sepsis.

Source: https://cdn1.sinobiological.com/styles/default/images/Cytokines/cytokines-in-sepsis-2.png.

Test Your Knowledge

1. How do infections progress to cause sepsis in the body?
2. What is the role of the immune response and inflammation in the development of sepsis?

6.2. Risk Factors for Sepsis

Learning Outcome

1. Define patient demographics and underlying conditions
2. Discuss the hospital-acquired versus Community-acquired sepsis
3. Identify the impact of invasive procedures and devices

Risk factors for sepsis extend beyond clinical signs to include a wide range of contributing health conditions and determinants of health. Diabetic, chronic obstructive pulmonary disease, and renal failure patients are more susceptible to infection, hence posing a greater risk of acquiring sepsis. In addition, the placement of invasive devices like catheters and ventilators creates an avenue for disease-causing agents to enter the body and hence further enhancing this risk. More precisely, Moore *et al.* (2025) emphasize the stark difference in sepsis outcomes between lower and upper socioeconomic groupings of children, highlighting the more profound role of environmental causes in health disparities. This means that while clinical vigilance is called for, a holistic approach considering the social determinants is most important in identifying populations at risk. Age is also an important risk factor in sepsis, with both the very young and the elderly particularly prone to severe infection and sepsis.

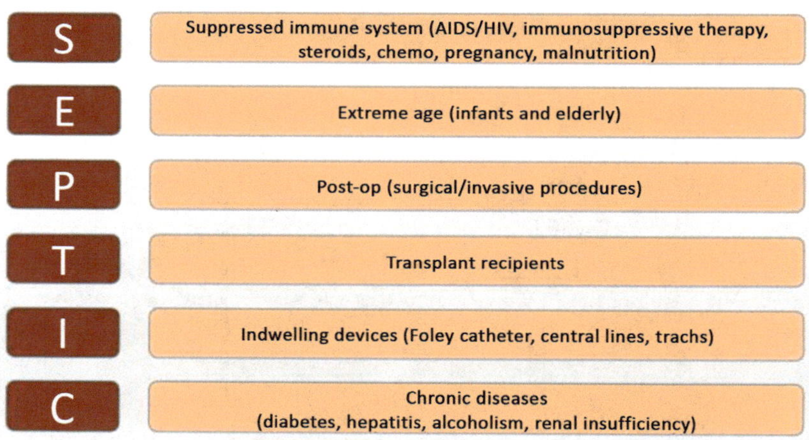

Figure 6.5. Risk factors for sepsis in adults.

Source: https://media.licdn.com/dms/image/v2/D4D22AQFqznpN_r8cGA/feedshare-shrink_800/B4DZPFb7v.HMAg-/0/1734184261197?e=2147483647&v=beta&t=FPnP9unKWq_zrvkGtmhxyEDTY61UcdofP3daWSP-wfA.

In children, immature immune systems might not suppress infections and hence lead to an increased likelihood of sepsis progression. In contrast, older individuals do acquire age-related impairments in immune function, and therefore, they are more prone to developing complications from infection. The intersection of these physiological susceptibilities underscores the need for targeted interventions and preventive actions employed in different age groups. Moreover, research on severe COVID-19 as a variant of viral sepsis describes how immune reactions that are implicated with increasing age can contribute to the risk of cardiovascular events and these are further compounded by the incidence of underlying medical conditions (Neu *et al.*, 2022).

Discovery and treatment approaches must be enhanced with regard to understanding complex risk factors of sepsis. Hospitalizations due to sepsis can further be complicated by comorbid interference, particularly with patients suffering from cardiovascular disease, which can exacerbate the course of sepsis and lead to disastrous outcomes, such as multi-organ dysfunction. Furthermore, cardiovascular risk factor evaluation becomes especially pertinent in the context of viral sepsis with COVID-19, wherein certain pathophysiological patterns become evident. The identification of these interlaced risk factors can inform clinical practice, emphasizing the need for an organized assessment in high-risk groups in both acute and post-acute phases of sepsis. The targeted, organized approach to treating these areas could have a significant role in decreasing morbidity and mortality from sepsis and sepsis-associated multi-organ dysfunction (Figure 6.5).

6.2.1. Patient Demographics and Underlying Conditions

It is significant to understand patient demographics and underlying illnesses while treating sepsis and associated multi-organ dysfunction. Incidence of sepsis relies heavily on demographic factors such as age, sex, and comorbidities. Older patients are particularly vulnerable and, in most instances, are accompanied by pre-existing illnesses that can trigger the progression of sepsis, ultimately impairing the host's immune ability. Because the immune system deteriorates with increasing age, it may be partly responsible for increased susceptibility not only to infection but also to severe sepsis consequences. Their identification might enhance clinical interventions and permit targeted interventions against individual vulnerability in each population (Jarczak *et al.*, 2021). Some underlying conditions, such as those related to chronic diseases, can greatly influence the course and severity of sepsis. For instance, subjects with chronic liver disorders such as cirrhosis possess an increased risk for adverse outcomes when they present with infection. The evidence reveals that cirrhotic patients possess significantly increased mortality related to infection, particularly COVID-19, with extreme increases in mortality seen with increasing severity of liver dysfunction, as graded by the Child-Pugh scoring system. Severe liver disease not only affects immune function but also makes the physiologic response to systemic infections more complex, thus increasing the overall risk for multi-organ dysfunction (Marjot *et al.*, 2020). This underscores the need for healthcare professionals to recognize and manage these predisposing conditions effectively. Interplay among demographics and underlying conditions underscores the necessity for effective risk assessment in clinical practice. For providers, awareness of the specific demographics of their patient population can lead to increased screening and preventive care for high-risk groups. In addition, recognition of comorbidities as powerful predictors of sepsis outcomes provides support for the integration of care approaches addressing both the infection and the broader systemic impact on health. With ongoing research, increasing the knowledge of patient demographics, comorbidities, and sepsis treatment will be crucial to creating effective treatment protocols to minimize morbidity and mortality related to multi-organ dysfunction (Jarczak *et al.*, 2021).

6.2.2. Hospital-Acquired Sepsis (HAS) Versus Community-Acquired Sepsis (CAS)

An understanding of the difference between HAS and CAS is necessary to facilitate effective diagnosis and management. HAS most often occurs in patients with a previous underlying medical condition, typically after invasive procedures or extended hospital stay. CAS occurs in patients who have not had a recent hospitalization, implying a community-acquired infection. The etiologic pathogens of HAS are normally not the same as those of CAS, the former having more antibiotic-resistant pathogens that complicate treatment plans and patient prognosis. HAS severity has a propensity to enhance the multifunctional organ dysfunction, which is an important factor because this disease enhances patient mortality. The distinctive characteristics of each of these two types of sepsis underscore the need for individualized management strategies based on each environment's own distinct pathogens and risk factors.

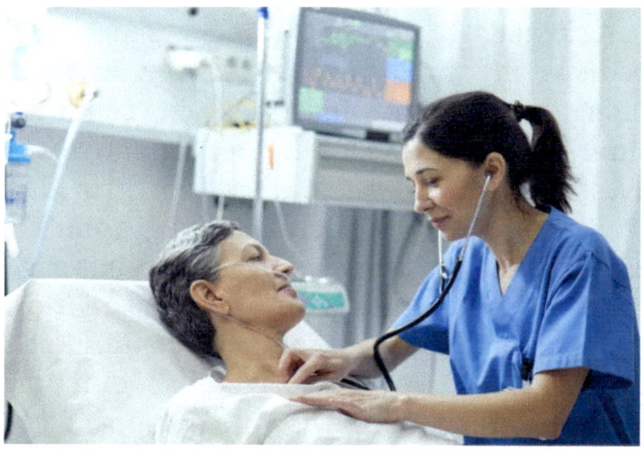

Figure 6.6. Hospital-Acquired Sepsis (HAS) Versus Community-Acquired Sepsis (CAS).

Source: https://res.cloudinary.com/highereducation/images/w_1024,h_683,c_scale/f_auto,q_auto/v1693924904/NurseJournal.org/Nurse-caring-patient-sepsis-monitor/Nurse-caring-patient-sepsis-monitor-1024x683.jpg.

The clinical presentation and consequences of sepsis also vary significantly between the hospital and community settings. CAS patients commonly present with less complicated symptoms representing usual infections, like pneumonia or urinary tract infection, and respond better to routine treatment regimens. Patients with HAS, on the other hand, may have more complicated and serious clinical presentations because of the compromise of more than one organ system. Literature suggests that severity scoring, like CURB-65 and qSOFA, are able to predict outcomes more accurately in community-acquired (Reddy *et al.*, 2024) (Figure 6.6).

Besides, CAS patients are more likely to receive early diagnosis, allowing immediate initiation of treatment, whereas this is less common for HAS patients. The latter might be exposed to long-term hospitalization complications, including additional infections, delayed care, and increased healthcare costs, thus becoming a significant issue for healthcare systems. Observation of biological markers also plays its crucial role in differentiating between HAS and CAS. For instance, procalcitonin (PCT) was identified as a valuable diagnostic indicator in the discrimination of sepsis from infections, particularly community-acquired pneumonia (AL-Banaa *et al.*, 2024).

This approach predicts the progression of sepsis and potential organ dysfunction. The diagnosis and treatment of sepsis are successfully made based on awareness of these indicators, which show the host's inflammatory response. Both clinical assessment and laboratory biomarkers are of primary importance in informing therapeutic choices, optimizing outcomes, and minimizing the impact of multi-organ dysfunction. With ongoing research seeking the subtleties of HAS and CAS, better diagnostic schema will eventually lead to targeted interventions and the aggregate care of sepsis across a wide range of clinical settings.

6.2.3. Impact of Invasive Procedures and Devices

The growing application of invasive devices and procedures in clinical medicine inevitably raises anxiety regarding their capacity to induce complications, particularly in sepsis and multi-organ failure. An illustration would be the application of intravascular catheters and ventilators in critically ill patients, which are frequently utilized but can become centers of infection. Such risk is particularly magnified in the setting of impaired immune response, where invasion by pathogens through such pathways can initiate an acute cascade of systemic inflammatory processes.

The consequences of such infections extend beyond localized complications and may contribute significantly to elevations in rates of morbidity and mortality among vulnerable populations. Thus, the determination of routes through which such equipment triggers sepsis is vital to the formulation of prevention strategies and mitigation of harm in patients with multi-organ dysfunction. Invasive procedures per se, while commonly life-saving, can also provoke a pro-inflammatory response, which exacerbates underlying pathophysiological conditions of sepsis.

Surgical operations, such as cholecystectomies and valve replacement, have been performed with improved outcomes when performed with special techniques, but are not free of risks. Pisano *et al.* (2020) point out that surgical procedures have to be optimized in a manner that prevents complications in high-risk patients. Without proper, careful attention to patient selection and postoperative treatment, the benefits from these operations get lost because of the complications arising from sepsis. Thus, doctors must walk a thin line between the necessity for invasive procedures and not inducing ensuing infections that would lead to multi-organ failure, highlighting the importance of stringent guidelines and protocols in surgery. Furthermore, as technology advances in the area of invasive devices, the need for updated clinical frameworks becomes increasingly apparent.

The Valve Academic Research Consortium's effort at standardization of definition and endpoints in clinical trials is part of a broader movement to optimize the safety and efficacy of medical devices. Philippe Généreux *et al.* (2020) present optimization of clinical endpoint definitions for transcatheter and surgical aortic valve intervention with continuous monitoring of device-related complications. Such systematic reanalysis not only allows for more accurate data reporting but also directs best practice intended to reduce the occurrence of infection that leads to sepsis. The medical community is thereby challenged to integrate new information in a continuous fashion, absorbing improved techniques and establishing a safety culture that optimizes patient outcomes while minimizing risks of invasive devices and procedures.

Test Your Knowledge

1. How do patient demographics and underlying conditions influence the risk of sepsis?
2. What are the key differences between hospital-acquired and community-acquired sepsis?

6.3. Clinical Manifestations of Sepsis

Learning Outcome

1. Identify the symptoms and signs of sepsis
2. Discuss the progression to septic shock
3. Explain the indicators of multi-organ dysfunction

The clinical picture of sepsis is extremely wide and reflects the underlying host dysregulation of the infection response. The presenting symptoms are typically fever, chills, and tachycardia, which can advance to more abrupt symptoms like hypotension and altered mental status. This progressive symptomatology is secondary to the body's attempt to clear the infective organism alongside experiencing systemic inflammatory response syndrome (SIRS). As sepsis advances, it may cause septic shock, characterized by the development of ongoing hypotension despite adequate fluid resuscitation, ultimately leading to multi-organ dysfunction. The variation in clinical manifestations renders diagnosis complicated and underscores the need for early detection and management, as delay in treatment can severely jeopardize patient outcomes and augment the risk of mortality. Recognition of these manifestations is critical for clinicians attempting to intervene in the sepsis continuum appropriately. Multi-organ dysfunction syndrome is a serious complication of sepsis due to the complex interaction between inflammation, microcirculatory dysfunction, and cellular injury. The heart, lungs, kidneys, and liver are most frequently affected, resulting in septic cardiomyopathy, acute respiratory distress syndrome, acute kidney injury, and hepatic failure. It is noteworthy that septic cardiomyopathy is directly implicated in cardiac dysfunction, placing patients at risk of cardiovascular collapse. The relationship between multi-organ failure and sepsis is potentiated by hyper-release of pro-inflammatory cytokines that can perpetuate tissue injury and lead to a cascade of dysfunction across various systems. With evaluation of the inter-relationship of such organs in sepsis, healthcare providers can better plan interventions targeted at both the causative infective organism and consequential organ dysfunction, thus improving patient prognosis and outcomes (Song *et al.*, 2023). Apart from the traditional clinical presentation of sepsis, similarities between sepsis and other conditions like COVID-19 have been highlighted in recent times, casting new light on their pathophysiologic processes. The two conditions have a common clinical presentation that includes consumptive thrombocytopenia, multi-organ dysfunction syndrome, and coagulopathy.

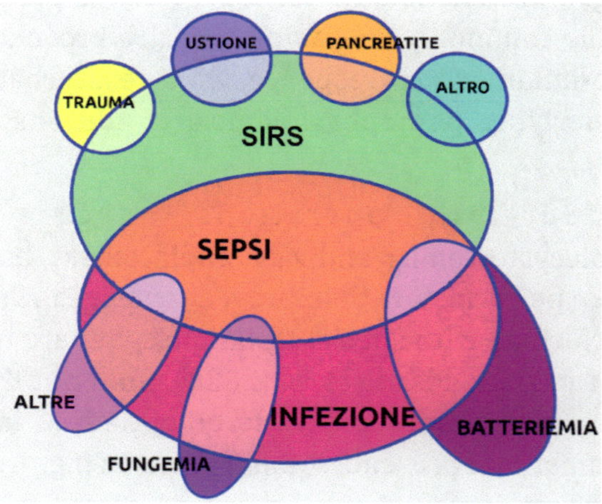

Figure 6.7. Systemic inflammatory response syndrome (SIRS).

Source: https://upload.wikimedia.org/wikipedia/commons/thumb/c/cf/Sepsi-SIRS.png/800px-Sepsi-SIRS.png.

The commonality of these signs calls for further investigation into the immunopathogenic processes underlying severe disease in both conditions (Olwal *et al.*, 2021). An understanding of these similarities is essential in designing treatment protocols that borrow from established sepsis care and adapt to fit new infectious diseases. Secondly, greater recognition of the clinical presentations can help to sensitize clinicians to early recognition and treatment of sepsis, particularly in co-infection scenarios. By analyzing these intersections, healthcare clinicians can develop a more integrated approach to the holistic nature of sepsis and its potential complications (Figure 6.7).

6.3.1. Symptoms and Signs of Sepsis

Diagnosis of sepsis is based on identifying a group of signs and symptoms of the body's deranged response to infection. Fever is one of the initial and most common presentations of sepsis, and it can also present as hypothermia in certain populations. Chills, tachycardia, and tachypnea are some of the symptoms that can be experienced by patients, and these are compensatory mechanisms when the body is attempting to cope with its systemic inflammatory response. As Gao *et al.* (2022) describe, this host response dysregulation can result in life-threatening organ dysfunction, and the early detection of these symptoms is thus of critical importance to the patient's survival. Moreover, confusion or altered mental status typically complicates the clinical presentation, which means the central nervous system is affected. This fever, tachycardia, and altered mental status combination demonstrates the severity of sepsis and the importance of early clinical intervention. With the classic presentation of infection, the presentation of organ failure can be dramatic in the septic patient. Hypotension is an interesting marker for septic shock that results from widespread vasodilation and fluid loss in the vascular compartment. Patients may present with signs of impaired organ perfusion, such as low urine output, indicating acute kidney injury. Furthermore, laboratory findings, such as an elevated lactate level, may be an indication of tissue hypoxia and necessitate immediate clinical intervention. The combination of these signs is compounded by the diverse etiology of infections that can cause sepsis, so proper clinical evaluation should be done in order to determine the offending factor. This presentation of symptoms across multiple organs necessitates an increased index of suspicion among healthcare providers, because timely diagnosis and intervention are paramount in the prevention of progression to multiorgan dysfunction (Chopra *et al.*, 2020).

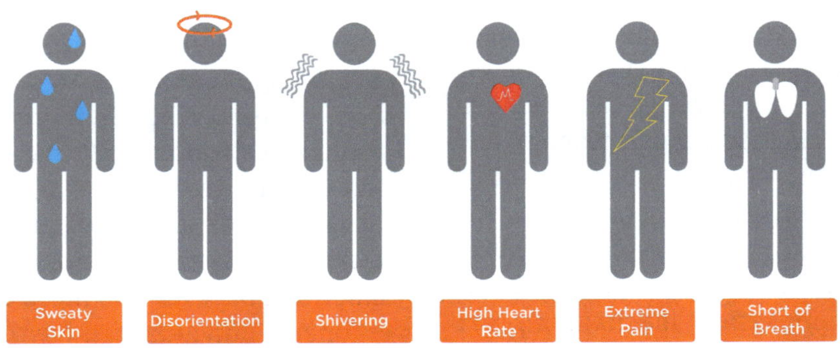

Figure 6.8. Signs and symptoms of Sepsis.

Source: https://www.steeperusa.com/SteeperGroup/media/SteeperGroupMedia/About%20Steeper/Insights/23-04Sepsis-signs-and-symptoms-01.jpg?ext=.jpg.

Sepsis presentations are usually non-specific and could be superimposed over other life-threatening conditions, necessitating differential diagnosis. An example includes gastrointestinal symptoms such as nausea, vomiting, and diarrhea, particularly with abdominal infections. Skin manifestations, including rash and mottled or pale skin, also indicate an extreme systemic response. The diverse symptoms can lead to sepsis being misdiagnosed if physicians fail to suspect sepsis in their differential diagnosis. The existing science of sepsis, including how regulatory T cells modulate the inflammatory response during sepsis, suggests a very complex interaction between the body's immune processes and the clinical presentation of sepsis (Gao *et al.*, 2022). Hence, the identification of the spectrum of signs and symptoms observed in sepsis is not only essential for immediate treatment but also for the establishment of intervention to avoid the long-term impact of this severe disease, ultimately improving the outcome of patients in the framework of sepsis and multi-organ failure (Figure 6.8).

6.3.2. Progression to Septic Shock

The progression to septic shock is the critical turning point in the continuum of sepsis, marked by an abrupt impairment of organ and hemodynamic function. Sepsis first develops as a consequence of an infection overwhelming local immune barriers and an ensuing induced systemic inflammatory response that can lead to multi-organ dysfunction. As the inflammation worsens, it can result in vasodilation, increased vascular permeability, and impaired immune microcirculation, all resulting in decreased perfusion and oxygenation of vital organs. This chain of pathophysiologic events paves the way for the onset of septic shock, where body compensation mechanisms are overpowered, causing continuous hypotension despite fluid resuscitation. It is necessary to understand how this transition is mediated in order that therapeutic interventions may be developed capable of restoring hemodynamic stability and preventing irreversible damage to organs. The clinical relevance of septic shock is immense, with unutterable implications for patient outcome. If a patient does advance to this point, mortality is significantly enhanced, highlighting the importance of early diagnosis and intervention. As underscored by current studies, the pro-inflammatory and anti-inflammatory reaction balance dictates septic shock development, so diagnosis as well as treatment becomes even more difficult. After initial resuscitation, the patient may experience chronic immune dysregulation, which derails the balance needed for recovery. This dysregulation not only contributes to the acute sepsis but also has a lasting effect on the immune system, enhancing susceptibility to secondary infection and contributing to prolonged hospitalization. Mitigation of this multi-dysregulation is required to improve not only the short-term survival of patients but also long-term health outcomes following sepsis. The treatment of septic shock is evolving, with emphasis on early recognition and targeted therapies. Improvements in intensive care have improved the approach to sepsis, enabling earlier intervention regimens to reduce the risk of mortality. Most survivors of septic shock, however, continue to experience chronic sequelae due to ongoing immune compromise and inflammation, both of which have been associated with long-term mortality beyond the acute phase. Studies have shown that such long-term immune function changes have the potential to predispose patients to repeated infections, thus complicating their course of recovery. While investigators continue to pursue immune modulatory treatments against these effects, focus is laid on the unscrambling of mechanisms underpinning the transition from sepsis to septic shock and beyond, into more efficient treatment regimens individualized for the patient (Delano *et al.*, 2016; Rosa *et al.*, 2017).

6.3.3. Indicators of Multi-Organ Dysfunction

The path of sepsis is usually concluded with multi-organ dysfunction, a key indicator of poor prognosis and mortality. Multi-organ dysfunction has some major indicators, such as organ-specific biomarker alterations, abnormal vital signs, and clinical findings. For instance, liver failure can be evidenced through laboratory parameters of elevated liver enzymes, and variations in creatinine are markers of renal failure. Additionally, patients also present with hypotension, an important vital sign that reflects inadequate delivery of oxygen and perfusion to the critical organs. As the condition worsens, multi-organ failure occurs, leading to a deteriorating clinical picture necessitating immediate medical intervention. Recognition of these signs is important for early treatment and diagnosis since early therapeutic interventions significantly alter the direction of sepsis and patient outcomes. Recognition of these markers enables clinicians to react with appropriate management strategies. Moreover, the presentation of patients who manifest signs of multi-organ dysfunction usually encompasses a constellation of symptoms not limited to failures within individual organs. These include changes in mental status, tachypnea, and peripheral edema as indicators of underlying system processes. Neurological impairment can present as confusion or lowered levels of consciousness, a reflection of the compromised state of the central nervous system due to systemic inflammation (Figure 6.9).

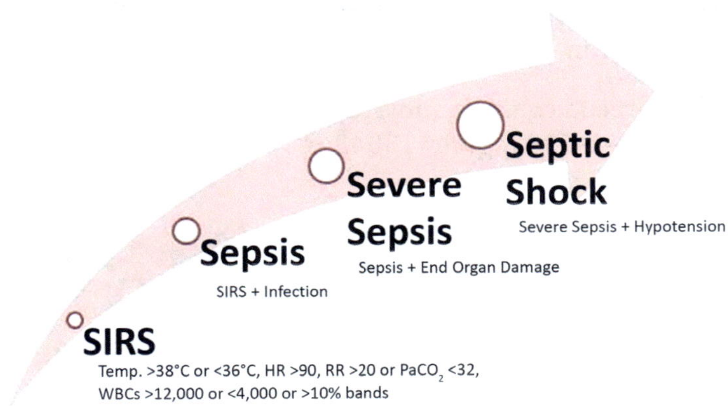

Figure 6.9. Stages of Sepsis.

Source: https://emedicalupdates.com/wp-content/uploads/2018/01/Stages-of-sepsis-image-photo-picture.jpg.

Similarly, respiratory distress, as observed by elevated respiratory rates and hypoxia, can signal pulmonary complications such as acute respiratory distress syndrome. Failure to notice these complex signs can have a long-lasting impact on the fate of a patient. Heightened awareness for such clinical indicators is necessary in sepsis treatment because their presence requires aggressive resuscitation efforts and may require augmented therapy to prevent organ injury. In sepsis-associated multi-organ dysfunction, recent research points to certain physiological mechanisms underlying organ failure and tissue damage. For instance, the release of inflammatory mediators such as cytokines may initiate a chain of events leading to endothelial dysfunction and impaired perfusion. Interestingly, studies suggest that processes like neutrophil extracellular traps (NETs) may be implicated in tissue injury in the setting of excessive inflammatory responses, as seen in diseases like COVID-19, which is implicated in lung damage and multi-organ failure pathophysiology

(Veras *et al.*, 2020). Such intricate processes must be elucidated to develop targeted therapy to minimize organ injury and improve recovery rates. The interaction between organ-directed injury, systemic inflammation, and treatment protocol reflects the intricacy of sepsis management and the need for interdisciplinary approaches to patient treatment (Figure 6.10).

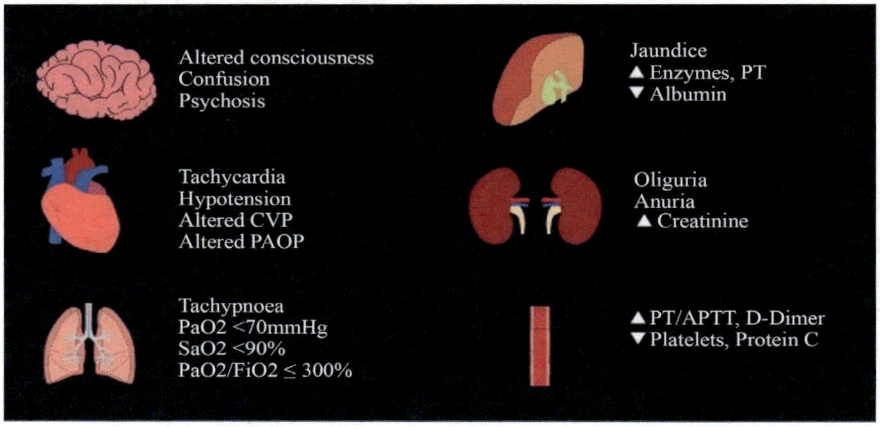

Figure 6.10. Organ dysfunction in severe sepsis.

Source: https://image.slidesharecdn.com/organdysfunctionsepsisgraceleo-170901111124/95/organ-dysfunction-in-sepsis-grace-leo-1-638.jpg?cb=1504264376.

Test Your Knowledge

1. What are the early symptoms and signs that suggest sepsis?
2. How does sepsis progress to septic shock in critically ill patients?

6.4. Diagnosis of Sepsis

Learning Outcome

1. Define clinical criteria and scoring systems
2. Explain the laboratory tests and imaging studies
3. Understand the challenges in early diagnosis

Sepsis diagnosis is a critical component of multi-organ dysfunction susceptible patients treatment. An early diagnosis of the disease can contribute significantly to patient outcomes, as a delay in its diagnosis would lead to progressive organ failure and mortality. Traditional methods for diagnosis include clinical examination and laboratory tests; however, a growing awareness is developing regarding the role of molecular diagnostics. Sepsis hub genes have been discovered in recent years, such as CD163, FCER1G, C3AR1, and ARG1.

They are strongly correlated with inflammatory responses and the dysregulation of the immune response in septic patients. Understanding these gene pathways not only enhances diagnostic accuracy but also offers insight into potential therapeutic interventions that may reverse the catastrophic effects of sepsis (Yu *et al.*, 2023) (Figure 6.11).

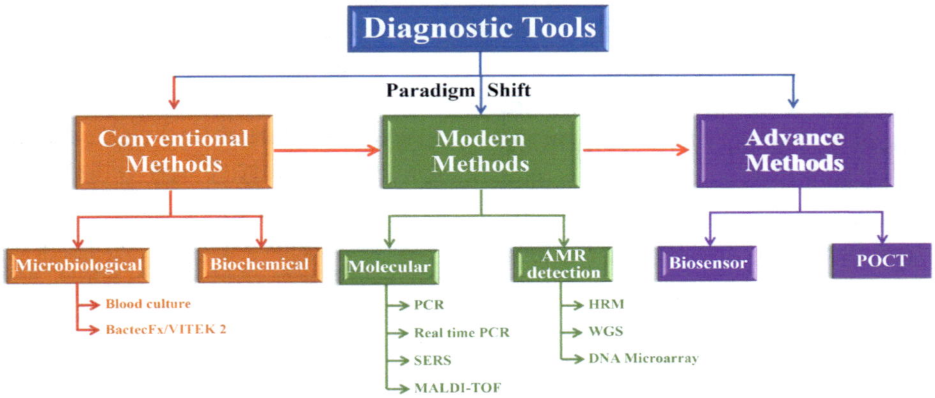

Figure 6.11. Schematic overview of the diagnostic methods.

Source: https://www.mdpi.com/2075-4418/13/2/277.

Diagnostic enhancement is particularly necessary since sepsis may manifest differently in populations of patients. Its presentation may range from low-grade fever to severe multi-organ dysfunction, and therefore, its diagnosis is difficult. For instance, sepsis can be caused by infections like scrub typhus, leading to serious complications such as acute respiratory distress syndrome (ARDS) and multi-organ dysfunction syndrome (MODS), as a demonstration of this difficulty in diagnosis.

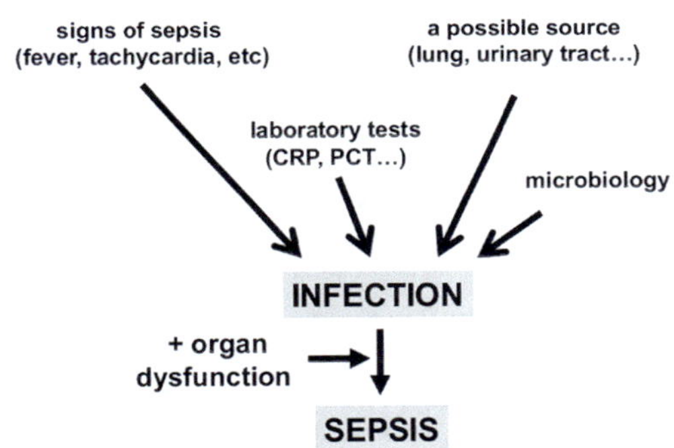

Figure 6.12. Diagnosing sepsis from infection.

Source: https://www.researchgate.net/figure/Diagnosing-sepsis-from-infection-An-infection-can-be-identified-from-clinical-signs-and_fig1_303320210.

A report of a patient of scrub typhus, who initially showed fever and subsequently developed MODS, underscores the importance of early diagnosis and treatment. The report indicates that the mortality rate, even with a range of 7% to 30% in untreated cases (Shah *et al.*, 2023), comes down significantly with prompt interventions. Therefore, enhanced understanding of the interconnectedness of infectious diseases and sepsis is vital in clinical practice to help achieve more rapid, accurate diagnoses. The landscape of sepsis diagnosis is evolving with the union of new molecular approaches and traditional methods. Identification of known hub genes reveals the complex connection between immune dysregulation and sepsis, which can assist clinicians in tailoring diagnostic tests and treatment protocols. With continued research breaking down the intricacies of sepsis pathways, it is evident that optimizing diagnostic precision is at the center of optimizing patient outcomes in sepsis and ensuing multi-organ dysfunction. Hence, continued research into genetic markers and their applications in the clinical setting is encouraging in optimising the efficacy of sepsis management regimens, overall reducing the impact of this life-threatening disease. Understanding the role of these genes in the immune response during infection can create the potential for the creation of targeted therapies that address the underlying causes of sepsis (Yu *et al.*, 2023) (Figure 6.12).

6.4.1. Clinical Criteria and Scoring Systems

In multi-organ dysfunction and sepsis, scoring systems and clinical scores are important tools for early detection and patient management with involvement. Scoring systems like Universal Vital Assessment (UVA), quick Sepsis-related Organ Failure Assessment (qSOFA), and Modified Early Warning Score (MEWS) are designed to enable quick assessment and risk stratification. These systems are particularly valuable in settings with limited resources, where clinicians will only have limited exposure to more advanced diagnostic technologies. Researchers, in a Ugandan study, identified that while such scoring systems can be precisely correlated with markers of immune activation and organ dysfunction, their content validity has not yet been investigated, more so in sub-Saharan Africa. Increased recognition of the transferability of these criteria to diverse populations and healthcare environments is essential to improving clinical outcomes in septic patients (Tiao *et al.*, 2025). Progress in information concerning scoring systems is reflected in ongoing research with the aim of maximizing their predictive power. It has recently been proven that multiple scoring systems demonstrate varying degrees of efficacy in assessing patient prognosis in acute respiratory failure due to sepsis (SA-ARF) (Figure 6.13).

The qSOFA score, which comprises of bedside clinical parameters, aims at identifying patients with sepsis who are at a higher risk for adverse outcomes.

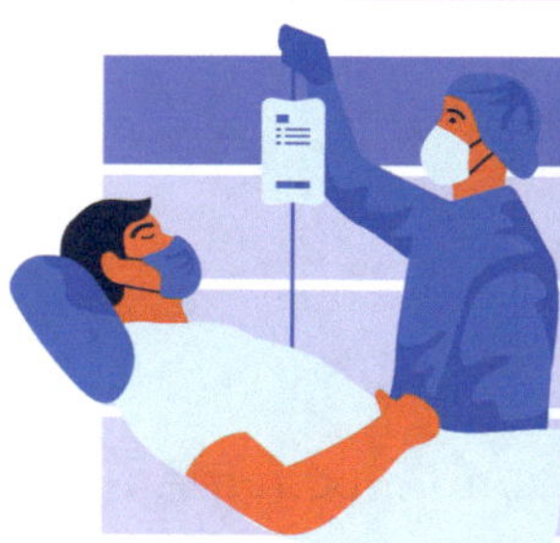

ASSESSMENT	SCORE
RESPIRATORY RATE > 22 breaths / min	1
SYSTOLIC BP < 100 mmHg	1
ALTERED MENTAL STATUS (GCS < 14)	1

qSOFA Scores of ≥2 is associated with a 3 to 14 fold increase in In-hospital mortality.

Figure 6.13. qSOFA SCORE - Quick Sequential Organ Failure Assessment score.

Source: https://www.openmed.co.in/2022/07/qsofa-score-quick-sequential-organ.html.

For instance, it was discovered that the Acute Physiology Score III (APS III) was a more accurate predictor of hospital deaths compared to a considerable number of established scoring systems, such as the Sequential Organ Failure Assessment (SOFA) and Simplified Acute Physiology Score II (SAPS II). MIMIC-IV database data analysis revealed that the area under curve (AUC) of APS III performed better compared to its alternatives, indicating that the addition of more sophisticated scoring parameters can significantly improve clinical decision-making in intensive care units. This focus on improving scoring systems serves to demonstrate their role in patient-specific treatment methods among multi-organ dysfunction patients (Fan *et al.*, 2024). Lastly, the integration of clinical criteria and scoring systems into daily practice is an important advancement in the management of sepsis and its resultant complications. Not only do these systems facilitate early recognition, but they also direct treatment pathways, allowing interventions that could be provided on time and improving patient outcomes. However, it becomes necessary to conduct additional research studies that validate these tools in different clinical settings, particularly in areas with unique healthcare challenges. Future studies should focus on developing a comprehensive understanding of the temporal relationship between host response dysregulation and organ dysfunction during sepsis, and this would inform further refinement of even improved scoring systems for specific patient cohorts. The goal remains to render clinical measurements not only precise and consistent but also responsive to the complex realities of global health (Fan *et al.*, 2024; Tiao *et al.*, 2025).

6.4.2. Laboratory Tests and Imaging Studies

Together with laboratory investigations and imaging procedures, their use is critical in the diagnosis of sepsis and multi-organ dysfunction (MOD). Routine laboratory evaluation typically includes complete blood counts, blood cultures, and biochemical panels to measure liver and renal function. Elevated inflammatory markers, such as procalcitonin and C-reactive protein, can indicate an ongoing infection and are correlated with sepsis severity. Furthermore, specific laboratory studies, like lactate, aid in the assessment of tissue perfusion and guiding resuscitation. Organ dysfunction can be detected early by these tests, and early detection can result in significant enhancements in clinical outcome, as prompt and targeted interventions are critical in this fatal state. Laboratory findings provide important information on patient's status, and therefore clinical decision-making must rely on wide testing. Imaging techniques are also crucial in sepsis and its complications, diagnosis, and treatment. Chest X-rays, for example, can reveal pulmonary infiltrates or signs of pulmonary involvement such as pneumonia, which commonly develops with sepsis. Computed tomography (CT) scans are more detailed examinations that can detect intra-abdominal infection or abscesses that are likely causing the patient's septic condition. For COVID-19, imaging findings can prove to be very valuable in identifying complications such as acute respiratory distress syndrome, leading to multi-organ failure as seen in recent research (Figure 6.14).

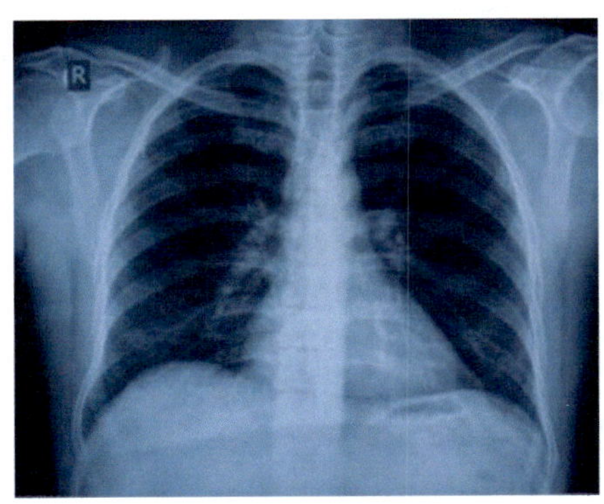

Figure 6.14. Chest X-rays.

Source: https://cdn.sepsis.org/wp-content/uploads/2017/12/iStock-92988886-300x245.jpg.

With developing diagnostic processes due to improved imaging techniques, the ability to observe systemic expressions of sepsis allows physicians to formulate treatment modalities appropriately and reduce morbidity and mortality due to the disease. Significance in correlating laboratory tests and imaging findings cannot be overstated, particularly with consideration for the complexity of sepsis. There is also some new evidence that certain biomarkers, such as neutrophil extracellular traps (NETs), are most likely to be at the core of sepsis pathophysiology since they can induce organ dysfunction via mechanisms of tissue damage (Veras *et al.*, 2020). Also, clinical presentations of pediatric COVID-19 indicate that multi-organ dysfunction would normally require a multifaceted process of diagnosis using both laboratory and imaging studies to determine the etiology (Dallan *et al.*, 2020). The combined approach enables a comprehensive appreciation of the patient's status, enabling clinicians to make intervention specific to the etiology of sepsis and complications, hence enhancing patient outcomes in the intensive care unit.

6.4.3. Challenges in Early Diagnosis

Early diagnosis of sepsis remains a pertinent issue in clinical practice since it is largely prompted by the nonspecific nature of its early symptomology. The patients typically report ill-defined fever, tachycardia, or malaise, which may readily be mistaken for other pathologies. This imprecision most commonly results in delayed therapies, thus enhancing potential organ dysfunction. Because sepsis progresses very rapidly, the delay produces grave consequences, including multi-organ dysfunction syndrome. Latest studies have evidenced the need for finding new predictive and diagnostic biomarkers that allow for early intervention in septic patients, pointing towards the possible role of serum concentrations of specific proteins as possible predictors of organ dysfunction (Jiang *et al.*, 2024). Yet, integrating these biomarkers into everyday clinical practice has additional hurdles, particularly across global availability and constraints in healthcare resources. Artificial intelligence (AI) technology is being proposed as a solution to bypass the early diagnosis of sepsis, bringing new possibilities for more accurate and timely detection. Machine learning algorithm advances are able to analyze large amounts of data, including laboratory results and clinical variables, to identify patterns that can forecast sepsis. But while AI holds promise, it is not without limitations. Current data can strengthen biases, which can affect the accuracy of the prediction. Further, healthcare practitioners may find it difficult to interpret outcomes generated by AI, thus resulting in resistance in applying these technologies in health practice. Thus, while AI holds promise in improving diagnostic performance, thorough understanding and application of these systems into existing frameworks are crucial for their success (Wang *et al.*, 2024). Finally, the conventional sepsis diagnosis approach relies on sole biomarkers, which are suboptimal for providing timely diagnoses. Instead of relying on a single marker, an integral approach based on a panel of biomarkers can offer greater diagnostic accuracy and prognostic value to clinicians. Scientific studies have indicated some serum proteins, such as Cathepsin B and S100-A9, which are found to be potential precise markers for preoperative assessment in septic patients (Jiang *et al.*, 2024). A combination of several biomarkers may not only enhance early diagnosis but also direct treatment regimens that address multi-organ dysfunction. However, verification of these markers in various patient groups would be needed in order to develop clinical practice guidelines that would direct diagnostic protocols. Thus, solving complex issues in early diagnosis becomes critical in order to improve sepsis and complicated patient outcomes.

Test Your Knowledge

1. What clinical criteria and scoring systems are commonly used to diagnose sepsis?
2. Which laboratory tests and imaging studies help confirm a diagnosis of sepsis?

6.5. Treatment Strategies for Sepsis

Learning Outcome

1. Define antibiotic therapy and its importance
2. Explain the supportive care and fluid resuscitation
3. Discuss the advanced therapies and emerging treatments

Effective treatment strategies for sepsis have seen significant modification in response to the multi-factorial nature of this potentially fatal condition, with its interaction with multi-organ dysfunction. Early detection and treatment initiation are critical components in the management of sepsis. Guidelines include the use of broad-spectrum antibiotics within a first-hour window following the diagnosis of suspected sepsis to counteract the responsible infection effectively. Additionally, fluid resuscitation remains a cornerstone of therapy as it aims to restore hemodynamic stability as well as sustain organ perfusion. These united efforts offer a fundamental strategy for the cessation of sepsis progression and the prevention of subsequent organ failure. Integrated clinical pathways that seek to enable the management of sepsis can further enhance patient outcomes, ensuring that early interventions are not only recommended but systematically carried out within medical institutions. Advances in diagnostic capacity have also transformed treatment strategies, with emphasis placed on the therapeutic potential of biomarkers for sepsis. Traditional markers like C-reactive protein and procalcitonin are greatly wanting, with research underway to explore new biomarkers with greater sensitivity and specificity. Emerging studies show the promise of emerging biomarkers like circular RNAs and microRNA-486-5p in facilitating early diagnosis and assessing treatment response. Such developments enable clinicians to tailor antibiotic therapy more effectively, particularly against multidrug-resistant organisms (MDROs) that complicate treatment regimens. Such precision medicine approaches, together with standard treatments, underscore the need for a multi-faceted perspective of sepsis so that outcome predictability and resource management can be done more effectively in critical care environments (Rong-He *et al.*, 2024). The appearance of multidrug-resistant organisms demands a shift in empirical treatment strategies against sepsis. Combination antibiotic therapy with drugs of various classes has come into the limelight as a strategy against MDROs and improved patient outcomes. It is particularly helpful when cultures may take longer to return, with effective and timely intervention being started in anticipation of final microbiological evidence. Further, point-of-care testing (POCT) devices to rapidly identify pathogenic organisms are a sepsis breakthrough that enables clinicians to successfully tailor treatment based on local resistance patterns (Kumar *et al.*, 2024). Such treatment advances, combined with efforts to inform healthcare workers regarding appropriate antibiotic stewardship, hold the potential for reduced recurrent sepsis rates and the economic cost of prolonged hospitalization and multi-organ dysfunction. In combination, these multidimensional approaches define an integrated strategy for addressing the sepsis challenges within the critical care setting (Figure 6.15).

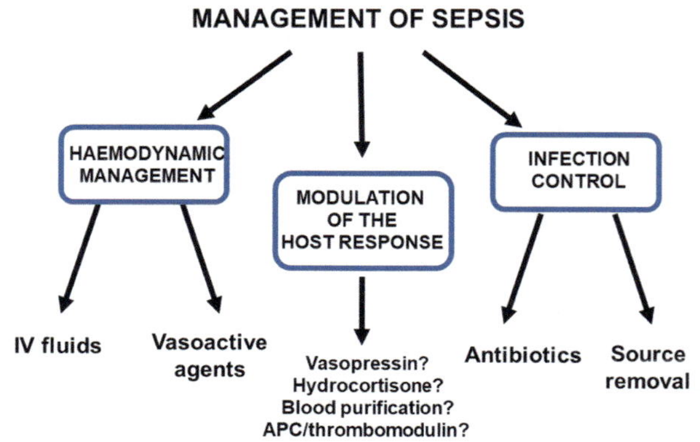

Figure 6.15. The three arms of sepsis management.

Source: https://www.thelancet.com/cms/10.1016/j.ebiom.2022.104318/asset/cab0a52f-5268-4da3-a497-fe4af9dadbcf/main.assets/gr1_lrg.jpg.

6.5.1. Antibiotic Therapy and Its Importance

Antibiotic therapy is an important aspect of sepsis management, which is lethal and is caused by the host response to infection that is dysregulated, leading to multi-organ failure. Early administration of antibiotics is crucial in sepsis-induced mortality prevention. Research indicates that for each hour of delay in beta-lactam antibiotic therapy, there is a 20% increased risk of 30-day mortality in post-operative sepsis patients and the need for early intervention (Singh *et al.*, 2025). In addition, studies demonstrate that the achievement of therapeutic levels of antibiotics within two hours significantly increases survival, which illustrates the importance of both the timing and adequacy of antibiotic dosing in sepsis treatment.

This association between optimal antibiotic treatment and favorable clinical outcomes supports the application of standardized guidelines to guide the timely administration of sepsis for various health care settings. Furthermore, the application of antibiotic therapy is not without difficulty; the problem of resistance to antibiotics has become a critical issue in the treatment of infections resulting in sepsis. Inappropriate or delayed use of antibiotics can result in the development of resistant organisms, thereby complicating follow-up treatments. This condition calls for careful consideration of antibiotic therapy, where practitioners need to weigh the need for treatment against the need to preserve the effectiveness of current antibiotics. Treatment of an elderly patient with Chlamydia psittaci infection provides an example and illustrates that multidrug treatments, including both antibiotic and antifungal treatments, may be required due to the presence of concurrent infections (Zhang *et al.*, 2024).

These intricacies highlight the imperative of ongoing education and adherence to evidence-based recommendations in minimizing resistance while optimally managing sepsis-related infection. Additionally, the importance of personalized antibiotic therapy cannot be overstressed in ensuring patients with sepsis receive the optimal outcome. The heterogeneity of patient response, comorbidities, and etiology of the infection necessitates tailored strategies with both pharmacokinetic and pharmacodynamic attention. For example, studies have revealed that some surgical groups could have a varied response to the administration and timing of antibiotics, which makes treatment even more complicated (Singh *et al.*, 2025). With the ongoing development of precision medicine, the integration of patient-specific factors into drug therapy will lead to improved outcomes in sepsis and multi-organ dysfunction patients. Health care providers are thus encouraged to adopt a multi-pronged strategy that includes early recognition of sepsis, timely administration of antibiotics, and treatment tailored to the individual to promote survival and minimize the sequelae of infection (Figure 6.16).

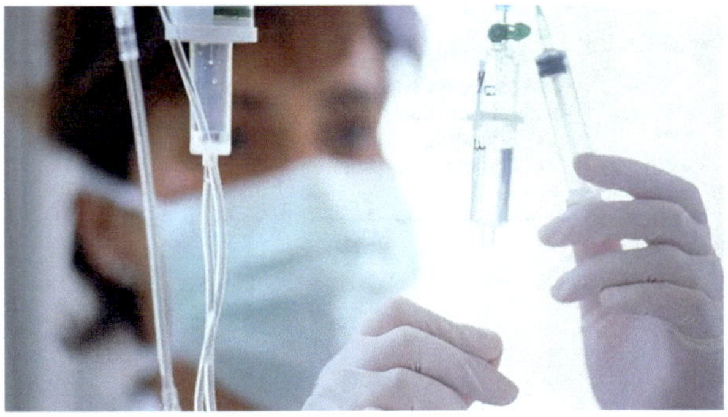

Figure 6.16. Antibiotic therapy.

Source: https://images.everydayhealth.com/images/infectious-diseases/sepsis/sepsis-treatment-rm-722x406.jpg?sfvrsn=52f3803_0.

6.5.2. Supportive Care and Fluid Resuscitation

The severity of sepsis necessitates an integrated approach to supportive care that is paramount to the patient's outcomes. The initial treatment protocols center on fluid resuscitation, with the goal of restoring intravascular volume and optimizing body perfusion of the vital organs. Research from studies confirms that the achievement of early fluid resuscitation significantly impacts mortality outcomes in sepsis, advocating for its priority in critical care. Importantly, fluid therapy must be tailored to the individual clinical status of the patient, as overfluid administration may result in complications including pulmonary edema or abdominal compartment syndrome. The delicate balance between successful resuscitation and potential fluid overload remains a focus for research interests, therefore emphasizing ongoing close monitoring and reassessment of the patient during treatment. By the application of a dynamic approach to fluid resuscitation, doctors are in a position to optimize organ function and decrease the formation of multi-organ dysfunction secondary to sepsis. Supportive care further entails other modalities in the treatment of sepsis and multi-organ dysfunction complex patient needs. These include analgesia, which minimizes pain and distress, thus allowing for better cooperation in treatment adherence by patients. Moreover, enteral nutrition takes precedence to ensure the preservation of gut integrity and immune function in the critically ill. The intimate relationship between nutrition and sepsis is, however, now better understood, and therefore favors early enteral nutrition whenever feasible. Patients with organ failure manifestations may also require tailored intervention, such as renal replacement therapy or respiratory therapy to restore their normal status. With the inclusion of these supportive interventions in an integrated care pathway, clinicians can devise an improved management plan considering both the short-term and the long-term consequences of sepsis. While supportive care and intravenous fluid resuscitation remain cornerstones of sepsis care, the emerging concept of immune dysregulation in sepsis challenges as well as provides opportunities.

The transition from the purely pathogen-centered approach to an appreciation of host reaction to infection necessitates reconsideration of the therapeutic approach. Current research suggests that disruption of specific immunological mechanisms could offer new avenues for intervention. However, the efficacy of supportive therapies like specific immunotherapy or hemoperfusion remains to be definitively established. This brings into focus the need for further research and clinical trials aimed at optimizing supportive care interventions in the treatment of the immune response in sepsis. Ultimately, expanding our knowledge about immune pathophysiology can lead to more specific interventions, thereby optimizing patient outcomes during sepsis and its severe complications, such as multi-organ dysfunction (Jarczak *et al.*, 2021; Szatmary *et al.*, 2022) (Figure 6.17).

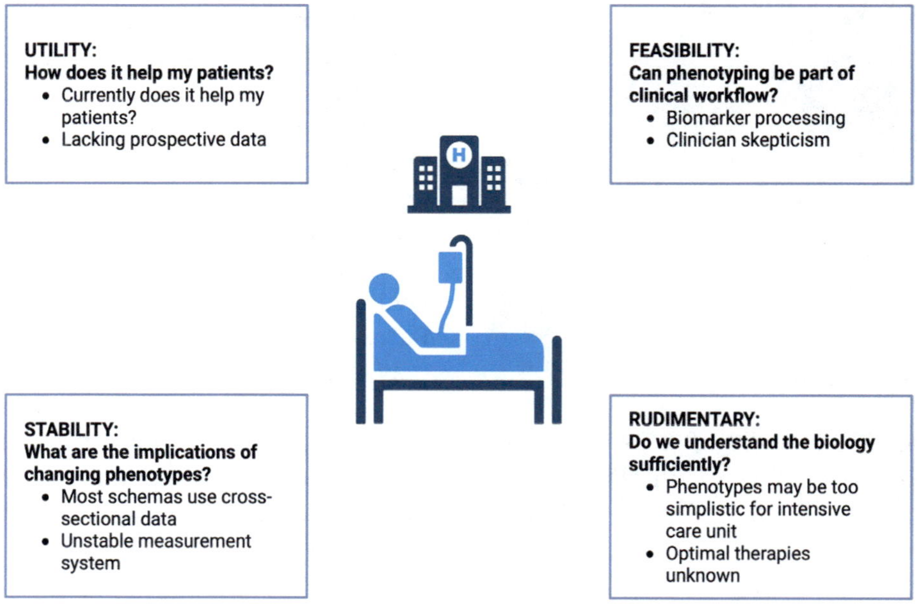

Figure 6.17. Evaluating Sepsis Phenotyping. This infographic details key considerations in sepsis phenotyping, divided into three aspects: UTILITY, questioning the immediate benefits for patient care; FEASIBILITY, addressing the practicality of incorporating phenotyping into clinical routines; and STABILITY, discussing the consistency of phenotypic classifications. A final note on RUDIMENTARY aspects suggests a need for deeper biological understanding to support phenotype-based treatments in intensive care settings.

Source: https://www.mdpi.com/2073-4409/13/5/439.

6.5.3. Advanced Therapies and Emerging Treatments

Treatment of sepsis and multi-organ dysfunction has so far relied on supportive therapy and broad-spectrum antibiotics. With the arrival of new therapies, the treatment paradigms are in the process of being re-evaluated. Novel immunomodulatory agents such as monoclonal antibodies with specificity for multiple mediators of inflammation hold promise to dampen the hyper-inflammatory process in sepsis. An interesting example is the anti-FABP4 monoclonal antibody ($6H_2$), which in experimental models was very effective. Several studies have demonstrated that treatment with 6H2 can inhibit systemic inflammation and enhance tissue protection across a number of organ systems, including the liver and kidney. These specific therapies offer the promise of a more refined approach to the management of sepsis, with the potential for reduced morbidity and mortality secondary to multi-organ dysfunction. With additional evidence for these therapies steadily accumulating, they soon may transition from experimental stages to mainstream clinical practice, marking a new era in the management of sepsis. Another fertile research area to treat sepsis comes from the recognition of the complex host-pathogen interactions underlying the disease. Personalized medicine that tailors intervention based on individual patient profiles and the respective microbial culprits is where research is currently focused. For example, identification of biomarkers for increased risk of sepsis can lead to early therapeutic intervention with certain therapies, such as certain antibiotics or immunomodulating therapy. Additionally, the timing and effectiveness of fluid resuscitation can have a significant impact on outcomes. As multi-organ failure typically follows a preceding septic insult, pairing advanced diagnostics with novel therapeutic agents could dramatically improve survival and quality of life in patients. This shift towards personalization not only optimizes care but also responds to the multifaceted nature of sepsis and its systemic effects. New therapies also include regenerative medicine modalities that attempt to restore damaged tissues as well as organ function. Mesenchymal stem cell methods have gained traction because they have anti-inflammatory properties as well as the ability to induce tissue regeneration. These cells can modulate the immune response and activate healing processes in injured organs, which qualifies them as prime candidates for sepsis-related complications. New clinical trials testing the use of stem cells to prevent organ injury and enhance recovery in critically ill patients are underway. In one case of severe paper wasp envenoming, aggressive treatment modalities were employed, like continuous renal replacement, symbolizing the need for newer therapeutic options in severe presentation with multi-organ failure (Lee *et al.*, 2025). With each passing day of advances in research work, it is imperative to study the inclusion of such treatments in our traditional sepsis management protocols, ultimately refining our methods against this critical clinical challenge (Ibrahim *et al.*, 2025).

Test Your Knowledge

1. What role does supportive care and fluid resuscitation play in treating sepsis?
2. What advanced therapies and emerging treatments are being explored for sepsis?

SUMMARY

The intersection of sepsis and multi-organ dysfunction is an intimidating critical care dilemma. Sepsis, characterized as an abnormal immune system response to infection, quickly progresses into multi-organ failure, with significant effects on patient morbidity and mortality rates. Understanding predisposing factors to both diseases such as comorbidities, infection types, and physiological response, is crucial in the formulation of effective management protocols. The findings of current studies underscore that chronic infections, in addition to background disease conditions, profoundly predispose to life-threatening complications, highlighting the need for heightened awareness among clinicians (Elfeky *et al.*, 2013). Awareness is not only required for immediate patient management but also for long-term outcome improvement. In addition, prompt detection of sepsis and associated organ dysfunction remains essential in an attempt to optimize clinical outcomes. Employing standardized assessment tools, such as the SOFA score, enables the health care team to formally evaluate patient status and risk. of particular interest are recent investigations focusing on the prognostic value of point-of-care ultrasound (POCUS) in evaluating physiologic markers such as tricuspid annular plane systolic excursion (TAPSE) in septic patients (Ali *et al.*, 2020). Though initial findings were not observed to be directly correlated with TAPSE values and patient outcomes, incorporation of such assessment could still have important roles in the treatment of individual patients. More study of such diagnostic measures must then become a top priority in making improved treatment protocols for sepsis-induced complications. Finally, the reversal of sepsis's impact on multi-organ dysfunction must entail a multi-faceted approach encompassing prevention, timely detection, and cautious treatment. Ensuring compliance with infection control procedures and promoting education to critical care teams will improve the capacity for effective treatment of patients (Elfeky *et al.*, 2013). Ongoing research into further understanding the pathophysiological processes where sepsis and organ dysfunction are related will inform future therapy. With the ever-changing field of healthcare, it will be increasingly important to prioritize both clinical education and innovative research studies to further enhance the management of sepsis and reduce its severe impact on multi-organ function. This comprehensive strategy will help to improve survival rates as well as enhance the quality of life for affected patients.

Over the past few years, the nature of sepsis as a clinical syndrome has become very prominent, particularly regarding its association with multi-organ dysfunction. Sepsis is largely characterized by an excessive and dysregulated inflammatory response to infection, leading to extreme tissue damage and failure of multiple organ systems. At the center of this cascaded failure is the activation of inflammatory mediators, such as fatty acid-binding protein 4 (FABP4). Current research indicates that FABP4 inhibition could be a new therapeutic approach to preventing the systemic inflammation and organ damage that typify sepsis. Research has shown that monoclonal antibodies against FABP4, including 6H2, have shown promising outcomes in animal models, decreasing tissue injury in various organ systems, such as the liver, lung, kidney, and heart (Ibrahim *et al.*, 2025). This emphasizes the promise of intensive interventions to improve outcomes in sepsis and sepsis-associated complications. The interplay between diabetes and hyperglycemia in multi-organ failure is worth investigating extensively, especially in the context of the importance of systemic inflammation in sepsis. Greater evidence is present to indicate that hyperglycemia might trigger organ-specific complications by inducing endothelial dysfunction and modifying leukocyte dynamics. Recent work employing single-cell RNA sequencing unraveled transcriptional remodeling in various tissues following hyperglycemia, which is a major step in the understanding of the onset of diabetic complications. Notably, organ-specific transcriptional responses occurred in major cell types such as macrophages and endothelial cells and revealed insight into the pathological mechanisms causing multi-organ failure. This evolving definition of diabetic complications is consistent with that of sepsis, requiring multidisciplinary efforts to manage patients with these interconnected pathologies (Braithwaite *et al.*, 2024). Finally, the solution to sepsis and multi-organ dysfunction requires more insight into common pathways and mechanisms of the two diseases. Research on the potential therapeutic application of agents like the anti-FABP4 monoclonal antibody reveals that the resolution of inflammation can cause considerable tissue integrity and organ function improvements in septic occurrences. Concurrently, the identification of hyperglycemia-induced transcriptional responses underscores the importance of early treatment in preventing the development of organ-specific diabetic complications in diabetes-related conditions. The intersections at which these processes overlap explain the requirement for an integrated approach to patient management, treating the immune response and metabolic dysregulation in harmony. These findings collectively form a critical point of intersection for future research into therapeutic intervention in sepsis and multi-organ dysfunction, driving the creation of improved clinical outcomes in targeted patient populations.

KEY TERMS FROM THIS CHAPTER

- Acute kidney injury (AKI)
- Antibiotic therapy
- Bacteremia
- Blood cultures
- Broad-spectrum antibiotics
- C-Reactive protein (CRP)
- Crystalloids
- Cytokine storm
- Endotoxins
- Fluid resuscitation
- Infection
- Lactate clearance
- Lactic acidosis
- Multi-organ dysfunction syndrome (MODS)
- Norepinephrine
- Organ dysfunction
- Organ perfusion
- Procalcitonin
- Sepsis
- Sepsis bundle

CRITICAL THINKING QUESTIONS

1. **According to the Sepsis-3 definition, sepsis is defined as:**
   a. Infection with high-grade fever
   b. Infection with hypotension
   c. Life-threatening organ dysfunction caused by a dysregulated host response to infection
   d. Bacteremia confirmed by blood culture
2. **Which scoring system is commonly used in the ICU to assess organ dysfunction in sepsis?**
   a. APGAR
   b. SOFA (Sequential Organ Failure Assessment)
   c. GCS (Glasgow Coma Scale)
   d. Wells Score
3. **What is the most important initial step in the management of suspected sepsis?**
   a. Start corticosteroids
   b. Administer vasopressors
   c. Obtain blood cultures and start broad-spectrum antibiotics
   d. Intubate and ventilate the patient
4. **Which organ system is typically the first to fail in sepsis-related MODS?**
   a. Renal
   b. Respiratory
   c. Hepatic
   d. Cardiovascular
5. **In septic shock, despite fluid resuscitation, the need for vasopressors and elevated lactate levels indicates:**
   a. Mild sepsis
   b. Chronic infection
   c. Multi-organ failure
   d. Persistent tissue hypoperfusion

Short Answer Questions

1. What is the current definition of sepsis according to the Sepsis-3 guidelines?
2. How does sepsis differ from septic shock in terms of clinical criteria and hemodynamic impact?
3. What is the role of the SOFA and qSOFA scores in the diagnosis and prognosis of sepsis?
4. What are the pathophysiologic mechanisms behind sepsis-induced organ dysfunction?
5. What is the significance of early identification of sepsis, and how does it impact outcomes?

Answer to Critical Thinking Questions

1. (c); 2. (b); 3. (c); 4. (b); 5. (d)

REFERENCES

1. Al-Banaa, J. S. J., Kadhum, N. H., Rahi, S. J., Alhibaly, H. A., & Aljanabi, M. A. (2024). The value diagnostic of procalcitonin and complete blood count in patients with sepsis due to community-acquired pneum*onia. Karbala Journal of M*edicine. https://www.semanticscholar.org/paper/24ca8a624ddb9e09b3f2bb70434ae598e2e5a135 (accessed on 22 May 2025).
2. Ali, Q., Fischetti, C., Fox, J. C., Lahha*m, S.,* et al. (2020). Tricuspid annular plane of systolic excursion for the evaluation of patients with severe sepsis and septic shock. https://core.ac.uk/download/286361891.pdf.
3. Braithwaite, N. A., Pezzolla, D., Paget, D., Krausgruber, T., Bock, C., Carnice*r, R.,* et al. (2024). Multi-organ single-cell RNA sequencing in mice reveals early hyperglycemia responses that converge on fibroblast dysregul*ation. The FASEB Jour*nal, 38. https://www.semanticscholar.org/paper/b8ffc4f9e166d7685bde698894250252c10f3e82 (accessed on 22 May 2025).
4. Castro, H. J., & Yousif, M. G. (2023). Cognizance of post-COVID-19 multi-organ dysfunction through machine learning ana*lysis. ArXiv, abs/230*9.16736. https://www.semanticscholar.org/paper/5314269e6729d34f193f509f102a46b14ed02bec (accessed on 22 May 2025).
5. Chopra, V., Flanders, S. A., O'Malley, M., Malani, A. N., & Prescott, H. C. (2020). Sixty-day outcomes among patients hospitalized with COV*ID-19. Annals of Internal Medic*ine, 174, 576–578. https://doi.org/10.7326/m20-5661.
6. Copaescu, A., Smibert, O., Gibson, A., Phillips, E. J., & Trubiano, J. A. (2020). The role of IL-6 and other mediators in the cytokine storm associated with SARS-CoV-2 infe*ction. Journal of Allergy and Clinical Immunolo*gy, 146(3), 518–534.e1. https://doi.org/10.1016/j.jaci.2020.07.001.
7. Dallan, C., Romano, F., Siebert, J. N., Politi, S., Lacroix, L., & Sahyoun, C. (2020). Septic shock presentation in adolescents with COV*ID-19. The Lancet Child & Adolescent H*ealth, 4(7), e21–e23. https://doi.org/10.1016/s2352-4642(20)30164-4.
8. Delano, M. J., & Ward, P. A. (2016). The immune system's role in sepsis progression, resolution, and long-term outcome. Immunological Reviews, 274, 330–353. *https://doi.org/10.11*11/imr.12499.
9. De Rosa, S., Samoni, S., Villa, G., & Ronco, C. (2017). Management of chronic kidney disease patients in the intensive care unit: Mixing acute and chroni*c illness. Blood Purificat*ion, 43, 151–162. https://doi.org/10.1159/000452650.
10. Du, X., Zhang, M., Zhou, H., Wang, W., Zhang, C., Zhang, L., Q*u, Y.,* et al. (2022). Decoy nanozymes enable multitarget blockade of proinflammatory cascades for the treatment of multi-drug-resistant bacterial se*psis. Researc*h, 2022. https://doi.org/10.34133/2022/9767643.
11. Elfeky, A., Mohammed, H., Abd El Aziz, F., & Mohammed, W. Y. (2013). Factors predisposing to organ(s) dysfunction among critically ill adult patients at a selected university hospital in Egypt. https://core.ac.uk/download/234686829.pdf.
12. Fan, S., & Ma, J. (2024). The value of five scoring systems in predicting the prognosis of patients with sepsis-associated acute respiratory fai*lure. Scientific Repo*rts, 14. https://www.semanticscholar.org/paper/24a1433cebfc7256ef19bc9d81390dbc500cad13 (accessed on 22 May 2025).
13. Gao, Y., Yao, Y., Zhang, X., Chen, F., Meng, X., Chen, X., Wang, *C. l.,* et al. (2022). Regulatory T cells: Angels or demons in the pathophysiology of se*psis? Frontiers in Immuno*logy, 13. https://doi.org/10.3389/fimmu.2022.829210.

14. Gebeyehu, G. M., Rashidiani, S., Farkas, B., Szabadi, A., Brandt, B., Pap, M., & Rauch, T. A. (2024). Unveiling the role of exosomes in the pathophysiology of sepsis: Insights into organ dysfunction and potential biomar*kers. International Journal of Molecular Scien*ces, 25. https://www.semanticscholar.org/paper/0338022da4e8760108a2c9d68245eea54eee9b82 (accessed on 22 May 2025).

15. Généreux, P., Piazza, N., Alu, M., Nazif, T., Hahn, R. T., Pîbarot, P., Bax, *J. J.,* et al. (2020). Valve Academic Research Consortium 3: Updated endpoint definitions for aortic valve clinical res*earch. European Heart Jour*nal, 42, 1825–1857. https://doi.org/10.1093/eurheartj/ehaa799.

16. He, R. R., Yue, G. L., Dong, M., Wang, J., & Cheng, C. (2024). Sepsis biomarkers: Advancements and clinical applications—A narrative r*eview. International Journal of Molecular Scien*ces, 25, 9010. https://doi.org/10.3390/ijms25169010.

17. Huang, Q., Ding, Y., Fang, C., Wang, H., & Kong, L. (2023). The emerging role of ferroptosis in sepsis: Opportunity or chal*lenge? Infection and Drug Resista*nce, 16, 5551–5562. https://doi.org/10.2147/idr.s419993.

18. Ibrahim, M. M., Li, C., Ma, Y., & Fang, C. (2025). Therapeutic effect of anti-FABP4 mAb (6H2) on systemic inflammation in sepsis: Insights from abdominal organ ana*lysis.* bioRxiv. https://www.semanticscholar.org/paper/421a55732e4e9b20a82e3963537a9e32af23957f (accessed on 22 May 2025).

19. Jarczak, D., Kluge, S., & Nierhaus, A. (2021). Sepsis—Pathophysiology and therapeutic con*cepts. Frontiers in Medi*cine, 8. https://doi.org/10.3389/fmed.2021.628302.

20. Jiang, L., Chen, S., Li, S., Wang, J., Chen, W., Shi, Y., Xion*g, W.,* et al. (2024). Exploring biomarkers for diagnosing and predicting organ dysfunction in patients with perioperative sepsis: A preliminary investig*ation. Perioperative Medi*cine, 13. https://www.semanticscholar.org/paper/1d34c02c6dbc6de90276abdd35e32d5659289728 (accessed on 22 May 2025).

21. Jiang, L., Tang, K., Levin, M., Irfan, O., Morris, S. K., Wilson, K. M., Klein, *J. D.,* et al. (2020). COVID-19 and multisystem inflammatory syndrome in children and adoles*cents. The Lancet Infectious Disea*ses, 20, e276–e288. https://doi.org/10.1016/s1473-3099(20)30651-4.

22. Kumar, T., Balraj, T. A., Kempegowda, S. N., & Prashant, A. (2024). Multidrug-resistant sepsis: A critical healthcare chal*lenge. Antibio*tics, 13, 46. https://doi.org/10.3390/antibiotics13010046.

23. Lee, J., Lee, S. K., & Lee, S. T. (2025). Case report: Multi-organ dysfunction in a dog following massive paper *wasp (Polistes r*othneyi) envenom*ation. Frontiers in Veterinary Scie*nce, 12. https://www.semanticscholar.org/paper/249f0932efed757a2ab7fc5c14623b3eba1b3660 (accessed on 22 May 2025).

24. Marjot, T., Moon, A. M., Cook, J., Abd-Elsalam, S., Aloman, C., Armstrong, M. J., Pos*e, E.,* et al. (2020). Outcomes following SARS-CoV-2 infection in patients with chronic liver disease: An international registry *study. Journal of Hepato*logy, 74, 567–577. https://doi.org/10.1016/j.jhep.2020.09.024.

25. Moore, R., Chanci, D., Brown, S. R., Ripple, M. J., Bishop, N. R., Grunwell, J., & Kamaleswaran, R. (2025). Association of the child opportunity index with in-hospital mortality and persistence of organ dysfunction at one week after onset of Phoenix Sepsis among children admitted to the pediatric intensive care unit with suspected infe*ction. PLOS Digital He*alth, 4. https://www.semanticscholar.org/paper/e171e81d0cae99afa3908fd73d8cbe9ec160b823 (accessed on 22 May 2025).

26. Murray, C. J. L., Ikuta, K. S., Sharara, F., Swetschinski, L. R., Robles Aguilar, G., Gray, A. P., Han, C., et al. (2022). Global burden of bacterial antimicrobial resistance in 2019: A systematic analysis. *The Lancet*, 399(10325), 629–655. https://doi.org/10.1016/s0140-6736(21)02724-0.

27. Neu, C., Baumbach, P., Scherag, A., Kortgen, A., Götze, J., & Coldewey, S. (2022). Identification of cardiovascular and molecular prognostic factors for the morbidity and mortality in COVID-19-sepsis (ICROVID): Protocol for a prospective multi-center cohort study. *PLoS ONE*, 17. https://www.semanticscholar.org/paper/6b79cff3cc6feaf43720e59ae2eaf5e837eeab2c (accessed on 22 May 2025).

28. Niu, Y., Liu, Y., Huang, L., Liu, W., Cheng, Q., Liu, T., Ning, Q., et al. (2024). Antiviral immunity of severe fever with thrombocytopenia syndrome: Current understanding and implications for clinical treatment. *Frontiers in Immunology*, 15. https://www.semanticscholar.org/paper/8de38cb9849d7c2390e8c3454ab557fe97d2f011 (accessed on 22 May 2025).

29. Olwal, C. O., Nganyewo, N. N., Tapela, K., Djomkam Zune, A. L., Owoicho, O., Bediako, Y., & Duodu, S. (2021). Parallels in sepsis and COVID-19 conditions: Implications for managing severe COVID-19. *Frontiers in Immunology*, 12. https://doi.org/10.3389/fimmu.2021.602848.

30. Osikov, M., Telesheva, L. F., Konashov, A., Gusev, A. V., & Konashov, V. (2024). Modern ideas of the role of the immune process and hemostasis in the pathogenesis of sepsis. *Acta Biomedica Scientifica*. https://www.semanticscholar.org/paper/e810bf069c33ac06f643c7bc08ccf69101cc030d (accessed on 22 May 2025).

31. Pisano, M., Allievi, N., Gurusamy, K. S., Borzellino, G., Cimbanassi, S., Boerna, D., Coccolini, F., et al. (2020). 2020 World Society of Emergency Surgery updated guidelines for the diagnosis and treatment of acute calculus cholecystitis. *World Journal of Emergency Surgery*, 15. https://doi.org/10.1186/s13017-020-00336-x.

32. Pratapa Reddy, D. V., Vijayakumari, V., Kumar, R. S., Bhushana Rao, C. H. R. N., Gowtham, S., & Perumal, S. (2024). Comparison of pneumonia-specific scores, sepsis score and generic score in predicting the severity of community-acquired pneumonia: A cross-sectional study. *Journal of Clinical and Diagnostic Research*. https://www.semanticscholar.org/paper/336c1a356d94645648b3f34761d3404c1784e8f7 (accessed on 22 May 2025).

33. Shah, B., Kumar, S. S., & Shah, S. (2023). A rare presentation of scrub typhus: Multi-organ dysfunction [acute kidney injury, hepatitis] and acute respiratory distress syndrome. *Asian Journal of Research in Infectious Diseases*. https://www.semanticscholar.org/paper/2bbea51f7dccf7e58c41bc5995e2efc8d3e1356d (accessed on 22 May 2025).

34. Shahid, A., Chambers, S., Scott-Thomas, A., & Bhatia, M. (2024). Gut microbiota and liver dysfunction in sepsis: The role of inflammatory mediators and therapeutic approaches. *International Journal of Molecular Sciences*, 25. https://www.semanticscholar.org/paper/5c07b10a416f9f6787833145713799168770ebd5 (accessed on 22 May 2025).

35. Singh, N., Rebello, A., Gill, J., & Goyal, S. (2025). The impact of beta-lactam antibiotic timing on patient outcomes in post-operative sepsis management: A multi-center analysis of orthopedic and general surgery cases. *Journal of Neonatal Surgery*. https://www.semanticscholar.org/paper/c8215f511924477aa6607099db70656160b99d70 (accessed on 22 May 2025).

36. Song, J., Fang, X., Zhou, K., Bao, H., & Li, L. (2023). Sepsis-induced cardiac dysfunction and pathogenetic mechanisms (Review). *Molecular Medicine Reports*, 28. https://doi.org/10.3892/mmr.2023.13114.

37. Srdić, T., Đurašević, S., Lakić, I., Ružičić, A., Vujovic, P., Jevđović, T., Dakić, *T.,* et al. (2024). From molecular mechanisms to clinical therapy: Understanding sepsis-induced multiple organ dysfunc*tion. International Journal of Molecular Scien*ces, 25. https://www.semanticscholar.org/paper/945a2f46bd282041ef519bfe3e8bafc105cb314b (accessed on 22 May 2025).

38. Szatmary, P., Grammatikopoulos, T., Cai, W., Huang, W., Mukherjee, R., Halloran, C., Beye*r, G.,* et al. (2022). Acute pancreatitis: Diagnosis and trea*tment. Dr*ugs, 82, 1251–1276. https://doi.org/10.1007/s40265-022-01766-4.

39. Tiao, B., Bakamutumaho, B., Owor, N., Kayiwa, J., Namulondo, J., Byaruhanga, T., Muwang*a, M.,* et al. (2025). Associations between organ dysfunction scoring systems and dysregulated host responses in adults with severe infection in Uganda: A prospective cohort *study. The American Journal of Tropical Medicine and* Hygiene. https://www.semanticscholar.org/paper/530e5302db19a29eb30d5022d8097aac5ea39b1d (accessed on 22 May 2025).

40. Veras, F. P., Pontelli, M. C., Silva, C. M., Toller-Kawahisa, J. E., de Lima, M., Nascimento, D. C., Schneider, *A. H.,* et al. (2020). SARS-CoV-2–triggered neutrophil extracellular traps mediate COVID-19 path*ology. The Journal of Experimental Medic*ine, 217(12). https://doi.org/10.1084/jem.20201129.

41. Wang, X., & Qi, W. (2024). Research progress of artificial intelligence technology in early diagnosis of sepsis [Research art*icle]. Zhonghua Wei Zhong Bing Ji Jiu Yi* Xue, 36(1), 98–101. https://www.semanticscholar.org/paper/123ca8e293da3206cdc94778e0a624a945f9ede7 (accessed on 22 May 2025).

42. Yu, Y., Li, J., Li, J., Zen, X., & Fu, Q. (2023). Evidence from machine learning, diagnostic hub genes in sepsis and diagnostic models based on Xgboost models, novel molecular models for the diagnosis of se*psis. Current Medicinal Ch*emistry. https://www.semanticscholar.org/paper/61d5c932cdc5c19d7e208dc4de4c923f42e5cc5c (accessed on 22 May 2025).

43. Zhang, M., Xu, Q., Zhang, H., Cao, Y. Y., & Lu, W. (2024). Multiple infections secondary to immunosuppression *after Chlamydia p*sittaci infection: A case r*eport. BMC Infectious Disea*ses, 24. https://www.semanticscholar.org/paper/42fc664a79ee9396288abdfea9299a2015a16cc5 (accessed on 22 May 2025).

ACUTE RESPIRATORY DISTRESS SYNDROME (ARDS)

7

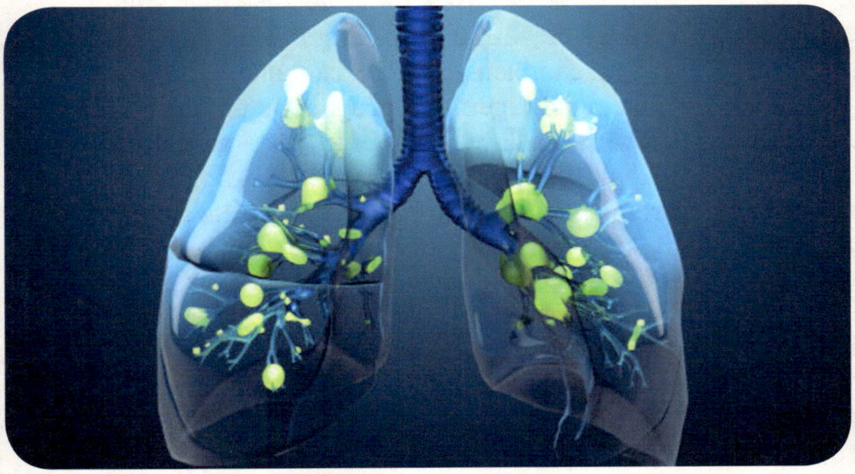

Introduction

Acute Respiratory Distress Syndrome (ARDS) is a critical pathophysiologic disorder with excessive respiratory failure that is typically caused by other primary diseases. ARDS results through inflammatory mechanisms leading to the increased permeability of the alveolar-capillary membrane, resulting in pulmonary edema and impaired gas exchange. The incidence of ARDS has been on the rise in recent years, particularly under viral pandemics such as COVID-19, which has stressed the need for appropriate treatment protocols to alleviate respiratory distress and lung failure among affected individuals (Amjadi *et al.*, 2025). Furthermore, illnesses like Chlamydia psittaci infection predispose a patient to developing ARDS, which further emphasizes the use of early diagnosis and treatment (Wang *et al.*, 2024). While clinicians attempt to optimize patient outcomes, comprehension of ARDS's multi-factorial etiology and its impact on therapy remains the top concern in the healthcare community.

LEARNING OBJECTIVES

After studying this chapter, you will be able to:

1. Describe pathophysiology of ARDS.
2. List the causes and risk factors.
3. Explore diagnosis and assessment.
4. Discuss about treatment and management.

Definition of Acute Respiratory Distress Syndrome (ARDS)

For one to understand the definition of ARDS, it is crucial to note the clinical progression of this disease. Initially considered acute respiratory failure due to noncardiogenic pulmonary edema, Ashbaugh *et al.* (1967) initially defined ARDS, but its definition drastically transformed with the publication of the Berlin definition in 2012, which standardized criteria for diagnosis and severity classification. Recent developments have threatened this definition in the context of embracing progress in clinical management, such as the use of high-flow nasal oxygen and ultrasound, particularly in low-resource settings. A forthcoming consensus conference among leading ARDS authorities aims at more clearly defining the condition with the perspective of making it remain practical and useful in a range of care environments (Matthay *et al.*, 2023). The dynamism in ARDS definitions is a reflection of the flexibility needed in diagnosis and treatment protocols in order to improve patient outcomes under critical care (Yıldırım *et al.*, 2022) (Figure 7.1).

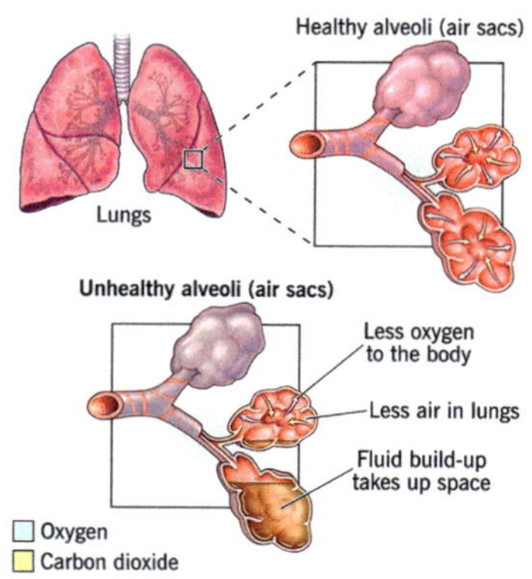

Figure 7.1. Acute respiratory distress syndrome (ARDS) happens when fluid builds up in the tiny air sacs in your lungs.

Source: https://my.clevelandclinic.org/-/scassets/images/org/health/articles/acute-respiratory-stress-syndrome.

Importance of Studying Acute Respiratory Distress Syndrome (ARDS)

Study of ARDS is of the utmost significance since it has a far-reaching impact on patient outcomes and the healthcare system, particularly in pandemics such as COVID-19. Study of clinical data indicates that most of the COVID-19 pneumonia patients develop ARDS, which comes with an extremely high mortality rate—more than 52% of cases in some research studies (Wu *et al.*, 2020). Understanding predictors and mechanisms of ARDS can enable improved clinical management, prognostic outcome, and prevention. Emerging predictive models that use gradient boosted trees, for example, offer promising results in predicting the development of ARDS, offering clinicians a valuable tool to intervene earlier and improve care for patients (Le *et al.*, 2020). Given the evolving health challenges, there is an urgent need to improve the understanding of ARDS to minimize its deadly impacts and improve survival among various populations.

Significance of Early Diagnosis

Early diagnosis of ARDS matters in terms to improving the prognosis of patients and reducing mortality rates for this lethal disease. Early recognition allows medical professionals to apply appropriate interventions, such as non-invasive ventilation or increased supportive care, which can have a great impact on respiratory function and general prognosis. The finding of serum markers, such as platelet-mononuclear cell aggregates (PMAs), has been a hopeful prospect for early diagnosis as indicative markers, and the significance of ongoing research into personalized biomarkers for ARDS, particularly sepsis-related ones (Huang *et al.*, 2024), is essential. Moreover, the effectiveness of various ventilation strategies in managing different levels of ARDS supports early diagnosis to provide an efficient therapeutic management

(Théo Battalian, 2024). Therefore, a concerted effort to optimize diagnostic accuracy will not only reduce treatment protocols but also create the impetus for targeted therapy to attenuate the impact of this serious illness.

Brief History of Acute Respiratory Distress Syndrome (ARDS) Research

Investigation into ARDS has been influenced over the years by seminal studies defining its pathophysiology and treatment. Originally described in the 1960s, the syndrome was originally conceptualized primarily in terms of trauma and pneumonia, leading to an increased understanding of the mechanisms of lung injury. Over several decades, breakthroughs in critical care accrued from the reduction of the etiology and therapeutic choices for ARDS. Above all, cases of opportunistic infections, like those of Pneumocystis jirovecii pneumonia (PJP), expanded research areas, highlighting particular at-risk patient groups, for instance, the immunocompromised (Hehsan, 2024). In addition, the complex interaction of genetic determinants, as seen in studies of X-linked inhibitor of apoptosis deficiency, has contributed to the knowledge of ARDS risk and severity (Kim *et al.*, 2024). Thus, ongoing research keeps designing therapeutic approaches, customized to the multifaceted character of ARDS (Figure 7.2).

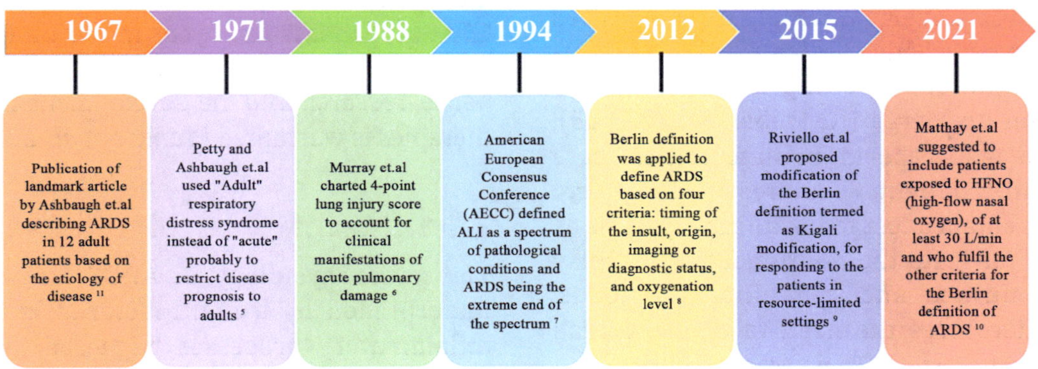

Figure 7.2. Overview of proposed refinements in Acute Respiratory Distress Syndrome (ARDS) definition.

Source: https://www.researchgate.net/figure/Overview-of-proposed-refinements-in-ARDS-definition-data-collected-from-references-5_fig1_360984297.

Current Statistics on Acute Respiratory Distress Syndrome (ARDS) Prevalence

It is necessary to know how prevalent ARDS is so that its enormous contribution to health can be addressed at an international level. Current evidence indicates that ARDS occurs in approximately 10%–20% of intensive care admissions, with varying rates according to underlying disease and population. It often follows pneumonia, sepsis, or trauma, highlighting the association with critical illness. Moreover, with the outbreak of the COVID-19 pandemic, there has been an increase in ARDS cases because the virus impacts respiratory function negatively. Specifically, evidence has shown that COVID-19 patients diagnosed with ARDS are subjected to prolonged ventilator usage and high mortality. The identification of effective treatments for ARDS, i.e., examination of ventilation modes like airway pressure release ventilation (APRV), underscores the necessity of new clinical guidelines in intensive care units (Aldhahir *et al.*, 2024; Amjadi *et al.*, 2025).

Impact of Acute Respiratory Distress Syndrome (ARDS) on Healthcare Systems

The influence of ARDS on the health system is multifaceted, with a significant impact on resource utilization, patient outcomes, and rehabilitation access. Since ARDS is a leading cause of increased ICU admission rates and mechanical ventilation, hospitals typically incur heavy burdens that outweigh available resources. For instance, the COVID-19 pandemic brought patients with ARDS issue to the fore, which laid bare the systemic vulnerabilities against disparities in rehabilitation access. Studies have shown that socio-economic determinants have a negative effect on ARDS patients' recovery because those under vulnerable circumstances are likely to experience difficulties during post-ICU rehabilitation, resulting in lower quality of life upon discharge (Kl Méber *et al.*, 2025). Also, even when the immediate critical care need of ARDS patients is addressed, long-term outcomes remain a test to healthcare systems as they must navigate the multi-faceted interplay of comorbidities and rehabilitation needs, which underscores the need to create overall healthcare strategies (Rana *et al.*, 2024).

7.1. Pathophysiology of Acute Respiratory Distress Syndrome (ARDS)

Learning Outcome

1. Understand the mechanisms of lung injury
2. Describe the role of inflammation in ARDS
3. Define alveolar-capillary membrane damage
4. Explain the surfactant dysfunction
5. Define impaired gas exchange
6. Identify the stages of ARDS development.
7. Understand the systemic effects of ARDS
8. Discuss biomarkers associated with ARDS
9. Explain the differences between ARDS and other respiratory conditions

The pathophysiology of ARDS is due to a severe inflammatory reaction that impairs the integrity of the alveolar-capillary membrane. The impairment may be due to direct lung injuries, e.g., pneumonia, or indirect impairment from disorders such as sepsis. Once the integrity of the alveolar-capillary membrane is impaired, it is leaky, and fluid penetration into the alveoli is encouraged, impairing gas exchange and leading to respiratory failure. The inflammatory processes also amplify lung injury through cell recruitment of inflammatory cells and release of cytokines, producing diffuse alveolar injury and hypoxemia, the latter being a vital aspect of ARDS and indicating severe tissue oxygenation deficiency (Hendrickson *et al.*, 2013). Interestingly, given the incidence of ARDS, which occurs in an estimated 150,000 patients each year in the United States, successful treatment regimens are lacking, and hence, research into the development of targeted therapies is warranted (Yunker *et al.*, 2014).

7.1.1. Mechanisms of Lung Injury

The pathophysiology of ARDS lung injury is underpinned by a multi-factorial interplay of inflammatory processes triggered by various insults, such as sepsis, pneumonia, and trauma. The centerpiece in this pathogenic process is endothelial cells (ECs), which are ideally placed to ensure the integrity of the pulmonary barrier. In sepsis, these cells become damaged, and therefore an increase in vascular permeability results in pulmonary edema, which is the hallmark of ARDS (Qiao *et al.*, 2024). In addition to that, there is also activation of the inflammatory process by various immune cells, and they inflict additional damage on the lungs through the release of pro-inflammatory cytokines, leading to extensive alveolar injury (Zheng *et al.*, 2024). In spite of much advancement in the knowledge of these mechanisms, therapeutic strategies are inefficient, and much larger efforts are needed to explore the underlying pathophysiology to find intervening potential for lung injury reduction in ARDS (Figure 7.3).

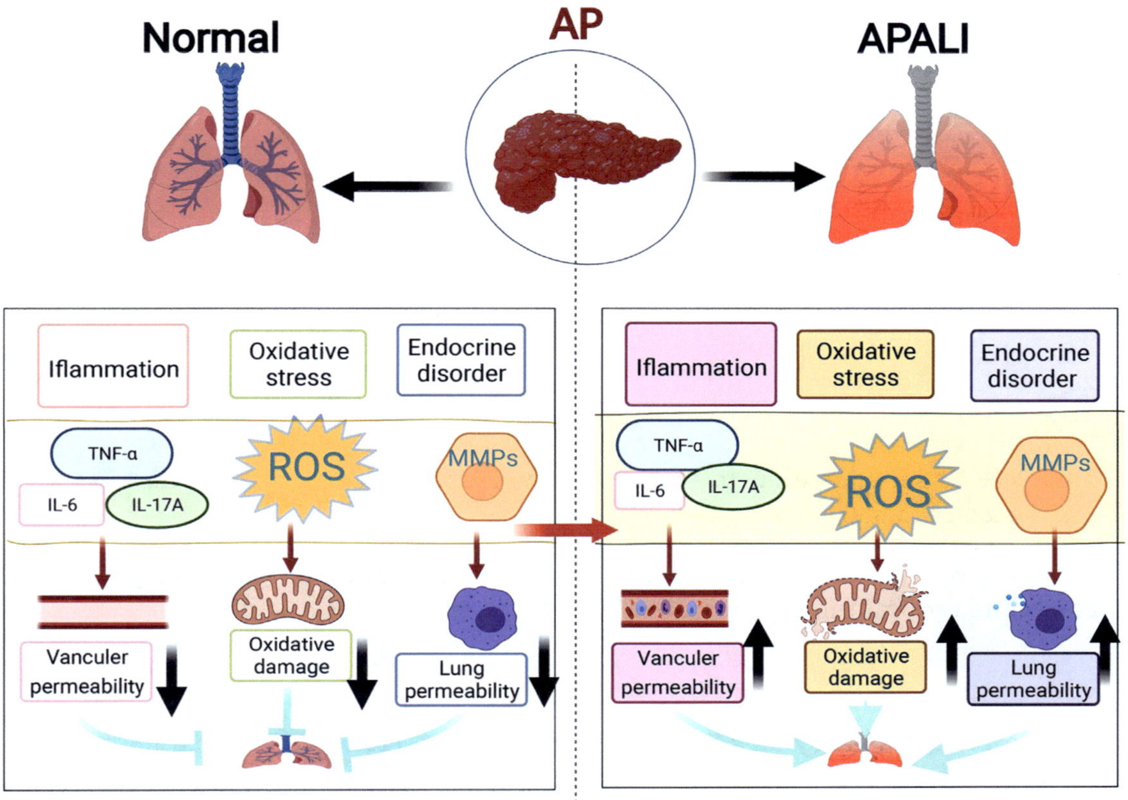

Figure 7.3. The three main mechanisms of lung injury in acute pancreatitis (AP).

Source: https://www.frontiersin.org/files/Articles/904078/fmed-09-904078-HTML/image_m/fmed-09-904078-g001.jpg.

7.1.2. Role of Inflammation in Acute Respiratory Distress Syndrome (ARDS)

The inflammatory component in ARDS is central, as it is behind the pathophysiological processes in the disease. ARDS is characterized by global inflammation that results in disruption of alveolar and microvasculature lung integrity and function, finally leading to hypoxemic respiratory failure. The disease has been attributed to uncontrolled systemic inflammation, predominantly in studies; hence the importance of learning more about inflammatory pathways in ARDS treatment (Fowler, 2024). Some of the consequences of inflammation include damage to endothelial as well as alveolar epithelial cells, which worsen lung pathology and complicate therapeutic approaches (Zhang *et al.*, 2024). Effective anti-inflammatory strategies, such as the potential use of vitamin C, may play an essential role in reducing lung damage by reversing such inflammatory processes. Thus, a unified understanding of the contribution of inflammation in ARDS is essential in the formulation of aimed therapeutic approaches (Figure 7.4).

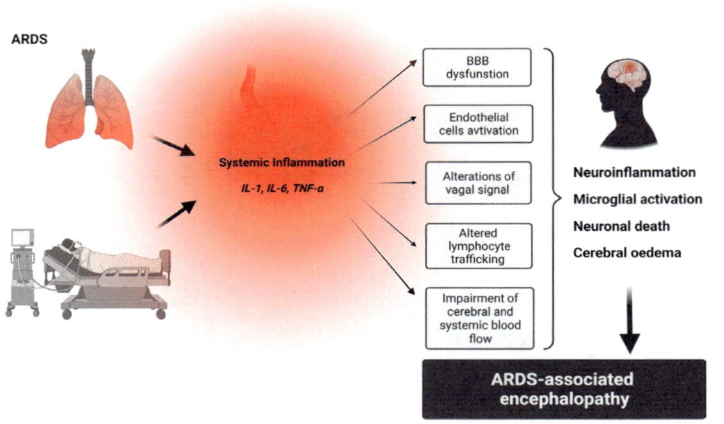

Figure 7.4. Role of inflammation in the development of acute respiratory distress syndrome (ARDS)-associated secondary brain injury.

Source: https://www.researchgate.net/figure/Role-of-inflammation-in-the-development-of-ARDS-associated-secondary-brain-injury_fig2_362679774.

7.1.3. Alveolar-Capillary Membrane Damage

The extent of alveolar-capillary membrane damage is a focal factor in ARDS pathophysiology and a principal cause of the syndrome's mortality and morbidity. The disruption of this membrane, a critical barrier to gas exchange, leads to increased permeability that enables protein and fluid leakage into the alveoli.

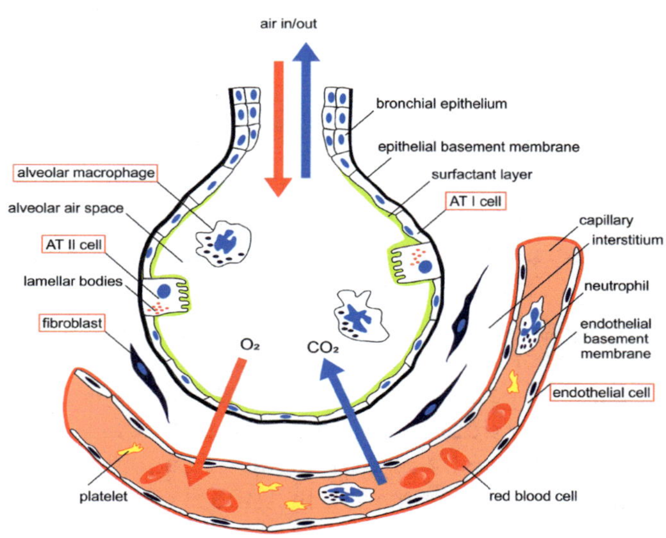

Figure 7.5. Schematic arrangement of alveolar-capillary membrane-related pulmonary cells.

Source: https://www.mdpi.com/1422-0067/20/4/831.

This is exacerbated in viral infection-induced ARDS, such as COVID-19 and Influenza A, wherein the pathological mechanisms can cause intense net damage to the membrane (Svraka *et al.*, 2025). Moreover, exposure to pneumotoxic agents has been observed to impair the barrier, precipitating the need for new therapeutic modalities for maintenance of membrane integrity and improved outcomes in these patients (Isabekov *et al.*, 2024). Knowledge of the exact processes of such damage is necessary for the creation of effective interventions and management strategies in ARDS patients (Figure 7.5).

7.1.4. Surfactant Dysfunction

Surfactant failure is a key element in the pathogenesis of ARDS since it disrupts alveolar surface tension, leading to collapse and instability. It is achieved through a surfactant protein-lipid imbalance, which is critical in the prevention of atelectasis and stability of the alveolus. Research demonstrates that etiologies of acute lung injury contribute significantly to surfactant dysfunction, increasing ARDS symptom severity (Dezfouli *et al.*, 2025). Moreover, inflammation in ARDS is linked to alterations in the surfactant system via pathways such as nuclear factor κB (NF-κB) that promote inflammation and endothelial barrier dysfunction (Zuo *et al.*, 2024). Thus, finding the pathophysiology of surfactant dysfunction becomes essential so that therapeutic strategies can be formulated that may restore normal lung mechanics and maximize patient outcomes in ARDS.

7.1.5. Impaired Gas Exchange

Gas exchange impairment syndrome is a characteristic of ARDS, with significant inflammation of the lung and failure of alveolar-capillary membranes. The resulting increase in permeability leads to filling of the alveoli with fluid, with significant inhibition of oxygen diffusion and removal of carbon dioxide. As reviewed in the literature, mechanical ventilation emerges as a central intervention for the management of these patients; however, issues like ventilator-induced lung injury and diminished respiratory muscle strength can complicate the process during the recovery stages (Jain, 2024). Moreover, the weaning process from controlled to assisted ventilation is especially challenging, e.g., maintaining adequate respiratory drive and methods to prevent self-inflicted lung injury (Battaglini *et al.*, 2024). Hence, an understanding of such dynamics is essential to the development of specifically targeted therapeutic strategies that will regain effective gas exchange with fewer side effects toward ultimately improving survival and enhancing the quality of treatment for ARDS patients (Figure 7.6).

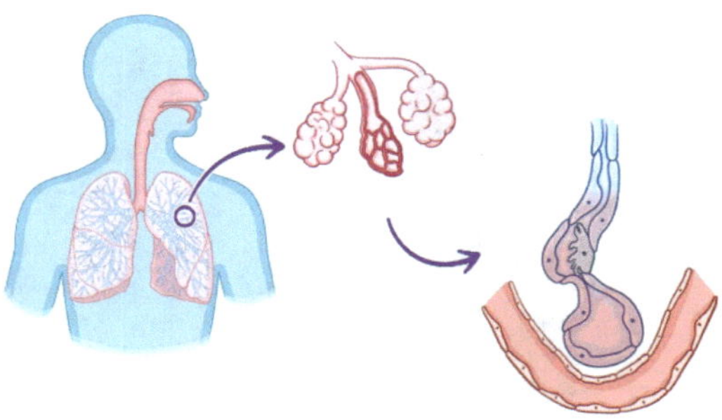

Figure 7.6. The phenomenon of impaired gas exchange is a hallmark of acute respiratory distress syndrome (ARDS).

Source: https://d16qt3wv6xm098.cloudfront.net/4u2XgGDST6a9HRxgrFTmhXj5Q1qc0F7r/_.jpg.

7.1.6. Stages of Acute Respiratory Distress Syndrome (ARDS) Development

It is worthwhile to appreciate the stages of ARDS in clinical care and intervention. ARDS will typically progress through three broad stages: the exudative, proliferative, and fibrotic stages. The exudative stage is marked by the migration of inflammatory cells into tissue with resultant vascular permeability and secondary pulmonary edema. This can begin early, typically a few hours following the precipitant, highlighting the imperative to treat. When the state evolves to the proliferative phase, there is a return to repair characteristic of alveolar epithelial cells and fibroblast proliferation. Inability to reverse inflammation, however, leads to the fibrotic phase when permanent injury is achieved, significantly impairing lung function. Latest research indicates the potential of mesenchymal stem cells (MSCs) in the prevention of ARDS-associated liver damage, opening up their application during such critical intervals (Redko *et al.*, 2023). In addition, novel machine learning techniques might enhance early prediction of ARDS development during admissions, crucial for early intervention (Lam *et al.*, 2021) (Figure 7.7).

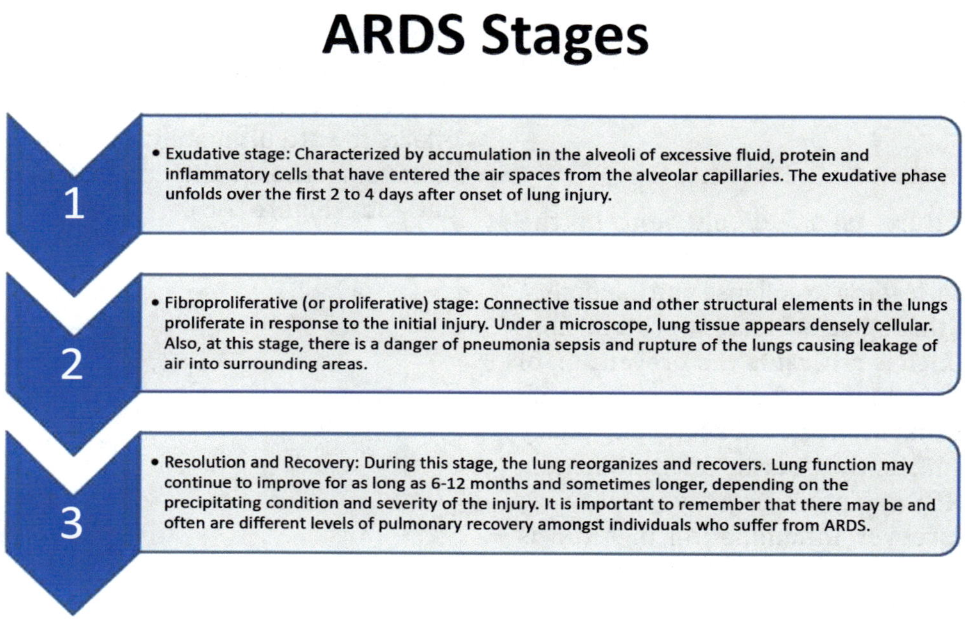

Figure 7.7. The three stages of acute respiratory distress syndrome (ARDS).

Source: https://sites.pitt.edu/~super1/lecture/lec33251/003.htm.

7.1.7. Systemic Effects of Acute Respiratory Distress Syndrome (ARDS)

The systemic implications of ARDS are extensive beyond the lungs and have a significant impact on the overall physiological condition of the victim. One of the primary features of ARDS is the induction of inflammatory mechanisms, leading to the release of a number of mediators that sustain a systemic inflammatory process. For instance, neutrophil elastase plays a central role in lung damage during sepsis, a common etiology of ARDS, through cell recruitment by inflammation and enhancement of pulmonary tissue injury (Ma *et al.*, 2023). Other novel therapies, such as primed MSCs, are also studied for their immunomodulation potential. These cells are capable of inhibiting inflammatory mediators and stimulating tissue repair, holding promise in controlling local as well as systemic features of the syndrome (Kong *et al.*, 2025). Thus, understanding the broader implications of ARDS is crucial for developing therapeutic measures that not only control lung pathology but also inhibit systemic sequelae.

7.1.8. Biomarkers Associated with Acute Respiratory Distress Syndrome (ARDS)

The identification of biomarkers of ARDS is important for the improvement of the diagnostic effectiveness and for guiding the choice of treatment. From the wide range of potential biomarkers, PMAs are significant markers for sepsis with ARDS. It has been found through studies that serum levels of PMAs are significantly higher in such patients and correlate positively with the Acute Physiology and Chronic Health Evaluation (APACHE) II score, a marker of illness severity (Huang *et al.*, 2024). Furthermore, the classification of ARDS into sub-phenotypes based on clinical as well as biomarker data is being explored, which could enhance a more tailored therapeutic strategy (Liu *et al.*, 2024). By introducing this biomarker-guided approach into clinical care, physicians may be able to diagnose patients earlier and enhance ARDS patients' management, thereby translating into improved patient outcomes (Figure 7.8).

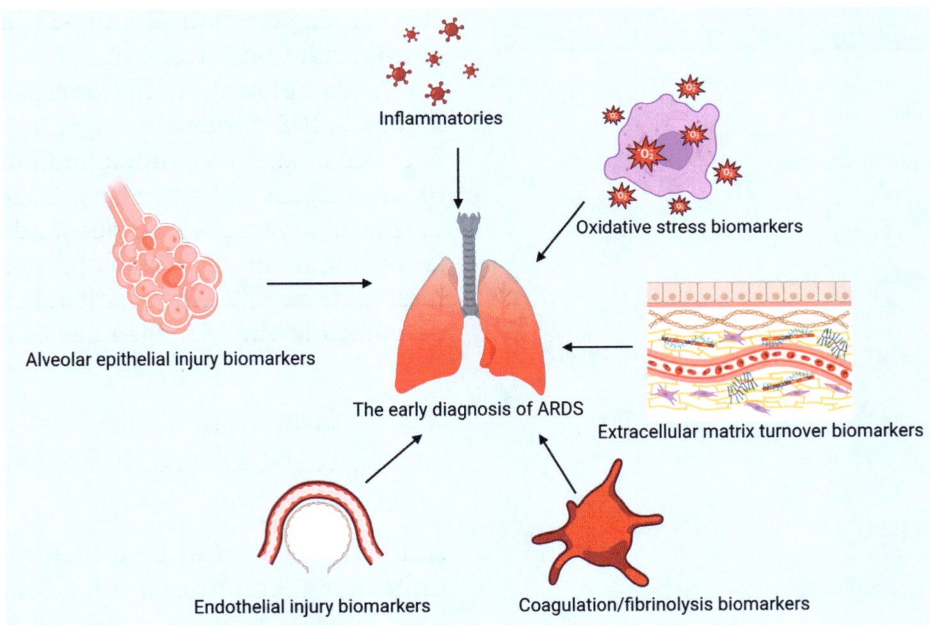

Figure 7.8. The classification of the biomarkers for ARDS.

Source: https://www.mdpi.com/2075-4418/13/21/3296.

7.1.9. Differences Between Acute Respiratory Distress Syndrome (ARDS) and Other Respiratory Conditions

It is important to realize how ARDS differs from other respiratory diseases so that appropriate diagnosis and treatment can be established. In contrast to chronic respiratory diseases such as asthma or chronic obstructive pulmonary disease (COPD), in which progression is slow and care can be managed over time, ARDS typically comes on abruptly following some precipitant event and is characterized by severe hypoxemia and pulmonary inflammation. Further, ARDS is also characterized by a reduction in lung compliance and a large drop in the functional residual capacity, basically altering gas exchange dynamics. Studies have confirmed that extrinsic factors such as vaccination status influence the causation of ARDS, with patients who are vaccinated showing a reduced risk for severe presentation compared to their unvaccinated peers (Madrid *et al.*, 2024). Second, hemoglobin's oxygen affinity plays an even more significant part in ARDS because impaired binding enhances hypoxemic conditions, and the detection of oxygen dynamics in acute and chronic respiratory impediments is a matter of paramount importance (Lopes *et al.*, 2024).

Test Your Knowledge

1. What are the primary mechanisms that lead to lung injury in ARDS?
2. How does inflammation contribute to the development and progression of ARDS?

7.2. Causes and Risk Factors

Learning Outcome

1. Identify the common causes of ARDS
2. Discuss the infectious agents leading to ARDS
3. Understand the non-infectious causes of ARDS
4. Describe risk factors associated with ARDS
5. Explain the role of pre-existing conditions
6. Analyze the environmental factors contributing to ARDS
7. Discuss the genetic predisposition to ARDS
8. Identify the impact of age and gender on ARDS risk
9. Discuss the prevention strategies for at-risk populations

ARDS is initiated by an enormous number of causes and risk factors responsible for its multifactorial pathophysiology. The major initiator among them is traumatic injury, which has been a well-documented cause of ARDS development for years. These wounds trigger an inflammatory response that can compromise pulmonary function, according to recent evidence demonstrating the efficacy of pentoxifylline in suppressing inflammation in trauma-related ARDS, despite no significant reduction in incidence of the syndrome itself (Shirzadeh *et al.*, 2024). Additionally, biomarkers such as angiopoietin-2 (Ang-2) have emerged as important prognostic markers, with elevated levels correlating with increased mortality among ARDS patients, suggesting a direct link between mediators of inflammation and severity of the disease (Zhang *et al.*, 2024). Detection of these diverse etiologies and risk factors is essential for the development of targeted interventions and improvement in world patient outcomes in the management of ARDS.

7.2.1. Common Causes of Acute Respiratory Distress Syndrome (ARDS)

ARDS can be caused by a number of different underlying conditions that lead to severe lung injury. Pneumonia, particularly viral and bacterial infection, is a frequent cause since it can lead to extreme inflammation and flooding of the alveoli with fluid, producing severe gas exchange impairments. Other diseases, such as sepsis and trauma, also lead to ARDS by initiating systemic inflammation and thus leading to lung damage. Notably, recent studies have also placed greater emphasis on COVID-19 as a prominent cause of ARDS development, considering the complexity of its pathophysiology and the potential for widespread organ involvement beyond the respiratory system (Sen *et al.*, 2021).

Finally, long-term consequences of ARDS can be observed in patient outcomes, where a notable percentage of survivors experience significant morbidity and mortality despite hospitalization (Chopra *et al.*, 2020). Familiarity with these common causes is crucial for early diagnosis and management in healthcare institutions (Figure 7.9).

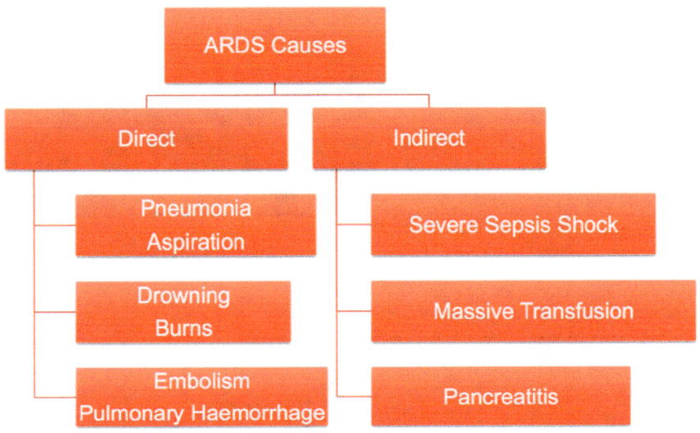

Figure 7.9. Causes of acute respiratory distress syndrome (ARDS).

Source: https://emergencypedia.com/wp-content/uploads/2016/03/ards-causes.png?w=748.

7.2.2. Infectious Agents Leading to Acute Respiratory Distress Syndrome (ARDS)

ARDS usually follows infections as an acute complication and is induced by different infectious agents, triggering its development. Respiratory viruses are among the most important ones, particularly influenza and SARS-CoV-2, both causing severe inflammatory reactions leading to acute lung injury. Influenza illness can lead to a cytokine storm because the pathogen-associated molecular patterns (PAMPs) stimulate an overexuberant immunological response, resulting in ARDS accompanied by severe hypoxemia and pulmonary edema. Moreover, the recent emergence of SARS-CoV-2 brought the viral-induced ARDS issues into focus and underlined the virus's new capability to impair respiratory function and contribute to systemic effects as noted during the COVID-19 pandemic (Hu *et al.*, 2020; Shirey *et al.*, 2021). Explaining the mechanisms by which these causative agents of infection lead to ARDS may contribute to designing targeted therapy aimed at alleviating the harmful consequences of these diseases.

7.2.3. Non-Infectious Causes of Acute Respiratory Distress Syndrome (ARDS)

ARDS can be caused by several non-infectious causes that significantly impair lung function. of these, trauma, aspiration, and chemical inhalation are significant offenders. Trauma is largely lung contusion, leading to inflammation and fluid buildup in the alveoli, resulting in less effective gas exchange. Aspiration of gastric content leads to chemical pneumonitis, with the result in ARDS due to direct alveolar injury and inflammation. Chemical inhalation, typically the product of industrial accidents or toxic fume exposure, also causes strong damage to the lungs, leading to an ensuing inflammatory response. Such an understanding of non-infectious aetiologies is required for the development of targeted treatment interventions. For instance, studies highlight that mechanical ventilation parameters and early interventions are crucial in determining ARDS patient survival, facilitating timely detection and management of non-infectious etiologies (Boada *et al.*, 2024; Liu *et al.*, 2024). Management of these underlying conditions can actually have a major impact on prognosis as well as overall patient care.

7.2.4. Risk Factors Associated with Acute Respiratory Distress Syndrome (ARDS)

ARDS is very reliant on many risk factors shared by pre-existing states and acute disease. Interestingly, preterm birth seems to be a determining risk factor in pediatric patients, and 67.13% of patients were preterm infants in one study, indicating a startling prevalence of ARDS within this vulnerable subgroup (Awan *et al.*, 2025). In another note, post-operative condition and more severe conditions like sepsis have also been identified to heighten the risk of ARDS, and studies where patients with higher SOFA scores and lactate levels not only met ARDS criteria but also had higher mortality rates (Bardají-Carrillo *et al.*, 2024). The interaction between mechanical ventilation, the need for advanced therapies, and baseline disease increases risk, and it is therefore crucial to have an intimate understanding of these dynamics to control ARDS occurrence as well as improve patient outcomes in pediatric and adult patients (Figure 7.10).

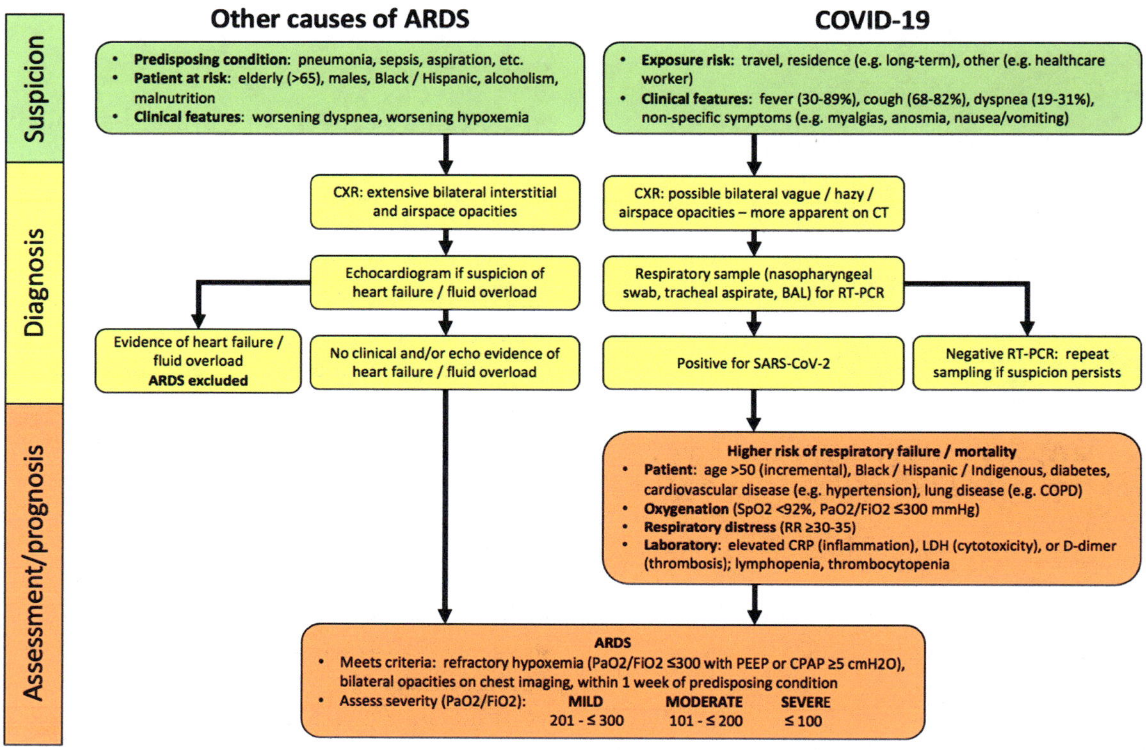

Figure 7.10. Algorithm for hospitalized patients at risk for acute respiratory distress syndrome (ARDS) and coronavirus disease 2019 (COVID-19).

Source: https://www.mdpi.com/diagnostics/diagnostics-10-01053/article_deploy/html/images/diagnostics-10-01053-g001.png.

7.2.5. Role of Pre-Existing Conditions

Pre-existing conditions contribute significantly to the pathogenesis and severity of ARDS and influence patients' outcomes as well as clinical management. Chronic underlying conditions such as respiratory disease, cardiovascular disease, or obesity carry an increased risk of developing ARDS and tend to have worse prognoses than those without these underlying conditions. These underlying conditions can exacerbate lung injury and limit respiratory reserve, complicating clinical presentation during acute attacks. For instance, coexisting pulmonary complications can hinder effective ventilation strategies, necessitating interventions like V-V ECMO to enable gas exchange in severe cases. It has been demonstrated that properly implemented strategies, including therapies such as prone positioning, greatly enhance the health of ARDS patients, particularly those that benefit from such therapy, as documented by recent studies on lung aeration augmentation (Huai *et al.*, 2024; K N *et al.*, 2024). Therefore, it is crucial to be aware of such conditions when outlining treatment plans for the care of ARDS (Figure 7.11).

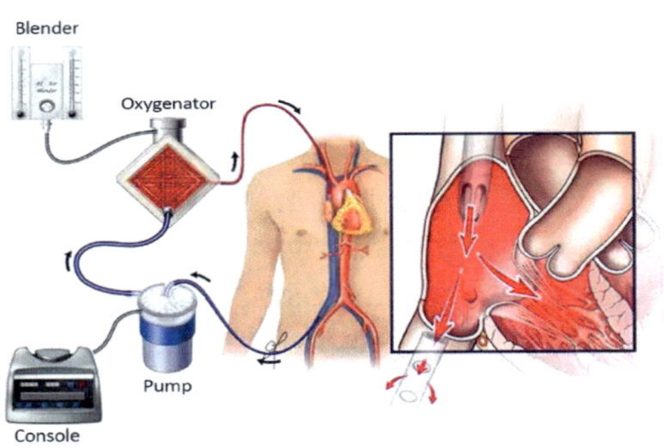

Figure 7.11. Venovenous (VV) extracorporeal membrane oxygenation (ECMO) is a temporary mechanical assistance device that allows for prolonged cardiopulmonary support.

Source: https://consultqd.clevelandclinic.org/venovenous-extracorporeal-membrane-oxygenation-for-lung-failure.

7.2.6. Environmental Factors Contributing to Acute Respiratory Distress Syndrome (ARDS)

Several environmental factors significantly contribute to ARDS development and severity, highlighting the intricacy of the relationship between the external environment and respiratory functions. Exposing oneself to airborne pollutants, allergens, and infectious particles can limit lung function and predispose a person to ARDS, particularly in susceptible populations. For instance, individuals with a history of respiratory conditions or inhabitants of urban areas with extensive industrial discharges may be more vulnerable, as harmful substances may trigger inflammatory responses in the lungs.

Additionally, there are particular risk populations, such as those under allogeneic hematopoietic stem cell transplantation, that possess certain risk profiles under environmental exposures throughout the treatment process, as noted in recent reports detailing differential ARDS presentations and clinical outcomes for these groups (Elendu *et al.*, 2024; Guo *et al.*, 2024). These existing factors require increased sensitivity and improved prevention strategies to counter the environmental stimuli associated with ARDS (Figure 7.12).

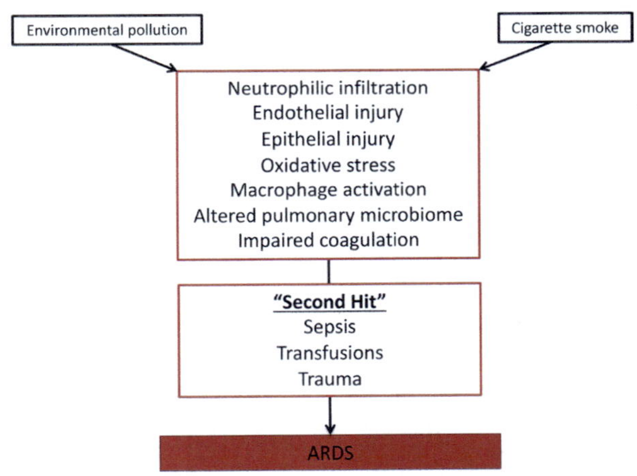

Figure 7.12. Pollution and/or cigarette smoke exposure likely predisposes the lung to severe injury in the presence of risk factors for ARDS such as trauma, sepsis, or multiple transfusions.

Source: https://www.criticalcare.theclinics.com/cms/10.1016/j.ccc.2021.05.002/asset/153645ee-ac70-4ad2-bf4f-70ebe4ea7849/main.assets/gr3_lrg.jpg.

7.2.7. Genetic Predisposition to Acute Respiratory Distress Syndrome (ARDS)

Knowledge of the genetic susceptibility to ARDS is important in evaluating the risk factors for the fatal condition. Studies have shown that genetic variations impact the immune response of the individual to make them susceptible to ARDS after infectious triggers, including influenza or bacterial pneumonia. For instance, in patients with influenza-associated ARDS, body mass index and co-infection status were significant risk factors, considering the complexity of genetic interactions in the severity of disease extent (Hsu *et al.*, 2024). In addition, the use of therapies such as venovenous extracorporeal membrane oxygenation (VV ECMO) has been under scrutiny with regard to genetic markers, suggesting that particular therapeutic strategies can contribute to improved patient outcomes, especially in those who are genetically predisposed (Li *et al.*, 2024). By recognizing these genetic determinants, focused interventions can indeed lower the incidence and improve the treatment of ARDS.

7.2.8. Impact of Age and Gender on Acute Respiratory Distress Syndrome (ARDS) Risk

Age and gender influence risk for the development of ARDS significantly, in a complex interaction that enhances vulnerability among diverse populations. Individuals who are younger, particularly children, develop ARDS following severe pneumonia, as per studies which reveal that age is of overriding significance in diagnosis as well as lung injury outcomes in pediatric patients (Mu *et al.*, 2024). In contrast, older patients tend to exhibit increased risk on the basis of age-related physiological compromise, such that their vulnerability to respiratory failure is heightened. Gender differences also contribute to this scenario, given research that suggests men could be more likely to experience severe forms of ARDS compared to women, possibly due to variations in biological and behavioral influences on immune mechanisms and comorbidities. It is necessary to comprehend such demographic variables to influence prevention and treatment strategies for ARDS across different age groups and genders to eventually improve patient outcomes.

7.2.9. Prevention Strategies for at-Risk Populations

Successful prevention strategies in risk groups are crucial in minimizing the occurrence and severity of ARDS. Directed interventions, such as rigorous monitoring and tailored therapy regimens, can significantly reduce ARDS risk in individuals with predisposing illnesses, such as patients undergoing allogeneic hematopoietic stem cell transplantation. Evidence indicates that factors like the Sequential Organ Failure Assessment (SOFA) score have been found to be predictive of in-hospital mortality among patients like these, demonstrating the need for tight clinical observations (Guo *et al.*, 2024). Furthermore, the use of lung-protective ventilation strategies is effective in reducing pneumothorax and pneumomediastinum complications among ARDS patients, hence recommending their use among vulnerable populations (Teo *et al.*, 2023). With these measures, medical professionals are able to enhance the outcome of patients and ultimately reduce the burden of ARDS on susceptible communities.

Test Your Knowledge

1. What are the primary mechanisms that lead to lung injury in ARDS?
2. How does inflammation contribute to the development and progression of ARDS?

7.3. Diagnosis and Assessment

Learning Outcome

1. Explain the clinical presentation of ARDS
2. Discuss diagnostic criteria for ARDS
3. Describe the role of imaging studies in diagnosis
4. Explain the laboratory tests used in ARDS assessment
5. Identify the differential diagnosis of ARDS
6. Discuss the severity classification of ARDS
7. Explain the importance of early recognition
8. Understand the challenges in diagnosing ARDS
9. Identify the use of scoring systems in ARDS evaluation

Accurate diagnosis and assessment of ARDS are integral components of care for this complex illness, as they guide therapeutic management and prognostication. Extensive clinical assessments, together with imaging techniques, have traditionally been the predominant methods of ARDS identification, but emerging modalities such as point-of-care ultrasound are taking on increased significance.

This point-of-care approach provides dynamic evaluation of the lung, right heart, and diaphragm and therefore facilitates real-time clinical decision-making in the intensive care unit. As implied in recent publications, the incorporation of ultrasound can significantly enhance diagnostic precision and monitoring, but must be used responsibly with clinical symptoms and other monitoring modalities because of their limitations (Zhang *et al.*, 2024). Moreover, failure predictors of non-invasive ventilation (NIV) would assist in the decision-making process of treatment, and evidence in the literature has determined worse outcome factors in ARDS patients (Battalian, 2024). Thus, the entire diagnostic process needs to be maximized for patient care (Figure 7.13).

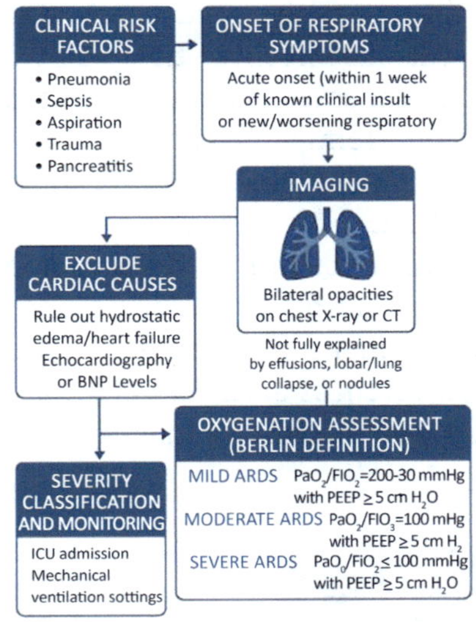

Figure 7.13. Diagnosis and assessment of Acute Respiratory Distress Syndrome (ARDS).

Source: https://sdmntprnorthcentralus.oaiusercontent.com/files/00000000-0354-622f-814a-c93c40085245/raw?se=2025-05-09T12%3A58%3A50Z&sp=r&sv=2024-08-04&sr=b&scid=00000000-0000-0000-0000-000000000000&skoid=bbd22fc4-f881-4ea4-b2f3-c12033cf6a8b&sktid=a48cca56-e6da-484e-a814-9c849652bcb3&skt=2025-05-09T11%3A23%3A16Z&ske=2025-05-10T11%3A23%3A16Z&sks=b&skv=2024-08-04&sig=XhOqQcmMVy0Thlr6nVRNJOtFRRCj-FGTAqDzepsOVxq0%3D.

7.3.1. Clinical Presentation of Acute Respiratory Distress Syndrome (ARDS)

Clinical presentation of ARDS is characterized by the rapid onset of severe respiratory distress, typically within hours to days after the offending insult. Patients can present with hypoxemia, tachypnea, and dyspnea, necessitating supplemental oxygen or mechanical ventilation to attain an adequate level of oxygenation. Bilateral infiltrates on chest imaging, such as X-ray or CT scan, help differentiate from other acute respiratory conditions like pneumonia or heart failure. For instance, a case of HAdV-induced severe pneumonia complicated by ARDS illustrates the syndrome's ability to be caused by various infective etiologies, warranting cautious clinical assessment (Zhang *et al.*, 2025). Moreover, differential diagnoses must consider atypical pathogens like *Chlamydia psittaci* in pediatric patients who present to the intensive care unit with critical respiratory failure, emphasizing the need for careful assessment and tailored treatment regimens (Marchese *et al.*, 2023). In summary, awareness of ARDS's clinical subtleties is important for successful management (Figure 7.14).

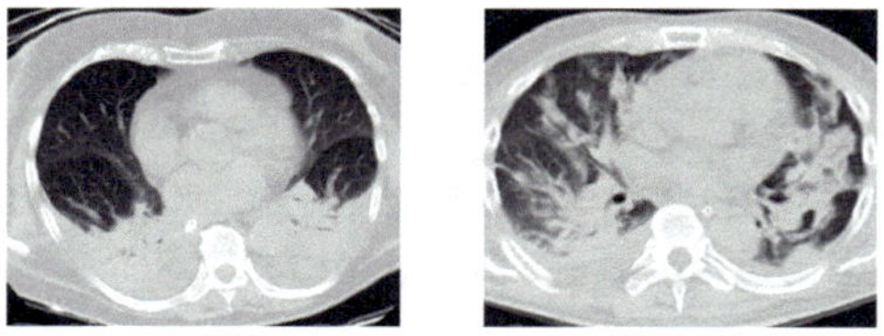

Figure 7.14. Two CT scans showing ARDS focal pattern on right panel and diffuse pattern on left panel.

Source: https://annalsofintensivecare.springeropen.com/articles/10.1186/s13613-021-00870-0.

7.3.2. Diagnostic Criteria for Acute Respiratory Distress Syndrome (ARDS)

Accurate diagnosis of ARDS is critical for effective management of patients, mainly due to existing consensual diagnostic criteria. The Berlin definition, a standardized method most frequently used in clinical settings, divides ARDS into three parameters: timing, imaging, edema source, and severity of hypoxemia. This approach is centered on the imperative for clinicians to recognize the condition early, with a focus on the need for robust identification systems within intensive care units. A study carried out at Hebei General Hospital recently showed that although there was an incidence rate of 3.4% of ARDS among ICU patients, clinical awareness varied significantly with severity (Yang *et al.*, 2024). Evidence suggests that while diagnostic vigilance and adherence to lung protective strategy are high in general, additional standardization and surveillance are needed to achieve optimal outcomes for ARDS patients (Cave *et al.*, 2024). Fine-tuning of diagnostic criteria, therefore, is a critical field of ongoing research and clinical interest.

7.3.3. Role of Imaging Studies in Diagnosis

Imaging diagnosis also has a key role in ARDS diagnosis, particularly with chest X-rays and CT scans, which provide critical information on lung pathology. Both imaging procedures allow medical practitioners to visualize the extent of pulmonary infiltrates and their presence, thus differentiating ARDS from other etiologies of respiratory failure and consequently guiding appropriate and timely treatment decisions. Recent advancements have seen the application of artificial intelligence (AI) in interpreting radiological images, where studies have demonstrated that AI algorithms can achieve accuracy levels higher than individual physicians, particularly in challenging cases of ARDS where uncertainty exists (Farzaneh *et al.*, 2025). This complementarity suggests the importance of hybrid diagnostic approaches with both AI potential and medical expertise, potentially augmenting clinical therapy for ARDS patients, as with trials assessing treatments such as sivelestat sodium (Wu *et al.*, 2025). Such integrative methods suggest a shift in the paradigm of the diagnostic approaches within critical care settings.

7.3.4. Laboratory Tests Used in Acute Respiratory Distress Syndrome (ARDS) Assessment

In ARDS management, laboratory testing is central to determining the severity of the disease, in the decision to treat, and in predicting outcomes. Key parameters measured are arterial blood gases (ABG), which indicate a patient's ventilation and oxygenation, and are central to determining the success of interventions like high-flow nasal cannula oxygen therapy. Research has indicated that scores such as the mROX score are highly predictive of clinical outcomes, for example, higher lactate and greater SOFA scores were found in one study to be predictive of failure of HFNC in ARDS patients (Wang *et al.*, 2024). Also, markers of inflammation, such as procalcitonin and interleukin-6, can reveal the cause of respiratory distress, giving valuable information for a tailored treatment approach. New techniques, including ultrasound, have also been found useful in lung recruitment evaluation, thereby broadening the scope of laboratory investigations in managing ARDS (Youssef *et al.*, 2023) (Figure 7.15).

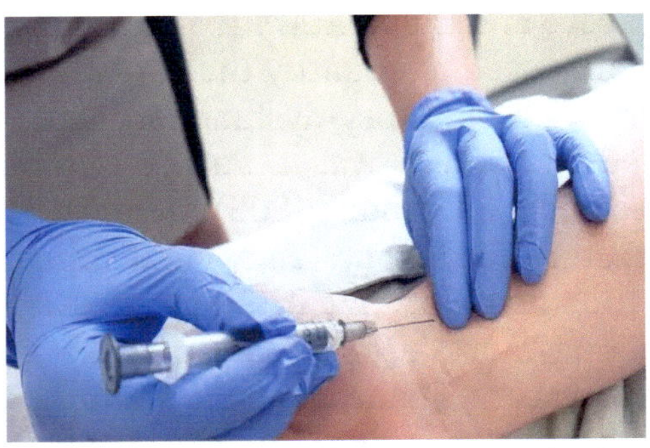

Figure 7.15. Arterial blood gas (ABG).

Source: https://stgaccinwbsdevlrs01.blob.core.windows.net/newcorporatewbsite/blogs/February2024/I4mOcCaagf4wIicEdqqU.webp.

7.3.5. Differential Diagnosis of Acute Respiratory Distress Syndrome (ARDS)

Differential diagnosis of ARDS is crucial in the clinical practice, as its presentation can be mimicked by many other conditions. Pulmonary infections like pneumonia are usually prime suspects, and they must be ruled out with complete scrutiny. Complicating systemic disease, such as sepsis, adds further complexity to the process of diagnosis. In particular, rare cases, such as ARDS due to Lyme disease, illustrate the importance of considering less common etiologies when standard etiologies are excluded, such as in a 70-year-old woman whose serial negative infectious workups foreclosed her diagnosis earlier (Magloire *et al.*, 2025). Furthermore, postoperative ARDS following minimally invasive cardiac surgery highlights that even routine surgery can lead to this devastating respiratory failure, again underlining the significance of thorough investigation and timely intervention to enable maximum outcomes (Nagase *et al.*, 2025). Thus, a thorough differential diagnostic approach is essential to treat ARDS effectively.

7.3.6. Severity Classification of Acute Respiratory Distress Syndrome (ARDS)

One of the primary keys to treating ARDS is the correct classification of its severity, a correct finding that has significant implications for both treatment and outcome. The Berlin definition offers a system of classification based on mild, moderate, and severe classification according to the degree of hypoxemia as quantified by the PaO_2/FiO_2 ratio. Interestingly, research indicates that the severity of ARDS is linked with declines in health-related quality of life (HRQL), particularly in children, in whom the likelihood of clinically significant HRQL deterioration was substantially less for those with more severe forms of ARDS (Killien *et al.*, 2024). Moreover, it has been observed that while ARDS mortality is age- and severity-related, the correlation is non-linear with greater mortality with increasing severity in all age groups (Patel *et al.*, 2024). Hence, severity-based classification not only guides the acute management but also the recovery profiles of patients in the long term.

7.3.7. Importance of Early Recognition

Early recognition of ARDS is essential in averting its typically catastrophic consequences. Early diagnosis also means early treatment, which can be very effective in improving patient outcomes, particularly in intensive care units. Cases such as those of neutropenic sepsis patients demonstrate the risks of delayed diagnosis, wherein such a condition may mask the appearance of ARDS symptoms, leading to catastrophic consequences if not addressed promptly enough (Pata *et al.*, 2024). Similarly, the complexity of circumstances under which chemical injuries cause ARDS points to the necessity of an early intervention to avoid aggravation of respiratory failure and complications (Francis *et al.*, 2024). By highlighting early detection, healthcare providers can initiate special therapies and supportive care that are essential to enhancing survival rates and the quality of treatment for ARDS patients. Therefore, a knowledgeable, conscious approach to the diagnosis of this syndrome's symptoms is required for effective management and better clinical outcomes.

7.3.8. Challenges in Diagnosing Acute Respiratory Distress Syndrome (ARDS)

ARDS diagnosis is complex and is challenging to clinical management and patient outcomes. ARDS diagnostic criteria, such as acute onset, bilateral pulmonary infiltrates, and hypoxemia, overlap with other respiratory conditions and can lead to misdiagnosis. A case of pneumonia caused by *Aeromonas jandaei*, which outlines the difficulty of diagnosing atypical sources of infection that can predispose to ARDS (Palanivel *et al.*, 2024). Moreover, viral infections, such as herpes simplex virus, can also obscure the clinical presentation, such as in a patient with neutropenic sepsis who, in the absence of an undetected viral etiology, progressed to ARDS (Pata *et al.*, 2024). Without an early and accurate diagnosis, clinicians are unable to implement specific treatments, further emphasizing the imperative need for improved diagnostic processes in ARDS management.

7.3.9. Use of Scoring Systems in Acute Respiratory Distress Syndrome (ARDS) Evaluation

In the evaluation of ARDS, scoring systems play a basic role in classifying the severity of illness and patient outcome. There are a number of clinical severities scoring systems, such as the SOFA score and the APACHE II score, which are commonly used to quantify the extent of organ failure and respiratory dysfunction. One study showed that there was a strong correlation between lung ultrasound (LUS) scores and these pre-existing scoring systems, vindicating their utilization in monitoring ARDS progression and estimating mortality risk (Basu *et al.*, 2023). Moreover, scoring indices like the Multiple Organ Dysfunction Score (MODS) and Lung Injury Score (LIS) have been successful in identifying clinical patterns and etiological determinants of ARDS outcomes, especially in regions where tropical disease is prevalent (Chabukswar *et al.*, 2018). Individually and together, these scoring indices enhance clinical decision-making and allow for specific interventions.

Test Your Knowledge

1. What diagnostic criteria are used to confirm a case of ARDS?
2. How do imaging studies and laboratory tests assist in the diagnosis and assessment of ARDS?

7.4. Treatment and Management

Learning Outcome

1. Describe the general principles of ARDS management
2. Discuss the mechanical ventilation strategies
3. Explain the pharmacological treatments for ARDS
4. Identify the role of corticosteroids in ARDS
5. Understand the supportive care measures
6. Describe the nutritional considerations in ARDS patients
7. Discuss the emerging therapies for ARDS
8. Explain the importance of multidisciplinary care
9. Analyze the long-term management and rehabilitation

Effective management and treatment of ARDS are based on a range of modalities consisting of supportive and pharmacological treatments. Traditional care has traditionally incorporated mechanical ventilation strategies that minimize ventilator-induced lung injury, combined with adjunctive therapy such as prone positioning and extracorporeal membrane oxygenation. Recent advancements have highlighted the role of glucocorticoids, specifically dexamethasone, in inflammation reduction but with dangerous side effects when administered for prolonged periods, especially in obese patients (Wu *et al.*, 2025). Recent advances, including polyethylene glycol conjugation of dexamethasone, have been found to have the ability to enhance the therapeutic index by having better pharmacokinetics and lesser toxicity (Wu *et al.*, 2025). Furthermore, ongoing research of biologics and new therapies aims to more precisely target the pathophysiology of ARDS, an indicator of increasing demand for personalized medicine in obtaining the best patient outcomes. Overall, these developments offer a promising new era in ARDS management.

7.4.1. General Principles of Acute Respiratory Distress Syndrome (ARDS) Management

Effective management of ARDS relies upon a variety of generalized principles focused on optimizing patient outcomes and influencing the complex nature of this severe disease. Fundamental to ARDS treatment is lung-protective mechanical ventilation, which avoids ventilator-induced lung injury by employing low tidal volumes and careful pressure control. Other strategies, including fluid restriction, are essential in limiting pulmonary edema, thus promoting enhanced gas exchange and augmented respiratory function.

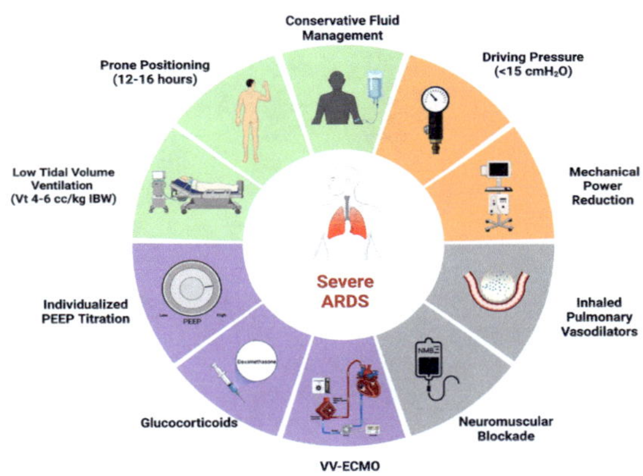

Figure 7.16. Severe acute respiratory distress syndrome (ARDS) treatments.

Source: https://ccforum.biomedcentral.com/articles/10.1186/s13054-023-04572-w.

The recent technological advances using Electrical Impedance Tomography (EIT) and Artificial Intelligence (AI) have encouraged more personalized management of ARDS through the facilitation of real-time data on lung physiology and modulation of ventilation adjustments (Cappellini *et al.*, 2024). Additionally, extracorporeal membrane oxygenation (ECMO) is a potential lifeline in the critically hypoxemic and hypercapnic patients, yet again bringing to the fore the significance of multimodal management of ARDS (Guru *et al.*, 2023). Both of these principles emphasize the core balance between intervention and patient care in ARDS management (Figure 7.16).

7.4.2. Mechanical Ventilation Strategies

Treatment for ARDS often involves the utilization of effective mechanical ventilation strategies to support respiratory function and improve outcomes in patients. With the heightened incidence of ARDS cases that have been induced by the COVID-19 pandemic, there has been a search for alternative modes of ventilation, like awake-prone positioning, that have been reported with promising results in improving patient oxygenation without the need for intubation. Observational research has reported that early application of this strategy among non-intubated patients is related to better clinical outcomes and reduced ICU transfers, although high-quality evidence is necessary to substantiate these findings. In addition, clinicians have to balance the benefits and risks of various modes of ventilation against potential harm, particularly as an evolving picture of SARS-CoV-2 and its effects on respiratory illness (Chen *et al.*, 2022; Hu *et al.*, 2020) remains. This suggests a continued need for rigorous studies to enhance mechanical ventilation techniques in ARDS therapy (Figure 7.17).

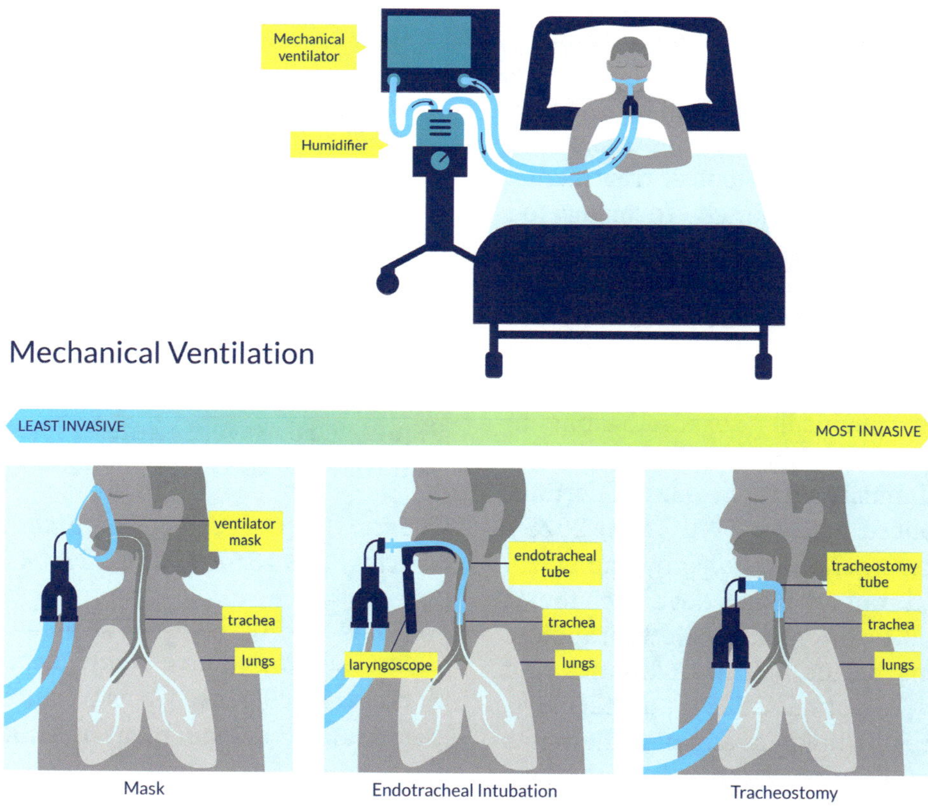

Figure 7.17. Mechanical ventilation procedures.

Source: https://scireproject.com/wp-content/uploads/2023/10/MechVent.png.

7.4.3. Pharmacological Treatments for Acute Respiratory Distress Syndrome (ARDS)

The treatment of ARDS continues to be challenging for clinicians primarily due to the absence of universally effective pharmacological interventions. Among the few pharmacologic therapies that have been made available, glucocorticoid therapy in the form of dexamethasone (DEX) has been a major therapeutic choice; however, its application is fraught with significant risks of side effects, particularly upon prolonged use (Wu *et al.*, 2025). Research has shown that augmentation of DEXs pharmacokinetics via chemical alteration, for example, conjugation with polyethylene glycol, can enhance its therapeutic index, maximizing effectiveness without increasing toxicity (Wu *et al.*, 2025). Moreover, the heterogeneity of ARDS requires a more sophisticated strategy towards management, with particular relevance to phenotyping patients to address interventions more effectively. This individualized strategy aims to delineate individualized subphenotypes of ARDS, ultimately optimizing therapeutic outcome by utilizing particular pharmacologic treatment strategies tailored to treat the patients' pathophysiologic patterns.

7.4.4. Role of Corticosteroids in Acute Respiratory Distress Syndrome (ARDS)

Use of corticosteroids in managing ARDS has gained prominence due to their capacity to suppress inflammation, a central factor in disease pathophysiology. Corticosteroids like dexamethasone are among drugs that are effective in dampening hyperinflammatory responses that are normally compounded by diseases like COVID-19, where there is an excessive cytokine storm. Evidence has revealed that corticosteroids enhance the survival of ARDS patients, but their side effects, like hyperglycemia and increased susceptibility to infection, make them a matter of serious consideration for their use. Early investigations emphasized the importance of identifying in distinct terms those subgroups of patients for whom this therapy would be most beneficial, since not all respond in an identical manner. With continued research, combining evidence from several trials will be essential in optimizing corticosteroid therapy in ARDS care, emphasizing the need for personalized strategies to this multi-factorial syndrome (Segú-Vergés *et al.*, 2023; Sinha *et al.*, 2024).

7.4.5. Supportive Care Measures

For ARDS, supportive care measures are a critical component of improving patient outcomes and lessening the devastating effects of the disease. The key measures include innovative mechanical ventilation tactics such as lung-protective ventilation, which assists in minimizing ventilator-related lung injury by employing lower tidal volumes and optimal levels of positive end-expiratory pressure (PEEP). In addition, body position maneuvers, like the prone position, are increasing due to their robust capacity to ensure oxygenation and increase functional residual capacity in ARDS patients (Habana *et al.*, 2024). Fluid therapy for supportive treatment also aims to prevent overhydration and dehydration, and pharmacologic treatment targets inflammation at its core and the complex syndrome pathophysiology, targeting key biomarkers like HMGB1 (Liu *et al.*, 2021). Through the unification of these strategies, healthcare providers are able to optimize patient safety and comfort while addressing challenges from ARDS.

7.4.6. Nutritional Considerations in Acute Respiratory Distress Syndrome (ARDS) Patients

Nutrition in the situation of ARDS is a significant patient care factor that can contribute largely to the success of recovery. Evidence on the influence of an interdisciplinary nutritional support team

(NST) showed that its implementation was associated with a remarkable 19% reduction in 30-day mortality among ARDS patients when compared to patients treated with usual care alone without assistance (Oh *et al.*, 2024). The function of NST involves tailored nutrition plans that address the augmented metabolic requirements and prevent malnutrition, important in realizing optimal healing for critically ill patients. Besides, factors of related conditions, such as burn injuries, have been established to further complicate ARDS cases, emphasizing the significance of comprehensive nutritional assessments that consider individual patient factors (Sim *et al.*, 2024). Generally, an organized nutrition program increases survival significantly and should be considered a priority in the management of ARDS.

7.4.7. Emerging Therapies for Acute Respiratory Distress Syndrome (ARDS)

The development of novel therapeutic approaches to ARDS is a significant breakthrough in critical care medicine. Standard treatment has long been supportive, with limited pharmacologic interventions for the comprehensive pathophysiology underlying the syndrome. Recent studies have elucidated the potential of biologic therapies, mesenchymal stem cells, and novel immunomodulatory therapies in the modulation of inflammatory processes underlying the pathogenesis of ARDS. Furthermore, research into the complement cascade has revealed its pivotal role in the disease's pathophysiology and emphasized the need for therapeutic interventions that mitigate its overactivation and subsequent lung injury (Yang *et al.*, 2023). Ongoing clinical trials into these avenues signal a paradigm shift towards precision medicine, to tailor therapies based on patient-specific profiles and disease pathways. Together, all these new treatments can improve patient outcomes and reduce ARDS mortality (Jain, 2024).

7.4.8. Importance of Multidisciplinary Care

Multidisciplinary treatment is essential in the management of ARDS because the condition typically presents with sophisticated physiological problems that require the services of multidisciplinary teams of professionals. Effective treatment programs need coordination among critical care physicians, respiratory therapists, nurses, and other specialists to address the multi-symptomatic problem of ARDS and its complications. For instance, in complex conditions such as bronchoesophageal fistula, a very rare condition leading to further compromise of respiration, early diagnosis and management become critical for survival in the patients, emphasizing the need for synergy in collaborative work among specialists to best craft management plans in accordance (Lee *et al.*, 2025). Second, beyond managing immediately life-threatening conditions, in complex medical presentations such as those caused by infectious diseases such as leptospirosis, recognition of interdisciplinary implications provides health care teams with the option to advance timely, integrated care, thereby improving both neonatal and maternal outcomes in pregnant patients (Singh *et al.*, 2024). Such integrated care ultimately raises the chances for improved outcomes among ARDS patients.

7.4.9. Long-Term Management and Rehabilitation

Long-term rehabilitation and management are crucial in the management of survivors of ARDS as the long-term health complications they develop upon discharge from the hospital. There is proof that the majority of individuals suffer from lasting physical, mental, and cognitive impairment known as Post-Intensive Care Syndrome (PICS) with a profound negative impact on their quality of life (Latronico *et al.*, 2024). Rehabilitation programs, including early pulmonary rehabilitation, are thus very crucial in helping patients recover. For instance, research identifies that timely pulmonary rehabilitation increases lung function, reduces complications, and enhances survival after invasive ventilation in ARDS patients (Da *et al.*, 2024). The treatment of muscle weakness, cognitive dysfunction, and psychiatric disorders with personalized therapeutic interventions can lead to improved outcomes. Thus, it is vital to utilize extensive rehabilitation protocols to facilitate recovery and achieve a high quality of life for ARDS survivors in the long run.

Test Your Knowledge

1. What are the general principles involved in the management of ARDS?
2. Which mechanical ventilation strategies are recommended for ARDS patients?
3. What pharmacological treatments, including corticosteroids, are used in ARDS management?

SUMMARY

In conclusion, ARDS remains a complex and severe disease in respiratory medicine, necessitating both advanced research and integrative clinical strategies. Recent studies highlight very significant biomarkers, including miR-193a-5p, whose suppression in ARDS inversely correlates with pro-inflammatory cytokines like IL-6 and TNF-α, and thus might be a promising therapeutic target for the treatment of neonatal ARDS (Zhu *et al.*, 2025). In addition, clinical predictors of survival in ARDS patients, in particular in COVID-19, underscore the need for personalized respiratory treatment and vigilant observation, as illustrated by predictors including mechanical ventilation and ICU length of stay (Boada *et al.*, 2024). Lastly, an integrated approach combining advancements in molecular medicine with robust clinical practices will be instrumental to improving treatment for patients with ARDS. Greater awareness and concerted research activity are necessary to stem the incidence of this debilitating condition.

ARDS is a multifactorial illness characterized by the acute presentation of severe respiratory failure due to multiple underlying etiologies, including sepsis, pneumonia, and trauma. Current studies have outlined critical mechanisms such as mitophagy and ferroptosis in sepsis-induced ARDS, and modulation of these processes can potentially enhance therapeutic interventions in affected patients (Cheng *et al.*, 2024). Besides, the European Society of Intensive Care Medicine (ESICM) has revised its ARDS guidelines, emphasizing the effectiveness of non-pharmacologic respiratory support interventions like the use of high-flow nasal oxygen and continuous positive airway pressure (Mansoor, 2024). This emphasizes the importance of an interdisciplinary approach to the treatment of ARDS, considering the central role of early intervention and individualized treatment in minimizing patient morbidity and mortality. Identification of these critical issues highlights the dynamic nature of ARDS management and the need for ongoing investigation to optimize therapeutic strategies.

KEY TERMS FROM THIS CHAPTER

- Acute lung injury (ALI)
- Barotrauma
- Bilateral infiltrates
- Driving pressure
- Low tidal volume ventilation
- Mechanical ventilation
- Non-cardiogenic pulmonary edema
- Permissive hypercapnia
- ARDS severity
- Berlin definition
- Compliance
- Hypoxemia
- Lung protective strategy
- Neuromuscular blockade
- Oxygenation index
- Plateau pressure

CRITICAL THINKING QUESTIONS

1. **What is the hallmark feature of ARDS on chest imaging?**
   a. Unilateral pleural effusion
   b. Focal lobar consolidation
   c. Bilateral pulmonary infiltrates
   d. Cardiomegaly
2. **According to the Berlin Definition, ARDS is characterized by all except:**
   a. Onset within one week of a known clinical insult
   b. Bilateral opacities on imaging
   c. PaO_2/FiO_2 ratio > 300 mmHg
   d. Respiratory failure not fully explained by cardiac failure or fluid overload
3. **Which of the following ventilator strategies is recommended in the management of ARDS?**
   a. High tidal volume ventilation
   b. Low tidal volume ventilation (6 mL/kg ideal body weight)
   c. Zero PEEP strategy
   d. Mandatory hyperventilation
4. **Prone positioning is recommended in patients with:**
   a. Mild asthma
   b. Moderate to severe ARDS with PaO_2/FiO_2 < 150 mmHg
   c. Chronic obstructive pulmonary disease (COPD)
   d. Pulmonary embolism
5. **Which of the following is not a common cause of ARDS?**
   a. Sepsis
   b. Pneumonia
   c. Pancreatitis
   d. Myocardial infarction

Short Answer Questions

1. What is the Berlin Definition of ARDS, and how are the severity categories (mild, moderate, severe) determined?
2. What are the major pathophysiological mechanisms leading to ARDS?
3. What is the role of increased alveolar-capillary membrane permeability in ARDS?
4. How does ARDS differ from cardiogenic pulmonary edema, and what tests help differentiate them?
5. What are some common direct (pulmonary) and indirect (extrapulmonary) causes of ARDS?

Answer to Critical Thinking Questions

1. (c); 2. (c); 3. (b); 4. (b); 5. (d)

REFERENCES

1. Aldhahir, A., Alqarni, A. A., Madkhali, M., Madkhali, H. H., Bakri, A. A., Shawany, M. A., Alasimi, A. H., *et al.* (2024). Awareness and practice of airway pressure release ventilation mode in acute respiratory distress syndrome patients among nurses in Saudi Arabia. *BMC Nursing, 23.* https://www.semanticscholar.org/paper/fa6a2541291620df6108c4822c2eff19cdd3ce19 (accessed on 22 May 2025).
2. Amjadi, A., Mohammadpour, M., Pouraghajan, K., Mahdiuni, H., Nezamabadi Farahani, L., Nadimi, M., Mohammadi, G. A., *et al.* (2025). Ameliorating COVID-19-related acute respiratory distress syndrome (ARDS) with the multi-target strategy utilizing natural supplements—from *in-silico* to a randomized controlled clinical trial. *International Journal of Ayurvedic Medicine.* https://www.semanticscholar.org/paper/f0a2049f3e720f03da8614fb867196b6c569a881 (accessed on 22 May 2025).
3. Awan, D. A., Sharif, Z., Naeem, U., Batool, T., Habib, G., & Shahzadi, K. (2025). Risk factors associated with acute respiratory distress syndrome in pediatrics. *Indus Journal of Bioscience Research.* https://www.semanticscholar.org/paper/9272d6b327b333e377e0099df9455963586f4e76 (accessed on 22 May 2025).
4. Bardají-Carrillo, M., Martín-Fernández, M., López-Herrero, R., Priede-Vimbela, J. M., Heredia-Rodríguez, M., Gómez-Sánchez, E., Gómez-Pesquera, E., *et al.* (2024). Post-operative sepsis-induced acute respiratory distress syndrome: Risk factors for a life-threatening complication. *Frontiers in Medicine, 11.* https://www.semanticscholar.org/paper/5b33fc8e26627763be4403733154749de496b9ca (accessed on 22 May 2025).
5. Basu, S., Verma, R. N., Joshi, A., Dwivedi, D., Mateen, M. A., & Bhatia, J. S. (2023). A prospective observational study to correlate lung ultrasound with clinical severity and prognosis score in patients with primary pulmonary pathology on invasive ventilatory support. *International Journal of Critical Illness and Injury Science, 13*, 151–158. https://www.semanticscholar.org/paper/5428385e21190f909d290474d72f28fbff385fd1 (accessed on 22 May 2025).
6. Battaglini, D., & Rocco, P. R. M. (2024). Challenges in transitioning from controlled to assisted ventilation in acute respiratory distress syndrome (ARDS) management. *Journal of Clinical Medicine, 13.* https://www.semanticscholar.org/paper/c30ba31b63bfca721ae62e9ad9e910f9e7301268 (accessed on 22 May 2025).
7. Battalian, T. (2024). Respiratory management of acute respiratory distress syndrome (ARDS) in the intensive care unit from early diagnosis: Narrative review. *Socratic Lectures, 10*(Part II). https://www.semanticscholar.org/paper/035f518f2cd92a0aeb7dc2e9076ee7f130e702ec (accessed on 22 May 2025).
8. Boada, P. N., Chamorro, K., & Ballaz, S. J. (2024). Survival analysis of COVID-19 versus non-COVID-19 patients requiring intensive care for acute respiratory distress syndrome: An observational retrospective study. *Canadian Journal of Respiratory Therapy: CJRT = Revue Canadienne de la Thérapie Respiratoire: RCTR, 60*, 112–121. https://www.semanticscholar.org/paper/4773db2d29a470a130202170196f64c302c68c1a (accessed on 22 May 2025).
9. Cappellini, I., Campagnola, L., & Consales, G. (2024). Electrical impedance tomography, artificial intelligence, and variable ventilation: Transforming respiratory monitoring and treatment in critical care. *Journal of Personalized Medicine, 14.* https://www.semanticscholar.org/paper/1386c4e368c925cc2b10bde06c3a99fe21feb597 (accessed on 22 May 2025).

10. Cave, C., Samano, D., Sharma, A. M., Dickinson, J. D., Salomon, J. D., & Mahapatra, S. (2024). EXPRESS: Acute respiratory distress syndrome: A review of ARDS across the life course. *Journal of Investigative Medicine: The Official Publication of the American Federation for Clinical Research*. https://www.semanticscholar.org/paper/ac52a1c775fa1216e5a2306d6055b7082b92ead1 (accessed on 22 May 2025).

11. Chabukswar, P. S., & Baviskar, J. (2018). Study of etiology and scoring system in acute lung injury and acute respiratory distress syndrome patients. *International Journal of Advances in Medicine*. https://www.semanticscholar.org/paper/dcff6fe29512f44a391c11187d5bca3ca06b71ce (accessed on 22 May 2025).

12. Chen, L., Zhang, Y., Li, Y., Song, C., Lin, F., & Pan, P. (2022). The application of awake-prone positioning among non-intubated patients with COVID-19-related ARDS: A narrative review. *Frontiers in Medicine, 9*. https://doi.org/10.3389/fmed.2022.817689.

13. Cheng, H., Wang, X., Yao, J., Yang, C., & Liu, J. (2024). Mitophagy and ferroptosis in sepsis-induced ALI/ARDS: Molecular mechanisms, interactions and therapeutic prospects of medicinal plants. *Journal of Inflammation Research, 17*, 7819–7835. https://www.semanticscholar.org/paper/6239f9be253b91d14b4621505017a3b7f1a2bf32 (accessed on 22 May 2025).

14. Chopra, V., Flanders, S. A., O'Malley, M., Malani, A. N., & Prescott, H. C. (2020). Sixty-day outcomes among patients hospitalized with COVID-19. *Annals of Internal Medicine, 174*, 576–578. https://doi.org/10.7326/m20-5661.

15. Da, L., & Zhang, K. (2024). Early pulmonary rehabilitation in ARDS patients: Effects on respiratory function and long-term outcomes: A retrospective study. *Medicine, 103*. https://www.semanticscholar.org/paper/10a5af953ba4f5f5a6c744135dd3ed02336a69d7 (accessed on 22 May 2025).

16. Djurdjevic Svraka, A., Švraka, D., Azaric, B., Malić, J., Barić, G., & Kovačević, P. (2025). What proteins and albumins in bronchoalveolar lavage fluid and serum could tell us in COVID-19 and influenza acute respiratory distress syndrome on mechanical ventilation patient—A prospective double center study. *The Journal of Critical Care Medicine, 11*, 64–69. https://www.semanticscholar.org/paper/bb30bfc74cb09e9b09e019dc50fb53982d8278fe (accessed on 22 May 2025).

17. Elendu, C., & Amaechi, D. C. (2024). Atrial flutter complicating acute respiratory distress syndrome (ARDS): A rare case report. *Medicine, 103*. https://www.semanticscholar.org/paper/571f7e8e2a9026fb699f383a8b27e4cb89eecfa2 (accessed on 22 May 2025).

18. Farzaneh, N., Ansari, S., Lee, E., Ward, K. R., & Sjoding, M. (2025). Optimizing AI-physician collaboration for enhanced diagnostic accuracy: A case study on acute respiratory distress syndrome detection using chest X-ray imaging. *Journal of Clinical and Translational Science, 9*, 7, 8. https://www.semanticscholar.org/paper/bbed253422299593015577fd93f7c052b2f8a2ed (accessed on 22 May 2025).

19. Filippini, D. F. L., Smit, M., & Bos, L. D. J. (2024). Sub phenotypes in acute respiratory distress syndrome: Universal steps toward treatable traits. *Anesthesia and Analgesia*. https://www.semanticscholar.org/paper/170cc870366f4ae173b1218ba7eeaed65270d457 (accessed on 22 May 2025).

20. Fowler, A. A. (2024). Vitamin C: Rationale for its use in sepsis-induced acute respiratory distress syndrome (ARDS). *Antioxidants, 13*. https://www.semanticscholar.org/paper/

a569da254fb79bf32b62e81ef59877c0021ff401 (accessed on 22 May 2025).

21. Francis, N., Asapu, P., Husain, M., & Jaiganesh, T. (2024). Severe hydrocarbon pneumonitis, a fatal complication of petroleum aspiration: A case report. *Saudi Journal of Emergency Medicine.* https://www.semanticscholar.org/paper/9f251f1e645603fc9232a290b0052b68fb45bd06 (accessed on 22 May 2025).

22. Guo, S., Xie, D., Gao, Y., Yang, L., Chen, J., He, Y., Sun, Y., *et al.* (2024). Risk factors for in-hospital mortality in recipients of allogeneic hematopoietic stem cell transplantation with acute respiratory distress syndrome: A retrospective study based on the 2023 new definition of acute respiratory distress syndrome. *BMC Pulmonary Medicine, 24.* https://www.semanticscholar.org/paper/347981c5af772792aa66ee19c5f0c3f5c1b294e5 (accessed on 22 May 2025).

23. Guru, P. K., & Sahoo, T. K. (2023). Finding the needle in haystack of questions: ECMO in hypoxemic respiratory failure. *Journal of Nepalese Society of Critical Care Medicine.* https://www.semanticscholar.org/paper/9a164d26be115e69292bb68f9247d5d326b5bc10 (accessed on 22 May 2025).

24. Habana, M. A. E., Germar, M. J. V., Aguilar, A. S., *et al.* (2024). A proof-of-concept study on the comfort and usability of a supportive pillow for pregnant patients with COVID-19 acute respiratory distress syndrome. *Acta Medica Philippina, 58,* 13–21. https://www.semanticscholar.org/paper/8c4ea93ad4412328c86515b7685b0f5e12b696b0 (accessed on 22 May 2025).

25. Hehsan, M. R. (2024). Severe acute respiratory distress syndrome with *Pneumocystis jirovecii* pneumonia in man-to-man sexual relations: A case report. *Asian Journal of Medicine and Biomedicine.* https://www.semanticscholar.org/paper/0141dff2fb35147b00d4560e23a7b0f5a58ee9dd (accessed on 22 May 2025).

26. Hendrickson, C. M., & Matthay, M. A. (2013). Viral pathogens and acute lung injury: Investigations inspired by the SARS epidemic and the 2009 H1N1 influenza pandemic. https://core.ac.uk/download/323072736.pdf.

27. Hsu, P. C., Lin, Y. T., Kao, K., Peng, C. K., Sheu, C., Liang, S., Chan, M., *et al.* (2024). Risk factors for prolonged mechanical ventilation in critically ill patients with influenza-related acute respiratory distress syndrome. *Respiratory Research, 25.* https://www.semanticscholar.org/paper/8cccd436d8315f01d2615161e12b99006ba1469e (accessed on 22 May 2025).

28. Hu, B., Guo, H., Zhou, P., & Shi, Z. L. (2020). Characteristics of SARS-CoV-2 and COVID-19. *Nature Reviews Microbiology, 19,* 141–154. https://doi.org/10.1038/s41579-020-00459-7.

29. Huai, J., & Ye, X. (2024). Lung ultrasound evaluation of aeration changes in response to prone positioning in acute respiratory distress syndrome (ARDS) patients requiring Veno venous extracorporeal membrane oxygenation: An observational study. *Cureus, 16.* https://www.semanticscholar.org/paper/eafe2294700dc27a64ef534d3e8c1ac1cdd399cc (accessed on 22 May 2025).

30. Huang, C., Li, J. J., & Wei, W. K. (2024). Clinical significance of platelet mononuclear cell aggregates in patients with sepsis and acute respiratory distress syndrome. *World Journal of Clinical Cases, 12,* 966–972. https://www.semanticscholar.org/paper/5f9fa5276636f5fbc437186d5df016edf38a3c50 (accessed on 22 May 2025).

31. Isabekov, N. R., Tonshin, A. A., & Bonitenko, E. (2024). Justification of the possibility of using liquid artificial lung ventilation for the treatment of acute respiratory distress syndrome of toxic genesis. *Russian Journal of Occupational Health and Industrial Ecology.* https://www.

semanticscholar.org/paper/22f293ea3096cc9f33419dadaeb7cee77893c157 (accessed on 22 May 2025).

32. Jain, A. (2024). Understanding and managing acute respiratory distress syndrome (ARDS): New pharmacological approaches reviewing recent developments in the pharmacological management of ARDS. *Innovations in Pharmacy Planet.* https://www.semanticscholar.org/paper/ea680bba85b0de2fa5b1e824770ef5fe60e54b2c (accessed on 22 May 2025).

33. Killien, E., Ohman, R., Dervan, L., Smith, M. B., Rivara, F. P., & Watson, R. S. (2024). Pediatric acute respiratory distress syndrome severity and health-related quality of life outcomes: Single-center retrospective cohort, 2011–2017. *Pediatric Critical Care Medicine.* https://www.semanticscholar.org/paper/2a81f595d87e3f056c19bc3da9c0b0c65e3b9efa (accessed on 22 May 2025).

34. Kim, D., Liu, S., Zolotov, E., & Padalkar, R. (2024). X-linked inhibitor of apoptosis (XIAP) deficiency complicated by hemophagocytic lymph histiocytosis on immunotherapy leading to acute respiratory distress syndrome and multiorgan failure secondary to opportunistic infections. *Cureus, 16.* https://www.semanticscholar.org/paper/b227bccfea81b08ebdf700c68b1e4c22a53d5fa1 (accessed on 22 May 2025).

35. Kléber, M., Meunier-Beillard, N., Fournel, I., Ksiazek, E., Jacquier, M., Ecarnot, F., Rigaud, J., *et al.* (2025). Barriers to and facilitators of rehabilitation according to socio-economic status, after acute respiratory distress syndrome due to COVID-19: A qualitative study in the RECOVIDS cohort. *PLOS One, 20.* https://www.semanticscholar.org/paper/1c931fb81fe564b8594684f337712f73534912ae (accessed on 22 May 2025).

36. Kong, T., Seo, S. K., Han, Y. S., Seo, W. M., Kim, B., Kim, J., Cho, Y. J., *et al.* (2025). Primed mesenchymal stem cells by IFN-γ and IL-1β ameliorate acute respiratory distress syndrome through enhancing homing effect and immunomodulation. *Biomolecules & Therapeutics, 33*, 311–324. https://www.semanticscholar.org/paper/c05fbec29ada66a796087de7042e99cbe83818d1 (accessed on 22 May 2025).

37. Lam, C. K., Tso, C., Green-Saxena, A., Pellegrini, E., Iqbal, Z., Evans, D., Hoffman, J., *et al.* (2021). Semi supervised deep learning techniques for predicting acute respiratory distress syndrome from time-series clinical data: Model development and validation study. *JMIR Formative Research, 5.* https://www.semanticscholar.org/paper/7aefdb814875712250d57df5e85d95cd8efee753 (accessed on 22 May 2025).

38. Latronico, N., Eikermann, M., Ely, E. W., & Needham, D. M. (2024). Improving management of ARDS: Uniting acute management and long-term recovery. *Critical Care, 28.* https://www.semanticscholar.org/paper/d0c4fe445e49d2169973ff39007665516959e9b3 (accessed on 22 May 2025).

39. Le, S., Pellegrini, E., Green-Saxena, A., Summers, C., Hoffman, J., Calvert, J., & Das, R. (2020). Supervised machine learning for the early prediction of acute respiratory distress syndrome (ARDS). *Journal of Critical Care, 60*, 96–102. https://www.semanticscholar.org/paper/bb6af404b7d68083dfd75969254913e26af89c73 (accessed on 22 May 2025).

40. Lee, S. J., Ng, B., & Thangavelautham, S. (2025). Diagnostic and therapeutic challenges of postoperative broncho esophageal fistula leading to acute respiratory distress syndrome. *Cureus, 17.* https://www.semanticscholar.org/paper/b98db49da2e64d38ed70926d90619a5ba7638a91 (accessed on 22 May 2025).

41. Li, W., Chen, Y., Li, D., Meng, X., Liu, Z., Liu, Y., & Fan, H. (2024). Hemadsorption in acute respiratory distress syndrome patients requiring Veno venous extracorporeal membrane oxygenation: A systematic review. *Respiratory Research, 25.* https://www.semanticscholar.org/paper/4bb699c96099e2ce19e45afa47d4483e2f689533 (accessed on 22 May 2025).

42. Liu, J., Sala, M., & Kim, J. (2021). Dampening the fire: A negative feedback loop in acute respiratory distress syndrome. *American Journal of Respiratory Cell and Molecular Biology, 64*, 158–160. https://www.semanticscholar.org/paper/cae9bb5dd1d54b2793a9b17fc5044379ee3a1c9f (accessed on 22 May 2025).

43. Liu, Y. F., Zhan, Q., Huang, X., Wu, D. W., Lu, H. N., Wang, D. X., Deng, W., *et al.* (2024). [Analysis of compliance with lung protective mechanical ventilation strategy in patients with acute respiratory distress syndrome]. *Zhonghua Jie He He Hu Xi Za Zhi, 47*(5), 419–429. https://www.semanticscholar.org/paper/4b58687df88b7a2d9b77b13f480e5e273b793968 (accessed on 22 May 2025).

44. Liu, Y. N., & Ma, X. C. (2024). [The precision medicine for the treatment of acute respiratory distress syndrome is based on identification of phenotypes]. *Zhonghua Yi Xue Za Zhi, 104*(15), 1253–1257. https://www.semanticscholar.org/paper/6af0310e8590d7ad5e8832313b3130d88a4f25cb (accessed on 22 May 2025).

45. Lopes, D. G., Jorge, T. T., Costa, F. F., & Jorge, S. (2024). Modulatory effects of Voxelotor and 5-HMF on hemoglobin affinity, heme-heme cooperativity and Bohr effect—Prospecting the use of these compounds in cases of hypoxemia, such as in the acute respiratory distress syndrome (ARDS). *Blood.* https://www.semanticscholar.org/paper/dbc24f1b39187297cf916f59dc061cb6986ddd11 (accessed on 22 May 2025).

46. Ma, S., Li, C., Gao, Z., Xie, J., Qiu, H., Yang, Y., & Liu, L. (2023). Effects of intravenous sivelestat sodium on prevention of acute respiratory distress syndrome in patients with sepsis: Study protocol for a double-blind multicenter randomized controlled trial. *BMJ Open, 13.* https://www.semanticscholar.org/paper/e9f3ce39b394e0b63ac5f2290b1be78de6590485 (accessed on 22 May 2025).

47. Madrid, J., Agarwal, P., Müller-Peltzer, K., Askani, M., Benning, L., Selig, M., Diehl, P., *et al.* (2024). Vaccination protects against acute respiratory distress syndrome (ARDS) in hospitalized patients with COVID-19. *Clinical and Experimental Medicine, 24.* https://www.semanticscholar.org/paper/98eead332408dd78cc95c6463b8174c8e29e308f (accessed on 22 May 2025).

48. Magloire, C., Aghabekyan, T., Morley, N. E., Turcan, S., Sexton, S., Khatoon, D., Okoye, C., *et al.* (2025). Severe acute respiratory distress syndrome in Lyme disease: A case report and review of the literature. *Cureus, 17.* https://www.semanticscholar.org/paper/9895f3ecf364ff0c4c9a128e7e7ec71071b22e40 (accessed on 22 May 2025).

49. Mansoor, F. (2024). "ESICM guidelines on acute respiratory distress syndrome 2023" –A short summary. *Anesthesia, Pain & Intensive Care.* https://www.semanticscholar.org/paper/7cce6a560c2d46357b178a7e709fb0f71cef19fb (accessed on 22 May 2025).

50. Marchese, S., Marchese, G., Paviglianiti, G., Lapi, M., Ottoveggio, G., Pipitone, G., & Corsello, G. (2023). A pediatric case of *Chlamydia psittaci* caused severe acute respiratory distress syndrome (ARDS) in Italy. *Italian Journal of Pediatrics, 49.* https://www.semanticscholar.org/paper/7124dd2d551e0204f0e03d4665bc6d59c574ff92 (accessed on 22 May 2025).

51. Matthay, M., Arabi, Y., Arroliga, A., Bernard, G., Bersten, A., Brochard, L., Calfee, C., *et al.*

(2023). A new global definition of acute respiratory distress syndrome. *American Journal of Respiratory and Critical Care Medicine, 209,* 37–47. https://www.semanticscholar.org/paper/a1460aa39563d339b120298e5952c0b4cf26e092 (accessed on 22 May 2025).

52. Mokhber Dezfouli, M., Eftekhari, Z., & Sadeghian Chaleshtori, S. (2025). The factors effect on natural lung surfactant content for the treatment of respiratory distress syndrome. *Iranian Journal of Veterinary Medicine.* https://www.semanticscholar.org/paper/f5bfaf29b0900cd6289bdd10a421dcb5e4341ba8 (accessed on 22 May 2025).
53. Mu, S., Zou, Y., Guo, Y., Yu, M., Huang, B., Gao, W., & Zhang, T. (2024). Early diagnostic and prognosis prediction of circ_0054633 for acute lung injury/acute respiratory distress syndrome in children with severe pneumonia. *Zhonghua Wei Zhong Bing Ji Jiu Yi Xue, 36*(9), 957–961. https://www.semanticscholar.org/paper/81248971da82739b3525054f919c5da7bcce715e (accessed on 22 May 2025).
54. N, K., Ramyea, R., Elumalai, R., Josika, T., Jothish, M., & Kirithick, S. (2024). Segmentation and classification of acute respiratory distress syndrome (ARDS) using deep learning. *2024 International Conference on Electronics, Computing, Communication and Control Technology (ICECCC).* https://www.semanticscholar.org/paper/202ac226ce1ed266e584b4fff6cceda09985eaf8 (accessed on 22 May 2025).
55. Nagase, T., Kashiyama, N., Ryugo, M., Monta, O., & Oda, S. (2025). Acute respiratory distress syndrome following minimally invasive cardiac surgery. *Cureus, 17.* https://www.semanticscholar.org/paper/19d3434f2b5084f2553a77cd835c78886fc6acdd (accessed on 22 May 2025).
56. Oh, T., Lee, K., Cho, J., & Song, I. (2024). Multidisciplinary nutritional support team and mortality in critically ill patients with acute respiratory distress syndrome. *Acta Anesthesiologic Scandinavica.* https://www.semanticscholar.org/paper/9c583bacd9c3f8762e3f38ccd4a49677859626d0 (accessed on 22 May 2025).
57. Palanivel, J., Upadhya, P., Mohapatra, M., Bagarhatta, P., & Karthikeyan, M. (2024). A rare case of community-acquired pneumonia complicated by severe acute respiratory distress syndrome in an immunocompetent male: *Aeromonas jandaei. Chest Disease Reports.* https://www.semanticscholar.org/paper/1ace25d3ebb5ed4efeb4c1bbece3590f64cf6836 (accessed on 22 May 2025).
58. Pata, R., Kosuru, B., & Kristeva, J. (2024). Herpes Simplex pneumonitis presenting as acute respiratory distress syndrome and septic shock. *Cureus, 16.* https://www.semanticscholar.org/paper/aa28ecae5180b124ffced4d848198ca0193ad274 (accessed on 22 May 2025).
59. Patel, B. M., Reilly, J. P., Bhalla, A., Smith, L., Khemani, R., Jones, T., Meyer, N., *et al.* (2024). Association between age and mortality in pediatric and adult acute respiratory distress syndrome. *American Journal of Respiratory and Critical Care Medicine.* https://www.semanticscholar.org/paper/c70ed5bdb2320b94b5e625f5b76461b78556f83a (accessed on 22 May 2025).
60. Qiao, X., Yin, J., Zheng, Z., Li, L., & Feng, X. (2024). Endothelial cell dynamics in sepsis-induced acute lung injury and acute respiratory distress syndrome: Pathogenesis and therapeutic implications. *Cell Communication and Signaling, 22.* https://www.semanticscholar.org/paper/865827f0549e821ceab8fa2a8db1fb0bbd20a3c8 (accessed on 22 May 2025).
61. Rana, R., & Akhtar, A. (2024). Retrospective comparison of influenza and COVID-19-associated

acute respiratory distress syndrome (ARDS): An experience from a tertiary care hospital. *Cureus, 16.* https://www.semanticscholar.org/paper/d156db191efc760573c125113f7c941e3cd077c4 (accessed on 22 May 2025).

62. Redko, O., & Dovhalyuk, A. (2023). Ultrastructural changes of liver in rats with induced acute respiratory distress syndrome and subsequent mesenchymal stem cell intervention during the initial stages of the experiment. *Clinical Anatomy and Operative Surgery.* https://www.semanticscholar.org/paper/e696827b9b2afd9869bc9d757020ce422d64a648 (accessed on 22 May 2025).

63. Segú-Vergés, C., Artigas, L., Coma, M., & Peck, R. (2023). Artificial intelligence assessment of the potential of tocilizumab along with corticosteroids therapy for the management of COVID-19 evoked acute respiratory distress syndrome. *PLOS ONE, 18.* https://www.semanticscholar.org/paper/3f6ef6912886047b9393178f256296c819291389 (accessed on 22 May 2025).

64. Sen, M., Honavar, S. G., Sharma, N., & Sachdev, M. S. (2021). COVID-19 and eye: A review of ophthalmic manifestations of COVID-19. *Indian Journal of Ophthalmology, 69,* 488–509. https://doi.org/10.4103/ijo.ijo_297_21.

65. Shirey, K. A., Blanco, J. C. G., & Vogel, S. N. (2021). Targeting TLR4 signaling to blunt viral-mediated acute lung injury. *Frontiers in Immunology, 12.* https://doi.org/10.3389/fimmu.2021.705080.

66. Shirzadeh, S., Omidkhoda, N., Mohammadpour, A., Mannani, R., & Jomehzadeh, V. (2024). Evaluation of preventive pentoxifylline effect on acute respiratory distress syndrome (ARDS) incidence in traumatic patients: A randomized triple-blind placebo-controlled trial. *Medical Journal of the Islamic Republic of Iran, 38.* https://www.semanticscholar.org/paper/d8dd602dcacc24cf4fa7fe6def9223abd0a4eb88 (accessed on 22 May 2025).

67. Sim, D., Subramanian, M., & Caffrey, J. A. (2024). Risk factors and in-hospital outcomes of acute respiratory distress syndrome (ARDS) in burn patients: An analysis of the National Trauma Data Bank (NTDB). *Plastic and Reconstructive Surgery Global Open, 12.* https://www.semanticscholar.org/paper/dfe8b5e1c880e625f96bd36325c47930cf85f87e (accessed on 22 May 2025).

68. Singh, S., Acharya, N., Karnik, M., Reddy, B. S. K., Waghe, T., & Beedkar, A. (2024). Leptospirosis-associated acute respiratory distress syndrome (ARDS) in pregnancy: A rare presentation. *Cureus, 16.* https://www.semanticscholar.org/paper/64d89b3ef87cfd4b25e3a28bd7a321166713a168 (accessed on 22 May 2025).

69. Sinha, S., Patnaik, R., & Behera, S. (2024). Steroids in acute respiratory distress syndrome: A panacea or still a puzzle? *World Journal of Critical Care Medicine, 13.* https://www.semanticscholar.org/paper/5f569c3da67bff8d872893e10cafec4208e22302 (accessed on 22 May 2025).

70. Teo, Y. X., Geetha, H. S., Mishra, A. K., & Lal, A. (2023). Pneumomediastinum and pneumothorax in acute respiratory distress syndrome (ARDS) patients: A narrative review. *Mediastinum, 8.* https://www.semanticscholar.org/paper/7b84ca49fa6282b8ba00c0a36d04cf2a399a8f34 (accessed on 22 May 2025).

71. Wang, D. X., Xiao, L. X., Deng, X. Y., & Deng, W. (2024). Omadacycline for the treatment of severe pneumonia caused by *Chlamydia psittaci* complicated with acute respiratory distress syndrome during the COVID-19 pandemic. *Frontiers in Medicine, 10.* https://www.semanticscholar.org/

paper/5972d7ab05df8bc50946909593a4e50a363160af (accessed on 22 May 2025).

72. Wang, X., Zhang, Z., & Cao, W. (2024). [Value of modified ROX index in predicting the outcome of patients with acute respiratory distress syndrome due to SARS-CoV-2 infection treated with high-flow nasal cannula oxygen therapy]. *Zhonghua Wei Zhong Bing Ji Jiu Yi Xue, 36*(6), 585–590. https://www.semanticscholar.org/paper/6410484a522d06f264a21a6de1361aea582696fc (accessed on 22 May 2025).

73. Wu, C., Chen, X., Cai, Y., Xia, J., Zhou, X., Xu, S., Huang, H., *et al.* (2020). Risk factors associated with acute respiratory distress syndrome and death in patients with coronavirus disease 2019 pneumonia in Wuhan, China. *The Journal of Emergency Medicine, 58*, 713–714. https://www.semanticscholar.org/paper/ae968d4d9c013c78c9cde788bc1085b380150d1e (accessed on 22 May 2025).

74. Wu, T., Wang, T., Jiang, J., Tang, Y., Zhang, L., Jiang, Z., Liu, F., *et al.* (2025). Effect of neutrophil elastase inhibitor (sivelestat sodium) on oxygenation in patients with sepsis-induced acute respiratory distress syndrome. *Journal of Inflammation Research, 18*, 4449–4458. https://www.semanticscholar.org/paper/95ed7f77b8fc8be06957f66a4cfeb5005bae3ad5 (accessed on 22 May 2025).

75. Wu, X., Guo, H., Hu, X., Li, Y., Kowalke, M. A., Zhang, W., Oh, J. H., *et al.* (2025). PEGylation improves the therapeutic index of dexamethasone to treat acute respiratory distress syndrome with obesity background in mouse. *Molecular Pharmaceutics.* https://www.semanticscholar.org/paper/fd2d7ac8a8d65f957a75298802199d86629c83bb (accessed on 22 May 2025).

76. Yang, Z., Nicholson, S. E., Cancio, T. S., Cancio, L., & Li, Y. (2023). Complement as a vital nexus of the pathobiological connectome for acute respiratory distress syndrome: An emerging therapeutic target. *Frontiers in Immunology, 14.* https://www.semanticscholar.org/paper/8bd339bed6c2cbe4b194edf86460fa3d12369fb9 (accessed on 22 May 2025).

77. Yang, Z., Zu, Y., Luo, Y., & Du, Q. (2024). [Analysis of clinical treatment of acute respiratory distress syndrome assisted by artificial intelligence]. *Zhonghua Wei Zhong Bing Ji Jiu Yi Xue, 36*(4), 369–376. https://www.semanticscholar.org/paper/f042ab3c30fc1add70cf3d34695128b977008102 (accessed on 22 May 2025).

78. Yıldırım, F., Gulhan, P., Karaman, I., & Kurutkan, M. N. (2022). Bibliometric analysis of acute respiratory distress syndrome (ARDS) studies published between 1980 and 2020. *Advances in Clinical and Experimental Medicine*. https://www.semanticscholar.org/paper/6e8c9e356ff15433fa9ae8ad040d36d038ffa79b (accessed on 22 May 2025).

79. Youssef, A., Essawy, T., Mohammad, K., & Abo-Youssef, S. (2023). The role of ultrasound in assessment of positive end-expiratory pressure-induced lung recruitment in acute respiratory distress syndrome patients. *The Egyptian Journal of Chest Diseases and Tuberculosis, 72*, 461–467. https://www.semanticscholar.org/paper/0cf27988a005a1618d0c45a870756e2669729726 (accessed on 22 May 2025).

80. Yunker, J. (2014). *Acute Respiratory Distress Syndrome.* https://core.ac.uk/download/144427769.pdf (accessed on 22 May 2025).

81. Zhang, H. L., & Shang, Y. (2024). The value of point-of-care ultrasound in the diagnosis and management of acute respiratory distress syndrome. *Zhonghua Yi Xue Za Zhi, 104*(15), 1225–1229. https://www.semanticscholar.org/paper/9670528c126adfe54b6bbdd968897a9e3fc6bf94 (accessed on 22 May 2025).

82. Zhang, L., Bai, X., Li, Y., Shui, P., Zhao, C., & Dai, J. (2024). [Study on the correlation between angiopoietin-2 and prognosis in patients with acute respiratory distress syndrome]. *Zhonghua Wei Zhong Bing Ji Jiu Yi Xue, 36*(9), 962–965. https://www.semanticscholar.org/paper/4e4752637d914fbef1624bc71e5daecffbae0f53 (accessed on 22 May 2025).

83. Zhang, L., Guo, Y., Wang, X., Gai, W., & Liu, L. (2025). Severe adenovirus pneumonia complicated by acute respiratory distress syndrome in immunocompetent patients: A case report and literature review. *Frontiers in Medicine, 12.* https://www.semanticscholar.org/paper/ec6c8625eff9990a3c26bcf2cfd0598e4239b573 (accessed on 22 May 2025).

84. Zhang, X., Su, L., & Pan, P. (2024). Advances and applications of lung organoids in the research on acute respiratory distress syndrome (ARDS). *Journal of Clinical Medicine, 13.* https://www.semanticscholar.org/paper/e064435b0d8cf6a7a67d8a0a2fe7d572a43f64db (accessed on 22 May 2025).

85. Zheng, Z., Qiao, X., Yin, J., Kong, J., Han, W., Qin, J., Meng, F., *et al.* (2024). Advancements in omics technologies: Molecular mechanisms of acute lung injury and acute respiratory distress syndrome (Review). *International Journal of Molecular Medicine, 55.* https://www.semanticscholar.org/paper/1fdab7810c4dcf7348f273c7003533542e90f824 (accessed on 22 May 2025).

86. Zhu, C., Zhang, L., Ma, H., Zhang, C., Cheng, F., An, H., & Zhu, W. (2025). Clinical diagnostic value of miR-193a-5p in neonatal acute respiratory distress syndrome and analysis of its effect on human lung epithelial cells. *Fetal and Pediatric Pathology*. https://www.semanticscholar.org/paper/021959de9baadf92f7d9ac198ed330f5b940838b (accessed on 22 May 2025).

87. Zuo, W., Tian, F., Ke, J., Jiang, C., Yang, Y., & He, C. (2024). Mechanisms and research progress of traditional Chinese medicine regulating NF-κB in the treatment of acute lung injury/acute respiratory distress syndrome. *Chinese Medicine and Natural Products.* https://www.semanticscholar.org/paper/fea56c61b8626a32d4b5f434b872cb22d6d32694 (accessed on 22 May 2025).

ACUTE RENAL FAILURE AND RENAL REPLACEMENT THERAPY

8

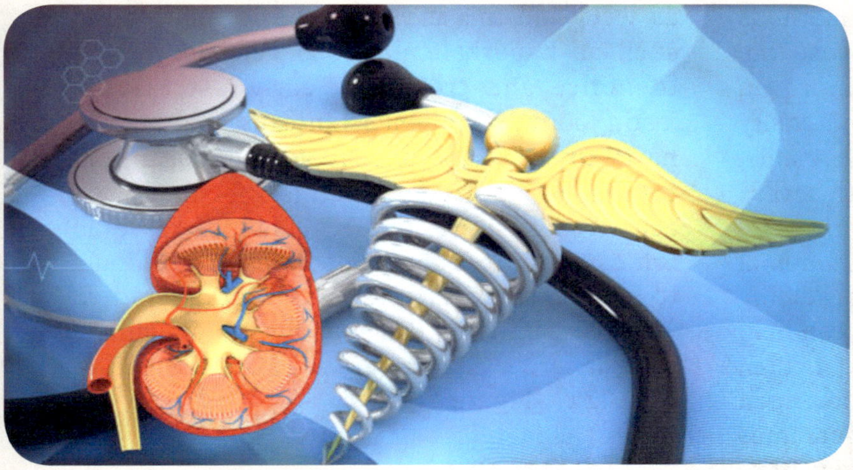

LEARNING OBJECTIVES

After studying this chapter, you will be able to:

1. List the causes of acute renal failure.
2. Define symptoms and diagnosis.
3. Explain pathophysiology of acute renal failure.
4. Elaborate the treatment options.
5. Explore the types of renal replacement therapy.
6. Focus on the complications and challenges.

Introduction

Acute renal failure (ARF), also known as acute kidney injury (AKI), is a critical and potentially reversible condition characterized by a sudden decline in kidney function, leading to an inability to maintain fluid and electrolyte balance. This impairment can occur due to various causes, including ischemia, nephrotoxins, or obstructive pathologies. Many clinical complications are linked to the development of ARF, such as fluid buildup, changes in metabolism, and higher death rates. It is very important to know that ARF has many causes, especially when treating people who are at high risk, such as those having surgery or with other health problems. As ARF is becoming more common worldwide, finding effective ways to treat it quickly becomes essential. Renal replacement therapy (RRT) stands as a cornerstone in the management of ARF, aimed at replacing renal function to maintain homeostasis in patients experiencing inadequate kidney performance. Various modalities of RRT exist, including intermittent hemodialysis, continuous renal replacement therapy (CRRT), and peritoneal dialysis. All these techniques have their pros and cons, usually depending on the patient's condition, blood pressure, and the extent of kidney failure. Recent studies, such as those evaluating the impact of early high-volume sodium bicarbonate infusion during CRRT, suggest that timely intervention can significantly improve patient outcomes, particularly in cases of sepsis-associated acute kidney injury (Ouyang *et al.*, 2025). This points out that customizing RRT strategies for each patient is important for better recovery. Because of better renal replacement methods and a clearer understanding of the disease, the outlook for patients with ARF has improved a lot. The ability to implement high-intensity CRRT protocols has shown promising results, particularly in critically ill patients with severe complications, such as paracetamol-induced acute liver failure and severe hyperammonemia (Chaba *et al.*, 2024). They suggest that catching the disease early and managing it well can help more patients avoid transplants. In particular, when treatment plans are created for each patient's unique needs, the clinical outcomes can be better. For this reason, it is important to keep researching RRT methods and ARFs to help patients recover and reduce health problems.

Definition of Acute Renal Failure (ARF)

ARF, which is now called AKI, describes a quick and usually temporary drop in kidney function that is shown by higher serum creatinine or less urine output. It may be caused by different factors which are grouped into prerenal, intrinsic, and postrenal causes. Prerenal failure is usually brought on by a lack of blood flow to the kidneys, which can happen due to severe dehydration, sepsis, or heart failure. Direct damage to the kidney tissue is the main intrinsic cause, and it is often seen in acute tubular necrosis or glomerulonephritis. When something blocks the urinary tract and urine cannot leave the body, it is called postrenal failure, and this is commonly due to kidney stones or tumors. It is very important to understand these classifications to design the best therapy for patients needing renal replacement therapy. Acute renal failure looks different in each patient, which makes it difficult to diagnose and treat. Some of the usual symptoms are feeling tired, swelling, changes in how much urine is passed, and high blood pressure. Laboratory tests can show that creatinine and blood urea nitrogen are higher than normal, which indicates kidney problems. Electrolyte disturbances can happen as well, and this may result in complications such as hyperkalemia. It is very important to notice and treat ARF early, since long-lasting kidney problems can cause permanent harm to the kidneys. It is very important to establish standard guidelines for handling acute renal failure. These guidelines serve as critical resources for healthcare professionals to ensure that best practices are adhered to while emphasizing the need for individualized patient care (Vahanian *et al.*, 2021; Visseren *et al.*, 2021) (Figure 8.1).

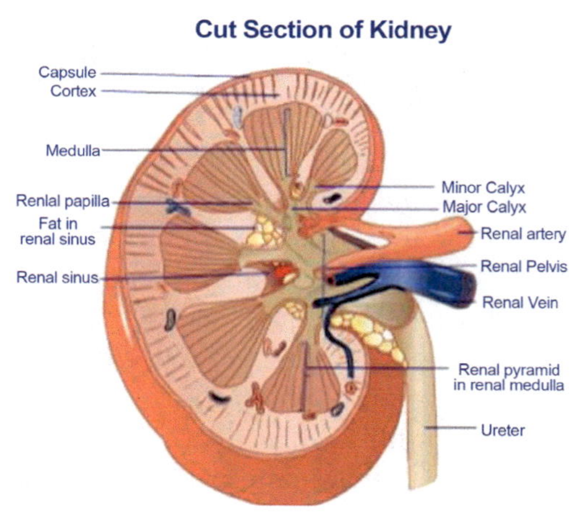

Figure 8.1. Acute renal failure (ARF).

Source: https://drsatishd.com/wp-content/uploads/2015/12/acute-renal-failure-1-728-copy.jpg.

In the context of renal replacement therapy, understanding the definition and implications of acute renal failure is vital. When kidney failure or AKI is so severe that recovery is unlikely, renal replacement therapy—dialysis and kidney transplantation—becomes very important for these patients. Many doctors disagree on the optimal timing for initiating renal replacement therapy, as some prefer clinical signs instead of strict laboratory tests. The overall health of the patient, what led to renal failure, and the chance of recovery all play a big role in choosing treatments. So, managing acute renal failure well requires a team effort involving nephrology experts to help design and carry out the best treatments for patients. Healthcare providers can only give complete and effective care to patients with ARF if they understand the details of the disease and its treatment.

Importance of Understanding Renal Failure

The understanding of renal failure, particularly ARF, plays a critical role in both clinical practice and patient outcomes. If renal failure occurs, waste products can build up rapidly and electrolytes become unbalanced, so quick action is needed to avoid permanent harm. Knowing the mechanisms of ARF allows healthcare professionals to provide the right treatments. It has been found that AKI can occur due to systemic diseases, injuries, or toxic drugs, which shows the importance of understanding a patient's general health. A strong understanding of kidney health allows clinicians to catch kidney problems early, which benefits the patient's health and reduces the effects of renal impairment in the long run. This knowledge becomes most important during emergencies because making quick decisions can greatly impact whether a patient's kidney function improves or worsens. In addition, renal failure has consequences for healthcare resources and the economy, not just for the patients themselves. For patients with advanced kidney failure, RRT such as dialysis and transplantation are important method of care. By knowing the different routes to renal failure, healthcare providers can manage resources and give patients the right treatments. According to the ESC/EAS Guidelines, strategies linked to effective management of renal failure can improve patient compliance while also reducing the burden of chronic renal diseases on healthcare systems (Mach *et al.*, 2019).

Since more people are requiring RRT, knowing about renal failure helps to create strategies and guidelines for early prevention and treatment that can improve patients' health. In addition, realizing that renal failure can result from acute situations such as viral infections like COVID-19 emphasizes how it can harm health. Research has revealed that AKI may occur in critically ill patients, exacerbating their overall health decline, as seen in the recent analysis of kidney abnormalities associated with COVID-19 (Su *et al.*, 2020).

Because viral infections can directly harm the kidneys, there is a need to consider renal health carefully when treating infections. Remembering that renal failure has many aspects is useful for handling emergencies and for guiding future studies and treatments. When healthcare practitioners understand renal failure well, they can help people with acute kidney problems and encourage better kidney health care.

Overview of Renal Replacement Therapy (RRT)

RRT encompasses a range of medical interventions designed to perform the essential functions of the kidneys in patients with ARF. Most importantly, RRT is used to correct electrolyte levels, eliminate toxins, and treat excessive fluid in the body that can happen in ARF. RRT is most frequently carried out using hemodialysis, peritoneal dialysis, and renal transplantation, which have their applications and effects on patients. Hemodialysis is usually used in emergencies since it quickly removes waste from the blood, but peritoneal dialysis is gentler since it uses the patient's peritoneum as a filter. The decision on which technique to use is influenced by the patient's overall health, any comorbidity , and the available resources , so each ARF case requires a customized approach. Starting RRT often requires a careful analysis of the reasons for renal failure.

Acute tubular necrosis might be managed differently than prerenal azotemia caused by a lack of fluid. Assessing the patient thoroughly helps decide on the urgency and form of RRT, since when RRT begins can greatly affect the patient's outcome. With management changes, there is now more attention on improving recovery after surgery, which is affecting RRT practices. Recent guidelines, such as those published by the Enhanced Recovery After Surgery Society, advocate for evidence-based protocols that optimize perioperative care, thereby minimizing the risk of renal damage during surgical interventions (Gustafsson *et al.*, 2018). It shows that surgical management and renal care are closely linked in patients with acute renal failure. New technologies and therapies are reshaping renal replacement therapy, which could affect how clinical practices are carried out. One example of this is nanomedicine, which uses nanotechnology to help deliver treatments more effectively to the kidneys. This method not only enables precise treatment but also mitigates potential side effects associated with more conventional therapies (Patra *et al.*, 2018). Researchers are exploring the use of nanoparticles for delivering renal protective drugs or new dialysis methods, which is a promising area in RRT. With the field growing, using both new and traditional therapies in RRT might result in better patient outcomes, less mortality, and a guide for tackling future cases of acute renal failure.

8.1. Causes of Acute Renal Failure (ARF)

Learning Outcome

1. Define pre-renal causes
2. Discuss the intra-renal causes
3. Explain the post-renal causes

Acute renal failure, or acute kidney injury (AKI), is characterized by a rapid decline in kidney function, which can be precipitated by various causes. Prerenal conditions are a main cause, and they happen when the kidneys are not getting enough blood due to things like low blood volume, dehydration, or low blood pressure. Severe diarrhea, using too many diuretics, or heart failure can result in low blood volume or pressure, which can decrease the flow of blood to the kidneys. When this happens during an acute illness, it is very concerning because early detection and treatment of prerenal causes often help the kidneys recover. When the main issues are not addressed, it can result in more serious kidney damage, so renal replacement therapy may be required to help recover function. Another important way acute renal failure can start is through intrinsic kidney problems. Direct harm to the renal parenchyma belongs to this category and may be caused by nephrotoxins, infections, or inflammation. For instance, the exposure to nonsteroidal anti-inflammatory drugs (NSAIDs), certain antibiotics, and radiocontrast agents can inflict cellular damage to renal tubules and interstitial tissue, leading to acute tubular necrosis (ATN). Another type of intrinsic cause is when systemic problems like glomerulonephritis or acute interstitial nephritis occur, which can make kidney failure worse. Usually, treating intrinsic renal causes involves identifying and stopping the agents that led to the problem, as well as giving supportive care. When kidney function declines greatly, renal replacement therapy might be needed to handle electrolyte problems and remove toxins from the blood. In most cases, acute renal failure caused by postrenal problems is due to obstruction of the urinary tract, which may occur at any point. Kidney stones, tumors, and enlarged prostates are common reasons for obstruction, which can cause high pressure inside the kidneys and damage to the kidneys.

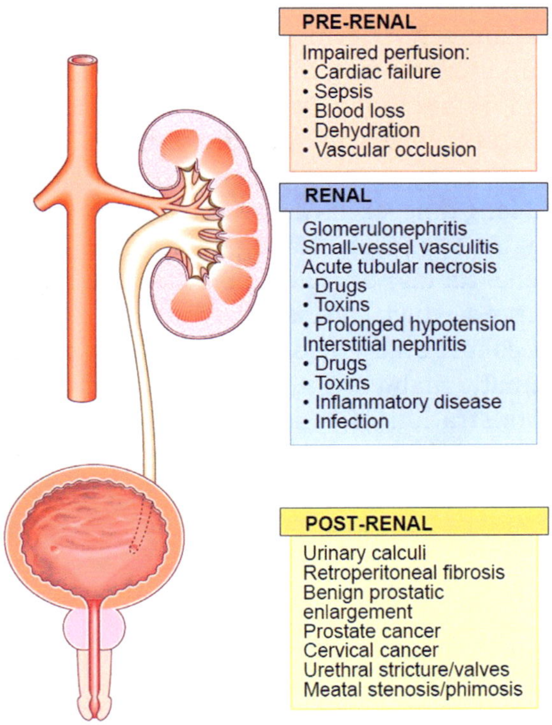

Figure 8.2. Causes of acute kidney injury (AKI).

Source: https://img.grepmed.com/uploads/3937/acute-kidney-injury-diagnosis-prerenal-original.jpeg.

A blocked urinary tract results in urine building up in the kidneys, which can harm the tissue unless the problem is treated. The main challenge for doctors is to detect the obstruction early, and imaging tests usually help. Most of the time, management means removing the blockage, which may involve surgery or placing drainage tools. In summary, recognizing the multifactorial causes of acute renal failure is vital for prompt intervention and can significantly influence patient outcomes, emphasizing the importance of tailored renal replacement therapy when necessary (Julien *et al.*, 2024; Karnina *et al.*, 2024) (Figure 8.2).

8.1.1. Pre-Renal Causes

Understanding pre-renal causes of acute renal failure is crucial for effective treatment and management of the condition. Pre-renal azotemia happens when blood flow to the kidneys is reduced, and this can happen for different reasons. Common reasons are when the body loses fluids due to dehydration, bleeding, or taking too many diuretics. Heart failure or sepsis may weaken the heart, which reduce blood flow to the kidneys. A drop in perfusion may lead to the activation of the renin-angiotensin-aldosterone system, which tries to maintain normal blood pressure and blood flow to the kidneys. If the main issue is not quickly handled, ongoing ischemia in the kidneys may result in permanent damage, so additional treatment such as renal replacement therapy may be required to handle renal failure. Systemic problems that change vascular resistance and blood volume are also major pre-renal causes. As an example, liver cirrhosis can result in hypovolemia because of splanchnic vasodilation, which makes the kidneys less efficient. In patients with nephrotic syndrome, too much protein in urine causes low oncotic pressure, which leads to more fluid being held in the body. Furthermore, the impact of NSAIDs and angiotensin-converting enzyme (ACE) inhibitors on renal perfusion is also noteworthy. They may interfere with the body's way of maintaining blood flow to the kidneys during a loss of blood, which can worsen acute renal failure. Knowing about these factors is important for both identifying the problem and designing treatments that can address pre-renal causes. Being able to spot the clinical signs and symptoms of pre-renal disorders helps ensure quick treatment. Patients with renal failure may experience reduced urine output, no urine at all, and signs of hypovolemia, which include a fast heart rate, low blood pressure, and dry mouth. Laboratory evaluations often reveal elevated blood urea nitrogen (BUN) and creatinine levels, along with an increased BUN-to-creatinine ratio, indicating pre-renal azotemia. When there is dehydration or bleeding, the main goal is to restore intravascular volume by giving fluids through resuscitation. Also, checking urine flow and urinary indices can be useful for telling apart pre-renal problems from renal failure, which helps the doctor choose the right treatment. Early identification and intervention can prevent the transition to more severe renal impairment, ultimately reducing the need for renal replacement therapies (Figure 8.3).

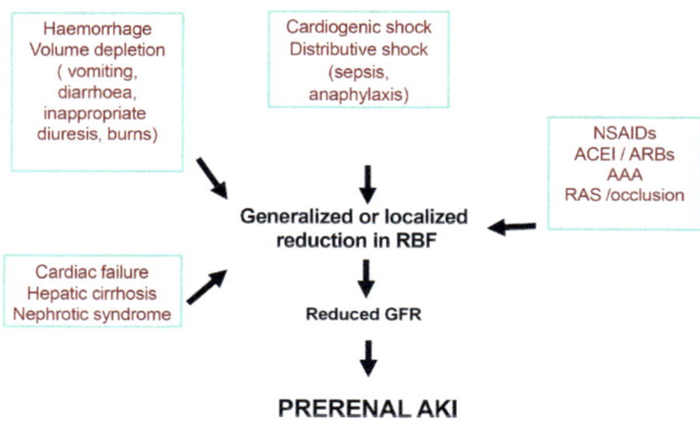

Figure 8.3. Pre-Renal Causes

Source: https://image.slidesharecdn.com/arf-101015091916-phpapp01/95/cme-acute-renal-failure-13-728.jpg?cb=1287134573.

8.1.2. Intra-Renal Causes

The etiology of intra-renal causes of ARF encompasses a diverse range of factors that directly affect the renal parenchyma. One of the most frequent intra-renal causes is acute tubular injury, which may happen due to ischemia, exposure to nephrotoxins, or infections. If there is prolonged hypotension or dehydration, the kidneys may not receive enough blood, which causes ischemic injury. Besides, some medications and substances found in the environment can be nephrotoxic and harm renal tubular cells, which may result in ATN. In tropical areas, leptospirosis is being noticed because it is linked to a high number of acute kidney injury cases, adding to the problem. Patient outcomes can vary significantly based on the timely identification and management of these intra-renal causes, influencing the decision-making process regarding renal replacement therapy (Julien *et al.*, 2024). Rhabdomyolysis, which happens when muscle tissue breaks down and myoglobin enters the blood, is another important reason for acute renal failure within the kidneys. It may be brought on by severe trauma, being immobilized for a long time, or having seizures or neuroleptic malignant syndrome. Myoglobinuria may result in renal tubular cells being blocked and directly damaged, which can lead to acute kidney injury. In a cohort study involving patients with non-traumatic rhabdomyolysis, it was noted that the administration of renal replacement therapy was indicated in cases where patients exhibited prolonged anuria or threatening hyperkalemia (Aboudar *et al.*, 2023) (Figure 8.4).

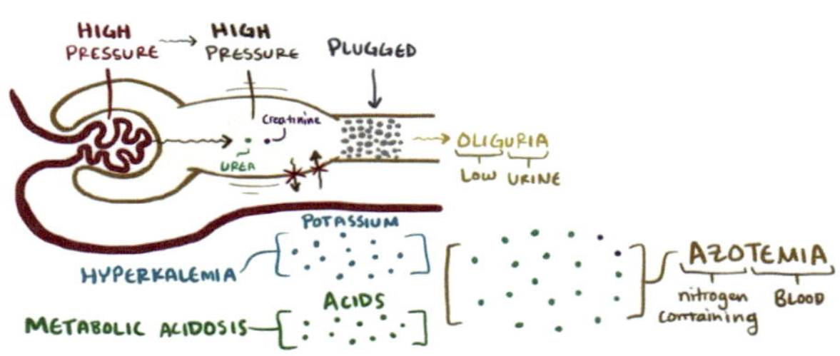

Figure 8.4. Intrarenal acute kidney injury (AKI).

Source: https://upload.wikimedia.org/wikipedia/commons/thumb/0/00/Intrarenal_acute_kidney_injury.webm/1812px--Intrarenal_acute_kidney_injury.webm.jpg.

The study suggests that early recognition and proper care of rhabdomyolysis are necessary because it greatly influences renal recovery and the need for renal replacement therapy.

Also, recognizing intra-renal causes includes understanding how systemic illnesses may indirectly harm the kidneys. Severe infections throughout the body can cause acute kidney injury by triggering sepsis, which leads to blood pressure changes and inflammatory substance release. Severe cases of sepsis can lead to acute renal failure, which is often found in multi-organ dysfunction syndrome. Because these systemic factors affect the kidneys, treatment plans become more complicated, and renal replacement therapy may be required in urgent situations. This rampancy of intra-renal causes necessitates a comprehensive understanding for clinicians, as timely intervention can greatly affect patient outcomes and reduce morbidity associated with acute renal failure (Julien *et al.*, 2024).

8.1.3. Post-Renal Causes

Post-renal causes of ARF arise from obstructions that occur downstream of the renal system, inhibiting the flow of urine and leading to increased intrarenal pressure. Such obstructions may be anatomical, for example, because of tumors or kidney stones, or functional, for example, because of muscle spasms or blood clots. It is very important to recognize these obstructions, since acting promptly can save the kidneys from serious and permanent damage. For example, when hydronephrosis is very severe and lasts a long time, it can make renal failure worse and make renal replacement therapy more difficult. Ultrasounds or CT scans are important for detecting these blockages, so that doctors can quickly start treatments to open the obstruction and help restore the kidneys' function. Other than anatomical problems, post-renal acute renal failure may also be caused by conditions such as neurogenic bladder dysfunction. The bladder cannot empty properly because of neurological problems, which results in a large amount of urine remaining in the bladder. Some causes are spinal cord injuries, multiple sclerosis, or diabetic neuropathy. Because of this dysfunction, the bladder can become overly full and block the ureters, which can interfere with how the kidneys function. It is very important to notice and treat these neurological problems to prevent post-renal failure from leading to severe kidney damage. Managing these cases may require catheterization, drugs that make the bladder contract better, or actions that lower the bladder volume, showing that several methods are needed to treat post-renal causes well. Besides affecting the kidneys, post-renal causes can also lead to complications for the patient and require careful attention in how treatment is planned. If these conditions are not diagnosed and managed promptly, they can cause additional stress on healthcare services, because patients might eventually need renal replacement therapy due to the obstructed kidneys.

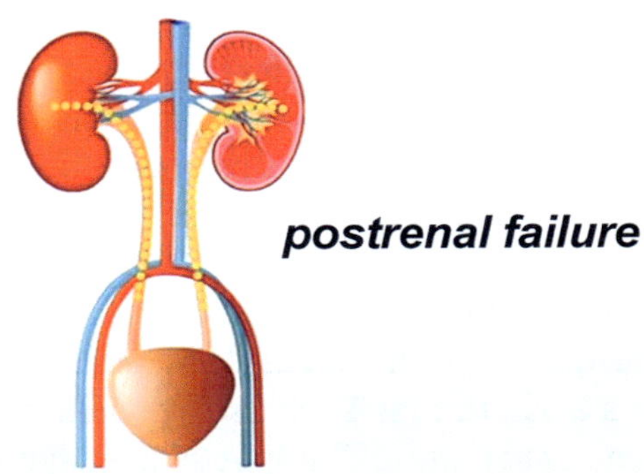

Figure 8.5. Postrenal failure.

Source: https://study.com/cimages/videopreview/acute-renal-failure-postrenal-failure-and-how-it-alters-the-body1_123871.jpg.

By seeing how post-renal causes affect the patient's health, healthcare workers can develop complete assessment and treatment strategies. Preventive methods can be used to lower the risk of urinary tract infections, and repeat imaging may be advised to monitor how the kidneys are functioning. Collaborating with specialists in urology and nephrology may also enhance patient outcomes, emphasizing the importance of an interdisciplinary approach in tackling the complexities of acute renal failure in post-renal situations (Mach *et al.*, 2019; Lorusso *et al.*, 2021) (Figure 8.5).

Test Your Knowledge

1. What are the common pre-renal causes of acute kidney injury (AKI)?
2. How do intra-renal causes differ from pre-renal and post-renal causes in terms of pathophysiology?

8.2. Symptoms and Diagnosis

Learning Outcome

1. Identify the common symptoms of acute renal failure.
2. Discuss the diagnostic tests and procedures.
3. Explain the importance of early diagnosis.

Depending on the reason for ARF and how much the kidneys are affected, the symptoms may be quite different. Typical signs are less urine produced, feeling tired, and confusion. In some more serious cases, patients can develop symptoms of fluid overload, for example, edema and hypertension. In addition, hyperkalemia often occurs and can result in serious arrhythmias such as slow heartbeat or sudden heart failure. The spectrum of symptoms emphasizes the need for clinicians to prompt recognition of ARF, as early intervention may be crucial in preventing further renal impairment and associated complications (Shah *et al.*, 2023). The appearance of these symptoms usually demands that doctors check the cause and severity of renal failure right away. A thorough clinical examination and laboratory tests are both used for ARF diagnosis. Usually, the first steps are to measure serum creatinine and blood urea nitrogen to check how the kidneys are working. Electrolyte panels are important for finding conditions like hyperkalemia, which is frequently linked to problems like blockages or damage to cells. Further details can be seen from urinalysis, pointing to whether the cause of acute failure is in the kidneys, the blood flow to the kidneys, or the urinary tract. For instance, the presence of nephritic sediments or eosinophils may suggest acute interstitial nephritis, while myoglobinuria can indicate rhabdomyolysis (Fujisawa *et al.*, 2023). If acute kidney injury is thought to be caused by an infection, such as a gastrointestinal infection, doctors usually order imaging and the proper culture tests to determine the pathogen. In some medical situations, especially when ARF is related to multiple organ failure or severe infections, quick diagnosis and treatment are essential. If a patient has acute kidney injury because of Legionnaires' disease, they should receive antibiotics and assistance from the kidney support team right away.

This can include continuous renal replacement therapy (CRRT), particularly when metabolic acidosis persists despite standard interventions (Fujisawa *et al.*, 2023). Also, realizing that acute renal failure can interact with other issues, such as non-occlusive mesenteric ischemia, highlights the importance of looking at all possible factors in diagnosis. A comprehensive understanding of symptomatology and diagnostic methodologies not only enhances clinicians' capacity to manage acute renal failure effectively but also improves patient outcomes by guiding timely and appropriate therapeutic strategies (Shah *et al.*, 2023).

8.2.1. Common Symptoms of Acute Renal Failure (ARF)

ARF, also termed AKI, presents with a variety of symptoms that can signal the underlying dysfunction of the renal system. One of the most common indicators is a significant decrease in urine output, often described as oliguria (less than 400 mL per day) or anuria (no urine output). These changes happen because the kidneys are not working properly, which can affect the body's ability to filter and get rid of fluids and electrolytes. Edema can also be a sign of fluid retention, which is caused by the kidneys not handling sodium and water properly. The presence of urinalysis abnormalities, such as hematuria or proteinuria, can indicate underlying damage to the renal tissues and will further guide diagnostic considerations related to acute renal failure, emphasizing the need for early identification and intervention (Evans *et al.*, 2021). Also, acute renal failure may lead to general symptoms such as tiredness, weakness, and confusion. Many patients develop metabolic problems such as too much urea and creatinine in their blood, which is called uremia. These symptoms, such as nausea, vomiting, and loss of appetite, may result from the buildup. Electrolyte imbalances, particularly hyperkalemia (elevated potassium levels), can pose severe cardiac risks, underscoring the significance of continuous monitoring in diagnosed individuals. Timely recognition and management of these symptoms are vital, as they can rapidly progress to life-threatening conditions if renal function is not restored and complications adequately addressed (Ronco *et al.*, 2020). It is very important to recognize the usual symptoms of acute renal failure to treat it properly. If patients having renal replacement therapy notice these symptoms, it can help doctors make better treatment choices earlier. Noticing changes in symptoms and getting a proper medical evaluation allows for a faster start to important interventions. Healthcare providers need to watch for sudden kidney changes, mainly in people with previous health problems or those who have sepsis or undergo major surgery. This proactive approach not only improves patient prognosis but also optimizes care delivery across multidisciplinary teams, marking an essential component of effective chronic kidney disease management (Evans *et al.*, 2021) (Figure 8.6).

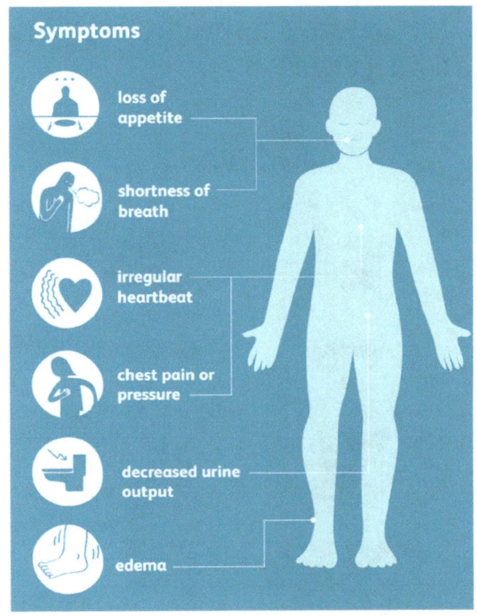

Figure 8.6. Symptoms of acute renal failure (ARF).

Source: https://www.verywellhealth.com/thmb/hbfKjTYzh6J1q2H4ASwzFTkB7A4=/1500x0/filters:no_upscale():max_bytes(150000):strip_icc()/acute-renal-failure-symptoms-5ae1f536ff1b780036287ecb.png.

8.2.2. Diagnostic Tests and Procedures

Diagnostic tests and procedures play a crucial role in the management of ARF and the subsequent decision-making process regarding renal replacement therapy (RRT). The first step is to take a detailed history and perform a physical exam, and then targeted laboratory tests are done to assess kidney function and find out what is causing the problem. Serum creatinine is a main test for kidney function, and BUN is also measured in key laboratory testing. Urinalysis can also give useful information about kidney disease, for example, by showing proteinuria, hematuria or the presence of casts, which may indicate damage to the glomerulus or tubules. This initial diagnostic work-up is essential in categorizing the type of acute kidney injury—prerenal, intrinsic, or postrenal—which is vital for guiding appropriate therapeutic interventions (Figure 8.7).

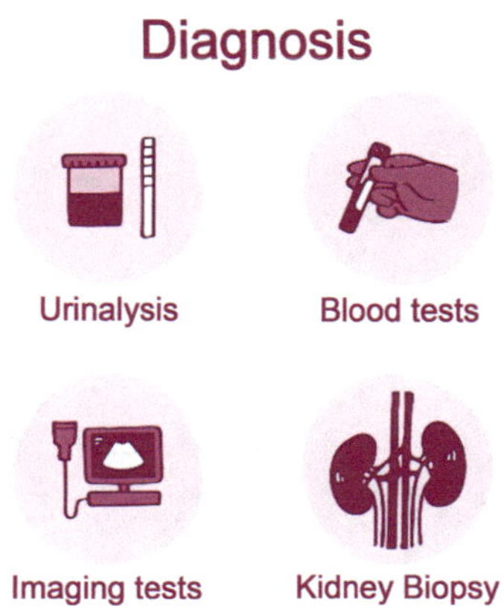

Figure 8.7. Diagnosis of acute kidney injury (AKI).

Source: https://www.consuremedical.com/wp-content/uploads/2023/02/tests-diagnosing-acute-kidney-injury.jpg.

Beyond basic laboratory tests, advanced diagnostic procedures are often utilized to elucidate the etiology of ARF. Imaging studies, such as ultrasound or computed tomography (CT), can assess anatomical abnormalities, such as obstructive uropathy or renal masses, that may contribute to renal dysfunction. Also, examining kidney tissue obtained from a biopsy can give clear answers when intrinsic kidney damage is suspected. This becomes very important in cases like acute interstitial nephritis or glomerulonephritis, as examining kidney tissue can guide the right therapy. All of these tests together help identify the main causes of ARF and also help decide whether dialysis is necessary, since some causes may be managed medically instead. It is very important to combine the results from diagnostic tests with what doctors observe in patients to manage acute renal failure and decide when renal replacement therapy is needed. If a patient has persistent low urine output or major electrolyte problems, it is usually important to begin RRT early to avoid major issues.

Also, CRRT is often used for critically ill patients because it maintains blood pressure better than standard intermittent hemodialysis. The clinical course and repeat laboratory tests are necessary to adjust RRT to a person's changing condition. Thus, a multifaceted approach involving diagnostic tests and close clinical evaluation is essential in optimizing outcomes for patients with acute renal failure and in determining when renal replacement therapy should be instituted, particularly in complex cases like those affected by COVID-19 and other underlying conditions (Northup *et al.*, 2020; Su *et al.*, 2020).

8.2.3. Importance of Early Diagnosis

The significance of early diagnosis in the context of ARF cannot be overstated. Quickly noticing renal dysfunction helps doctors take action to prevent serious problems like the requirement for renal replacement therapy. If kidney damage is found early, healthcare providers can use treatments that help stop the disease from getting worse, which improves the patient's outlook.

According to studies, noticing AKI early helps reduce mortality and serious health complications, because it allows for early treatment before the kidneys fail. For example, early interventions can stop complications such as too much fluid in the body and electrolyte imbalances, which are very dangerous for patients, proving that an early approach to diagnosis is necessary for proper renal care. Besides affecting patients, late detection of renal problems puts a great burden on the healthcare system. The high prevalence of chronic kidney disease (CKD) underscores the pressing need for proactive diagnostic measures. Not identifying kidney dysfunction early increases the expenses for treating advanced CKD and related health problems. Without early diagnosis, CKD can cause severe health problems that might have been prevented. It is clear from a complete analysis of CKD's economic impact that regular screening for kidney dysfunction can help save a lot of healthcare costs. By reducing the progression to kidney failure, healthcare systems can allocate resources more effectively while improving patient quality of life, thus underscoring the critical importance of routine early diagnosis as advocated by initiatives like (García Sánchez *et al.*, 2021). In cases where acute renal injury is associated with conditions such as acute promyelocytic leukemia (APL), early diagnosis takes on an even more pressing urgency. Findings indicate that patients undergoing certain chemotherapy regimens face risks of acute kidney injury secondary to differentiation syndrome, leading to high rates of early mortality and decreased long-term survival (Shen *et al.*, 2025). For this reason, clinicians should be very aware of renal impairment in people at risk, so they can respond promptly. More attention and regular monitoring of kidney function can result in better outcomes because healthcare teams can take steps to protect the kidneys. Therefore, establishing systematic approaches for early diagnosis in vulnerable cohorts serves not only to improve individual patient trajectories but also contributes to an overarching strategy for improved health outcomes amid complex medical therapies (Figure 8.8).

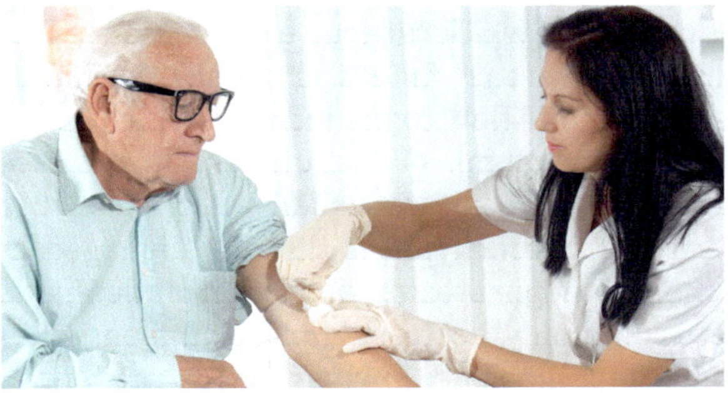

Figure 8.8. Early diagnosis in the context of ARF.

Source: https://www.niddk.nih.gov/-/media/Images/Health-Information/Kidney/TW_AUG20_KidneyDisease_TwitterCard_TestingforKidneyDisease.png.

Test Your Knowledge

1. What are the common symptoms associated with acute renal failure?
2. Which diagnostic tests and procedures are commonly used to confirm acute renal failure?

8.3. Pathophysiology of Acute Renal Failure

Learning Outcome

1. Discuss the mechanisms of kidney injury
2. Identify the impact on homeostasis
3. Explain the consequences of prolonged renal failure

There are many complex reasons why acute kidney injury or ARF causes damage to the kidneys. ARF may start due to problems before the kidneys, within the kidneys, or after the kidneys, all of which can lead to decreased kidney function. Prerenal failure is usually caused by reduced blood flow to the kidneys, which can be due to hypovolemia or heart failure. In this case, intrinsic renal failure usually happens when the renal parenchyma is directly damaged by ischemia, nephrotoxins or glomerulonephritis. Less commonly, postrenal failure happens when something blocks the urinary tract, preventing normal urination. The interplay of these factors ultimately results in a disturbance of the glomerular filtration rate (GFR), leading to the accumulation of waste products in the bloodstream, electrolyte imbalances, and adverse impacts on bodily homeostasis. If not managed well, ARF can become CKD. A significant contributor to this transition is contrast-induced nephropathy (CIN), a form of acute kidney injury frequently observed following intravascular contrast media administration during diagnostic procedures. People with pre-existing CKD, diabetes mellitus, or dehydration are more likely to develop CIN. Pathophysiologically, CIN arises through mechanisms such as direct tubular toxicity, intrarenal vasoconstriction, and excessive production of reactive oxygen species (ROS). As a result, renal function is reduced, and this may eventually cause lasting harm, requiring permanent renal replacement therapy. Understanding these mechanisms can inform preventive strategies and optimize management, ensuring better outcomes for those at risk of developing ARF and its complications (Kusirisin *et al.*, 2020). Because COVID-19 often causes kidney problems in infected individuals, it has made acute renal failure more difficult to understand. In some cases, the severe effects of COVID-19 may cause acute kidney injury, which may need renal replacement therapy. It appears that several factors, for instance, systemic inflammation, lack of oxygen, and the virus itself, contribute to renal impairment. Those with severe COVID-19 can have kidney problems that vary from mild proteinuria to complete acute renal failure. Since there are no specific treatments for COVID-19-related AKI, it is very important to understand its underlying causes. Identifying patients at risk and adapting management strategies based on emerging evidence enhances the potential for effective treatment, underscoring the need for collaborative research efforts to address these contemporary challenges in renal health (Ronco *et al.*, 2020).

8.3.1. Mechanisms of Kidney Injury

The mechanisms underlying kidney injury are multifaceted, with acute renal failure often arising from a combination of pathological events. CIN is a major reason for kidney failure, and it usually appears after contrast media is given for imaging or interventions. This kind of injury is more likely to affect people with CKD, diabetes, and those who are dehydrated. CIN mainly occurs when the kidneys are directly damaged, blood vessels in the kidneys narrow, and there is an increase in reactive oxygen species. All these processes together cause kidney tissue to stop functioning properly and, in the worst cases, can lead to permanent kidney damage, so patients might need long-term dialysis. Understanding these mechanisms is crucial to developing effective prevention strategies and improving clinical outcomes for at-risk patients (Kusirisin *et al.*, 2020). In addition to CIN, AKI is frequently associated with severe systemic illnesses, exemplified by the outbreak of coronavirus disease 2019 (COVID-19). It has been found that in COVID-19 patients, kidney problems may be as minor as proteinuria or as severe as AKI that requires RRT. Experts are still trying to understand the reasons behind kidney injury in this situation, and it is thought that systemic inflammation, reduced blood flow, and viral infections in the kidneys may be involved. Severe COVID-19 can lead to several organ failures, which makes kidney problems more noticeable. Currently, management is mainly about supporting patients, with a special emphasis on spotting those at greater risk. There is an urgent need for collaborative research that can provide robust evidence to guide clinical practices concerning AKI linked to COVID-19 (Ronco *et al.*, 2020) (Figure 8.9).

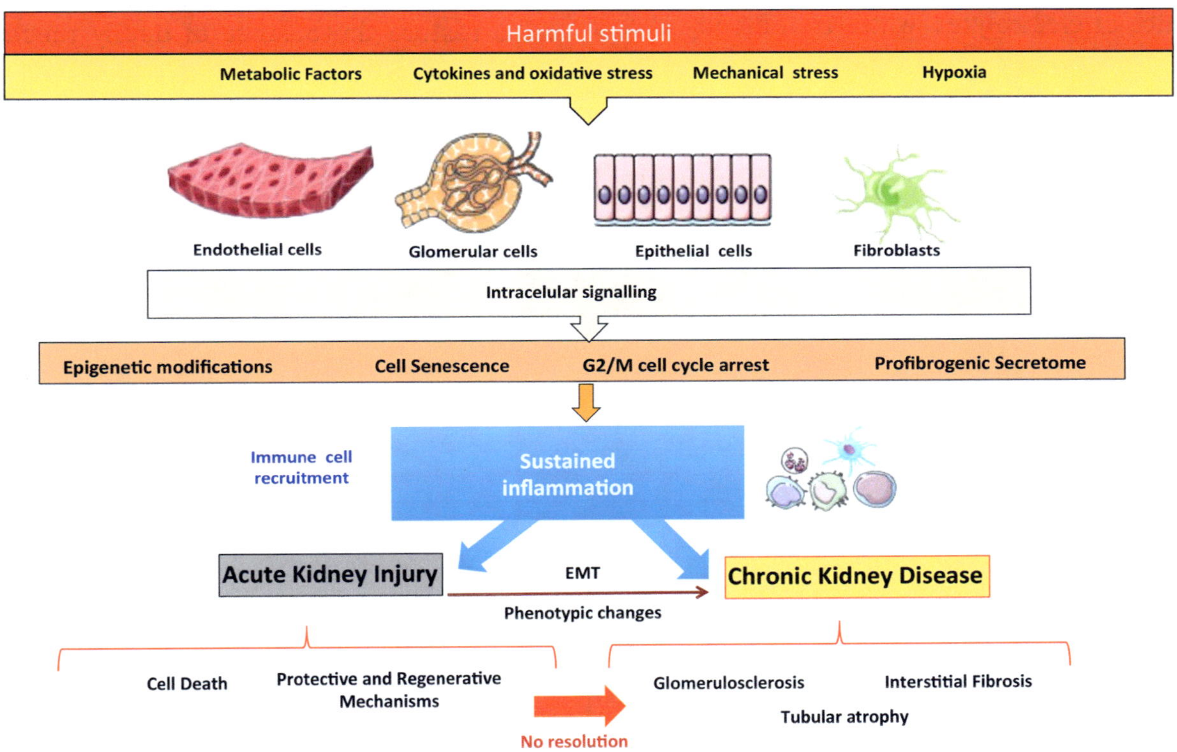

Figure 8.9. Mechanisms of kidney injury and repair.

Source: https://www.mdpi.com/ijms/ijms-23-01542/article_deploy/html/images/ijms-23-01542-g001.png.

Also, because kidney injury can have many different causes, it makes both diagnosing and treating the condition more difficult. Several factors, such as drug effects, oxygen shortage, and general inflammation, make it difficult to treat patients who might develop acute renal failure. Treatments that protect kidney function, such as those that control oxidative stress or raise renal blood supply, are another option being explored. Also, it is very important to use preventative methods such as picking the right contrast agents and handling fluids carefully in those who might be at risk. Ultimately, a comprehensive understanding of the mechanisms of kidney injury not only enhances diagnostic accuracy but also informs the development of targeted interventions, potentially reducing the incidence of AKI and improving patient outcomes in clinical settings (Kusirisin *et al.*, 2020).

8.3.2. Impact on Homeostasis

Homeostasis, the body's ability to maintain a stable internal environment, is significantly compromised in ARF. The kidneys help clean the blood, remove waste, and control the balance of electrolytes, water in the body, and blood pressure. If acute renal failure happens, these functions are interrupted, which causes negative changes in the body. Too much urea and creatinine in the blood can result in azotemia and disrupt acid-base balance, which can lead to acidosis. Also, when electrolytes, mainly potassium, are not regulated well, it can cause hyperkalemia, which can be very dangerous and lead to cardiac arrhythmias and electrical problems. In other words, acute renal failure is a major disturbance to homeostasis, which means effective interventions like renal replacement therapy are necessary. RRT, such as CRRT, helps restore the balance of bodily functions in patients who have acute renal failure.

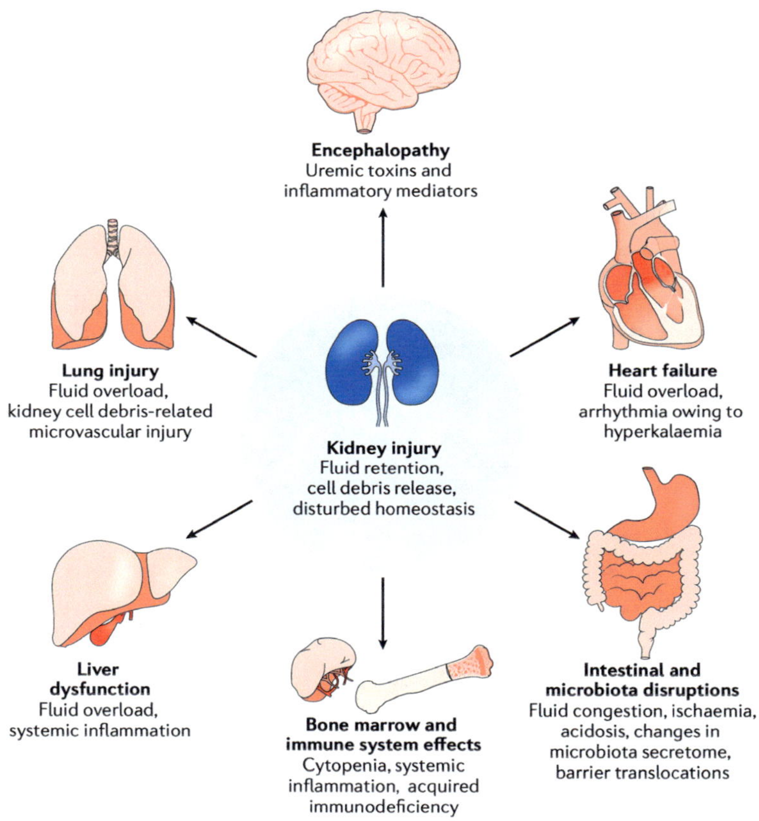

Figure 8.10. The kidneys maintain homeostasis; hence, acute kidney injury (AKI) affects almost all systems of the body, albeit in different ways. Fluid retention affects especially the lungs and the heart, frequently with clinical signs of respiratory or circulatory failure.

Source: https://www.researchgate.net/figure/The-kidneys-maintain-homeostasis-hence-acute-kidney-injury-AKI-affects-almost-all_fig3_353294748.

It helps eliminate toxins, corrects the levels of electrolytes, and may stabilize blood pressure. RRT started early has been linked to better outcomes because it helps reduce deaths from serious electrolyte and metabolic issues. Using sodium bicarbonate with CRRT in patients with sepsis-related acute kidney injury can cut the 28-day mortality rate by a significant amount. Specifically, the early high-volume sodium bicarbonate infusion has demonstrated its role as a protective factor, enhancing shock reversal rates, which are critical for maintaining adequate tissue perfusion and metabolic function during acute renal failure (Ouyang *et al.*, 2025). With these interventions, RRT helps restore normal body functions. Moreover, the health of a patient's nutrition plays a big role in their recovery after acute renal failure treatment. The prognostic nutritional index (PNI), which integrates albumin levels and lymphocyte counts, has been identified as a predictor of RRT-free survival and mortality rates among critically ill patients. Higher PNI scores correlate with improved survival rates and better recovery outcomes, highlighting the importance of maintaining adequate nutrition during treatment (Lee *et al.*, 2024). The link between nutrition, kidney function, and maintaining balance in the body shows that managing acute renal failure is not simple. Ultimately, addressing both the technical aspects of renal replacement therapy and the patient's nutritional needs can facilitate a more comprehensive restoration of homeostasis, improving overall prognosis and quality of life for affected individuals (Figure 8.10).

8.3.3. Consequences of Prolonged Renal Failure

The consequences of prolonged renal failure extend beyond immediate physiological disruptions, significantly impacting various organ systems and overall patient health. As the kidneys stop working properly, the buildup of waste in the blood causes uremia, which is marked by tiredness, nausea, and confusion. If this condition is not handled quickly, it can become very dangerous. In addition, the kidneys are responsible for keeping fluid and electrolytes balanced, so renal failure can lead to problems such as hyperkalemia and hyponatremia, which can cause serious heart problems. The situation is worsened by metabolic acidosis, which disrupts many functions in the body and makes it harder to treat patients with acute kidney injury, so urgent treatment and dialysis are necessary to avoid severe outcomes. Acute cardiorenal syndrome clearly demonstrates that when renal function is impaired for a long time, it can make heart failure worse, and the same is true in the other direction. When heart failure is acute, poor blood flow to the kidneys can cause them to function less well, which in turn makes the patient's overall health worse. Patients experiencing this syndrome typically present with elevated N-terminal Pro-B-type Natriuretic peptide (NT-proBNP) levels, indicating heart stress, alongside deteriorating kidney function. A recent study emphasized the relationship between CKD stages and acute cardiorenal syndrome, highlighting that higher stages of CKD significantly increase the risk of developing acute complications in heart failure patients (Aletras *et al.*, 2025). Because these conditions are connected, doctors should manage both the kidneys and the heart to help the patient recover. Another important complication of long-lasting renal failure is electrolyte disturbances, which must be managed carefully in patients. It is the kidneys that control the levels of potassium, sodium, and calcium in the body. When the kidneys fail, the body can develop dangerous imbalances in electrolytes, especially too much potassium (hyperkalemia), which can cause heart rhythm problems or even stop the heart if not treated. Furthermore, problems with metabolism, such as acidosis, can lead to muscle weakness and a greater chance of falling and breaking bones because of changes in calcium and phosphate levels. Renal replacement therapy emerges as a crucial therapeutic modality in such cases, aiding in the correction of these disturbances and alleviating the metabolic consequences of renal failure (Muaddi *et al.*, 2022). In general, removing toxic waste and balancing electrolytes with renal replacement therapy is necessary to improve patient safety and quality of life in acute renal failure.

Test Your Knowledge

1. What are the main mechanisms that contribute to kidney injury at the cellular and systemic levels?
2. How does kidney injury affect the body's ability to maintain fluid, electrolyte, and acid-base balance?

8.4. Treatment Options

Learning Outcome

1. Understand the medical management
2. Define renal replacement therapy overview
3. Explain the supportive care strategies

The management of ARF should be planned according to the cause, the patient's health, and the chance of renal function recovery. In the beginning, doctors look for and fix any reversible problems that lead to ARF, including dehydration, shock from infection, or urinary obstructions. It is very important to provide fluids, especially when someone is in hypovolemic shock, as it helps the kidneys get enough blood flow. There is now more evidence that dynamic assessments are effective in managing fluids, as studies have shown that methods like passive leg raising help find out if a patient is fluid responsive. Research indicates that this approach can lead to improved outcomes in patients with septic shock by reducing the need for RRT while promoting hemodynamic stability and enhancing kidney function (Douglas *et al.*, 2020). So, the best way to deal with ARF is to act quickly and use personalized fluid therapy. If conservative care does not work for patients with severe ARF, RRT steps in, mainly using dialysis. When patients have severe electrolyte imbalances, cannot be helped by diuretics, or show uremic symptoms, RRT is often started. CRRT is often helpful for critically ill patients as it slowly removes fluids, which helps keep blood pressure stable. Additionally, intermittent hemodialysis (IHD) can be employed in more stable patients (Figure 8.11).

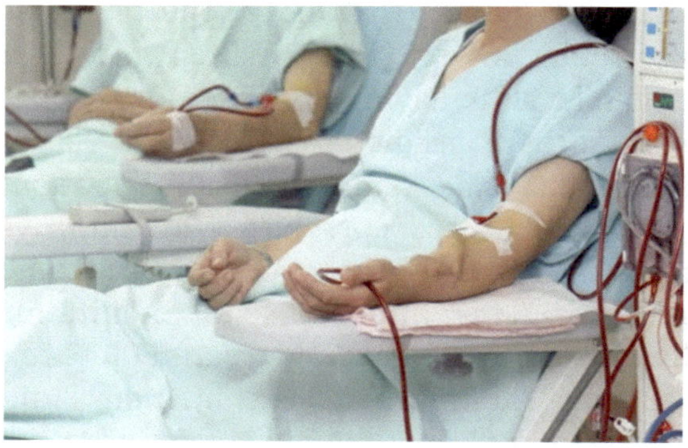

Figure 8.11. Renal replacement therapy (RRT).

Source: https://d2jx2rerrg6sh3.cloudfront.net/image-handler/picture/patient%20monitored%20by%20electronic%20sphygmomanometer%20during%20dialysis%20session-Picsfive_thumb.jpg.

Each modality presents unique advantages and drawbacks, necessitating careful consideration of the patient's overall condition and the urgency of therapy. The timing of RRT initiation remains contentious; however, recent evidence suggests that early initiation of RRT can improve survival rates, particularly in cases complicated by the systemic inflammatory response (Mach *et al.*, 2019). Making RRT decisions that fit each patient's situation helps improve the results. Along with fluid management and RRT, giving supportive care is very important in treating ARF. This means overseeing and managing problems such as metabolic acidosis, hyperkalemia, and phosphate imbalances, which might happen because the kidneys are less able to keep the body balanced. Patients often need more nutrition during acute illness, so nutritional care is very important. Giving proper nutrition can reduce the breakdown of tissues and support the kidneys in recovering.

The use of diuretics, antihypertensive drugs, and kidney-supporting agents should be carefully considered, so as not to put more stress on the kidneys. Continuous observation of how the kidneys are functioning and frequent evaluation of how treatment is working are necessary for success. Treating ARF and renal replacement therapy patients with a plan that covers all these factors gives the best chance for them to recover.

8.4.1. Medical Management

Managing acute renal failure is very important since the kidneys interact with other health systems in the body. Dehydration, sepsis, and exposure to nephrotoxic agents are some of the causes of AKI, so it needs to be recognized and treated quickly. The best management strategies should handle the causes of kidney disease and also work to keep kidney function intact.

The main elements of this strategy are handling fluids, checking electrolytes, and using medicines appropriately. CRRT becomes an important option when other dialysis methods are not enough or are not suitable. Evidence suggests that CRRT not only aids in volume control but also offers an ultrafiltration mechanism that can improve overall patient prognosis by removing toxic substances and reducing inflammatory responses (Karnina *et al.*, 2024). In the context of acute renal failure, it is imperative to consider the implications of cardiorenal syndrome (CRS), which complicates the clinical landscape. Patients with heart failure can develop acute kidney injury because of their heart's deterioration, which can increase their chances of becoming seriously ill and dying. Since heart and kidney problems often go together, doctors should treat them together with a coordinated plan. By using continuous renal replacement therapy, the kidneys and heart of these patients are likely to function better. By addressing excess fluid and electrolyte imbalances, CRRT can contribute to improved hemodynamic stability, which is often a crucial goal in the management of patients suffering from CRS (Karnina *et al.*, 2024).

It demonstrates the need for teams of different specialists to manage acute renal failure, since various problems can occur at the same time. The exploration of alternative therapies such as therapeutic plasma exchange (TPE) and continuous venovenous hemodiafiltration (CVVHDF) further enriches the medical management of acute renal failure. In those with multiple organ failure, advanced techniques have shown good results. Latest research finds that TPE helps remove harmful substances from the blood, which can help protect kidney function. If TPE is performed along with continuous renal replacement therapy, the combination can greatly improve liver function and the overall health of patients, mainly those who have acute liver failure. The combination of these approaches highlights the need to always improve renal replacement methods, which demonstrates a commitment to helping people with acute renal failure live longer and better. As these methods continue to evolve, further research is necessary to validate their effectiveness across diverse patient populations and clinical settings (Figure 8.12).

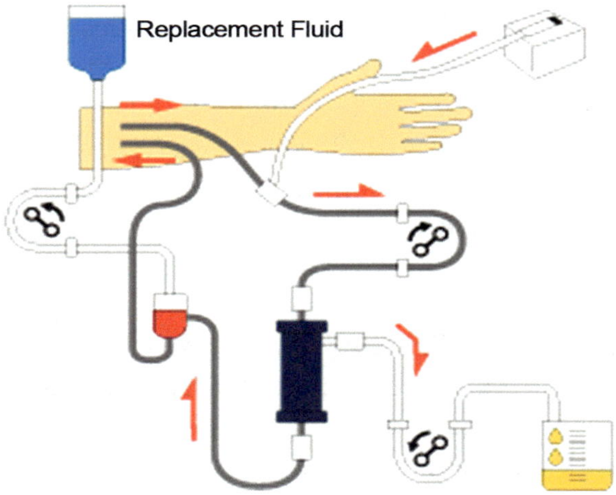

Figure 8.12. CRRT (Continuous renal replacement therapy).

Source: https://prime.horizonhospital.com/wp-content/uploads/2018/08/crrt-2.gif.

8.4.2. Renal Replacement Therapy Overview

RRT serves as a crucial intervention in managing patients with acute renal failure, particularly when kidney function fails to restore naturally. RRT mainly involves hemodialysis, peritoneal dialysis, and CRRT, and each has different ways it is used in clinical practice. A hemodialysis machine is used to take out waste, electrolytes, and extra fluid from the blood, whereas peritoneal dialysis relies on the patient's peritoneal membrane as a filter. CRRT is intended for patients who are very ill and may not be able to handle regular hemodialysis because their blood pressure is unstable. Its gentler approach allows for gradual removal of solutes and fluids, making it a favorable option in pediatric intensive care settings where renal support is often imperative (Cortina *et al.*, 2023). Knowing about these treatments is necessary to improve outcomes for people with acute renal failure. Usually, RRT is started after the cause of acute renal failure is assessed and the patient's overall condition is considered. If someone has sarcoidosis, kidney involvement could result in granulomatous interstitial nephritis, which could cause kidney failure and require RRT. Early diagnosis and timely intervention with corticosteroids can improve prognosis, yet there are instances where severe cases warrant immediate renal support (Calatroni *et al.*, 2023). Because care can be quite complicated, it is important to use a team approach to provide each patient with the right therapy for their particular needs. It is important to keep monitoring and evaluating patients in RRT to prevent complications and help them move to recovery or long-term dialysis if required. Besides, decision-makers should also think about the short-term and long-term effects of RRT on patients. It has been found that RRT can save lives, but it may also result in infections, problems with vascular access, and possible long-term kidney problems in people who survive AKI. Knowing about these risks helps nephrologists and healthcare providers plan the best care for patients after initiating RRT. Also, public health efforts that address AKI risk factors and fast referrals to specialized clinics can greatly improve patient outcomes and healthcare efficiency. Education about RRT options helps patients become involved in their care and prepares them for the difficulties of renal recovery, which improves outcomes for those with acute renal failure.

8.4.3. Supportive Care Strategies

In the context of acute renal failure, supportive care strategies play a pivotal role in improving patient outcomes while addressing the underlying conditions contributing to renal impairment. Managing these patients well usually involves a team effort that focuses on keeping their blood pressure and kidney function in good shape. This may require controlling fluids to prevent too much fluid from accumulating in the body, as it can worsen kidney injury, and giving medications that help improve blood flow to the kidneys, such as inotropes, when the heart is not functioning well. The goal is to keep the patient stable and prevent more harm to the kidneys, so they can be ready for renal replacement therapy if it is required. Supportive care is integral to enhancing resilience against further insults and may facilitate a quicker recovery in patients with acute kidney injuries, particularly those stemming from conditions like sepsis and hypovolemia, where early intervention can significantly alter the clinical trajectory (Lorusso *et al.*, 2021). It is also very important to have careful monitoring systems in place when managing acute renal failure. Assessing kidney function with serum creatinine, urine output, and electrolyte balances regularly allows doctors to notice any worsening soon and take action quickly. Technological devices such as continuous renal replacement therapy monitors help doctors make quick changes to treatment plans to maintain the right balance of fluids and electrolytes in the body. In addition, tailored nutrition plans that address calorie and protein needs help the body repair and support general health, which lowers the risk of catabolism caused by illness. Adapting supportive strategies according to each patient's unique pathophysiological status not only addresses renal failure but also enhances overall recovery potential, underscoring the importance of a tailored approach in acute care settings (Lorusso *et al.*, 2021). It is also important to use palliative care ideas in supportive care, mainly for patients with acute renal failure, since decisions about their treatment can be very challenging. Nephrologists, nurses, and palliative care specialists work together to provide emotional and social support to patients and their families during illness. . This becomes very important when patients are not expected to recover or when dialysis is not a good option for them. Supportive care strategies aim to manage symptoms, improve quality of life , and help with planning, so that patients' dignity is safeguarded when they are critically ill. As such, the amalgamation of physical and emotional support forms a comprehensive approach that is essential for those navigating the challenging landscape of acute renal failure and its associated therapies (Ronco *et al.*, 2020) (Figure 8.13).

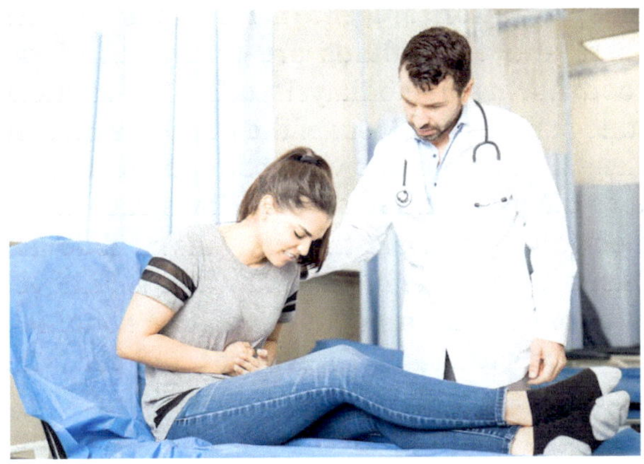

Figure 8.13. Supportive care strategies.

Source: https://img.freepik.com/free-photo/beautiful-young-woman-having-severe-stomach-ache-visiting-doctor-treatment_662251-540.jpg?t=st=1746797189~exp=1746800789~hmac=52081a69d7b83c3540553a71fdeda83d429dc85916fcb05ca004fe8d5e30e37f&w=740.

Test Your Knowledge

1. What are the key components of medical management in patients with acute or chronic kidney failure?
2. What are the main types of renal replacement therapy, and when are they typically initiated?

8.5. Types of Renal Replacement Therapy (RRT)

Learning Outcome

1. Discuss the hemodialysis
2. Explain the peritoneal dialysis
3. Define kidney transplantation

RRT serves as a critical intervention in the management of acute renal failure, offering various modalities to sustain bodily functions. Hemodialysis, peritoneal dialysis, and kidney transplantation are the main types of RRT. Waste and extra fluids are taken out of the blood during hemodialysis using an artificial kidney or dialyzer. Most of the time, this method takes place in a clinic with patients needing to go to dialysis centers several times each week. In peritoneal dialysis, the lining of the abdomen is used to filter the blood, and waste is removed by a special solution put into the abdomen. Since every therapy has its pros and cons, the decision is mostly based on the patient's age, any other health conditions, and what they prefer. Kidney transplantation is a main form of renal replacement therapy that helps patients recover from acute renal failure for a long time. A diseased kidney is removed and replaced with a healthy kidney provided by a donor. Unlike dialysis, a transplant may help people with renal failure by easing many long-term problems, such as needing to follow a special diet and having to attend regular treatments. Still, there are many difficulties with organ transplants because it is tough to find suitable donors, and patients must take immunosuppressive drugs for life to prevent their body from rejecting the organ. In addition, patients must go through a thorough evaluation to make sure they are aware of the possible risks and benefits before being considered for transplantation. Because of this, it is important to understand the details of each therapy to make the best decisions in acute renal failure. Appropriate renal replacement therapy is chosen after reviewing clinical guidelines and the patient's situation. Professional healthcare organizations have built detailed systems for making these choices, highlighting that each patient should be treated individually. For example, hemodialysis is often used in emergencies because it works fast on fluid and electrolytes, whereas peritoneal dialysis is better for those who want to be in charge of their treatment at home. In addition, if a patient has diabetes or cardiovascular disease, these conditions can be very important since certain treatments may make them worse or better. For this reason, healthcare providers should use evidence-based guidelines and tailor their care to each patient's situation to get the best results in acute renal failure management. This approach ultimately underscores the individualized nature of renal replacement therapy, wherein collaborative decision-making aligns with persistent advancements in both practice and research (Cosentino *et al.*, 2019; Davies *et al.*, 2018) (Figure 8.14).

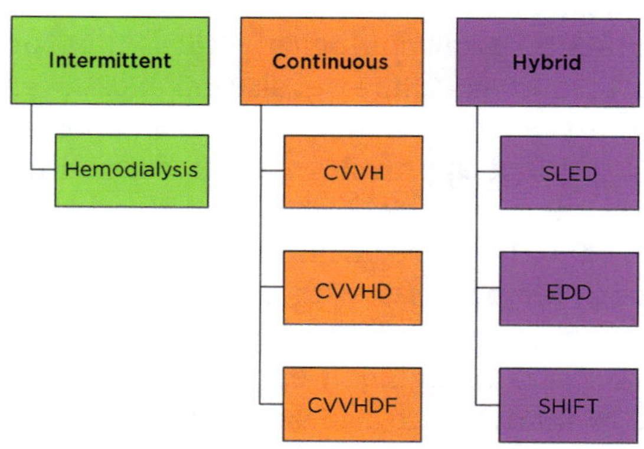

Figure 8.14. Types of renal replacement therapy (RRT) in the acute kidney injury (AKI).

Source: https://pharmacylibrary.com/do/10.21019/aki_figure_RRTModalities/full/.

8.5.1. Hemodialysis

Acute renal failure, characterized by a rapid decline in kidney function, often necessitates renal replacement therapy to manage the complexities associated with this condition. In hemodialysis, a machine is used to clean the blood by removing waste and extra fluid, since the kidneys are not working properly. It is very important for homeostasis, mainly in those who have severe electrolyte imbalances or too much fluid in their bodies. An external circuit is used in hemodialysis to eliminate urea and creatinine, which build up in the blood because the kidneys are not working properly. For this reason, starting hemodialysis promptly is necessary, since it greatly helps patients with acute renal failure and stops the development of metabolic acidosis and uremia. Whether to start hemodialysis depends on the reason for acute renal failure, how the patient is feeling, and if there are any additional health problems. For example, people with severe sepsis or cardiovascular disease are more likely to die and could need immediate renal help with hemodialysis. According to studies, using CRRT, such as hemodialysis, can help critically ill patients live longer, as it removes fluids and electrolytes more gently than intermittent hemodialysis. Additionally, the efficacy of hemodialysis in managing acute renal failure is further underscored in cases of autosomal dominant polycystic kidney disease (ADPKD), where timely therapy can mitigate the progression to end-stage kidney disease and subsequent dependence on dialysis for survival, presenting significant implications for patient management strategies (Wu *et al.*, 2024). Also, the relationship between renal failure and liver function highlights the many difficulties patients on hemodialysis may encounter. Studies have found that markers of liver function can predict outcomes for patients receiving continuous renal replacement therapy, which underlines the need to monitor both the liver and the kidneys. For critically ill patients on hemodialysis, higher total bilirubin levels have been connected to a higher risk of death. Because liver function has a major impact on patient outcomes, the interdisciplinary management of acute renal failure should include careful assessments of both the kidneys and the liver. Integrating these considerations into clinical practice is essential for optimizing treatment approaches and enhancing patient survival, particularly among those experiencing multifactorial causes of acute renal failure, including sepsis and cardiovascular complications (Nishino *et al.*, 2024) (Figure 8.15).

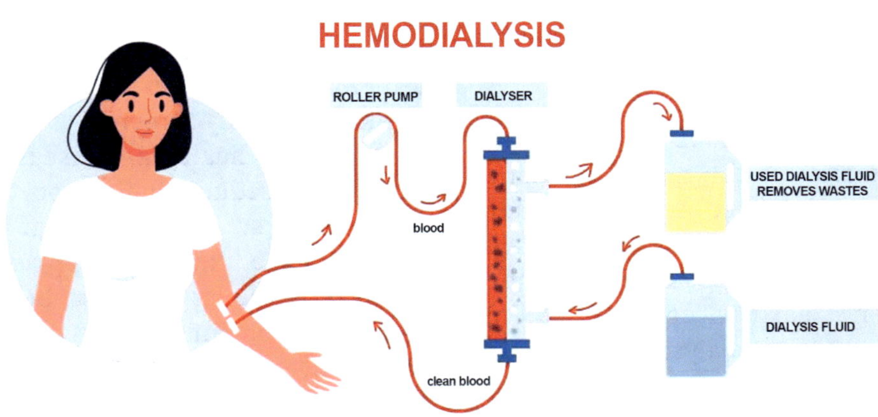

Figure 8.15. Hemodialysis.

Source: https://assets.lybrate.com/imgs/tic/enadp/causes-and-symptoms-of-hemodialysis.jpg.

8.5.2. Peritoneal Dialysis (PD)

In the context of acute renal failure, PD serves as a vital modality for renal replacement therapy. The peritoneal cavity is used as a membrane, and waste products, electrolytes, and extra water are removed from the blood by mixing with the dialysate. When vascular access for hemodialysis is hard in patients who are critically ill or have systemic illnesses, PD is very beneficial. Because PD is flexible, it can be used either all the time or just occasionally, which fits different medical needs. As it utilizes the patient's peritoneal lining as a natural filtering surface, PD can often be less invasive and more comfortable compared to hemodialysis, making it an essential option for those experiencing acute kidney injury (Thakare *et al.*, 2020). Even though it has many advantages, using peritoneal dialysis during acute renal failure brings some difficulties. A main worry is the chance of peritonitis, which may make dialysis less effective. For PD to work well, staff in acute care need to be well-trained because they might not be used to this technique. Also, the need to frequently change the dialysate can put extra pressure on healthcare resources, mainly in places with many patients and high levels of sickness. As healthcare systems grapple with the increasing burden of acute renal failure, the integration of PD into treatment protocols must be carefully managed to optimize outcomes while minimizing associated risks (Goldfarb *et al.*, 2020). Due to recent global health issues such as the COVID-19 pandemic, using peritoneal dialysis is now more important. Because of a sharp increase in acute kidney injury among COVID-19 patients, peritoneal dialysis is now seen as a good choice when hemodialysis is not easily accessible. Where there are not enough hemodialysis resources or skilled staff, institutions have switched to PD to handle the kidney problems caused by severe viral infections. But, because of this change, it is important to develop a strategy to make sure that patients and healthcare teams are well-prepared for the challenges of peritoneal dialysis in emergencies. Ensuring a robust supply chain for dialysis supplies and fostering cross-training among healthcare providers will be critical in optimizing the efficacy and safety of this essential treatment modality (Thakare *et al.*, 2020).

8.5.3. Kidney Transplantation

Acute renal failure patients are now more often treated with kidney transplantation when dialysis is either not enough or not suitable. The goal is to replace the damaged kidney with a new one, either from a living person or a deceased one, to help the patient's kidneys work normally and improve their life. Kidney transplantation helps solve the urgent problems of acute kidney injury and also manages the ongoing risks and complications of chronic kidney disease. Moreover, new developments in immunosuppressive therapy have greatly improved how long transplanted kidneys last, showing how important it is for transplant management to influence patient outcomes in renal failure treatment. Thus, kidney transplantation is widely considered the best choice, mainly because it helps people live longer and avoid the complications of dialysis. There is more to kidney transplantation than the surgery; it also involves a detailed check before the transplant and careful management afterward. Those who want a kidney transplant are first carefully screened to determine if they meet the age, health, and disease requirements for the procedure. It is important to do this assessment so that transplant recipients can tolerate the immunosuppressive therapy that stops the organ from being rejected. It is also important to focus on post-operative care, since transplant recipients can develop rejection episodes and infections, which are still major concerns. With personalized medicine and progress in transplant immunology, new immunosuppressive methods can be used, so patients have better outcomes and fewer side effects. For this reason, it is very important to use both pre- and post-operative strategies to get the most from a kidney transplant. As kidney transplantation advances, it becomes an attractive method for dealing with acute renal failure in renal replacement therapy. Studies are showing that transplants are more effective in restoring kidney function, which greatly improves patients' overall health and well-being. It is important to understand the role of transplantation in this group, as diabetes and hypertension, the main causes of renal failure, are becoming more common. Also, the limited number of donor organs and the rising number of patients on the waiting list highlight the need for better coordination of transplantation. Recent findings from Werbel *et al.* (2021) suggest that improving educational outreach concerning organ donation could enhance donor rates and subsequently influence outcomes positively. Moreover, Biggins *et al.* (2021) indicates that tailored post-transplant protocols contribute crucially to the long-term success of kidney transplantation, emphasizing the need for continued innovation in surgical and therapeutic techniques (Figure 8.16).

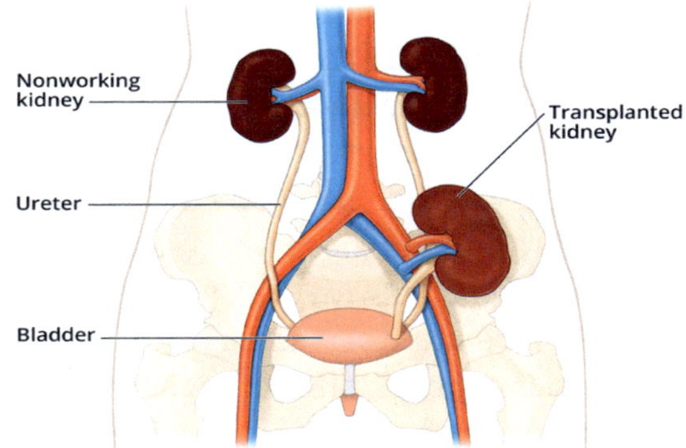

Figure 8.16. Surgeon connects the transplanted kidney to blood vessels and bladder. Blood flows through an artery into the transplanted kidney, and a vein takes filtered blood out. Urine flows through a transplanted ureter to bladder.

Source: https://www.niddk.nih.gov/health-information/kidney-disease/kidney-failure/kidney-transplant.

Test Your Knowledge

1. How does hemodialysis remove waste products and excess fluid from the blood?
2. What are the main differences between peritoneal dialysis and hemodialysis in terms of procedure and patient suitability?

8.6. Complications and Challeges

Learning Outcome

1. Discuss the complications associated with renal replacement therapy
2. Identify the psychological and social impacts
3. Analyze the long-term management considerations

The management of ARF presents a series of complications and challenges that significantly impact patient outcomes. A major issue is the quick worsening of kidney function, which may result in multiple organ failure if not treated promptly. AKI in critically ill patients may occur in 3%–15% of cases, depending on what caused the illness and any medications that could harm the kidneys. Because of AKI, patients may experience problems such as electrolyte imbalances and excess fluid, which make treatment more complicated. Also, the use of RRT brings up new challenges, for example, choosing the right patients, deciding when to begin the procedure, and the chance of problems such as infections and changes in blood pressure during the procedure. Because of these complexities, it is necessary to use a variety of approaches to handle ARF well. Along with the urgent health concerns, how ARF affects people over the long run is also very concerning. Patients with AKI may recover fully or have lasting kidney problems, and some may even be more likely to develop chronic kidney disease. Nearly 30% of those who get through an episode of AKI end up with CKD, underlining the risk of permanent kidney damage. In addition, the difficulties of hospitalization, concerns about another cancer, and managing ongoing medical care lower a person's quality of life. It is very important to watch over and manage patients during rehabilitation, but this is often difficult because of a lack of resources in health care settings. It is important to educate patients about renal health and changes in lifestyle, which makes addressing ARF even more difficult. Difficulties in treating ARF are worsened by the ongoing global health crisis, mainly during the COVID-19 pandemic. The virus can impact kidney function in different ways, causing extra problems for patients with kidney problems and those who develop AKI from COVID-19, which occurs in 3%–9% of cases. Because kidney problems can occur, these patients may have a higher risk of death, and acute kidney injury is an additional factor. With many COVID-19 patients in hospitals, the distribution of resources for renal replacement therapies becomes very important. When managing a new viral infection, healthcare professionals must address the challenges of keeping kidney function normal, which highlights the strong link between overall health and kidney health. The combined challenges of ARF and COVID-19 require innovative strategies to optimize care and ensure favorable patient outcomes, as reflected in recent guidelines and clinical recommendations (Naicker *et al.*, 2020; Williams *et al.*, 2018).

8.6.1. Complications Associated with Renal Replacement Therapy (RRT)

The implementation of RRT is often necessitated by acute renal failure, yet it is not without significant complications that can impact patient outcomes. Among the many complications, AKI is one of the most common, and it is often made worse by other health problems, how severity of the renal failure, and the need for further treatment. Studies indicate that patients undergoing procedures like extracorporeal membrane oxygenation (ECMO) are at high risk for both AKI and fluid overload (FO) during their treatment. This relationship between RRT modalities and the development of AKI necessitates a deeper understanding of how these therapies can both manage renal insufficiency and simultaneously introduce new complications, as highlighted in recent multicenter studies that catalog outcomes in patients undergoing concurrent CRRT on ECMO (Gist *et al.*, 2024). Also, issues with RRT can cause more than renal problems; they can spread to other parts of the body. A major risk of long-term RRT is the chance of metabolic problems, mainly in people with conditions such as methylmalonic aciduria. When this happens, serious complications may develop, and managing them with intermittent hemodialysis or similar treatments stabilizes the patient. Treating these metabolic problems while stopping any additional kidney damage is crucial, because poor management can lead to chronic kidney disease, which might require stronger RRT in the future. Consequently, effective interdisciplinary management is crucial to mitigate the impact of these complications and improve patient prognosis (Pintus *et al.*, 2024). Technical and logistical problems are another major factor in the complications of renal replacement therapy in acute care units. Using CRRT during ECMO treatment makes people wonder about the best timing and how to handle fluid management. There is a clear need for more studies that determine the best way to start CRRT, especially by figuring out how fast fluid should be taken out to reduce the risk of hypotension and electrolyte imbalances. These issues highlight the importance of developing standardized protocols that can both minimize the risks of complications while maximizing the efficacy of RRT in treating acute renal failure, thus fostering better patient outcomes across various clinical scenarios (Gist *et al.*, 2024) (Figure 8.17).

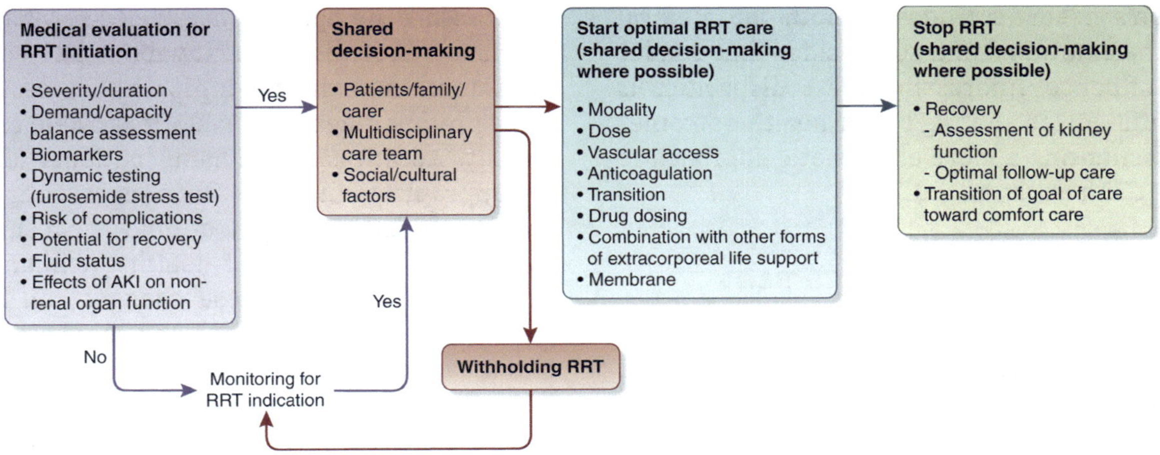

Figure 8.17. Schematic diagram of renal replacement therapy (RRT) decisions in acute kidney injury (AKI).

Source: https://www.researchgate.net/figure/Schematic-diagram-of-renal-replacement-therapy-RRT-decisions-in-acute-kidney-injury_fig1_340962271.

8.6.2. Psychological and Social Impacts

The diagnosis of ARF and the subsequent need for RRT can significantly affect an individual's psychological well-being. Many patients have feelings like anxiety, depression, and fear about their health and what may happen next. The stress can grow when the diagnosis is sudden and the changes in lifestyle are required by the treatment. Having a condition can make patients feel that they cannot do much, which can lead to loneliness and isolation. Also, since RRT continues over time, people need to fit these treatments into their daily routines, which can cause stress about time and sticking to the therapy, affecting their mental health and quality of life. ARF and RRT can influence how families and social relationships are affected, not only the person with the disorder. If family members become caregivers, their relationships may suffer, which can cause caregiver exhaustion and less social support for the patient. Many patients also tend to avoid social events because they feel tired or because they are embarrassed by their illness. Treatment costs may lead patients to struggle with their jobs and the ability to pay for needed care which can affect their social lives. Such factors lead to less social connection and may keep distress going. It is very important for healthcare providers to understand the social impacts of ARF, as these can play a big role in how patients follow treatment and what their outcomes are. It is important to consider gender when talking about the mental and social effects of ARF and RRT. It is clear from evidence that men and women may respond differently to health problems, which can affect their emotional response to being diagnosed and treated. For instance, women may exhibit greater resilience and utilize social networks more effectively during times of crisis, while men may display increased vulnerability to mental health challenges, particularly if they have pre-existing conditions that complicate their prognosis (Jarvis *et al.*, 2020). This shows that support should be designed to fit each person's needs, considering both the medical and the emotional and social sides that gender can influence. Addressing these disparities is essential for promoting better health outcomes and facilitating a more empathetic approach to care (Gebhard *et al.*, 2020).

8.6.3. Long-Term Management Considerations

Effective long-term management of patients who have experienced acute renal failure necessitates a multifaceted approach that includes careful monitoring and lifestyle modifications. After an episode of acute renal failure, it is necessary to monitor renal function regularly since some patients may continue experiencing renal problems. Regularly monitoring serum creatinine, electrolytes, and urinalysis helps clinicians make decisions to stop the kidneys from getting worse. Understanding the reason for acute renal failure is crucial; using ischemic, nephrotoxic, or obstructive factors as a guide will influence the treatment plan. For example, if the renal failure was secondary to hypotension or sepsis, continued management of these underlying conditions through appropriate medications and lifestyle changes can promote renal recovery and prevent recurrence . Along with using medicines and monitoring, patients should learn why they need to change their diets and watch their fluid intake for long-term care. Eating a diet low in protein, sodium, and potassium can help improve kidney function, so this is often suggested. Changing your diet in this way takes some of the burden off the kidneys and helps ensure the right balance of electrolytes and nutrients. Informing patients about electrolyte imbalances and their symptoms is necessary, since prompt diagnosis makes it possible to act quickly. Additionally, advising patients about the appropriate intake of fluids is essential, as how much and what type of fluid is consumed can greatly impact renal health (Williams *et al.*, 2018). Following these changes can help patients care for their health and could support better kidney function over time. Last but not least, managing acute renal failure over time should include helping patients cope emotionally and considering any remaining complications. Many people who recover from cancer still deal with anxiety and depression because of what they went through and the worry of the illness returning. When people have access to mental health resources, their well-being and ability to stick with treatment can improve a lot. In addition, some patients can develop hypertension and chronic kidney disease, which require careful long-term management. Ongoing follow-ups that check heart health are necessary to help prevent future problems linked to earlier renal failure. Therefore, a comprehensive and multidisciplinary approach to post-acute care can enhance not only kidney recovery but also the overall quality of life for these patients, reflecting a commitment to enduring health outcomes.

Test Your Knowledge

1. What are the common medical complications associated with long-term renal replacement therapy?
2. How can renal replacement therapy affect a patient's psychological well-being and social life?

SUMMARY

Because ARF involves many aspects, one must understand its causes, how it is diagnosed, and the main treatments, especially RRT. As shown, several causes can lead to ARF, including issues before the kidneys, within the kidneys, and after the kidneys, and each requiring its own approach to diagnosis and treatment. When the kidneys cannot function properly, RRT becomes very important for providing the necessary support to the body. So, choosing the right RRT method—hemodialysis, peritoneal dialysis or continuous renal replacement therapy—depends on the patient's medical situation and health history. All in all, understanding these details allows healthcare providers to give patients with ARF better and more appropriate care. Also, using clinical guidelines helps ensure the best possible outcomes for patients with ARF. Well-defined guidelines go further than just being followed; they allow health professionals to base their decisions on the latest evidence and known best practices. The ESC and EAS guidelines make it clear that clinicians should take into account many aspects when deciding, including the patient's overall health and the features of renal impairment. The responsibility falls on healthcare providers to balance these guidelines with the nuances of each patient's situation, ensuring decisions are made collaboratively and ethically, thereby enhancing the quality of care delivered to patients with acute renal failure (Cosentino *et al.*, 2019; Mach *et al.*, 2019). The fact that treatment methods and technologies in renal medicine are always changing points to the active nature of handling acute renal failure. With new research, practitioners should stay alert to update their knowledge and skills to use these developments in their daily work. Patient education and involving patients and their families in making decisions are now important parts of treatment. When patient opinions are considered along with strict medical knowledge, the results can be improved treatment adherence and better outcomes. Both following established guidelines and providing personalized care are important in managing ARF, which means healthcare providers must keep learning to handle the challenge.

It is very important to understand the various ways through which ARF and RRT are interconnected , especially during today's medical challenges like COVID-19. A sudden drop in kidney function, ARF, can cause serious health problems and higher death rates. Inflammation triggered by various pathogens, such as the novel coronavirus, is a significant contributor to ARF. Patients with COVID-19 and acute kidney injury are at a much higher risk of dying, so urgent treatment is required. So, we must pay attention to the relationship between systemic illness and renal health, as this helps doctors decide on the best treatments and stresses the need for early diagnosis. When acute kidney injury is very severe, renal replacement therapy is necessary for patients. RRT supports people whose kidneys are not functioning well enough by using either hemodialysis or peritoneal dialysis. Since patients with ARF and multiple causes, such as dehydration or failure of several organs, may require RRT, it is clear that specific patient care is required. Furthermore, ensuring optimal fluid status is essential in mitigating the risk of acute kidney injury, as improper fluid management can exacerbate existing renal dysfunction (Horby *et al.*, 2020). As a result, regularly assessing and planning during RRT can influence how patients do and how many survive, especially in cases of infectious diseases such as COVID-19. While caring for ARF patients, receiving RRT, patient-centered communication is very important. Discussing risks and treatment plans with patients and their families helps everyone grasp the difficulties of their condition. By using this approach, anxiety about the diagnosis is reduced, and patients can choose the best treatment for themselves. It is very important to explain the need for RRT when someone has acute renal failure, especially when they are ill with other conditions, to help build trust and teamwork between healthcare providers and patients. By integrating effective communication strategies with evidence-based interventions, the healthcare community can enhance the management of ARF and optimize outcomes following renal replacement therapy (Horby *et al.*, 2020).

KEY TERMS FROM THIS CHAPTER

- Acute kidney injury (AKI)
- Acute renal failure (ARF)
- Anuria
- Azotemia
- Blood urea nitrogen (BUN)
- Creatinine clearance
- Dialysate
- Dialyzer
- Fluid overload
- Fractional excretion of sodium (FENa)
- Hemodialysis
- Hyperkalemia
- Intermittent hemodialysis
- Intrarenal (intrinsic) kidney injury
- Metabolic acidosis
- Oliguria

CRITICAL THINKING QUESTIONS

1. **Which of the following is the most common cause of acute kidney injury (AKI) in critically ill patients?**
   a. Obstructive uropathy
   b. Glomerulonephritis
   c. Acute tubular necrosis (ATN) due to ischemia or nephrotoxins
   d. Chronic kidney disease
2. **A rise in serum creatinine by ≥0.3 mg/dL within 48 hours is diagnostic of:**
   a. End-stage renal disease
   b. Stage 2 chronic kidney disease
   c. Acute kidney injury (AKI)
   d. Normal renal aging
3. **Which of the following is an absolute indication for initiating renal replacement therapy in ICU patients?**
   a. Mild metabolic acidosis
   b. Hypernatremia
   c. Refractory hyperkalemia
   d. Elevated blood urea nitrogen
4. **In critically ill patients, continuous renal replacement therapy (CRRT) is preferred over intermittent hemodialysis when:**
   a. Rapid clearance of toxins is needed
   b. The patient is hemodynamically unstable
   c. There is no access to dialysis machines
   d. The patient has normal blood pressure
5. **Which of the following parameters is most useful in distinguishing prerenal AKI from intrinsic renal failure?**
   a. Serum potassium level
   b. Urine output
   c. Fractional excretion of sodium (FeNa)
   d. Blood pH

Short Answer Questions

1. What is the definition of Acute Renal Failure (ARF), and how does it differ from chronic renal failure?
2. What are the three major categories of ARF, and how do they differ in terms of etiology and pathophysiology?
3. What is the RIFLE criteria, and how is it used in the classification and staging of acute kidney injury (AKI)?
4. What is the KDIGO (Kidney Disease: Improving Global Outcomes) classification, and how does it differ from RIFLE in staging AKI?
5. What is the difference between prerenal, intrinsic, and postrenal causes of AKI, and what are some common examples of each?

Answer to Critical Thinking Questions

1. (c); 2. (c); 3. (c); 4. (b); 5. (c)

REFERENCES

1. Aboudar, Z., Masrour, S., Chettati, M., Fadili, W., & Laouad, I. (2023). #6665 Non traumatic rhabdomyolysis and acute renal failure: Which indications of renal replacement the*rapy? Nephrology Dialysis Transplan*tation. https://www.semanticscholar.org/paper/c968c7ae0cdced20e50c8c15fa8a4df4c5a7edff (accessed on 22 May 2025).
2. Aletras, G., Bachlitzanaki, M., Stratinaki, M., Lamprogiannakis, E., Panagoutsos, S., Kantartzi, K., Georgopoulou, *T.,* et al. (2025). Unraveling acute cardiorenal syndrome: Predictors and consequences in acute heart fail*ure. Journal of Clinical Medic*ine, 14. https://www.semanticscholar.org/paper/fd2656d708d7f702089a1287ec2870c1d98799ae (accessed on 22 May 2025).
3. Biggins, S. W., Angeli, P., García-Tsao, G., Ginés, P., Ling, S. C., Nadim, M. K., Wong, *F.,* et al. (2021). Diagnosis, evaluation, and management of ascites, spontaneous bacterial peritonitis and hepatorenal syndrome: 2021 practice guidance by the American Association for the Study of Liver Dise*ases. Hepatolo*gy, 74, 1014–1048. https://doi.org/10.1002/hep.31884.
4. Calatroni, M., Moroni, G., & Ponticelli, C. (2023). Renal replacement therapy in sarcoid*osis. Frontiers in Medic*ine, 9. https://www.semanticscholar.org/paper/bb14398e8686a43021b0e6f11620384a2193c252 (accessed on 22 May 2025).
5. Chaba, A., Warrillow, S., Fisher, C., Spano, S., Maeda, A., Phongphithakchai, A., Pattamin*, N.,* et al. (2024). Severely hyperammonemia acute liver failure due to paracetamol overdose: The impact of high-intensity continuous renal replacement the*rapy. Blood Purifi*cation. https://www.semanticscholar.org/paper/114879a07fcd6d7df580e0b52aaab1ce5eac11c6 (accessed on 22 May 2025).
6. Colak, M., & Ocak, I. (2024). Management of pediatric liver failure with therapeutic plasma exchange and continuous renal replacement therapy: A retrospective observational *study. Medicin*e, 103. https://www.semanticscholar.org/paper/17625f147a6ffacf78e3ad02dec57b9baf40b062 (accessed on 22 May 2025).
7. Cortina, G., Daverio, M., Demirkol, D., Chanchlani, R., & Deep, A. (2023). Continuous renal replacement therapy in neonates and children: What does the pediatrician need to know? An overview from the Critical Care Nephrology Section of the European Society of Pediatric and Neonatal Intensive Care (ESP*NIC). European Journal of Pediatric*s, 183, 529–541. https://www.semanticscholar.org/paper/166b66ad784dff834216fa7c9a5020cfee6207d1 (accessed on 22 May 2025).
8. Cosentino, F., Grant, P. J., Aboyans, V., Bailey, C. J., Ceriello, A., Delgado, V., Federici*, M.,* et al. (2019). 2019 ESC guidelines on diabetes, pre-diabetes, and cardiovascular diseases developed in collaboration with the *EASD. European Heart Journ*al, 41, 255–323. https://doi.org/10.1093/eurheartj/ehz486.
9. Davies, M. J., D'Alessio, D. A., Fradkin, J., Kernan, W. N., Mathieu, C., Mingrone, G., Rossing, *P.,* et al. (2018). Management of hyperglycemia in type 2 diabetes, 2018: A consensus report by the American Diabetes Association (ADA) and the European Association for the Study of Diabetes (E*ASD). Diabetes Ca*re, 41, 2669–2701. https://doi.org/10.2337/dci18-0033.
10. Douglas, I. S., Alapat, P., Corl, K., Exline, M. C., Forni, L. G., Holder, A. L., Kaufman, D*. A.,* et al. (2020). Fluid response evaluation in sepsis hypotension and s*hock. CHES*T, 158, 1431–1445. https://doi.org/10.1016/j.chest.2020.04.025.

11. Evans, L., Rhodes, A., Alhazzani, W., Antonelli, M., Coopersmith, C. M., French, C., Ribeiro Machado*, F.,* et al. (2021). Surviving Sepsis Campaign: International guidelines for management of sepsis and septic shock *2021. Critical Care Medic*ine, 49, e1063–e1143. https://doi.org/10.1097/ccm.0000000000005337.

12. Fujisawa, Y., Miyanaga, T., Takeji, A., Shirota, Y., & Ueda, Y. (2023). A lethal combination: Legionnaires' disease complicated by rhabdomyolysis, acute kidney injury, and non-occlusive mesenteric isch*emia. The American Journal of Case Repor*ts, 24, Article e940792. https://www.semanticscholar.org/paper/c7fbd64eee572f154be9d58afbe96c6405b647df (accessed on 22 May 2025).

13. García Sánchez, J. J., Sultan, A., Ärnlöv, J., Cabrera, C., Card-Gowers, J., Nicola, L., Halimi*, J.,* et al. (2021). MO498INSIDE CKD: Modelling the clinical and economic impacts of targeted urinary albumin-to-creatinine ratio screening in European count*ries. Nephrology Dialysis Transplantati*on, 36. https://www.semanticscholar.org/paper/53d58855c7cdf342366dcb8362ca8746c53ce374 (accessed on 22 May 2025).

14. Gebhard, C., Regitz-Zagrosek, V., Neuhauser, H., Morgan, R., & Klein, S. L. (2020). Impact of sex and gender on COVID-19 outcomes in Eu*rope. Biology of Sex Differenc*es, 11. https://doi.org/10.1186/s13293-020-00304-9.

15. Gist, K. M., Bastero, P., Ricci, Z., Kaddourah, A., Strong, A., Chanchlani, R., Steflik, H*. J.,* et al. (2024). Acute kidney injury, fluid balance, and continuous renal replacement therapy in children and neonates treated with extracorporeal membrane oxygenat*ion. Intensive Care Medicine–Pediatric and Ne*onatal. https://www.semanticscholar.org/paper/bdedcbc01a567cc532ec1cc8b3a1452991ed5183 (accessed on 22 May 2025).

16. Goldfarb, D. S., Benstein, J. A., Zhdanova, O. I., Hammer, E. J., Block, C. A., Caplin, N., Thompson*, N.,* et al. (2020). Impending shortages of kidney replacement therapy for COVID-19 pati*ents. Clinical Journal of the American Society of Nephrolo*gy, 15, 880–882. https://doi.org/10.2215/cjn.05180420.

17. Gustafsson, U., Scott, M. J., Hübner, M., Nygren, J., Demartines, N., Francis, N., Rockall*, T.,* et al. (2018). Guidelines for perioperative care in elective colorectal surgery: Enhanced Recovery After Surgery (ERAS®) Society recommendations: *2018. World Journal of Surge*ry, 43, 659–695. https://doi.org/10.1007/s00268-018-4844-y.

18. Horby, P., Lim, W. S., Emberson, J., Mafham, M., Bell, J., Linsell, L., Staplin*, N.,* et al. (2020). Dexamethasone in hospitalized patients with COVI*D-19. New England Journal of Medicin*e, 384, 693–704. https://doi.org/10.1056/nejmoa2021436.

19. Julien, M., Lombardi, Y., & Rafat, C. (2024). #236 Immediate or delayed initiation of renal replacement therapy in patients with leptospirosis and acute kidney injury: A target trial emula*tion. Nephrology Dialysis Transplan*tation. https://www.semanticscholar.org/paper/d5a2b8c969934eede1ece4c1e3aef324486e8225 (accessed on 22 May 2025).

20. Karnina, R., Irawany, V., Manggala, S., Aulya, J. U., & Faruk, M. (2024). The role of continuous renal replacement therapy in the management of cardiorenal syndrome involving acute myocardial infarction with concomitant pneumonia: Case re*port. The Pan African Medical Journ*al, 49. https://www.semanticscholar.org/paper/98c272db70b11558bbce5a95e3e3e7433baf4987 (accessed on 22 May 2025).

21. Kusirisin, P., & Chattipakorn, N. (2020). Contrast-induced nephropathy and oxidative stress:

Mechanistic insights for better interventional approaches. *Journal of Translational Medicine*, 18. https://doi.org/10.1186/s12967-020-02574-8.

22. Lebreton, G., Schmidt, M., Ponnaiah, M., Folliguet, T., Para, M., Guihaire, J., Lansac, E., et al. (2021). Extracorporeal membrane oxygenation network organization and clinical outcomes during the COVID-19 pandemic in Greater Paris, France: A multicenter cohort study. *The Lancet Respiratory Medicine*, 9, 851–862. https://doi.org/10.1016/s2213-2600(21)00096-5.

23. Lee, Y. F., Lin, P. R., Wu, S. H., Hsu, H. H., Yang, S. Y., & Kor, C. T. (2024). Impact of the prognostic nutritional index on renal replacement therapy–free survival and mortality in patients on continuous renal replacement therapy. *Renal Failure*, 46. https://www.semanticscholar.org/paper/0bc43ddd1af4e4e5e07ffde072adac8e4eb0dc59 (accessed on 22 May 2025).

24. Lorusso, R., Shekar, K., MacLaren, G., Schmidt, M., Pellegrino, V., Meyns, B., Haft, J. W., et al. (2021). ELSO interim guidelines for Veno arterial extracorporeal membrane oxygenation in adult cardiac patients. *ASAIO Journal*, 67, 827–844. https://doi.org/10.1097/mat.0000000000001510.

25. Mach, F., Baigent, C., Catapano, A. L., Koskinas, K. C., Casula, M., Badimón, L., Chapman, M. J., et al. (2019). 2019 ESC/EAS guidelines for the management of dyslipidemias: Lipid modification to reduce cardiovascular risk. *European Heart Journal*, 41, 111–188. https://doi.org/10.1093/eurheartj/ehz455.

26. Mauvais-Jarvis, F., Bairey Merz, C. N., Barnes, P. J., Brinton, R. D., Carrero, J. J., DeMeo, D. L., De Vries, G. J., et al. (2020). Sex and gender: Modifiers of health, disease, and medicine. *The Lancet*, 396, 565–582. https://doi.org/10.1016/s0140-6736(20)31561-0.

27. Muaddi, L., Ledgerwood, C., Sheridan, R., Dumont, T., & Nashar, K. (2022). Acute renal failure and its complications, indications for emergent dialysis, and dialysis modalities. *Critical Care Nursing Quarterly*, 45(3), 258–265. https://www.semanticscholar.org/paper/7345ef3642541aa0e9025b36271972c4edecb687 (accessed on 22 May 2025).

28. Naicker, S., Yang, C. W., Hwang, S. J., Liu, B. C., Chen, J., & Jha, V. (2020). The novel coronavirus 2019 epidemic and kidneys. *Kidney International*, 97, 824–828. https://doi.org/10.1016/j.kint.2020.03.001.

29. Nishino, T., Kubota, Y., Kashiwagi, T., Hirama, A., Asai, K., Yasutake, M., & Kumita, S. (2024). Hepatic function markers as prognostic factors in patients with acute kidney injury undergoing continuous renal replacement therapy. *Renal Failure*, 46. https://www.semanticscholar.org/paper/5a5840899bd81e7e7dfa2c155c776f047fe8a523 (accessed on 22 May 2025).

30. Northup, P. G., García-Pagán, J. C., García-Tsao, G., Intagliata, N. M., Superina, R., Roberts, L. N., Lisman, T., et al. (2020). Vascular liver disorders, portal vein thrombosis, and procedural bleeding in patients with liver disease: 2020 practice guidance by the American Association for the Study of Liver Diseases. *Hepatology*, 73, 366–413. https://doi.org/10.1002/hep.31646.

31. Ouyang, L., Pan, Y., Wu, Y. F., Tang, Q., Wang, D., & Lou, N. (2025). Early and high-volume administration of sodium bicarbonate in sepsis-associated acute kidney injury in patients with malignancies, during continuous renal replacement therapy. *Renal Failure*, 47. https://www.semanticscholar.org/paper/5439faaf4e3f337d8f8f9eabaf66b938bb094871 (accessed on 22 May 2025).

32. Patra, J. K., Das, G., Fraceto, L. F., Campos, E. V. R., Rodriguez-Torres, M. d. P., Acosta-Torres, L. S., Díaz-Torres, L. A., et al. (2018). Nano based drug delivery systems: Recent developments

and future prospects. *Journal of Nanobiotechnology*, 16. https://doi.org/10.1186/s12951-018-0392-8.

33. Pintus, G., Vitturi, N., Carraro, G., Lenzini, L., Gugelmo, G., Fasan, I., Madinelli, *A.,* et al. (2024). Renal replacement therapy in methylmalonic aciduria-related metabolic failure: Case report and literature review. *Journal of Clinical Medicine*, 13. https://www.semanticscholar.org/paper/d8988971d134befc53f522b042297dc849e3bdd3 (accessed on 22 May 2025).

34. Ronco, C., Reis, T., & Husain-Syed, F. (2020). Management of acute kidney injury in patients with COVID-19. *The Lancet Respiratory Medicine*, 8, 738–742. https://doi.org/10.1016/s2213-2600(20)30229-0.

35. Selby, N. M., Forni, L. G., Laing, C., Horne, K., Evans, R., Lucas, B., & Fluck, R. (2020). COVID-19 and acute kidney injury in hospital: Summary of NICE guidelines. BMJ. https://doi.org/10.1136/bmj.m1963.

36. Shah, M., Palani, A., Hashemi, A., & Shin, J. (2023). Bradycardia, renal failure, atrioventricular nodal blockade, shock and hyperkaliemia syndrome involving digoxin toxicity: A case report. *Heart International*, 17(1), 60–62. https://www.semanticscholar.org/paper/a9426396d9323dcf1b9d8b198ae17826a0074ed2 (accessed on 22 May 2025).

37. Shen, K., Yang, C., Huang, J., Shuai, X., Niu, T., & Ma, H. (2025). The clinical characteristics and implications of acute kidney injury during induction therapy for acute promyelocytic leukemia. *Frontiers in Pharmacology*, 16. https://www.semanticscholar.org/paper/6f57c970d9348c9d5d5e4055e3c6c6cb26441281 (accessed on 22 May 2025).

38. Su, H., Yang, M., Wan, C., Yi, L. X., Tang, F., Zhu, H. Y., Yi, *F.,* et al. (2020). Renal histopathological analysis of 26 postmortem findings of patients with COVID-19 in China. *Kidney International*, 98, 219–227. https://doi.org/10.1016/j.kint.2020.04.003.

39. Thakare, S., Gandhi, C., Modi, T., Bose, S., Deb, S., Saxena, N., Katyal, *A.,* et al. (2020). Safety of remdesivir in patients with acute kidney injury or CKD. *Kidney International Reports*, 6, 206–210. https://doi.org/10.1016/j.ekir.2020.10.005.

40. Vahanian, A., Beyersdorf, F., Praz, F., Milojevic, M., Baldus, S., Bauersachs, J., Capodanno, *D.,* et al. (2021). 2021 ESC/EACTS guidelines for the management of valvular heart disease. *European Heart Journal*, 43, 561–632. https://doi.org/10.1093/eurheartj/ehab395.

41. Varga, Z., Flammer, A. J., Steiger, P., Haberecker, M., Andermatt, R., Zinkernagel, A. S., Mehra, M. *R.,* et al. (2020). Endothelial cell infection and endotheliosis in COVID-19. *The Lancet*, 395, 1417–1418. https://doi.org/10.1016/s0140-6736(20)30937-5.

42. Visseren, F. L. J., Mach, F., Smulders, Y. M., Carballo, D., Koskinas, K. C., Bäck, M., Bénétos, *A.,* et al. (2021). 2021 ESC guidelines on cardiovascular disease prevention in clinical practice. *European Heart Journal*, 42, 3227–3337. https://doi.org/10.1093/eurheartj/ehab484.

43. Wei, P. F. (2020). Diagnosis and treatment protocol for novel coronavirus pneumonia (Trial Version 7). *Chinese Medical Journal*, 133, 1087–1095. https://doi.org/10.1097/cm9.0000000000000819.

44. Werbel, W. A., Boyarsky, B. J., Ou, M. T., Massie, A. B., Tobian, A. A. R., Garonzik-Wang, J., & Segev, D. L. (2021). Safety and immunogenicity of a third dose of SARS-CoV-2 vaccine in solid organ transplant recipients: A case series. *Annals of Internal Medicine*, 174, 1330–1332. https://doi.org/10.7326/l21-0282.

45. Williams, B., Mancia, G., Spiering, W., Agabiti Rosei, E., Azizi, M., Burnier, M., Clement, D. *L.,* et al. (2018). 2018 ESC/ESH guidelines for the management of arterial hyperten*sion. European Heart Journ*al, 39, 3021–3104. https://doi.org/10.1093/eurheartj/ehy339.

46. Wu, M. J., Chen, C. H., & Tsai, S. (2024). Effectiveness of tolvaptan on renal replacement therapy in patients with autosomal dominant polycystic kidney disease: A retrospective cohort study from the TriNetX global collaborative net*work. Renal Failu*re, 46. https://www.semanticscholar.org/paper/e46d4ed3a2826845ad4dc98b21e3544eea905f14 (accessed on 22 May 2025).

NEUROLOGICAL MONITORING AND MANAGEMENT IN CRITICAL CARE

9

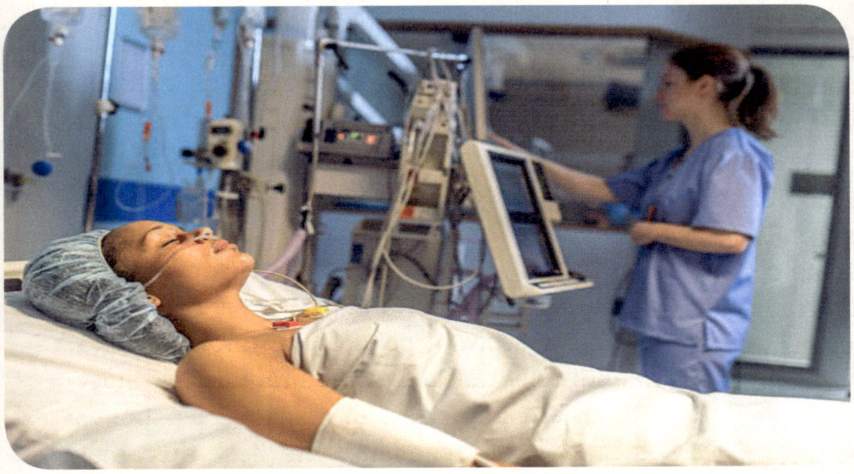

LEARNING OBJECTIVES

After studying this chapter, you will be able to:

1. Explain the types of neurological monitoring.
2. Describe indications for neurological monitoring.
3. Explore the techniques for neurological monitoring.
4. Focus on the challenges in neurological monitoring.
5. List the management strategies in critical care.

Introduction

The complexities of neurological conditions necessitate robust monitoring and management protocols within critical care settings. Neurological monitoring helps find and manage serious issues such as strokes, traumatic brain injuries, and seizures early. Because neurological disorders are happening more often, it is important to have real-time monitoring that gives quick updates on a patient's neurological health. For instance, studies have highlighted the dramatic rise in incident strokes globally, with over 12 million cases reported in 2019 alone, indicating an urgent need for effective monitoring to facilitate proper management and rehabilitation strategies (Feigin *et al.*, 2021). So, critical care areas should use new technologies and procedures to decrease the serious health problems or death of the patients. Managing neurological patients in critical care also requires to knowing about the risk factors and the ways to prevent complications. With the identification of high systolic blood pressure and obesity as leading contributors to stroke incidents, healthcare providers must tailor their management techniques accordingly (Feigin *et al.*, 2021). Therefore, it calls for using risk assessment tools and monitoring the neurological state of the patient at all times. It is also important to use clinical guidelines, so that treatments are given based on best practices and patient's health. Recent advice stresses that healthcare professionals should still use their professional judgment when making treatment plans for every patient.

It helps improve the care patients get and encourages different health professionals to cooperate. Also, since neurological conditions change along with population and healthcare trends, the methods for monitoring and treatment must be updated frequently. Neurological problems cause major challenges, mainly in poorer regions where healthcare and advanced tools are hard to find. The gap between high-income and low-income countries regarding stroke mortality rates illustrates the urgency for resource allocation and the establishment of evidence-based preventive strategies (Feigin *et al.*, 2021). Tackling these differences needs the effort of countries working together and making changes locally in healthcare systems. Developing a thorough and updated knowledge of neurological monitoring and management can help improve patient outcomes in critical care, which leads to better overall care for this group.

Definition of Neurological Monitoring

Neurological monitoring is a critical component of patient care in various clinical settings, especially within critical care environments. It requires checking and observing a patient's neurological state to find out if their condition is getting better or worse. Neurological monitoring is used to check important signs, level of awareness, movement, and other neurological aspects. This observation is essential for detecting brain ischemia, intracranial pressure (ICP) changes, or the onset of seizures, all of which can significantly impact clinical decision-making and treatment strategies. When neurological changes are recognized fast in acute cases, it may allow for urgent steps that help prevent more brain damage and improve the patient's condition. Critical care teams depend on a variety of methods and tools to monitor the nervous system. Techniques range from simple assessments, such as the Glasgow Coma Scale (GCS), to advanced imaging modalities and electroencephalography (EEG) for detecting seizure activity.

The use of technology, such as bedside monitors, for intracranial pressure and cerebral perfusion pressure , helps the healthcare team react quickly to changes in the patient's neurological condition. Using comprehensive neurological assessments helps doctors to decide immediate treatment and also supports the ongoing care of people with brain injuries or conditions that affect the brain. Using these methods are important for managing a patient's health and for choosing the best therapies for each person. Neurological monitoring is important not only for patient care but also for research and making critical care better. The combination of different monitoring methods allows healthcare workers to observe trends in neuronal activity, check the success of different treatments, and help to form evidence-based practices in critical care. Research projects use the data from neurological tests to know the effectiveness of the treatments and to understand the causes of brain disorders. As a result of these studies, we could improve how critical care is monitored, treated, and managed, which would show the progress in this field. Hence, neurological monitoring emerges not only as a foundational element of patient management but also as a critical enabler of research and educational advancements in the field of neurology and critical care (Figure 9.1).

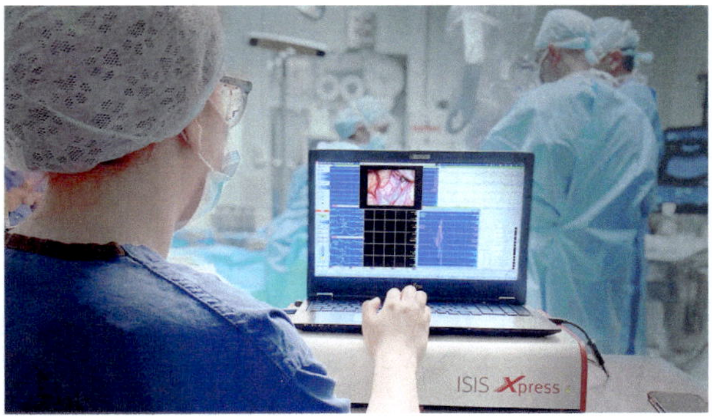

Figure 9.1. Neurological monitoring.

Source: https://www.en.inomed.com/fileadmin/media/produkte/Intraoperatives_Neuromonitoring/Neurophysiologisches_Monitoring/Neurophysiologisches-Monitoring-inomed-isis-xpress.png.

Importance in Critical Care Settings

In critical care settings, neurological monitoring is indispensable for optimizing patient outcomes, particularly in cases of severe brain injury and stroke. Conditions such as traumatic brain injury (TBI) and ischemic strokes necessitate careful observation of cerebral physiology to avert secondary complications. Regular assessment of ICP, as recommended in pediatric TBI guidelines, helps prevent further brain damage by managing elevated ICP and ensuring cerebral perfusion (Kochanek *et al.*, 2019). In short, fast monitoring of the brain provides vital information that guides immediate treatment, which can greatly affect patients' outcomes showing the importance in critical care. Also, new neurological monitoring technology closely and accurately track changes in patient health in critical care. Non-invasive monitoring methods in addition to the usual methods, give healthcare workers continuous updates without needing to be very invasive. This way of care improves comfort for patients and also helps to detect worsening health problems sooner. So, clinical teams can provide timely care, which leads to better patient care and results in the long run. The use of technology in neurocritical care demonstrates that management approaches must be flexible to meet the unique needs of each patient, which is very important in this field. Also, having a clear picture of how neurological diseases are spreading can influence the use of resources and planning of care in critical areas. For example, since stroke is becoming more common worldwide and TBIs can affect people differently, special preventive efforts are required. Specific data on incidence and mortality rates, as highlighted by global health assessments, assist healthcare institutions in tailoring interventions and allocating resources effectively (Feigin *et al.*, 2021). For this reason, using research-based knowledge in clinical settings improves how care is given in critical environments and encourages teams of different specialists to cooperate, which raises the level of care for people at risk.

9.1. Types of Neurological Monitoring

Learning Outcome

1. Discuss the continuous electroencephalography (EEG)
2. Define intracranial pressure (ICP) monitoring
3. Explain the neurological assessment scales (e.g., GCS)

Neurological monitoring is important in critical care since it helps detect and assess any neurological problems. One prominent method utilized in this realm is electroencephalography (EEG), which captures the brain's electrical activity. Because of new technologies, multi-view information fusion methods are now used to boost the EEG signals are processing. They use data from several channels, which helps to give a more detailed picture of brain activity than single-channel approaches. For this reason, multi-view information fusion in applications has led to more accurate seizure detection and assessments of cognitive state. Nevertheless, challenges such as data heterogeneity and high computational demands remain, underscoring the need for further innovations in EEG methodologies that can harness the power of artificial intelligence to optimize neurological diagnostic accuracy in critical care settings (Patir *et al.*, 2025). Another significant type of neurological monitoring is intracranial pressure (ICP) monitoring, which is essential for patients exhibiting potential intracranial hypertension, commonly seen in traumatic brain injuries or strokes. Regular measurements of ICP reveal the state of the brain, so doctors can decide quickly for treatment options. Recent studies suggested that using advanced imaging, hemodynamic support, and ICP monitoring together helps doctors to give better treatments for decompression and proper blood supply to the brain. This allows doctors to choose the correct treatments and reduce the risks that can arise from the late treatment. As a result, the incorporation of ICP monitoring into critical care emphasizes the necessity for prompt decision-making based on real-time data (Sandarage *et al.*, 2025). Additionally, neuromuscular monitoring, particularly through the use of electromyography (EMG) and nerve conduction studies, has gained prominence in critical care environments. They help healthcare professionals determine if the central and peripheral nervous systems are working correctly. In particular, EMG helps to find neuromuscular transmission problems and analyze muscle function in patients who are very ill. Also, using neuromuscular monitoring can greatly improve the understanding of neurological problems and their treatments. As we learn more about these monitoring methods, the chances for personal care rise, which can lead to better results in critically ill people. By assessing both muscular and neurological responses, caregivers can adjust treatment tactics more effectively, thereby maximizing recovery potential in critical care contexts (Sandarage *et al.*, 2025).

9.1.1. Continuous Electroencephalography (EEG)

In the context of critical care, continuous EEG offers a transformative approach to neurological monitoring, particularly for patients with acute brain injuries or disorders of consciousness (DoC).

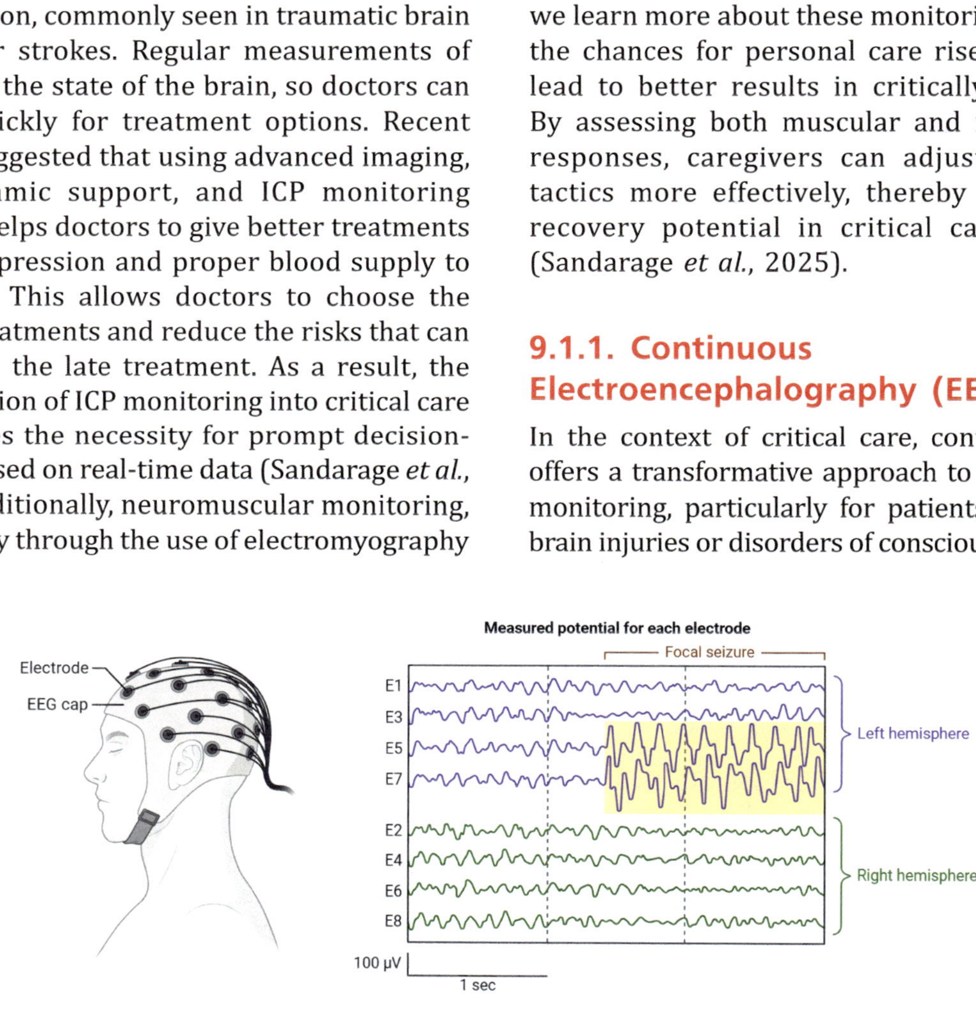

Figure 9.2. Electroencephalography (EEG) recording.

Source: https://external-content.duckduckgo.com/iu/?u=https%3A%2F%2Fwww.verywellhealth.com%2Fthmb%2FcGLVsyR-_yBenHLf1IEddKky2f8%3D%2F1500x0%2Ffilters%3Ano_upscale()%3Amax_bytes(150000)%3Astrip_icc()%2Feeg-601235088-5a524fdef1300a0037eeebe5.jpg&f=1&nofb=1&ipt=11693bc9cb0a746485965034b23c731ffde0d285c964b5047712dbce4eeebb12.

The usual EEG assessments done at intervals may not pick up brief and important neurological events that can happen in critical care. EEG monitoring over a long period provides doctors real-time data on brain activity and allows them to notice seizures or problems that might not be seen in a regular EEG. In addition, combining continuous EEG with full neurological examination helps doctors to make better decisions, for the benefits of the patients. As highlighted in recent guidelines, EEG monitoring should be a key component of neurological management protocols in intensive care units, serving as an essential adjunct to bedside evaluations and imaging modalities (Kondziella *et al.*, 2020) (Figure 9.2).

The implementation of continuous EEG monitoring is particularly crucial in evaluating patients with altered levels of consciousness. New EEG technology allows doctors to detect sleep stages such as rapid eye movement sleep and slow-wave sleep, which give important clues about a patient's neurological health. Knowing these patterns can help healthcare professionals tell apart coma, vegetative state, and minimally conscious state. Because of constant monitoring, clinicians are able to respond quickly to changes and treat the complexities of severe brain injuries. Also, using data analytics and machine learning with EEG analysis is gaining importance. These innovations facilitate the automatic identification of significant neurological patterns, thereby augmenting traditional assessment techniques and enhancing the overall efficacy of critical care management (Ravi Dì *et al.*, 2016). There are some difficulties associated with using continuous EEG monitoring in critical care. Such issues includes technical difficulties, need for trained personnel to interpret the data, and making sure the equipment keeps working in tough conditions. Also, it is important for care teams to be alert to any misinterpretation of EEG results, since this could result in unnecessary treatments or actions. For this reason, a team of neurologists, critical care doctors, and data analysts is needed to use continuous EEG to its fullest. By fostering collaboration across specialties, healthcare providers can better interpret EEG findings and tailor individualized treatment plans, ultimately enhancing patient care in neurological critical care settings (Kondziella *et al.*, 2020; Ravi Dì *et al.*, 2016).

9.1.2. Intracranial Pressure (ICP) Monitoring

ICP monitoring is a critical component in the management of patients suffering from severe neurological injuries, particularly traumatic brain injury (TBI) and other conditions that can lead to cerebral edema. Proper measurement of ICP is important, since high levels may show thecomplications and the quick action is needed to protect the brain. Often, clinicians insert intraparenchymal or ventricular catheters to get real-time information about a patient's ICP. Regular monitoring is necessary to plan treatment, since the severity and duration of the elevated ICP can strongly affect the outcome for the patient. So, knowing how ICP changes helps doctors handle critical cases more effectively. Proper management of increased ICP depends on knowing the various treatments and the reasons for cerebral edema. The current advice is to use hyperosmolar agents such as mannitol and hypertonic saline, which help reduce ICP by encouraging osmosis and moving fluid from inside cells to the blood vessels. Although these treatments can successfully lower ICP, studies suggest that their effect on overall neurological outcomes is not clear, which means personalized care is necessary. Since these agents can have side effects, it is very important to watch for any signs of harm while using them. Therefore, clinical teams must remain vigilant in their assessments and possess extensive knowledge regarding the use of these therapies in acute situations, as referenced in the emerging guidelines on cerebral edema management (Cook *et al.*, 2020).

Further complicating the management of ICP is the diverse clinical scenarios that require tailored treatment protocols, particularly in the case of severe traumatic brain injury (sTBI). Recently, experts have come to an agreement that monitoring ICP should be a main part of any management algorithm. They group interventions by risk and evidence, which helps doctors use a step-by-step plan to manage high ICP. They allow clinicians to use evidence when making choices and encourage consistency in how care is provided in different places. The algorithms advocate for a range of interventions, from basic physiological assessments to more aggressive treatments, which reflect the complex nature of managing sTBI while respecting individual patient needs (Hawryluk *et al.*, 2019). Consequently, these comprehensive strategies highlight the importance of collaborative clinical decision-making in optimizing neurological outcomes in critically ill patients (Figure 9.3).

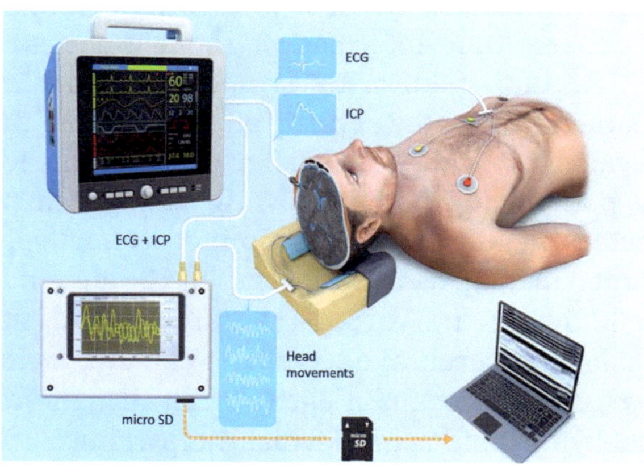

Figure 9.3. Intracranial pressure monitoring device.

Source: https://www.researchdive.com/blogImages/ehugRBH4iO.jpeg.

9.1.3. Neurological Assessment Scales (e.g., Glasgow Coma Scale (GCS))

Neurological assessment scales, especially the GCS, are essential for assessing patients in critical care who might have neurological problems. The GCS is used to determine the level of consciousness in trauma patients, which helps doctors assess them quickly and correctly. Using the GCS, doctors can assess the main areas of neurological function by measuring eye opening, speech, and movements. This scale is especially useful for managing severe TBI because it helps monitor how the patient changes over time, which guides the decisions and treatments used. Moreover, the GCS can identify trends that may necessitate modifications in therapeutic approaches, enhancing the overall management of patients in these high-stakes environments, as highlighted in the updated guidelines for pediatric TBI management (Kochanek *et al.*, 2019). Even though the GCS is still used, its weaknesses have encouraged the creation of new tools and techniques to help with more accurate neurological assessments. The GCS has been criticized because it is not always able to detect small changes in the brain that may show a patient's condition is getting worse. If patients have intubation or severe problems with speech, the GCS alone may not capture their true neurological state, which could result in an underestimation. So, clinicians can use additional methods such as ICP monitoring and neuroimaging, in addition to the GCS. These additional assessments can yield valuable information that assists in managing complex cases where GCS scores alone may provide an incomplete picture of the patient's condition, thereby improving outcomes in critical care settings (Afshari *et al.*, 2017). Using the GCS and modern monitoring methods together demonstrates why it is important to use a complete approach in managing neurological care in critical care. Because of this approach, it is possible to help patients quickly, which is important for preventing secondary brain injuries that can happen when consciousness is impaired for a long time. Clinicians can use regular monitoring and evaluatetreatments and make necessary changes using the most recent data. As a result, better management of neurological status in critically ill patients supports both quick responses to changes and better long-term outcomes. As further research continues to refine assessment methods, integrating various scales and monitoring tools into standard practice will be essential for advancing critical care protocols for neurological patients (Kochanek *et al.*, 2019) (Figure 9.4).

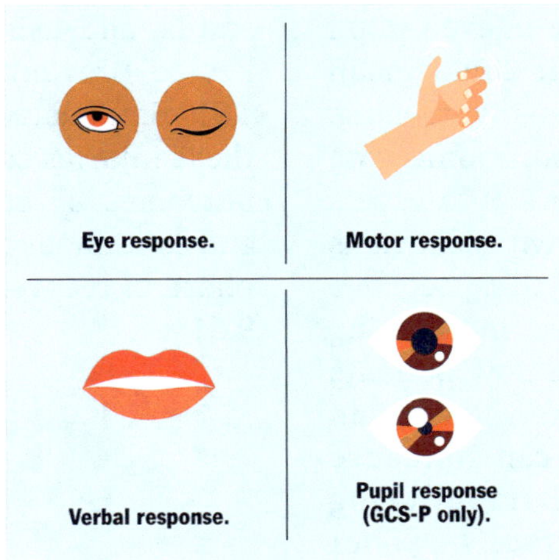

Figure 9.4. Glasgow coma scale (GCS).

Source: https://my.clevelandclinic.org/-/scassets/images/org/health/articles/24848-glasgow-coma-scale.

Test Your Knowledge

1. What is the role of continuous EEG in monitoring critically ill patients with neurological conditions?
2. How is intracranial pressure (ICP) monitored, and what are the clinical implications of elevated ICP?

9.2. Indications for Neurological Monitoring

Learning Outcome

1. Discuss the traumatic brain injury (TBI)
2. Define stroke management
3. Explain the post-operative neurosurgical patients

In the critical care setting, neurological monitoring is indispensable for patients with conditions that pose an imminent risk to cerebral function. These are some of the reasons monitoring is needed: changes in mental state, sudden neurological problems, or signs of further brain injury. If a patient shows signs of confusion, disorientation, or agitation, immediate neurological assessment is often needed because these can progress to a coma. Also, patients with ischemic stroke or intracerebral hemorrhage should be closely watched to detect any changes in their condition and receive appropriate treatment. Taking such actions helps prevent major neurological damage and improves the outcomes for patients. Neurological monitoring is also important for patients having surgery that carries a high risk, especially procedures on the central nervous system. To catch problems such as intracranial hypertension or hematomas, those who have undergone neurosurgery, for example, decompressive craniectomy or tumor resection, must be checked by neurologists frequently. If a patient shows an uneven pupil or any changes in movement, it could mean that their intracranial condition is worsening, so, quick action is needed. Also, monitoring protocols often involve checking ICP to assess brain health during recovery, allowing clinicians to respond and react quickly if anything negative occurs. Strictly following these monitoring guidelines can play a big role in how patients recover after surgery in neurology. When certain medicines or treatments that can influence brain function, neurological monitoring becomes very important. Those receiving a lot of corticosteroids or undergoing thrombolysis for stroke should be carefully watched, as the treatment may cause intracranial pressure to rise or cause severe changes in consciousness. When using high-risk treatments, neuroscience nurses or critical care teams must always watch for changes in a patient's neurological condition. These observations can be informed by clinical guidelines, such as those outlined by the International Society of Ultrasound in Obstetrics and Gynecology (ISUOG) for systematic evaluations. Effective neurological monitoring not only enhances patient safety but also provides a framework for timely intervention, ultimately improving outcomes in critical care scenarios (Honavar, 2021; Lees *et al.*, 2020).

9.2.1. Traumatic Brain Injury (TBI)

TBI is a significant public health concern, particularly in the context of critical care. Because TBI can be very serious and complicated, it requires unique neurological care to help patients recover well. Both mild and severe TBIs, such as concussions, can result in neurological problems that must be cared for right away and in a thorough manner. In these settings, healthcare providers have to address the health problems of TBI as well as the emotional and social effects on the patient and the family. Because of this, keeping an eye on intracranial pressure, checking neurological status, and using rehabilitation strategies are key to preventing long-term problems from TBI. Emphasizing specialized care units for these injuries can significantly improve clinical outcomes by ensuring targeted interventions and continuous monitoring throughout the acute phase of recovery (Valenti *et al.*, 2023) (Figure 9.5).

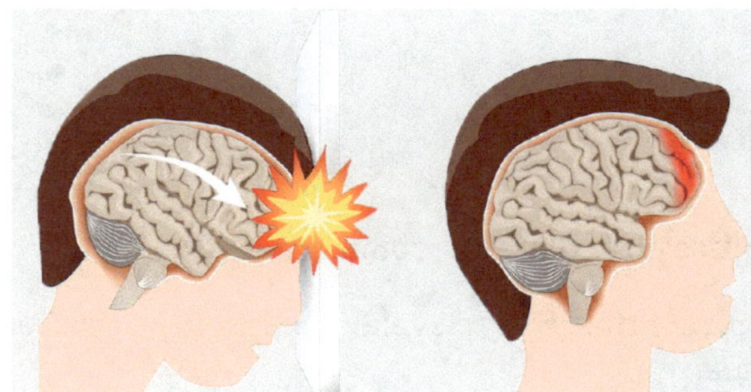

Figure 9.5. Traumatic brain injury (TBI).

Source: https://qureshi-neurosurgery.com/wp-content/uploads/2022/05/image-tbi.png.

A team of neurologists, neurosurgeons, rehabilitation specialists, and critical care physicians is important for managing patients with TBI. They collaborate to solve the different problems that TBI creates, which may include urgent complications as well as lasting functional disabilities. In particular, acting quickly and adjusting therapies correctly is linked to a better recovery process. Evidence suggests that outcomes for TBI patients can be enhanced through consistent monitoring, early rehabilitation strategies, and family support (Bartman *et al.*, 2018). Because TBI can be very mild or very severe, it is important to personalize care for each patient. Tailored care and a caring healthcare setting can help survivors of any age achieve better health and enjoy life more.

Changing from acute care to rehabilitation for TBI patients is difficult, especially where resources are limited. Because many individuals with TBI can have lasting problems with their abilities, it is important to keep providing rehabilitation. Current data indicate that many patients are not adequately referred for rehabilitation services, which may exacerbate the burden on families and increase societal costs (Bartman *et al.*, 2018). Public health strategies should consist of good rehabilitation programs, community support, and education about how to manage TBI for effective critical care. By prioritizing the implementation of structured rehabilitation pathways and addressing gaps in existing infrastructure, healthcare systems can facilitate recovery and significantly improve outcomes for TBI patients over the long term (Valenti *et al.*, 2023).

9.2.2. Stroke Management

Effective stroke management is crucial in critical care settings, where timely interventions can significantly impact patient outcomes. Rapidly restoring blood flow to the brain is the main aim in stroke management to prevent serious neurological problems. Intravenous thrombolysis using tissue plasminogen activator (tPA) is a common treatment for acute ischemic stroke, provided it is administered within the appropriate time window following symptom onset. Also, mechanical thrombectomy is now often used as an endovascular procedure for patients with large vessel occlusions when tPA does not work well enough. For these procedures to work well, healthcare providers must coordinate closely, pointing to the need for a team approach that can deliver the best care for stroke patients and watch for any changes in their condition. Since the COVID-19 pandemic began, there have been new issues in stroke management, especially around anesthesia during endovascular therapy. It is important for experts to ensure the best neurological results and to keep risks low for healthcare workers, which highlights the need for thoughtful anesthetic choices. Administration of general anesthesia or monitored anesthesia care should be chosen based on each patient's needs and the resources that are still available. Institutions should adjust the recommendations to fit their situations, which might differ depending on local customs and infection control standards. By developing guidelines that ensure both patient safety and provider protection, healthcare teams can navigate the complexities of stroke treatment amidst ongoing operational challenges brought on by the pandemic (Sharma *et al.*, 2020). Always being alert to possible complications after a stroke is necessary to manage the condition completely.

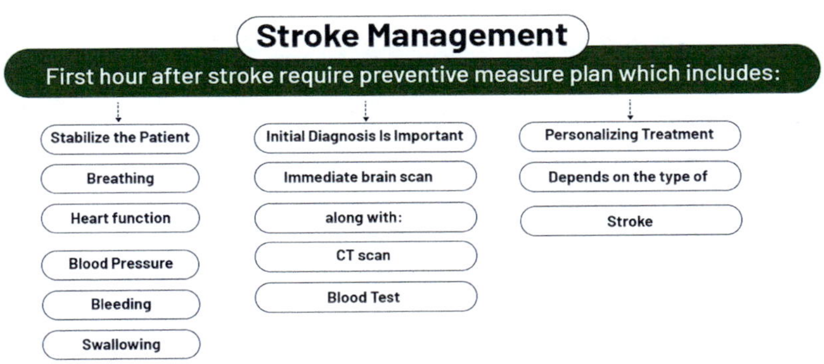

Figure 9.6. Different methods of stroke management.

Source: https://neurolifebrainandspine.com/wp-content/uploads/2022/02/Stroke-Management.jpg.

Patients who have experienced a stroke are at increased risk for subsequent events, including venous thromboembolism (VTE), which can lead to serious morbidity or mortality if left unaddressed. Doctors must consider a patient's condition and risk profile before giving anticoagulants as a preventive measure. Because COVID-19 can lead to coagulopathy and other problems, healthcare providers should be aware of new information and how it affects anticoagulation. Engaging in ongoing research and adapting guidelines for managing such complexities can help refine stroke management strategies, ultimately enhancing patient care and outcomes in the critical care environment (Wichmann, 2020) (Figure 9.6).

9.2.3. Post-Operative Neurosurgical Patients

The post-operative management of neurosurgical patients necessitates comprehensive neurological monitoring to ensure optimal recovery and identify complications early. After surgery, these patients may experience motor, speech, or consciousness problems, which can seriously influence their rehabilitation. It is important to use advanced tools such as ICP monitoring to constantly watch cerebral hemodynamics and avoid brain injury. Critical care teams are expected to quickly interpret information from their equipment to handle any unusual situations. The integration of evidence-based guidelines, such as those found in Hoh *et al.* (2023), can provide clinicians with a framework for managing complications related to aneurysmal subarachnoid hemorrhage, guiding interventions that enhance patient safety and comfort during the recovery process. The care of post-operative neurosurgical patients also covers dealing with complications like coagulopathy and post-traumatic bleeding. Many patients can have several issues, and their neurological problems can increase their risk of bleeding, which can make recovery more difficult. Implementing early diagnostic strategies and therapeutic interventions, as emphasized in Rossaint *et al.* (2023), is essential in identifying patients at risk for traumatic coagulopathy. For example, following standardized guidelines can help avoid many deaths caused by major bleeding by ensuring the right and timely care is given. With a multidisciplinary approach, healthcare providers can handle the needs of neurosurgical patients after surgery and also help to improve their recovery in the long run followed by better trauma care plans and decision-making paths. Additionally, care should be centered on the patient to meet all the needs of someone after neurosurgery. Involving patients and their families in the treatment plan encourages them to follow the plan and gives them comfort during a tough recovery.

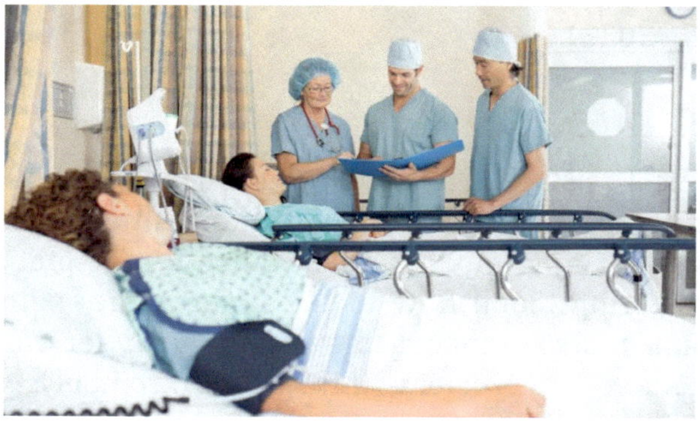

Figure 9.7. Post-Operative Neurosurgical Patients.

Source: https://res.cloudinary.com/du3lqn1yz/image/upload/c_limit,w_3840/f_auto/q_75/v1/volumes/ATLAS/1-PRINCIPLES_OF_CRANIAL_SURGERY/25-Postoperative_Care/PCS_Postop_01?_a=BAVFB+By0.

It is very important for healthcare professionals and patients to communicate well to ensure they both have realistic ideas about recovery and possible outcomes. When families are involved in rehabilitation, patients usually cope better and are more satisfied with the care they receive. Caring for the mind and body of neurosurgical patients is in line with modern care ideas and helps them recover their abilities and enjoy a better quality of life. As the medical community continues to refine management strategies, ongoing research and clinical education will remain pivotal in defining best practices in neurological monitoring and management in critical care (Figure 9.7).

Test Your Knowledge

1. What are the primary goals of initial management in patients with traumatic brain injury (TBI)?
2. What are the key differences in the acute management of ischemic stroke versus hemorrhagic stroke?

9.3. Techniques for Neurological Monitoring

Learning Outcome

1. Define non-invasive methods and Invasive methods
2. Explain the emerging technologies in monitoring

Proper neurological monitoring is very important for patients in critical care, especially those who have suffered major neurological damage. Pupillometry, a non-invasive technique, is being used more often to measure pupil reactions. It helps to more accurately measure nociception by watching how the pupil changes size in response to different stimuli, allowing for differences in central processing. Pupillometry helps doctors monitor pain and check the neurological condition of patients who cannot speak or communicate such as those under anesthesia. Using portable automated pupillometers, doctors can check and analyze light reflexes and pupil responses, which helps them choose the right analgesic approach for patients in the intensive care unit. Such advancements underscore the importance of utilizing pupillary metrics for tailored pain management and neurological assessments in critically ill patients (Packiasabapathy *et al.*, 2021). Another essential technique for neurological monitoring in critical care is the utilization of advanced imaging modalities, such as computed tomography (CT) and magnetic resonance imaging (MRI). They help doctors review the blood supply to the brain and the brain's structure in real time, which is very important for patients with acute ischemic stroke or traumatic brain injury. Easy access to imaging during critical care helps doctors decide on the best surgical or medical actions in a short time. Besides, these techniques can outline regions of ischemia, bleeding, and swelling and help determine what is causing neurological problems. Effective anesthetic management during imaging procedures is paramount. As highlighted during the COVID-19 pandemic, careful consideration of anesthetic techniques can optimize neurological outcomes while minimizing risks to healthcare professionals (Sharma *et al.*, 2020). Because imaging technologies can be used in many ways and are very specific, they are essential for monitoring the nervous system in critical care. Besides pupillometry and advanced imaging, continuous EEG is now a key part of monitoring critically ill patients in the neurology field. A continuous EEG is useful for catching non-convulsive seizures and for determining how deep a coma is and whether someone has encephalopathy. For patients who are very sick, this method is very useful since it allows doctors to observe brain activity without the need for surgery. The information collected can help decide when and what treatments to use, which may improve how patients do. Also, when EEG results are combined with other monitoring methods, healthcare providers can better understand the patient's brain health. By using multiple approaches, neurological monitoring supports patient management and adds to the overall understanding of neurological problems, which helps to create customized treatments for critical care patients.

9.3.1. Non-Invasive Methods

In the realm of neurological monitoring and management in critical care, non-invasive methods play a pivotal role in enhancing patient assessment while minimizing discomfort. Pupillometry is now a key method for assessing nociception in patients who have trouble communicating because of altered consciousness or serious disease. It measures how pupils react to painful stimuli, which helps understand a patient's pain and how well painkillers are working. Automated pupillometers, as mentioned in recent studies, can accurately measure reflexes of the pupils, such as the light reflex and the response to dilation. This makes pupillometry an advantageous non-invasive technique, particularly beneficial in perioperative and intensive care settings, thereby empowering clinicians to tailor pain management strategies effectively while ensuring patient comfort (Packiasabapathy *et al.*, 2021). Besides pupillometry, non-invasive monitoring also covers other assessments such as heart rate variability and checking blood pressure. They allow doctors to assess the patient's autonomic nervous system, which is important for treating critically ill patients. Regular, non-invasive monitoring allows medical staff to identify changes in a patient's condition quickly, which helps with making better decisions. This allows healthcare providers to know what is happening with a patient without causing them more stress or requiring invasive actions. The incorporation of these non-invasive methods aligns with the ethical imperative to prioritize patient comfort while still delivering high-quality medical care, particularly in critical settings where patient stability can rapidly fluctuate (Ricco *et al.*, 2017).

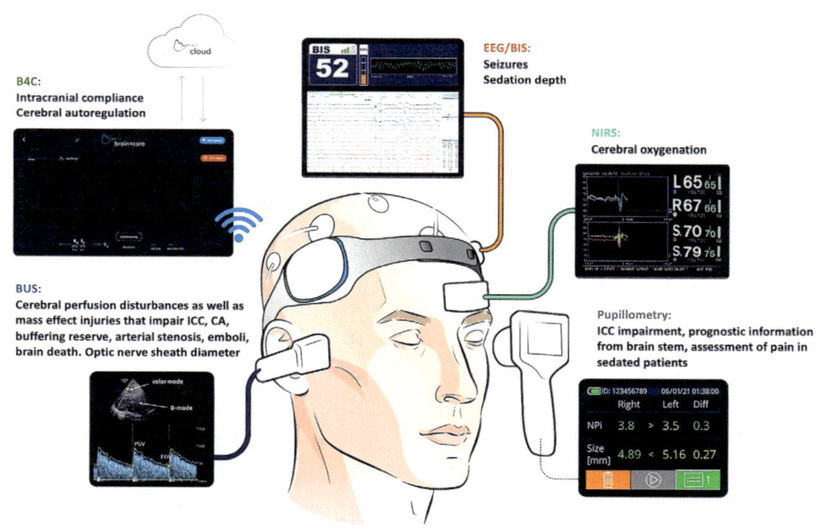

Figure 9.8. Multimodal noninvasive neuromonitoring tools currently used in the neurocritical care settings.

Source: https://link.springer.com/article/10.1007/s00134-024-07406-7/figures/1.

The development of neurological monitoring leads to more research on how advanced non-invasive techniques can help in critical care. New technologies such as advanced brain imaging and wearables that monitor brain functions create great chances for improving patient care. By combining these technologies, doctors could offer more personalized care and easily change the plan based on what the patient's brain is doing at the time. So, the use of non-invasive techniques highlights a complete approach to patient care, ensuring safety and well-being while dealing with the challenges of critical illness. Ongoing studies and clinical trials are essential to validate the efficacy of these techniques and to expand their application in diverse patient populations, ultimately advancing the standard of care in neurological monitoring (Packiasabapathy *et al.*, 2021) (Figure 9.8).

9.3.2. Invasive Methods

Invasive methods play a critical role in neurological monitoring and management within critical care settings, allowing for precise assessment and intervention in patients with acute neurologic conditions. ICP monitoring is done by inserting a catheter into the head, which provides instant information about pressure inside the skull. It is very important to monitor ICP when treating traumatic brain injuries, strokes, and similar conditions that can cause cerebral edema. The purpose is to ensure enough blood goes to the brain, avoid additional brain damage, and decide on appropriate treatments to handle possible complications. As demonstrated in various studies, timely interventions based on ICP readings have improved outcomes in critically ill patients, illustrating the importance of these invasive monitoring techniques in the management of serious neurological emergencies (Murray *et al.*, 2022). Using advanced imaging and neuromonitoring, along with invasive approaches, leads to better results. With continuous EEG, it is possible to find changes in electrical activity, especially in coma patients or those who might have seizures. Subclinical seizures can be found through continuous EEG monitoring, which are often missed by traditional methods, so therapy can be tailored to the patient's needs.

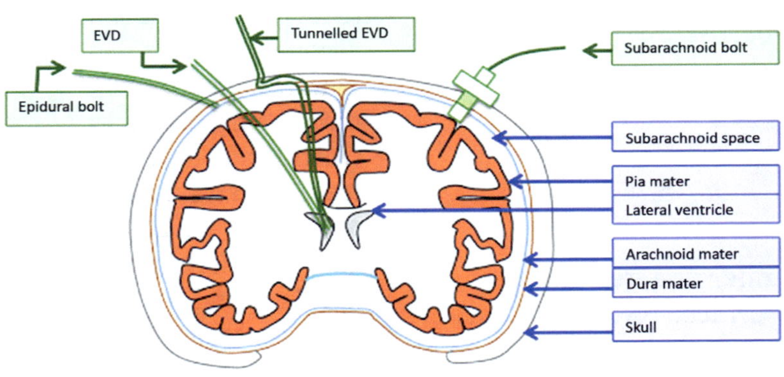

Figure 9.9. Intracranial pressure monitoring.

Source: https://lh4.googleusercontent.com/proxy/cxrfR9HdeF9Mo2nlhBt3Qr3xW0HJpJ3Z97G9Fik9K1SeNHhlQItsoOQIfZNvurGIq-CQ8iFiP6SAh2u9WL9fxia2VC6I-XNxfTFcIEgw.

Also, invasive neuromonitoring tools help to accurately measure the changes in brain metabolism, for example, the use of oxygen and glucose. These results showed that the therapies are effective and if they should change the treatment plan. The emphasis on these advanced invasive methods reflects a shift towards precision medicine in critical care, particularly in the context of neurological monitoring and management (Anger *et al.*, 2019). Yet, using invasive methods can raise issues and possible complications, so a careful approach to patient care is needed. The decision should consider the risks of infection, bleeding, or problems with the implanted hardware. Also, the issue of patient consent and the amount of monitoring or treatment should be considered, especially if the patient cannot make decisions for themselves. The team in critical care needs to consider how useful these methods are compared to the risks they may cause. Regular education, training, and following set procedures are necessary to prevent risks from invasive monitoring. As the field of neurological monitoring evolves, further research is essential to optimize these invasive techniques, ensuring the safest and most effective approaches for patient care in critical settings (Murray *et al.*, 2022) (Figure 9.9).

9.3.3. Emerging Technologies in Monitoring

The evolution of emerging technologies in monitoring plays a critical role in enhancing neurological assessment and management in critical care settings. Using advanced methods like continuous EEG, doctors can find out about subtle seizures or other brain activity that could indicate a patient's brain is deteriorating. Because these technologies give immediate updates, doctors can take action promptly to help patients. Furthermore, the integration of artificial intelligence (AI) into monitoring systems facilitates predictive analytics, which can identify patients at risk for complications before symptoms manifest. This proactive approach not only enhances patient safety but also optimizes resource allocation in intensive care units (ICUs), where swift decision-making is essential for managing complex neurological cases. As the volume of hospital admissions for neurological disorders, including epilepsy and stroke, continues to rise, adopting these technologies provides a roadmap for improving care delivery in critical care environments (Feigin *et al.*, 2021). With the introduction of wearable devices and remote monitoring, it is now possible to watch neurological parameters more closely. Now, devices that track heart rate variability and oxygen saturation also use data analytics to check neurological function. With telemonitoring, healthcare workers can watch patients from a distance, which helps them notice any neurological changes or risks sooner. This continuity of care can be particularly beneficial for post-intensive care syndrome (PICS) survivors, who often experience lingering neurological impairments after critical illness. Therefore, integrating these technologies into rehabilitation protocols directly supports recovery and rehabilitation strategies in patients recovering from severe neurological events (Falvey *et al.*, 2020). By using technology for monitoring, patients are given more control, which is also in line with modern healthcare trends that aim at better patient involvement and value. Advances in monitoring technology are also helping to solve the problem of having standard metrics in neurological care. Innovations in data interoperability allow for the seamless integration of monitoring systems with electronic health records (EHRs), enabling a holistic view of patient history and care plans. Collecting all the data from various sources helps different healthcare teams to communicate well and manage a patient's neurological condition together. Using big data analytics, healthcare professionals in critical care can spot patterns and relationships that guide their decisions and change the rate of survival and illness in their patients. Given the alarming statistics surrounding neurological incidents, such as the rising number of strokes and associated disabilities, the implementation of emerging technologies in monitoring can significantly reduce the burden of these conditions and improve long-term patient care outcomes (Feigin *et al.*, 2021) (Figure 9.10).

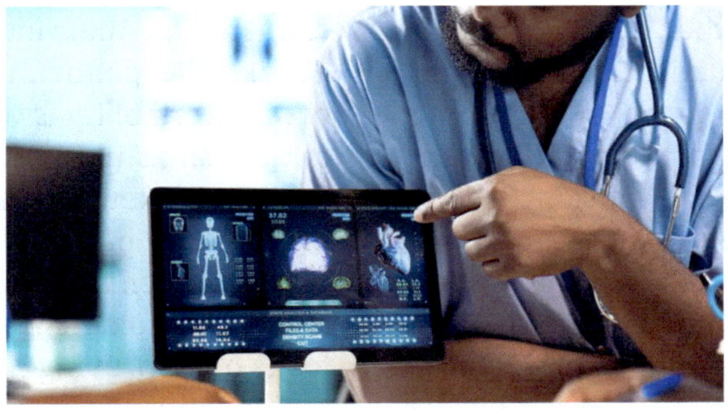

Figure 9.10. Emerging technologies in monitoring.

Source: https://www.healtharc.io/wp-content/uploads/2025/04/Top-Emerging-Technologies-Driving-the-Future-of-Remote-Patient-Monitoring.webp.

Test Your Knowledge

1. What are some commonly used non-invasive methods for monitoring vital signs and organ function in critically ill patients?
2. What invasive monitoring techniques are used in critical care, and what specific parameters do they measure?

9.4. Challenges in Neurological Monitoring

Learning Outcome

1. Discuss the patient variability and response
2. Define equipment limitations and complications
3. Explain the interpretation of monitoring data

The landscape of neurological monitoring in critical care presents numerous challenges that significantly impact patient outcomes. A big challenge is that patients with neurological disorders often show different symptoms. Examples like Sanfilippo syndrome, which is a progressive brain disorder, show the complexity of these issues by involving both mental and physical symptoms. There are no standard guidelines for such rare conditions around the world, which makes it difficult to monitor and treat patients consistently in different healthcare settings. A multidisciplinary approach is essential, yet the lack of universally accepted protocols often results in delayed diagnosis and suboptimal care delivery, ultimately hindering effective monitoring practices in critical care environments (Muschol *et al.*, 2022). A further problem in neurological monitoring is blending and understanding data from several monitoring methods. In cases of severe traumatic brain injury (sTBI), for instance, clinicians are often faced with the dilemma of navigating complex management algorithms that lack a robust evidence base. Since clinical consensus plays a key role in making protocols for sTBI patients with ICP monitoring, it is clear that creating uniform care is not easy. While following the experts' advice, these guidelines should be adjusted to fit each patient because neurological responses vary. This challenge is further compounded by the potential for miscommunication among the multidisciplinary teams engaged in a patient's care, often leading to fragmented monitoring efforts that can jeopardize patient safety (Hawryluk *et al.*, 2019). Still, the technical parts of neurological monitoring bring their own set of challenges that must be addressed continuously. Better monitoring technology can improve accuracy and dependability, but the complexity of these systems can make it hard to use in critical care. Professionals in healthcare should regularly learn new things to stay current with the latest advancements in technology, which are important for using monitoring data correctly. Also, problems with finances and inconsistent resources among institutions make it harder for some regions to use advanced monitoring tools. It is important to provide training and ongoing education to healthcare providers so they can use these technologies well. In short, handling the various problems in neurological monitoring means we must always work to improve both our clinical work and the technology we use.

9.4.1. Patient Variability and Response

In the realm of critical care, understanding patient variability and response is crucial for effective neurological monitoring and management. Every patient's body is different, which can impact the way they respond to different treatments and the outcomes. Age, having other diseases, genetic background, and mental state all play a role in making the disease different for each person. Elder patients might not react to sedatives the same way younger people do, since their pharmacokinetics are different. The psychological condition of a patient, especially in critical care, can change their physical reactions. Because there are differences among patients, anesthesia management should be adjusted to help patients and decrease risks related to neurological procedures. Noticing how these elements interact, healthcare providers are able to customize their methods to fit each patient's needs. The pandemic has made it clear that patient variability is very important in managing critical care situations. During the pandemic, the Society for Neuroscience in Anesthesiology and Critical Care published guidelines to handle the variation seen in endovascular therapy for acute ischemic stroke. They point out that we should focus on improving neurological results as well as deal with the special problems raised by the crisis. In addition, they suggest using strategies that can adjust to the differences in care and resources available. Following protocols that take into account individual patient details allows clinicians to give proper treatment without slowing down operations. Such efforts are pivotal not only to patient recovery but also in reducing the potential risk factors associated with broader healthcare challenges during unprecedented times like the pandemic (Sharma *et al.*, 2020). Also, checking how patients react during critical care situations can help with neurological monitoring decisions. It appears that how institutions operate can also affect response variability, which is why local assessments are important to consider the needs of patients and the resources available. Following protocols that consider these differences, healthcare facilities can follow guidelines and still give each patient the care they need. It is very important to be flexible, especially when trying to offer the same care to all patients despite their differences. Dynamic monitoring systems are necessary to gain detailed information on how individuals respond, so healthcare providers can adjust their care in real time. Ultimately, a thorough understanding of patient variability not only elevates the standard of care within critical settings but also fosters safety and enhanced outcomes for patients in need of neurological management (Williams *et al.*, 2018).

9.4.2. Equipment Limitations and Complications

In the context of neurological monitoring and management in critical care, equipment limitations can significantly impede the delivery of optimal care. Using MRI and CT scans is very important for managing and diagnosing brain and nerve conditions, but the access and performance of these tools may differ in different healthcare settings. When imaging results are delayed, it can stop doctors from giving prompt treatment which can worsen the patient's health. Because these machines are used so much, it is important for medical staff to be properly trained, since using them incorrectly can cause important information to be misunderstood. Having different and uneven equipment makes it more difficult to monitor and manage patients, especially in areas where the tools are not up to standard which can result in unreliable neurological assessments. Fixing these problems is important for improving care in critical care units and making sure patients get the needed treatments promptly. Besides, the use of neurophysiological monitoring equipment adds more difficulties to critical care. It is possible for devices measuring intracranial pressure, EEG and neuroimaging to give incorrect readings which may make it harder for doctors to decide on treatment. When equipment fails, either due to malfunction or mistakes by staff, it may hide the real neurological condition of patients which can result in the wrong diagnosis or wrong treatment. So, critical care teams should create detailed plans and protocols to deal with any equipment-related issues. Ensuring monitoring devices are regularly tested and staff are educated is important to avoid risks. Because equipment failure can impact clinical care, it is important to manage equipment in critical care areas in an organized way to ensure accurate and reliable neurological assessments. Also, the fact that neurological monitoring equipment has some drawbacks can be a major challenge when managing critically ill patients for a long time. As indicated in the literature, a multidisciplinary approach to treatment is essential, particularly in the context of complex conditions like infective endocarditis, where both diagnostic and therapeutic challenges abound (Baddour *et al.*, 2015). Since neurocritical care covers many areas, and equipment is limited, it is necessary for healthcare teams to cooperate to design personalized care plans. This collaboration is paramount, as the guidelines provided by professional organizations emphasize the importance of integrating various specialties in managing critical conditions (Habib *et al.*, 2015). Ultimately, overcoming equipment-related complications is not just an issue of technology; it significantly influences the trajectory of patient care, necessitating a cohesive effort to ensure that equipment not only functions optimally but is also adaptable to the rapidly evolving demands of critical care (Figure 9.11).

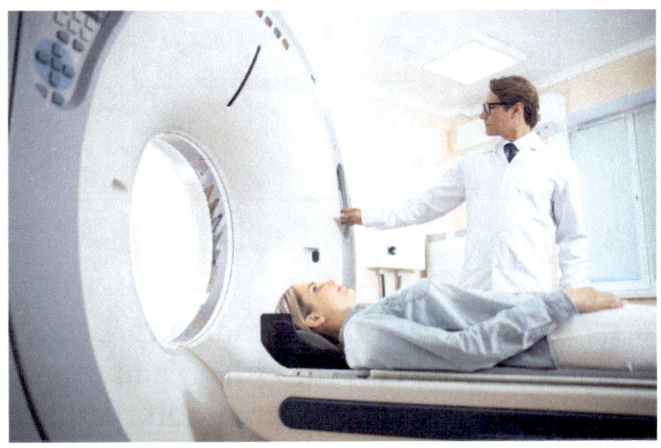

Figure 9.11. Neurological monitoring and management.

Source: https://neurologyoffice.com/wp-content/uploads/MRI-scaled.jpeg.

9.4.3. Interpretation of Monitoring Data

Effective interpretation of monitoring data is crucial in the realm of neurological management, particularly within critical care environments. This data often includes various parameters such as ICP, cerebral perfusion pressure (CPP), and neurological scoring systems. By reviewing these metrics correctly, healthcare providers can spot trends and respond right away to changes in the patient's health. If intracranial pressure (ICP) rises, it could signal worsening, so immediate actions are needed to prevent more harm to the brain. Doctors should always use the patient's history, demographic details, and the situation in the clinic to help them interpret the data. Frequently collected information on neurological incidents and the success of treatments supports better care for patients in critical care. Moreover, the integration of diverse data sources underlines the importance of a multidisciplinary approach to patient management in these high-stakes scenarios (Feigin *et al.*, 2021) (Figure 9.12).

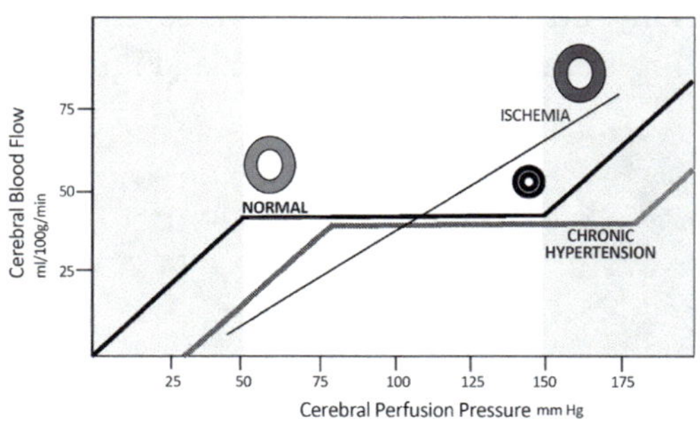

Figure 9.12. Idealized relationship between cerebral perfusion pressure (CPP) and cerebral blood flow (CBF). The normal autoregulation curve maintains a constant CBF over a range of CPP.

Source: https://www.researchgate.net/publication/318511917/figure/fig3/AS:11431281244108398@1715858165111/Idealized-relationship-between-cerebral-perfusion-pressure-CPP-and-cerebral-blood-flow.tif

Data monitoring with advanced technology has made it much easier to interpret information in critical care. For example, techniques like brain tissue oxygenation and EEG constantly monitor the brain and give data that helps with fast clinical decisions. They allow medical staff to notice changes that may happen before a patient's condition becomes noticeably worse. Advanced algorithms and data analysis tools help caregivers rapidly review and process a lot of data from monitoring. Yet, clinicians have to relate the data from monitoring to clinical signs to avoid misunderstanding. Training staff well and following evidence-based guidelines are necessary to get accurate results from data. As the field evolves, collaboration among practitioners utilizing these sophisticated tools and techniques will continue to enhance understanding of neurological status and patient management in critical settings (Lees *et al.*, 2020). Data interpretation from monitoring can guide immediate care and also help predict the patient's neurological condition in the future. If critical parameters change, it may point to possible complications or how the patient is recovering, which helps with discussions about the patient's outlook and deciding on the best care. Besides, when different experts share their views on the data, it gives a complete picture of the patient's health. It is especially important in critical care, since quick decisions can influence the results a lot. Besides, the discussions on data interpretation help manage patients and also support more research into the best ways to treat them. As the landscape of neurological monitoring continues to advance, a strong emphasis on interpreting monitoring data effectively will be paramount in achieving positive clinical outcomes in critical care environments (Feigin *et al.*, 2021).

Test Your Knowledge

1. How does patient variability affect the response to monitoring and treatment in critical care settings?

What are common limitations and complications associated with monitoring equipment in the ICU?

9.5. Management Strategies in Critical Care

Learning Outcome

1. Discuss the pharmacological interventions
2. Defile surgical interventions
3. Explain the multidisciplinary team approach

In critical care, effective strategies consider many aspects to help patients with neurological conditions have the best possible outcomes. The main focus is on regularly checking important neurological signs, so that doctors can notice any changes as they occur. Using ICP monitoring and EEG is essential for managing traumatic brain injury and stroke. They give important information about brain activity, which helps doctors act quickly to reduce the risk of further brain injuries. Moreover, integrating the measurement of circulating lactate as a diagnostic tool has proven essential in assessing patients' metabolic status and overall tissue oxygenation, thereby supporting clinical decision-making in rapidly evolving critical situations (Belu *et al.*, 2025). Using evidence-based protocols is another important part of management in critical care. Using clinical pathways to treat neurological patients can improve the quality of care, reduce mistakes, and save resources. For example, ICUs have started using early mobilization protocols, which have been shown to help patients recover faster and prevent weakness caused by their stay in the ICU. Additionally, the incorporation of AI in analyzing complex patient data can support personalized management strategies that consider each patient's unique physiological responses (Mehta, 2023). Using AI with traditional methods of monitoring helps managers to make decisions more easily and identify issues ahead of time. In addition, it is very important for different experts to collaborate in critical care management. Many neurological patients benefit from the care of neurologists, neurosurgeons, and rehabilitation therapists. Holding daily rounds with different specialists helps the team work better together, share important updates, and make sure everyone is on the same page with patient care. In addition, the teamwork helps everyone stay informed about the latest methods in critical care management. As the landscape of neurological monitoring and management evolves, ongoing training in emerging technologies and data integration will remain vital for enhancing patient outcomes and driving innovations in care practices (Belu *et al.*, 2025).

9.5.1. Pharmacological Interventions

In critical care, using drugs is very important for managing and monitoring neurological problems. Such interventions are used to manage different problems related to neurological conditions, mainly following brain tumor resection surgery. After surgery, doctors create strategies to manage the balance between intracranial pressure and blood flow to the brain, which can be affected by the procedure. In the ICU, giving corticosteroids and osmotic diuretics to patients, is important for reducing edema and inflammation, which is necessary for their stabilization. The implementation of evidence-based protocols is essential to optimize these interventions, as they can lead to improved neurological recovery and minimize the potential for long-term complications, a necessity highlighted in current literature surrounding postoperative management in brain surgery patients (Kusumawardani *et al.*, 2024). Cerebral edema is a major issue for critical care and usually requires the use of specific drugs. When fluid collects in the brain parenchyma to a large extent, it can cause the pressure inside the skull to go up, so prompt action is needed. Mannitol and hypertonic saline are examples of osmotic agents that help remove fluid from the brain, which lessens edema and protects against complications. Corticosteroids may be used to control inflammation that occurs after a brain injury or surgery. Anesthesiologists and critical care providers need to work together in monitoring how the patient responds to these drugs to manage cerebral edema and related issues. This approach underscores the importance of a multidisciplinary protocol in enhancing patient care and addressing the unique challenges posed by neurological conditions (Maciej Świercz *et al.*, 2024). In addition, the use of medication in critical care covers treating cerebral edema as well as managing seizures and offering neuroprotection. A seizure may occur in patients in the ICU because of brain injury or changes in their metabolism. The strategic use of antiepileptic drugs (AEDs) is essential for preventing seizure-related complications that could exacerbate existing neurological deficits. Also, drugs called NMDA receptor antagonists and therapeutic hypothermia are given to protect neurons from the effects of ischemia.

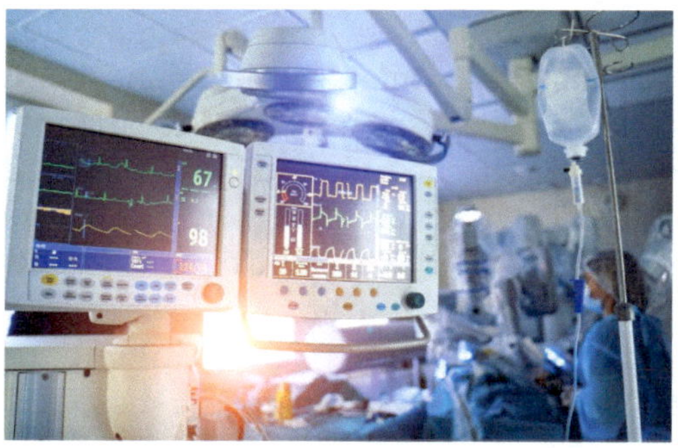

Figure 9.13. Managing and monitoring neurological problems.

Source: https://www.britishjournalofnursing.com/media/fw1bayw2/adobestock_337969744.jpg.

Treatment plans should be tailored to each patient and the reason for their neurological problems. By maintaining vigilance in monitoring and adjusting pharmacological therapies, healthcare providers can more effectively manage neurological conditions in the critical care environment, optimizing both immediate and long-term patient outcomes (Kusumawardani *et al.*, 2024; Maciej Świercz *et al.*, 2024) (Figure 9.13).

9.5.2. Surgical Interventions

In the context of neurological monitoring and management in critical care, surgical interventions play a pivotal role in addressing acute brain injuries (ABI). Immediate and strong action is usually required to prevent lasting neurological problems. Among the surgical procedures are decompressive craniectomy and clot evacuation, which help reduce pressure inside the skull and improve blood flow to the brain. These interventions are very important for patients who have serious brain swelling or bleeding strokes. If these surgeries are done too late, the patient may suffer permanent brain damage, which is why it is important to act quickly. Adding surgery to the care plan can help patients with serious neurological problems achieve better results and a higher quality of life. Even though neurosurgery can help, it should be part of a larger plan that includes checking the patient's neurological condition. Recent studies based on international agreement highlight that patients with ABI should be intervened with quickly after support from ECMO. Using advanced imaging and careful neurological exams helps identify patients who need surgery as soon as possible. Together, neurosurgeons, intensivists, and nurses ensure that any changes in the patient's condition are handled promptly, which increases the chance of a successful surgery. Taking a multidisciplinary approach to care is necessary for those facing complicated neurological problems in critical care, which greatly influences the rates of morbidity and mortality. It is also very important to have evidence-based guidelines for surgical procedures. There is a shortage of strong clinical evidence for ABI treatment during ECMO, which means more research and data are needed to guide the best practices. According to experts, filling the gaps in understanding surgical procedures and their timing is very important for designing effective treatment plans. By working together, the team seeks to improve how surgery is done and also increase the quality of care for critically ill neurological patients. It is important to keep monitoring patients after surgery and make adjustments in their care, since this helps healthcare providers know if the surgery was successful and take any needed actions. In this manner, surgical interventions become an integral component of a holistic approach to neurological management in critical care, ultimately striving for optimal patient outcomes and recovery (Figure 9.14).

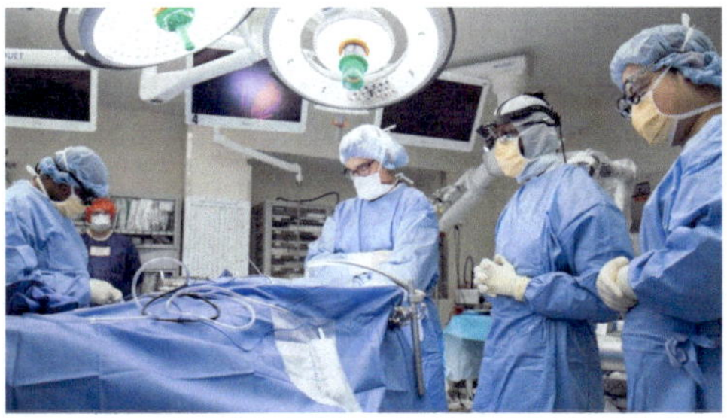

Figure 9.14. Surgical interventions.

Source: https://www.healthcareradius.in/cloud/2022/07/12/WYR5QxLz-fortis-brain-1200x676.jpg.

9.5.3. Multidisciplinary Team Approach

Using a multidisciplinary team in critical care greatly improves the care of neurological patients. Because neurology, intensive care, nursing, and rehabilitation are involved, this teamwork allows for a customized plan that meets each patient's needs. Since many patients have difficult neuromedical conditions such as traumatic brain injuries or severe strokes, it is very important to have a united approach. This method of working helps team members communicate well, so different skills can combine to benefit patients. Having standard protocols and regular team meetings encourages everyone to cooperate and respond promptly to any changes in a patient's condition, which boosts the quality and safety of care. A multidisciplinary team plays an important role in managing rare neurological disorders like Sanfilippo syndrome. The best way to handle these conditions is by involving experts from different areas who can offer special knowledge about diagnosis and care. It is clear from existing clinical practices that best practice guidelines are developed more successfully when a variety of specialists are involved, which helps with early detection and suitable treatments. For example, families dealing with rare diseases gain from teamwork among specialists that provides insights that fit their situation. As guidelines are made for Sanfilippo syndrome and similar conditions, families and local care providers have important tools to help manage these diseases, making the multidisciplinary approach very important. Moreover, contemporary challenges, such as the rise in incidences of infections like rhino-orbito-cerebral mucormycosis (ROCM), highlight the necessity for an agile multidisciplinary team in critical care settings. Because ROCM progresses quickly, it needs to be treated right away and aggressively, which is best done by a team working together. Specialists in infectious disease, neurology, and surgery must cooperate to ensure both diagnosis and treatment are done efficiently. It requires early detection of symptoms and signs, which is made possible by advanced imaging and microbiological tests. Because of evidence-based guidelines from different experts, treatment for critically ill patients is more effective, helping them survive longer. When teams work together, they can make better decisions and act quickly to manage serious neurological conditions in critical care, which demonstrates the significant benefits of a multidisciplinary system.

Test Your Knowledge

1. What are the primary goals of pharmacological interventions in the management of critically ill patients?
2. In what situations are surgical interventions necessary in critical care, and what are their potential risks?

SUMMARY

The main point of the essay on neurological monitoring and management in critical care is that following careful and evidence-based procedures improves patient outcomes. It is evident from looking at different therapies, such as ketogenic diet and hyperosmolar agents, that expert recommendations and clinical guidelines should be used. Evidence suggests that ketogenic diet therapies can be both safe and effective in managing conditions such as drug-resistant epilepsy in adults, while also highlighting the need for tailored approaches that account for the differences between pediatric and adult populations (Cervenka *et al.*, 2020).

It is very important to make these distinctions because they greatly affect the way these patients are treated and their outcomes. Also, handling cerebral edema and increased intracranial pressure demonstrates the importance of understanding neurocritical care well. It is important to regularly check how well and safely hyperosmolar agents like mannitol and hypertonic saline work. Guidelines that recommend specific interventions for conditions such as subarachnoid hemorrhage and traumatic brain injury emphasize a proactive and informed approach to treatment (Cook *et al.*, 2020). Regularly evaluating care helps patients and also leads to the creation of better practices in neurocritical care. In short, since neurological problems in critical care are complex, it is important to use different approaches backed by evidence. When new research and clinical findings appear, it is important to keep adapting how we manage patients to improve their care and results. It is very important for healthcare professionals to collaborate and combine their insights when making treatment plans. In the end, putting quality research and clinical studies first will help improve neurological care, so that patients can get the best and most personalized care.

In the realm of critical care, particularly for patients undergoing extracorporeal membrane oxygenation (ECMO), effective neurological monitoring and management are paramount. Recent guidelines highlight five important clinical topics that are important for ABI patients. The areas are neurological monitoring to detect early problems, post-cannulation physiological targets for proper cerebral blood flow, and neurological therapies that cover both medical and surgical approaches. They also stress that correct neurological predictions and regular follow-up help provide thorough care to patients. Collectively, these recommendations underscore the necessity of a multidisciplinary approach to the management of neurological health in the ECMO context, thus serving as critical tools for improving patient outcomes and reducing morbidity and mortality associated with ABI in this vulnerable population (Cho *et al.*, 2024).

Continuous electroencephalogram (EEG) monitoring has emerged as a vital component in the management of neurocritically ill patients. With more research in critical care EEG, our awareness of cerebral function grows, and it plays a key role in the early detection of seizures and different encephalopathies. The American Clinical Neurophysiology Society has established rules for using EEG, stressing that it is a non-invasive and real-time form of monitoring. The main reasons to use EEG in critical care are to find electrographic seizures, examine special brain disorders, and measure brain function for the prediction of outcomes. Moreover, neurologists need to be adept in interpreting critical care EEG data, as they provide necessary input for therapeutic strategies that can significantly affect patient management (Yoshimura, 2024). Working neuromonitoring technologies and strategies into critical care ensures better patient safety and better results. The recommendations from experts emphasize dealing with gaps in knowledge about neurological care, especially for ECMO patients with ABI. Finding and treating problems early helps reduce lasting damage to brain function. Using a systematic approach helps critical care teams to use more advanced strategies and monitor the patient's condition in detail. Consequently, advancing the understanding of neurological monitoring and care presents significant implications for improving overall survival rates and quality of life for individuals with complex neurological needs in the intensive care setting (Cho *et al.*, 2024).

KEY TERMS FROM THIS CHAPTER

Acute ischemic stroke management
Brain death
Cerebral autoregulation
Cushing's reflex
Glasgow coma scale (GCS)
ICP monitoring
(Intracranial pressure (ICP)
Neurological examination
Barbiturate coma
Brain injury
Cerebral perfusion pressure (CPP)
Electroencephalogram (EEG)
Hemorrhagic stroke
Intracerebral hemorrhage (ICH)
Ischemic stroke
Neurological monitoring

CRITICAL THINKING QUESTIONS

1. **Which of the following is a common indication for the use of intracranial pressure (ICP) monitoring in critically ill patients?**
   a. Traumatic brain injury (TBI) with Glasgow Coma Scale (GCS) ≤ 8
   b. Acute ischemic stroke without loss of consciousness
   c. Seizure without any neurologic deficit
   d. Persistent hypotension despite adequate fluid resuscitation
2. **In patients with acute subarachnoid hemorrhage, the first-line treatment to prevent rebleeding is:**
   a. Anticoagulation therapy
   b. Surgery or endovascular coiling
   c. Hyperventilation
   d. Mannitol administration
3. **What is the primary goal of managing elevated intracranial pressure (ICP) in critically ill patients?**
   a. To prevent ischemic stroke
   b. To maintain cerebral perfusion pressure (CPP) within a normal range
   c. To increase brain oxygenation
   d. To reduce the risk of seizures
4. **The use of sedation in neurological critical care is primarily aimed at:**
   a. Reducing the risk of infection
   b. Preventing movement-induced ICP fluctuations
   c. Enhancing brain oxygenation
   d. Reducing the need for mechanical ventilation
5. **A sudden decrease in the Glasgow Coma Scale (GCS) score in a comatose patient, particularly with dilated, non-reactive pupils, suggests:**
   a. Hypoxia
   b. Brain herniation
   c. Hypoglycemia
   d. Drug intoxication

Short Answer Questions

1. What are the key principles behind neurological monitoring in the intensive care unit (ICU)?
2. What are the reasons for keeping neurological monitoring on patients in critical condition?
3. What are the limitations of traditional neurological assessment tools like the Glasgow Coma Scale (GCS) in critically ill patients?
4. What is the role of continuous electroencephalography (EEG) in neurological monitoring, and when is it indicated?
5. How can intracranial pressure (ICP) monitoring be performed, and what are the normal and abnormal ICP values?

Answer to Critical Thinking Questions

1. (a); 2. (b); 3. (b); 4. (b); 5. (b)

REFERENCES

1. Afshari, A., Ageno, W., Ahmed, A., Duranteau, J., Faraoni, D., Kozek-Langenecker, S. A., Llau, J. V., *et al.* (2017). European guidelines on perioperative venous thromboembolism prophylaxis. *European Journal of Anesthesiology, 35*, 77–83. https://doi.org/10.1097/eja.0000000000000729.

2. Anger, J. T., Lee, U., Ackerman, A. L., Chou, R., Chughtai, B., Clemens, J. Q., Hickling, D., *et al.* (2019). Recurrent uncomplicated urinary tract infections in women: AUA/CUA/SUFU guideline. *The Journal of Urology, 202*(2), 282–289. https://doi.org/10.1097/ju.0000000000000296.

3. Baddour, L. M., Wilson, W. R., Bayer, A. S., Fowler, V. G., Tleyjeh, I. M., Rybak, M. J., Baršić, B., *et al.* (2015). Infective endocarditis in adults: Diagnosis, antimicrobial therapy, and management of complications. *Circulation, 132*(15), 1435–1486. https://doi.org/10.1161/cir.0000000000000296.

4. Bartman, T., & Brilli, R. (2018). Variability reduction—An essential aspect of quality. *Pediatric Critical Care Medicine.* https://www.semanticscholar.org/paper/6821452438b57954a25fbe0106b89137ae3906fe (accessed on 22 May 2025).

5. Belu, A., Filip, N., Trandafir, L., Spoială, E., Ţarcă, E., Zamosteanu, D., Ghiga, G., *et al.* (2025). Lactate, an essential metabolic marker in the diagnosis and management of pediatric conditions. *Diagnostics, 15.* https://www.semanticscholar.org/paper/8d04b8aecc0cc2215b736abf77cac8f36c4bae62 (accessed on 22 May 2025).

6. Cervenka, M. C., Wood, S. M., Bagary, M., Balabanov, A., Bercovici, E., Brown, M. G., Devinsky, O., *et al.* (2020). International recommendations for the management of adults treated with ketogenic diet therapies. *Neurology Clinical Practice, 11*(4), 385–397. https://doi.org/10.1212/cpj.0000000000001007.

7. Cho, S. M., Hwang, J., Chiarini, G., Amer, M., Antonini, M. V., Barrett, N., Belohlavek, J., *et al.* (2024). Neurological monitoring and management for adult extracorporeal membrane oxygenation patients: Extracorporeal Life Support Organization consensus guidelines. *Critical Care, 28*(1). https://www.semanticscholar.org/paper/d32892ca3dc9207c9024080894998be9c0ff08bc (accessed on 22 May 2025).

8. Cho, S. M., Hwang, J., Chiarini, G., Amer, M., Antonini, M. V., Barrett, N., Belohlavek, J., *et al.* (2024). Neurological monitoring and management for adult extracorporeal membrane oxygenation patients: Extracorporeal Life Support Organization consensus guidelines. *ASAIO Journal, 70*(2), e169–e181. https://www.semanticscholar.org/paper/60d856dc64331873b2916b466193e00e8dc4e23b (accessed on 22 May 2025).

9. Cook, A. M., Jones, G. M., Hawryluk, G. W. J., Mailloux, P., McLaughlin, D., Papangelou, A., Samuel, S., *et al.* (2020). Guidelines for the acute treatment of cerebral edema in neurocritical care patients. *Neurocritical Care, 32*, 647–666. https://doi.org/10.1007/s12028-020-00959-7.

10. Falvey, J. R., & Ferrante, L. E. (2020). Flattening the disability curve: Rehabilitation and recovery after COVID-19 infection. *Heart & Lung, 49*(5), 440–441. https://doi.org/10.1016/j.hrtlng.2020.05.001.

11. Feigin, V. L., Stark, B., Johnson, C. O., Roth, G. A., Bisignano, C., Gebreheat, G., Abbasifard, M., *et al.* (2021). Global, regional, and national burden of stroke and its risk factors, 1990–2019: A systematic analysis for the Global Burden of Disease Study 2019. *The Lancet Neurology, 20*(10), 795–820. https://doi.org/10.1016/s1474-4422(21)00252-0.

12. Habib, G., Lancellotti, P., Antunes, M. J., Bongiorni, M. G., Casalta, J.-P., Del Zotti, F., Dulgheru, R., *et al.* (2015). 2015 ESC Guidelines for the management of infective endocarditis. *European Heart Journal, 36*, 3075–3128. https://doi.org/10.1093/eurheartj/ehv319.

13. Hawryluk, G. W. J., Aguilera, S., Büki, A., Bulger, E. M., Citerio, G., Cooper, D. J., Diaz Arrastia, R., *et al.* (2019). A management algorithm for patients with intracranial pressure monitoring: The Seattle International Severe Traumatic Brain Injury Consensus Conference (SIBICC). *Intensive Care Medicine, 45*, 1783–1794. https://doi.org/10.1007/s00134-019-05805-9.

14. Hoh, B. L., Ko, N., Amin-Hanjani, S., Chou, S., Cruz-Flores, S., Dangayach, N., Derdeyn, C. P., *et al.* (2023). 2023 guideline for the management of patients with aneurysmal subarachnoid hemorrhage: A guideline from the American Heart Association/American Stroke Association. *Stroke, 54*. https://doi.org/10.1161/str.0000000000000436.

15. Honavar, S. G. (2021). Code Mucor: Guidelines for the diagnosis, staging and management of rhino-orbito-cerebral mucormycosis in the setting of COVID-19. *Indian Journal of Ophthalmology, 69*(5), 1361–1365. https://doi.org/10.4103/ijo.ijo_1165_21.

16. Kochanek, P. M., Tasker, R. C., Carney, N., Totten, A. M., Adelson, P. D., Selden, N. R., Davis-O'Reilly, C., *et al.* (2019). Guidelines for the management of pediatric severe traumatic brain injury, third edition: Update of the Brain Trauma Foundation guidelines. *Pediatric Critical Care Medicine, 20*(3S Suppl 1), S1–S82. https://doi.org/10.1097/pcc.0000000000001735.

17. Kondziella, D., Bender, A., Diserens, K., van Erp, W. S., Estraneo, A., Formisano, R., Laureys, S., *et al.* (2020). European Academy of Neurology guideline on the diagnosis of coma and other disorders of consciousness. *European Journal of Neurology, 27*, 741–756. https://doi.org/10.1111/ene.14151.

18. Kusumawardani, D. I., & Adiyanto, B. (2024). Post-operative protocol for brain tumor surgery in intensive care unit: A literature review. *Journal of Advanced Research in Medical and Health Science*. https://www.semanticscholar.org/paper/2f0f748e2609ba54830a7d0a2f130fd058bf81fc (accessed on 22 May 2025).

19. Lees, C., Stampalija, T., Baschat, A., da Silva Costa, F., Ferrazzi, E., Figueras, F., Hecher, K., *et al.* (2020). ISUOG practice guidelines: Diagnosis and management of small-for-gestational-age fetus and fetal growth restriction. *Ultrasound in Obstetrics and Gynecology, 56*, 298–312. https://doi.org/10.1002/uog.22134.

20. Mach, F., Baigent, C., Catapano, A. L., Koskinas, K. C., Casula, M., Badimón, L., Chapman, M. J., *et al.* (2019). 2019 ESC/EAS Guidelines for the management of dyslipidemias: Lipid modification to reduce cardiovascular risk. *European Heart Journal, 41*, 111–188. https://doi.org/10.1093/eurheartj/ehz455.

21. Mehta, V. (2023). Artificial intelligence in medicine: Revolutionizing healthcare for improved patient outcomes. *Journal of Medical Research and Innovation*. https://www.semanticscholar.org/paper/7dfa7d32d8ffa777095e6aa56aa629bc80742dd1 (accessed on 22 May 2025).

22. Murray, C. J. L., Ikuta, K. S., Sharara, F., Swetschinski, L. R., Robles Aguilar, G., Gray, A. P., Han, C., *et al.* (2022). Global burden of bacterial antimicrobial resistance in 2019: A systematic analysis. *The Lancet, 399*, 629–655. https://doi.org/10.1016/s0140-6736(21)02724-0.

23. Muschol, N., Giugliani, R., Jones, S., Muenzer, J., Smith, N., Whitley, C. B., Donnell, M., *et al.* (2022). Sanfilippo syndrome: Consensus guidelines for clinical care. *Orphanet Journal of Rare Diseases, 17*(1). https://doi.org/10.1186/s13023-022-02484-6.

24. Packiasabapathy, S., Rangasamy, V., & Sadhasivam, S. (2021). Pupillometry in perioperative medicine: A narrative review. *Canadian Journal of Anesthesia / Journal canadien d'anesthésie, 68*(5), 566–578. https://doi.org/10.1007/s12630-020-01905-z.

25. Patir, B., Jyoti, C., Kumar, Bora, P., & Hazarika, A. (2025). Multi-view information fusion for EEG signal in health care monitoring: A systematic review for modeling new strategies. *Journal of Information Systems Engineering and Management.* https://www.semanticscholar.org/paper/ec379bd93280881a21845f10fb6b216c7f068e1c (accessed on 22 May 2025).

26. Ravì, D., Wong, C., Deligianni, F., Berthelot, M., Andreu-Pérez, J., Lo, B., & Yang, G. Z. (2016). Deep learning for health informatics. *IEEE Journal of Biomedical and Health Informatics, 21*, 4–21. https://doi.org/10.1109/jbhi.2016.2636665.

27. Ricco, J. B., Bartelink, M. L., Björck, M., Brodmann, M., Cohnert, T., Czerny, M., De Carlo, M., *et al.* (2017). 2017 ESC guidelines on the diagnosis and treatment of peripheral arterial diseases, in collaboration with the European Society for Vascular Surgery (ESVS). *European Heart Journal, 39*(26), 763–816. https://doi.org/10.1093/eurheartj/ehx095.

28. Rossaint, R., Afshari, A., Bouillon, B., Černý, V., Cimpoeşu, D., Curry, N., Duranteau, J., *et al.* (2023). The European guideline on management of major bleeding and coagulopathy following trauma: Sixth edition. *Critical Care, 27*(1). https://doi.org/10.1186/s13054-023-04327-7.

29. Sandarage, R. V., Nashed, J. Y., & Tsai, E. C. (2025). Time is spine: Critical updates for the intensivist. *Current Opinion in Critical Care, 31*(2), 117–122. https://www.semanticscholar.org/paper/f63967a9a9a6665f24c2050e56f0c5c26eee00b7 (accessed on 22 May 2025).

30. Sharma, D., Rasmussen, M., Han, R., Whalin, M. K., Davis, M., Kofke, W. A., Venkatraghvan, L., *et al.* (2020). Anesthetic management of endovascular treatment of acute ischemic stroke during COVID-19 pandemic: Consensus statement from Society for Neuroscience in Anesthesiology & Critical Care (SNACC). *Journal of Neurosurgical Anesthesiology, 32*, 193–201. https://doi.org/10.1097/ana.0000000000000688.

31. Świercz, M., Markowiak, S., Wardęszkiewicz, M., Jabłońska, W., Kasprzak, A., Truchta, M., Mańkowska, A., *et al.* (2024). Anesthetic strategies in cerebral edema: Navigating neurological challenges amid trauma, tumors and therapeutic advances. *Journal of Education, Health and Sport.* https://www.semanticscholar.org/paper/4fcf0ca354b7c5cc0ab3209aaa37e5f9e8844a4c (accessed on 22 May 2025).

32. Valenti, R., Caruso, A., Scotto Di Luzio, A. E., Accavone, D., Cagliarelli, M. G., Chiti, G., Grassi, E., *et al.* (2023). Stroke unit and neurocritical care unit for acute neurological diseases in the USL Toscana Centro: A pilot model of Santo Stefano Hospital in Prato. *Frontiers in Stroke.* https://www.semanticscholar.org/paper/9cfe98e3ccea6ef5f98db5f518cde20e0a162ce9 (accessed on 22 May 2025).

33. Wichmann, D. (2020). Autopsy findings and venous thromboembolism in patients with COVID-19. *Annals of Internal Medicine, 173*, 1030. https://doi.org/10.7326/l20-1206.

34. Williams, B., Mancia, G., Spiering, W., Agabiti Rosei, E., Azizi, M., Burnier, M., Clement, D. L., *et al.* (2018). 2018 ESC/ESH Guidelines for the management of arterial hypertension. *European Heart Journal, 39*, 3021–3104. https://doi.org/10.1093/eurheartj/ehy339.

35. Yoshimura, H. (2024). [Utility of EEG in neurological emergencies and critical care]. *Rinsho Shinkeigaku = Clinical Neurology.* https://www.semanticscholar.org/paper/98d0a326be8c6d7e999fc22ea24d3a15e067603b (accessed on 22 May 2025).

INFECTION CONTROL AND MANAGEMENT IN THE ICU

10

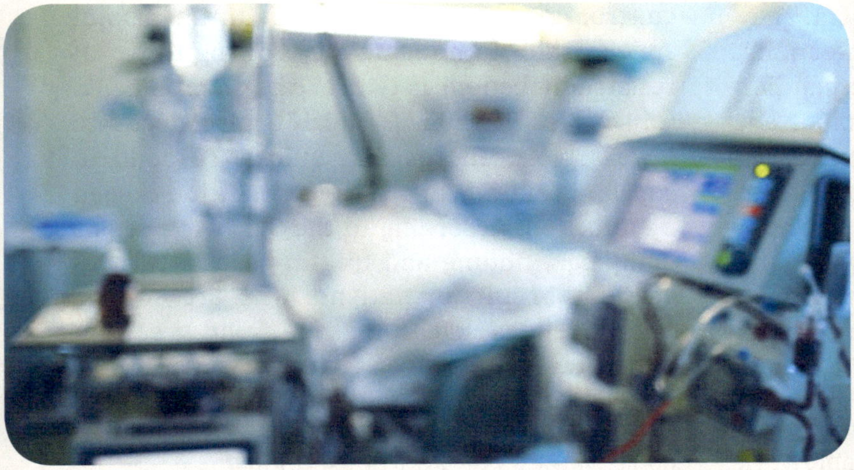

LEARNING OBJECTIVES

After studying this chapter, you will be able to:

1. List the types of infections common in the ICU.
2. Elaborate the risk factors for infections in the ICU.
3. Explain the infection prevention strategies
4. Define the role of antibiotics in infection management
5. Explain monitoring and surveillance of infections
6. Focus on the education and training for healthcare staff.

Introduction

The intensive care unit (ICU) represents a critical environment where patients are at heightened risk for infections due to their compromised health status and the invasive procedures often employed. It is important to maintain strict hygiene measures in the ICU and also to learn about the causes behind the high infection rates. Strong management strategies depend on the knowledge and views of healthcare professionals, especially the nurses, who plays important role in infections prevention. A recent study indicates that the perception of the importance of patient safety management significantly correlates with the direct performance of infection control interventions by ICU nurses, underscoring the need for continuous education and training in this area (Park *et al.*, 2025). Also, the way infection control is viewed in healthcare organizations has a big impact on infection managements. Nursing professionalism and a strong grasp of patient safety can increase direct and indirect results in infection control. Because managing critically ill patients is so complicated, it is necessary to outline the roles of healthcare providers in preventing infections. By fostering a culture that prioritizes infection control with interventions aligned to enhance awareness among ICU staff, there is potential for significant improvements in patient outcomes (Park *et al.*, 2025). Since medical practices and technologies are advancing, so, managing infections in the ICU requires new guidelines that balance between conservative and aggressive actions. Using advanced tools for monitoring and diagnosis helps catch infections early, which guides the choice of treatment. They represent a new way of handling infections, which is more like how infections are handled in today's medical practices. It is very important to learn different treatment methods, including surgery, that can change patients' outcomes to improve current strategies. Since ICU infection control and management are changing, the researchers and healthcare professionals must take care of the most at-risk patients.

Definition of Infection Control

Infection control is a comprehensive framework utilized in healthcare settings, particularly in the ICU, aimed at preventing the transmission of infectious agents among patients, healthcare personnel, and visitors. This multifaceted approach encompasses standard precautions, such as personal protective equipment (PPE) and appropriate hand hygiene practices, as well as more advanced measures like the sterile technique during invasive procedures. The primary objective of infection control is to minimize hospital-acquired infections (HAIs), which pose significant threats to patient safety, especially in vulnerable populations. Infection control decreases both the health problems and deaths caused by HAIs, as well as the stress on healthcare resources, which is very important for helping patients in critical care units. Integral to the definition of infection control is the understanding of antimicrobial resistance (AMR), which complicates treatment protocols and necessitates heightened preventive measures within the ICU. If bacteria become resistant to antibiotics, AMR occurs, and this makes treating infections more difficult, keeps patients in the hospital longer, and leads to a higher number of deaths. Because of this phenomenon, it is important to have strong infection prevention and control measures, as recent estimates have shown that millions of deaths worldwide in 2019 were due to bacterial AMR. These findings highlight the importance of precise surveillance, judicious antibiotic use, and enhanced infection control protocols tailored to antimicrobial stewardship to mitigate the growing threat of resistant infections in critical care environments (Murray *et al.*, 2022). The ICU also needs to have set procedures that quickly respond to sepsis, a common and serious condition caused by infection. According to the Surviving Sepsis Campaign, finding and treating sepsis early is very important for patients who are at risk. The guidelines suggest that the broad-spectrum antibiotics can be given right away, along with actions to keep the patient's blood pressure and heart rate stable. They guide healthcare workers to use a multidisciplinary strategy by offering training on infection control, raising awareness of sepsis symptoms, and setting up rapid response teams. By fostering a culture of vigilance and compliance with infection control measures, ICUs can significantly reduce the incidence of sepsis and improve overall patient care (Evans *et al.*, 2021).

Importance of Infection Control in the Intensive Care Unit (ICU)

The critical role of infection control in the ICU cannot be overstated, as HAIs significantly impact patient outcomes. The immune systems of ICU patients are usually weak, which makes them more likely to get infections. So, it is very important to follow strict infection prevention measures to reduce this risk. Using evidence-based practices such as proper hand washing, using PPE, and careful use of antibiotics can greatly lower the number of HAIs. In addition, closely monitoring infection rates in the ICU by collecting data is very important for making these protocols better. Understanding the burden of infections, particularly those stemming from antimicrobial resistance, is crucial for developing strategies that prioritize patient safety and optimize resource management in critical care settings (Murray *et al.*, 2022). Infection control steps help protect patients and also keep healthcare workers in the ICU safe. In the COVID-19 pandemic, it was especially important to have strong safety measures. Because healthcare workers were more likely to be exposed to infectious diseases, following infection control measures became necessary to stop the spread of diseases within hospitals. According to reports, following the correct use of PPE and maintaining good hand hygiene protects healthcare workers in high-risk areas. Case evidence illustrates that a significant number of healthcare workers were able to avoid infection during encounters with COVID-19 patients by employing thorough protective measures, demonstrating the effectiveness of well-established infection control protocols (Ng *et al.*, 2020). It shows that ICU staff should always be educated and trained on how to prevent infections. In addition to keeping patients and healthcare workers safe, infection control in the ICU affects the health of the general public. The emergence of AMR is a major problem that impacts healthcare everywhere. Strong infection control steps can stop multidrug-resistant organisms from spreading in ICUs, which improves the use of antimicrobials. When infections are prevented and less broad-spectrum antibiotics are needed, healthcare facilities can give better care to patients and save money. This highlights the importance of adopting a comprehensive infection control framework in the ICU that incorporates ongoing research and development of new guidelines to tackle emerging infectious threats and ensure optimal management of critically ill patients (Murray *et al.*, 2022).

10.1. Types of Infections Common in the Intensive Care Unit (ICU)

Learning Outcome

1. Explain the ventilator-associated pneumonia (VAP)
2. Discuss the catheter-associated urinary tract infections (CAUTI)
3. Explain the central line-associated bloodstream infections (CLABSI)

Infections commonly encountered in the ICU setting predominantly include ventilator-associated pneumonia (VAP), bloodstream infections (BSIs), and urinary tract infections (UTIs). VAP is especially important, as it often happens in patients who need mechanical ventilation and have tubes in their airways, which can lead to microbial growth. It is shown by studies that *Pseudomonas aeruginosa* and *Staphylococcus aureus* are the most common pathogens in VAP, and these multidrug-resistant organisms make the illness more severe and increase the risk of death in patients. Strictly following infection control measures and ventilator care bundles can greatly decrease the chance of VAP. Realizing the significance of these infections supports better treatment methods and encourages steps that prevent them, which helps patients in the ICU. Many BSIs in the ICU are caused by catheters, central lines, and invasive monitoring devices. Foreign objects in the body can make it easier for pathogens to enter the blood, which can cause sepsis. Common pathogens are typically Gram-positive cocci (e.g., *Staphylococcus epidermidis*) and Gram-negative rods (e.g., *Klebsiella pneumoniae*), with an alarming rise in antibiotic-resistant strains greatly complicating treatment regimens. To manage BSIs, one must be careful when placing and maintaining vascular access devices and quickly identify and treat infections. The use of antimicrobial stewardship programs is pivotal in this setting, optimizing antibiotic use and thereby mitigating the escalating issue of antimicrobial resistance, which poses a significant threat not only in the ICU but across broader healthcare contexts (Chopra *et al.*, 2020). Many ICU patients develop UTIs, mainly when they have urinary catheters or other procedures done on their urinary tract. The risk of getting a UTI goes up as catheterization lasts longer, and there are risks involved in managing the urinary tract. *Escherichia coli* is the main cause of these infections, but the rise of resistant strains means, cultures and susceptibility tests should be done regularly to guide the right treatment. It is very important to use sterile methods and keep catheters in place for a short time to reduce the risk of UTIs in critically ill patients. Additionally, the implementation of multidisciplinary teams focusing on infection prevention and control strategies can foster enhanced monitoring and surveillance of these infections, significantly improving overall patient care within the ICU setting (Murray *et al.*, 2022).

10.1.1. Ventilator-Associated Pneumonia (VAP)

Many patients in ICUs who are on mechanical ventilation for a long time often experience VAP. As a result, patients feel more ill, ICU stays are longer, and healthcare expenses rise. VAP is diagnosed by finding new infiltrates in the lungs, fever, an increase in white blood cells, and purulent tracheobronchial secretions, which all point to an infection in the lungs. Because of the many aspects of this diagnosis, medical staff are more likely to focus on prevention to avoid both invasive ventilation and respiratory infections. The implications of VAP are profound, as it complicates the clinical course of critically ill patients and can necessitate a shift in treatment protocols to address this growing concern (Figure 10.1).

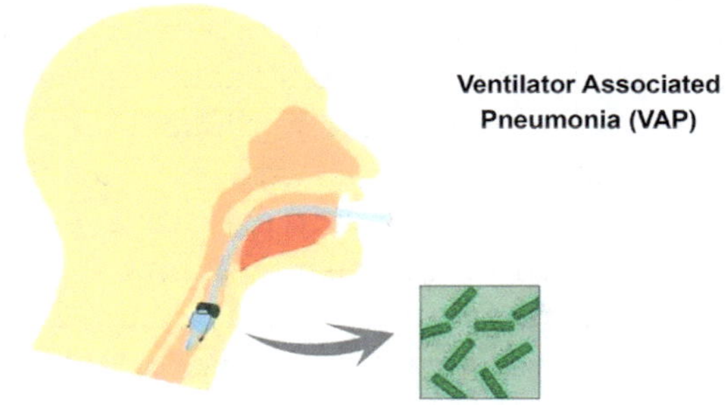

Figure 10.1. Ventilator-associated pneumonia (VAP).

Source: https://stgaccinwbsdevlrs01.blob.core.windows.net/newcorporatewbsite/blogs/June2024/2dQb3MjKXmtujgKSkoY5.webp.

Most of the bacteria that cause VAP are gram-negative and *Pseudomonas aeruginosa* is the most common one. The consequences of such infections extend beyond treatment challenges, often leading to severe complications such as acute respiratory distress syndrome (ARDS) and sepsis. Studies reveal that patients who get VAP tend to stay on mechanical ventilation and in the ICU for a much longer time, which increases the need for healthcare. This situation is made more difficult by the presence of multidrug-resistant organisms, which raises important concerns about using antibiotics in the ICU. Regular learning and strict following of infection control measures help to lower VAP cases and improve patient's recovery. Fighting VAP requires strong infection control measures. Some strategies are to maintain oral hygiene, keep the head of the bed elevated, and put ventilator-associated pneumonia bundles in place. Applying these preventive steps beforehand matches studies that show a lower risk of VAP in ICUs that strictly follow such guidelines. Additionally, emerging treatments such as intravenous immunoglobulin (IVIG) have shown promise in improving clinical outcomes, notably when administered early in the course of severe infections (Xie *et al.*,

2020). Implementing these measures not only addresses the direct impacts of VAP but also creates a more conducive environment for overall infection control and management within the ICU setting (Othman *et al.*, 2017).

10.1.2. Catheter-Associated Urinary Tract Infections (CAUTI)

CAUTIs are a major problem for patients in ICUs. Medical experts often believe that these infections are the result of extended use of urinary catheters, which are common in critically ill patients to help manage their fluids. Using and caring for these catheters increases the chance of urinary tract infections, which may cause severe health problems and keep patients in the hospital longer. So, it is important to have strong infection control to lessen CAUTIs and help patients recover well in the ICU. The high prevalence of CAUTI highlights the urgent need for healthcare facilities to adopt comprehensive protocols aimed at minimizing catheter use and optimizing catheter care (Sharma *et al.*, 2023) (Figure 10.2).

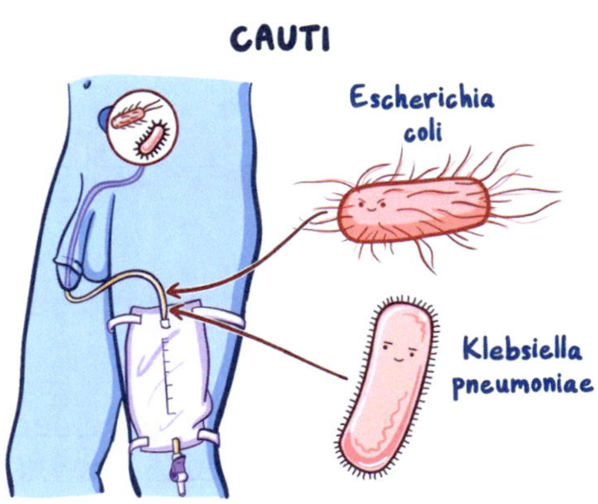

Figure 10.2. Catheter-associated urinary tract infection.

Source: https://www.osmosis.org/_next/image?url=https%3A%2F%2Fd16qt3wv6xm098.cloudfront.net%2FyEaRWOZiRtudrdVBOW9jevhiSQKLgu2j%2F_.jpg&w=3840&q=75.

The presence of biofilm on urinary catheters greatly increases the difficulties in managing and stopping CAUTIs. After forming, biofilms house many bacteria surrounded by a protective layer, which makes it harder to get rid of them with antibiotics. This complication necessitates a multifaceted approach to infection management. Strategies should make sure that catheter insertion and maintainace are performed aseptically and catheter is regularly checked and reviewed for its need and the duration. Recent reviews emphasize the importance of innovation in the design of catheters and the development of novel antimicrobial coatings that disrupt biofilm formation, thus reducing the risk of CAUTIs in critically ill patients (Sharma *et al.*, 2023). When strict infection control procedures are followed along with these new advancements, ICU infection outcomes may be greatly improved. It is important to monitor healthcare-associated infections, such as CAUTI, to assess how well infection control is working in ICUs. Gathering correct data is important for knowing the impact of CAUTI and deciding how to address it. The World Health Organization underscores the importance of standardized definitions and surveillance methodologies to guide research and inform public health strategies (Murhekar *et al.*, 2022). In several regions, especially where people are poor, CAUTI rates are very high because of the large number of multidrug-resistant organisms and inadequate use of infection prevention measures. Because CAUTI is so common in healthcare, more effort is needed to prevent infections in ICU settings. Keeping a close watch and using data helps reduce CAUTI, improve patient care, and create a safer environment in healthcare. Healthcare professionals who handle CAUTI management can improve patients' outcomes and decrease the overall number of healthcare-associated infections.

10.1.3. Central Line-Associated Bloodstream Infections (CLABSI)

Managing CLABSI is very important in the ICU because patients are especially at risk. The invasiveness of central venous catheters can cause these infections, which may result in more health problems, more deaths, and longer hospital stays. Data from surveillance programs show that CLABSI happens frequently in healthcare settings, and this is more common in low- and middle-income countries, where the rates of infection are much higher than in high-income regions. For instance, studies indicate that the pooled rates of CLABSI range from 5.1–4.3 per 1,000 central line days in various settings, underscoring the need for robust infection control strategies tailored to both the clinical environment and the available resources (Murhekar *et al.*, 2022). Therefore, having set guidelines for CLABSI prevention is very important, as they can be prevented by strict infection control . To prevent CLABSI, evidence-based techniques and changes in the hospital's system is needed. It is very important to use strict aseptic techniques when inserting catheters, but this should be supported by regular staff training and standard protocols to avoid infections. Infection control programs should regularly check infection rates so that any trends can be spotted and steps can be taken to decrease CLABSI cases. Also, regularly updating staff and having infectious disease specialists in the ICU can help improve infection control. Organizations like the World Health Organization emphasize that structured surveillance is essential for monitoring infection prevalence and guiding local practices (Buetti *et al.*, 2022). The use of such strategies is important for making the ICU a safer place for patients and lowering the risk of CLABSI. Also, using technology and data analytics in CLABSI prevention can lead to better patient outcomes. For instance, the implementation of electronic health records (EHR) can streamline documentation and alert clinicians to potential infection risks, enabling timely intervention. Automated data collection systems also help to improve surveillance, making it possible to track infection data as it occurs . Explaining the risks of central venous catheters to patients and their families helps them to be more careful in preventing infections. While resources may vary across healthcare systems, investing in continuous improvement strategies for CLABSI prevention can lead to significant reductions in infection rates and overall healthcare costs (Murhekar *et al.*, 2022). The intersection of technology, education, and patient engagement ultimately forms a comprehensive defense against CLABSI in the ICU setting (Figure 10.3).

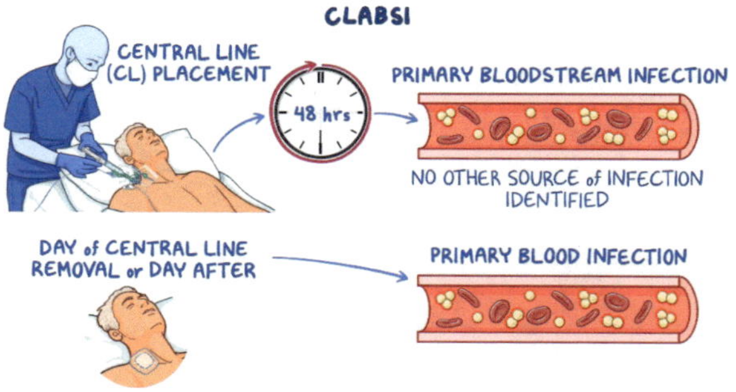

Figure 10.3. Central line-associated bloodstream infection.

Source: https://d16qt3wv6xm098.cloudfront.net/YkyemncZSrKU3teOU7-2E8LgQLuwAQQP/_.jpg.

Test Your Knowledge

1. What are the key preventive strategies for reducing the risk of ventilator-associated pneumonia (VAP)?
2. How can healthcare providers minimize the occurrence of catheter-associated urinary tract infections (CAUTI)?

10.2. Risk Factors for Infections in the Intensive Care Unit (ICU)

Learning Outcome

1. Explain the patient-related factors in the ICU
2. Discuss the environmental factors in the ICU
3. Describe the healthcare provider-related factors

It is a major issue in the ICU that critically ill patients are more likely to get infections. Patients in the ICU become more vulnerable because of their serious conditions, the complicated treatments they receive, and the common use of invasive procedures. Those with a weak immune system, those having surgery, and people with ongoing diseases are more likely to get infections. Besides, using invasive devices such as central venous catheters and endotracheal tubes increases the risk of infection by offering chances for microbes to enter the patient.

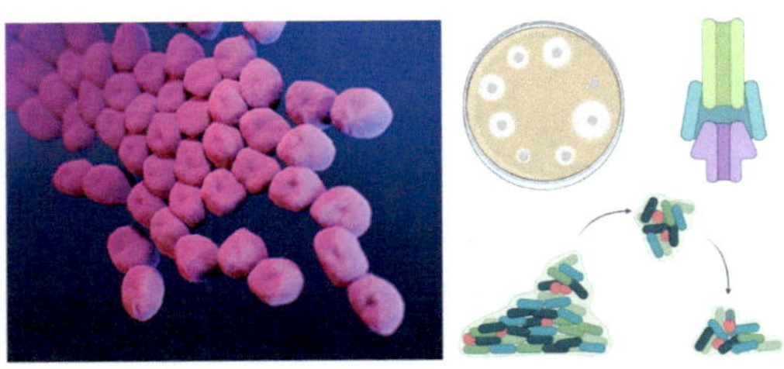

Figure 10.4. Carbapenem-resistant *Acinetobacter baumannii* (CRAB).

Source: https://microbenotes.com/wp-content/uploads/2022/09/Carbapenem-Resistant-Acinetobacter-baumannii-CRAB.jpg.

Because of these devices, there are more chances of infection with foreign bodies and increased colonization by organisms that are resistant to many drugs, which leads to more complications, more illness, and a higher death rate. Antimicrobial resistance (AMR) represents another critical risk factor in the ICU environment, complicating infection management significantly. Pathogens such as carbapenem-resistant Acinetobacter baumannii (CRAB) have emerged as formidable threats due to their resistance to commonly used antibiotics, which significantly limits treatment options (Figure 10.4).

Research has found that being male, having used carbapenems before, and having invasive devices are all independent reasons for getting CRAB bloodstream infections, which are linked to poor outcomes and higher death rates. These findings underscore the pressing need for infection control protocols and antibiotic stewardship strategies in the ICU, particularly as the reliance on broad-spectrum antibiotics can inadvertently contribute to the rise of resistant organisms, making effective infection management even more challenging (Liu *et al.*, 2020; Tabah *et al.*, 2022).

A long stay in the ICU increases the chances of getting hospital-acquired infections. Being in the hospital for a longer period increases the risk of infection, mainly because patients have many invasive procedures and their immune systems are weakened. Those who remain in the ICU for a long time are more prone to get catheter-related infections and ventilator-associated pneumonia, which are common complications there.

That is why it is important to have good infection control measures, such as washing hands often and removing invasive devices promptly. Also, by constantly monitoring and assessing risks, doctors can make changes to treatment plans early on, which can help critically ill patients in the ICU. Such comprehensive strategies are vital to address the multifaceted nature of infection risks and enhance patient care in this high-stakes environment (Figure 10.5).

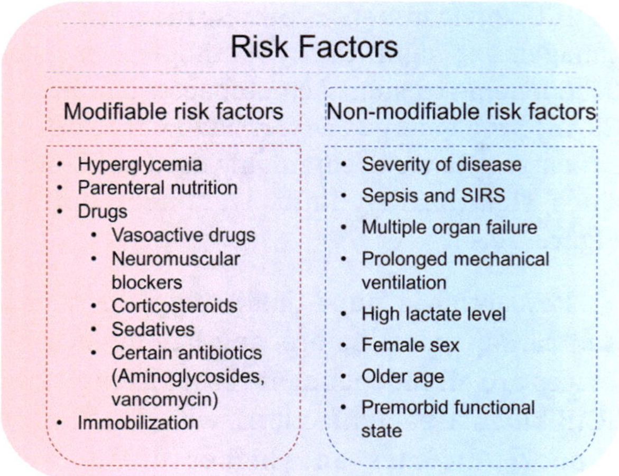

Figure 10.5. Risk factors for ICU-AW. The identified factors were classified as modifiable and non-modifiable.

Source: https://www.researchgate.net/figure/Risk-factors-for-ICU-AW-The-identified-factors-were-classified-as-modifiable-and_fig1_373494336.

10.2.1. Patient-Related Factors

Many patient-related factors play a big role in managing infections in the ICU. The health conditions of patients, for example, diabetes, can greatly affect their risk of getting infections, especially BSIs. Diabetes patients experience changes in their immune system and have trouble healing wounds which makes them more likely to get infections after being admitted to the ICU. Data indicate that patients undergoing Extracorporeal Membrane Oxygenation (ECMO) support, a critical intervention often seen in ICUs, experience a BSI incidence of approximately 20.34%. The interplay between prolonged ECMO catheter indwelling and heightened levels of inflammatory markers in diabetic patients suggests that effective infection control strategies must prioritize the management of underlying chronic conditions to mitigate infection risks in this population (Kang *et al.*, 2025). The time spent performing medical interventions, especially invasive ones, is also very important. Having catheters in place for a long time, which is often needed for treatment, makes it more likely for infection to develop due to bacteria forming biofilms on the catheters. The data from ICU studies underscore that longer catheterization correlates with increased procalcitonin and C-reactive protein levels, indicating a higher inflammatory response associated with infections (Kang *et al.*, 2025). This means it is important to weigh the urgent medical care of critically ill patients against the possible dangers of invasive procedures that last a long time.

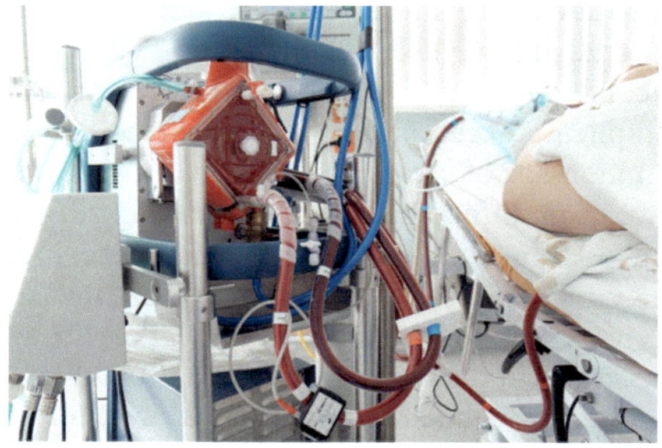

Figure 10.6. Basics of extracorporeal membrane oxygenation (ECMO).

Source: https://www.nursingcenter.com/getattachment/d91f7536-5f34-4003-9405-bb05d1722a86/The-Basics-of-Extracorporeal-Membrane-Oxygenation.aspx.

Keeping catheterization as short as possible and using strict infection control, such as thorough sterilization, are essential for preventing hospital-acquired infections in the ICU. Also, a patient's age, whether they are immunocompromised, and any other medications they are taking can affect their risk of infection and how it is managed. People who are older or have weak immune systems from cancer or medications are especially at risk of getting infections. They might need closer observation and specific infection control plans. It is also highlighted in the consensus statement that patients with unmanaged risk factors may have difficulty in achieving the best health outcomes, especially when dealing with infections. Therefore, understanding these patient-related factors is crucial for developing effective strategies for infection control and management in the ICU setting, ultimately fostering better patient outcomes and reducing morbidity associated with nosocomial infections (Figure 10.6).

10.2.2. Environmental Factors

How well infection control measures work in the ICU depends largely on the environment, which includes the physical setting, cleanliness, and infrastructure of the hospital. An optimized environment can diminish the risk of hospital-acquired infections (HAIs), particularly among patients with compromised immune systems. Air filtration, humidity control, and the types of surfaces all help to stop the spread of infections. Also, the layout of the ICU should ensure that patient beds are far enough apart so that clinicians can move easily and prevent cross-contamination. Because of these points, integrating evidence-based practices in the ICU is very important for improving patient safety and infection control. AMR makes it harder for ICU staff to manage patients, so, it is important to understand how the environment can cause resistant pathogens to multiply. It has been found that inadequate upkeep of infrastructure and insufficient sanitation can encourage multidrug-resistant organisms, which are very common in ICUs. The burden of AMR is underscored by alarming statistics, with millions of deaths attributed to bacterial resistance, indicating that continued surveillance and targeted interventions are crucial in controlling its impact (Murray *et al.*, 2022). It is also important to ensure the availability of antibiotics and to encourage it's proper use , which underlines the need for a well-kept and supportive ICU environment. Because of the COVID-19 pandemic, attention is being given to environmental factors in infection control in the ICU. The highly contagious nature of SARS-CoV-2 highlights the importance of maintaining optimal ventilation and air quality standards to prevent airborne transmission among critically ill patients (Wiersinga *et al.*, 2020). In many ICU areas, using negative pressure rooms and HEPA filters is now common to help stop the spread of viruses and bacteria. Also, strictly following cleaning guidelines, especially for the materials often touch by the people , is important for preventing the spread of viruses. Therefore, a comprehensive approach that encompasses well-structured environmental factors is crucial for effective infection control and management within the ICU, particularly during public health crises like the COVID-19 pandemic (Figure 10.7).

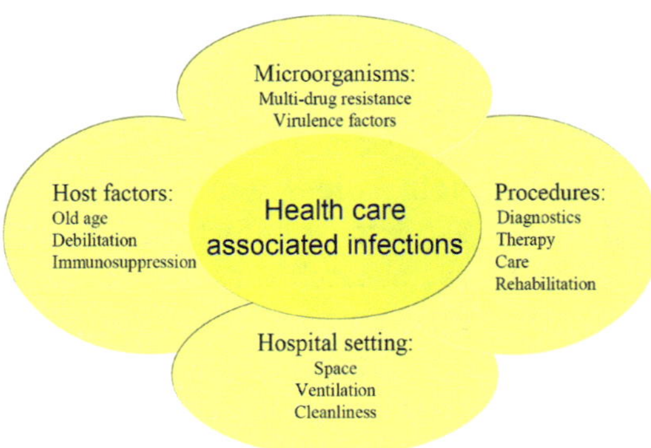

Figure 10.7. Factors determining health care associated infections.

Source: https://www.researchgate.net/figure/Factors-determining-health-care-associated-infections_fig4_221925213.

10.2.3. Healthcare Provider-Related Factors

Within the realm of ICUs, healthcare provider-related factors play a pivotal role in shaping infection control and management strategies. All of these factors include the skills, training, and ability to communicate of healthcare professionals, which are essential for making infection prevention protocols successful. For instance, the adherence to established guidelines often hinges on a provider's understanding of the multi-faceted nature of infection control, including the use of personal protective equipment (PPE) and the implementation of aseptic techniques. If staff are more aware and knowledgeable, they are more likely to use these protocols in the same way, which helps reduce nosocomial infections. Furthermore, ongoing training and education must be prioritized to ensure that all healthcare providers are equipped with up-to-date information regarding emerging pathogens and resistance patterns, as highlighted by the substantial burden of antimicrobial resistance in ICUs (Murray *et al.*, 2022). How healthcare providers work together is just as important for infection control in ICUs. Working together in teams encourages nurses, physicians, and ancillary staff to communicate and share the best ways to care for patients. Having a team approach means that everyone understands their roles, which helps keep an eye on all aspects of infection control. It allows providers to catch any problems with the protocol right away and start resolving them immediately. Also, having multidisciplinary rounds in the ICU helps everyone agree on patient care, making it easier to discuss and improve infection control measures. Such collaborative efforts contribute to a culture of safety that is essential in the high-stakes environment of the ICU, potentially reducing infection rates and improving patient outcomes, as reiterated in primary studies examining post-discharge outcomes among ICU patients (Chopra *et al.*, 2020). The way leaders and managers act in ICUs plays a big role in shaping how healthcare providers deal with infection control. Good leadership helps motivate infection prevention efforts by outlining what is needed and setting a good example. Leaders help create a culture in the organization that puts safety first, which motivates healthcare providers to stick to infection control guidelines. In addition, with feedback mechanisms, providers can identify areas where they can improve and notice when they are doing well in managing infections. Making sure staff feel appreciated and supported helps maintain a good attitude and proper infection control. Ultimately, by addressing the healthcare provider-related factors through robust training, effective teamwork, and inspiring leadership, ICUs can enhance their infection control strategies, leading to better patient care and outcomes in the face of increasing challenges posed by infections in critically ill patients (Murray *et al.*, 2022) (Figure 10.8).

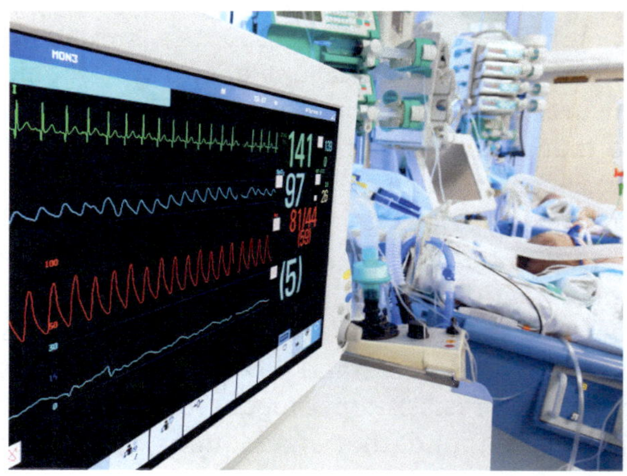

Figure 10.8. Healthcare provider-related factors.

Source: https://cdn.apollohospitals.com/health-library-prod/2019/06/Critical-Care-Unit.jpg.

Test Your Knowledge

1. What patient-related factors in the ICU increase vulnerability to complications such as infections or poor outcomes?
2. How do environmental factors within the ICU setting affect patient safety and recovery?

10.3. Infection Prevention Strategies

Learning Outcome

1. Define hand hygiene protocols
2. Explain the use of personal protective equipment (PPE) in infection control
3. Discuss sterilization and disinfection practices

It is essential to use infection prevention strategies in the ICU because patients are more likely to get infections in the hospital. It is very important for healthcare workers to practice strict hand hygiene. Following proper handwashing and using alcohol-based sanitizers after meeting patients greatly decreases the chance of spreading multidrug-resistant organisms. In addition, having hand sanitizing stations in the ICU makes it easier for everyone to use and follow the rules.

This multifaceted approach not only minimizes the risk of cross-contamination but also cultivates a culture of safety and vigilance in infection prevention, aligning with best practices as outlined in current literature on ICU management (Chopra *et al.*, 2020). PPE should be used because it acts as a shield against infections. In the context of the COVID-19 pandemic, the emphasis on appropriate PPE usage has magnified due to the airborne nature of the virus, demanding high-level protections such as N95 respirators or powered air-purifying respirators (PAPRs) for frontline healthcare workers. These protective measures work well only if staff are trained and follow the set procedures. Frequent tests of competency help staff to become skilled at donning and doffing, which greatly reduces the chance of them becoming contaminated. As hospitals continue to navigate infectious challenges, the application of stringent PPE protocols remains a cornerstone of effective infection prevention in the ICU (Wiersinga *et al.*, 2020). Antimicrobial stewardship is also important to ensure the antibiotics are used correctly to preventantibiotic-resistant infections in ICUs. It requires picking the right agents after testing culture results and sensitivity to provide targeted treatment.

Using methods that encourage reducing therapy when appropriate improves patient safety and helps address the problem of antibiotic resistance. Having regular multidisciplinary meetings to check on the treatment effectiveness and ongoing necessity support patients monitoring and adjust their care. By fostering a collaborative environment among healthcare teams and instituting robust stewardship programs, ICUs can effectively mitigate the risks associated with drug-resistant infections and promote better clinical outcomes for patients (Chopra *et al.*, 2020).

10.3.1. Hand Hygiene Protocols

Hand hygiene protocols are foundational to infection control practices, particularly in the ICU, where patients are vulnerable to HAIs. Taking care of hand hygiene helps to stop the spread of pathogens, for protecting patients whose immune systems are weak. The ways to do so are to use alcohol-based hand sanitizers and wash your hands with soap and water, especially when they are dirty. It is very important to follow these protocols because research has found that not doing so can result in more infections, longer hospital stays, and higher mortality rates among critically ill patients. For this reason, health organizations recommend that proper hand hygiene is very important in managing infections. Without the implementation of rigorous hand hygiene protocols, the risk of outbreaks, especially in the context of antimicrobial resistance, escalates dramatically (Murray *et al.*, 2022) (Figure 10.9).

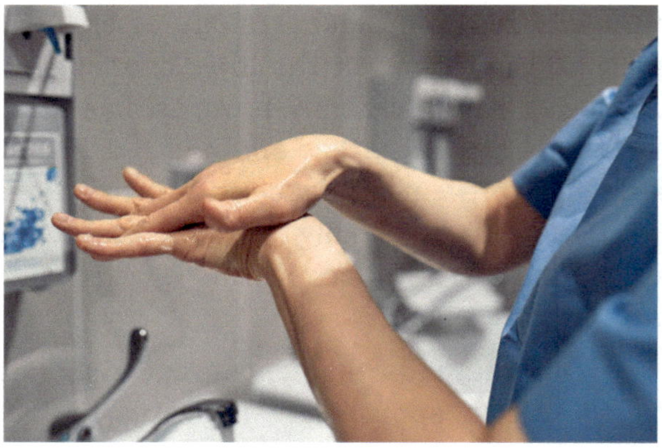

Figure 10.9. Hand hygiene protocols.

Source: https://hospitalprofessionalnews.ie/wp-content/uploads/2020/10/ICU-Hand-Hygiene-Toolkit-002.jpg.

The World Health Organization (WHO) emphasizes the importance of education and training related to hand hygiene protocols for all healthcare professionals in the ICU. The protocols tell you when to wash your hands, like before and after seeing a patient, after touching body fluids, and before doing any aseptic work. If healthcare workers are aware of these important moments, it can help boost compliance and improve patient' outcomes. Also, regularly checking and guiding staff on hand hygiene can encourage a safe environment in healthcare facilities. Multidisciplinary teams should continue their education, and reminders such as signs in the ICU can help everyone follow these protocols. Such measures are particularly relevant in the context of managing infectious diseases, where stringent hand hygiene practices are imperative for limiting the spread of pathogens, including those responsible for severe respiratory infections (World Health Organization, 2020). Advanced technology helps to ensure hand hygiene is followed in the ICU. Wearable sensors and cameras can give healthcare workers feedback on their hand hygiene as it happens. Because of these innovations, it is easier to identify non-compliance and take prompt action. Using artificial intelligence, it is possible to compare infection rates with hand hygiene compliance, helping to evaluate the effectiveness of existing protocols. As healthcare moves toward using data more, using technology to support hand hygiene may greatly improve how infections are controlled. Analyzing the relationship between hand hygiene practices and infection rates further underscores the need for continuous enhancement of these protocols, thereby contributing to more effective infection control strategies in the ICU environment (Murray *et al.*, 2022) (Figure 10.10).

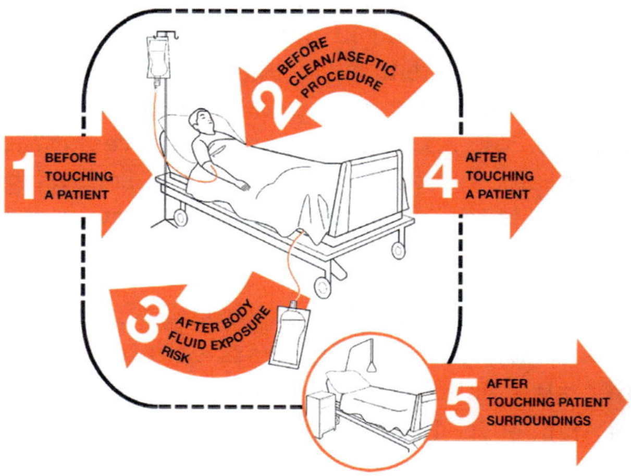

Figure 10.10. The five moments of hand hygiene.

Source: https://www.researchgate.net/figure/The-My-5-Moments-of-Hand-Hygiene_fig1_333718313.

10.3.2. Use of Personal Protective Equipment (PPE)

The utilization of PPE has emerged as a critical component in infection control and management within the ICU. The pandemic has clearly shown that the quality of PPE greatly affects the safety of healthcare workers and the number of patients affected. Since patients in the ICU are more likely to be at risk due to comorbidities and many medical procedures, using PPE properly is very important to prevent nosocomial infections. PPE keeps pathogens from reaching healthcare workers and also helps them feel secure in their work environment. As mandated by health authorities, including the World Health Organization, the adherence to PPE protocols has garnered attention to address ongoing shortages and ensure adequate protection for those at the frontline (Dykes *et al.*, 2020). Problems with PPE include not only having enough, but also making sure train people to follow the guidelines. Healthcare institutions should design strict training sessions to help staff handle PPE correctly. If the right steps for putting on and taking off PPE are not followed, there is a risk of contamination and higher chances of infection. Various healthcare systems have noted that even with PPE, using it incorrectly is a big issue, mostly because of the stress and time pressure in many procedures. Looking after patients with high-risk conditions during a pandemic adds more stress, and this stress can lead to mistakes in PPE use.

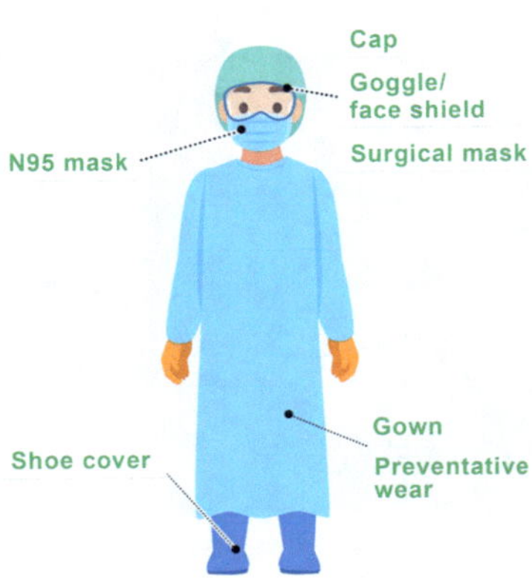

Figure 10.11. Impact of personal protective equipment on surgical performance during the COVID-19 pandemic.

Source: https://www.hogy.co.jp/english/images/products/ppe/01_sp.jpg.

Therefore, institutions must emphasize the importance of continual education and bolster psychological support for staff to ensure compliance and optimal protection during routine and crises (Buising *et al.*, 2020) (Figure 10.11).

Furthermore, the design and functionality of PPE play a crucial role in its effectiveness and acceptance among ICU staff. Fabrics that allow air to circulate and proper sizing can make healthcare workers more comfortable, which often leads to better compliance. During the pandemic, instances of healthcare worker infections were partly attributed to inadequate PPE availability and misapplication due to discomfort and fatigue (Buising *et al.*, 2020). Innovations to come in PPE should be designed with these factors in mind, so that important items are both safe and fit with the demanding routines in ICUs. This aligned focus on technological design and usability can contribute substantially to infection control, allowing healthcare providers to focus on patient care without the constant concern of personal safety, thereby enhancing the overall quality of care in ICUs (Dykes *et al.*, 2020).

10.3.3. Sterilization and Disinfection Practices

The implementation of effective sterilization and disinfection practices is paramount in the management of infections within the ICU. Because patients in the ICU are very sick and often have invasive procedures, the environment is very susceptible to HAIs. To address the dangers from these infections, all medical instruments and surfaces must be sterilized properly. People recognize that using steam sterilization in autoclaves is reliable and effective in killing many types of microorganisms. Also, using new disinfection methods such as vaporized hydrogen peroxide and UV light has become important for improving infection control. Using a combination of classic and modern sterilization techniques, ICUs can significantly lower HAIs and improve patient. Even though traditional sterilization is important, the rise of antimicrobial resistance makes it necessary to use strong disinfection methods in the ICU. If HAIs are not controlled, patients may stay in the hospital longer, medical costs may rise, and more patients may die. New disinfection technologies are helping to deal with this issue. Using antimicrobial coatings on surfaces and devices that are often handled can give an additional defense against the spread of pathogens. Moreover, studies highlight that healthcare staff should be trained regularly about sterilization, so they continue to follow the set guidelines. Risk assessments and standard operating procedures, used systematically, can make the ICU safer for all involved. It is important to use new and traditional methods together to keep infection control in risky areas. Using monitoring and feedback can help in evaluating sterilization and disinfection methods. Failures in disinfection can lead to outbreaks of resistant organisms, which shows the importance of reporting in the ICU. Effective infection prevention and control (IPC) programs must include regular assessments of high-level disinfection and sterilization practices, as these directly correlate with the rates of HAIs. Recent findings indicate a concerning gap in IPC programs, particularly in low- and middle-income regions, where only 60% of surveyed hospitals reported having structured IPC protocols in place (Castillo *et al.*, 2025). Also, half of the facilities did not have proper training in sterilization, showing that better educational programs are needed. By closing these gaps, ICUs can enhance their disinfection strategies, ultimately leading to improved patient safety and a reduction in the spread of resistant infections (Patiño-Marín *et al.*, 2025) (Figure 10.12).

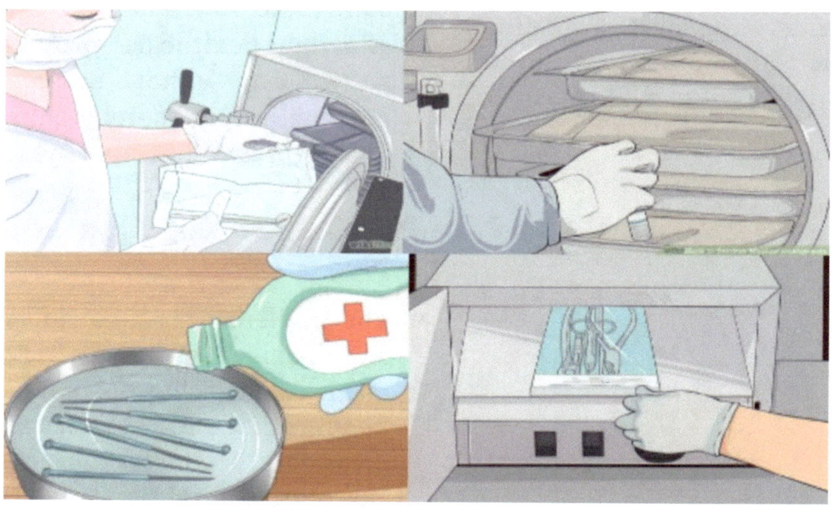

Figure 10.12. Sterilization process.

Source: https://www.slideshare.net/slideshow/sterilization-process/169862664.

Test Your Knowledge

1. Why is strict adherence to hand hygiene protocols critical in preventing healthcare-associated infections?
2. How does proper use of personal protective equipment (PPE) reduce the risk of transmission in clinical settings?

10.4. Role of Antibiotics in Infection Management

Learning Outcome

1. Discuss the guidelines for antibiotic use
2. Identify the antibiotic resistance issues
3. Explain the importance of antibiotic stewardship

Treating infections in the ICU often depends on the proper use of antibiotics, which are necessary for treating the common bacterial infections seen in critically ill patients. Many patients in the ICU can develop ventilator-associated pneumonia, bloodstream infections, or urinary tract infections, which can worsen their current health. Antibiotics are needed to clear these infections and also stop them from getting worse. The challenge, however, lies in selecting the appropriate antibiotics. Since antimicrobial resistance is a major issue in ICUs, it is very important to take into account both the local resistance patterns and the clinical features of the patient. Effective antibiotic stewardship becomes key in this context to minimize resistance development while ensuring effective infection control (Murray *et al.*, 2022). Also, when antibiotics are given is very important for the results in the ICU. If antibiotics are not started promptly, the chances of death increase, mainly in severe sepsis and septic shock. It has been shown that giving antibiotics within the first hour of severe infections in ICUs can greatly decrease the risk of death and help patients recover sooner. Treating patients with the wrong antibiotics can increase the time they have to stay in the hospital and raise the overall healthcare costs because of their prolonged illness. Therefore, an aggressive and informed approach to antibiotic therapy, including the use of intravenous antibiotics when necessary, is essential in managing complex infections prevalent in the ICU environment (Xie *et al.*, 2020). The situation is made more complicated in the ICU by the rise of AMR. AMR reduces the effectiveness of common antibiotics and also leads to patients staying in the hospital for a longer time and dying more often. Given that AMR-related infections accounted for nearly 5 million deaths in 2019, addressing this issue within the ICU is of utmost importance (Murray *et al.*, 2022). The main goal should be to apply strict infection control, use antibiotics judiciously and efficiently, and help create a setting that allows infections to be promptly recognized and treated, thereby minimizing unnecessary antibiotic use. These strategies are crucial in maintaining the efficacy of available antibiotics, ensuring that patients receive the most effective care possible during critical condition (Xie *et al.*, 2020).

10.4.1. Guidelines for Antibiotic Use

The judicious use of antibiotics is paramount in the ICU, where patients are often immunocompromised and vulnerable to complex infections. The rules for antibiotic use in the ICU are meant to stop resistance and treat infections effectively. The guidelines emphasize the need to find and treat certain pathogens early by using susceptibility testing. For example, empirical therapy is often used for critically ill patients, but the antibiotics must be changed if the culture results show something different to avoid unnecessary broad-spectrum use. According to recent studies on severe COVID-19, many patients develop secondary bacterial infections, highlighting the importance of strictly follow antibiotic stewardship. This ensures not only the treatment efficacy but also the minimization of potential side effects and the battle against antimicrobial resistance in this vulnerable population (Pourajam *et al.*, 2022). Along with using targeted therapy, ICU staff to engage in continuous learning and adhere to up-to-date guidelines. The WHO and various epidemiological studies advise that all healthcare professionals involved in prescribing antibiotics receive regular training on antimicrobial stewardship. It should clearly emphasize the importanceof correct antibiotic dosing, appropriate duration of use, , and the risks associated with exposing critically ill patients to unnecessary antibiotics. Because multidrug-resistant organisms are behind many hospital infections, it is important to stick to these guidelines. Studies indicate that the misuse of antibiotics significantly impacts the emergence of resistance, which complicates infection management in the ICU and can lead to increased mortality rates among patients who develop secondary infections due to resistant pathogens (Murray *et al.*, 2022) (Figure 10.13).

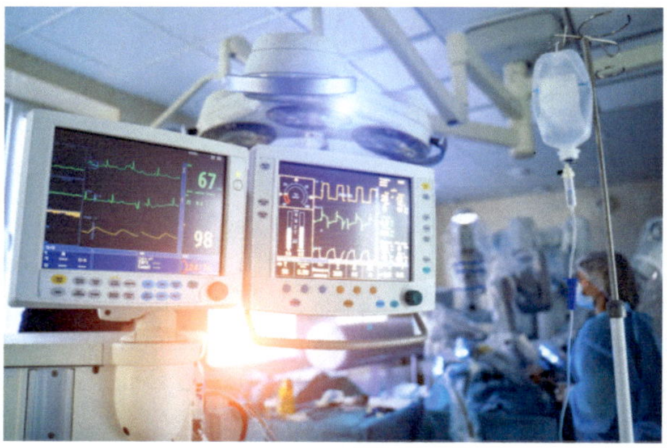

Figure 10.13. Antibiotic dosing technology speeds recovery of ICU patients.

Source: https://www.uq.edu.au/news/filething/get/319644/MED%20dosing%20Adobe%20620W.png.

Healthcare teams to work in collaboration to support the use of antibiotic guidelines in the ICU. Antibiotic selection and monitoring should be done by physicians, pharmacists, and infection control specialists. Because of this approach, doctors can discuss patient responses to antibiotics in different situations, which helps them to improve treatment strategies. When guidelines are implemented, it becomes important to establish protocols that involve regular review of treatment plans and adherence to the local antibiogram, which enlists the hospital's resistance patterns. Because the risk of infection is higher in the ICU, using these methods is significant for controlling antibiotic resistance. Ultimately, adhering to stringent antibiotic use guidelines within this setting can significantly improve patient outcomes and reduce the burden of antimicrobial resistance (Murray *et al.*, 2022; Pourajam *et al.*, 2022).

10.4.2. Antibiotic Resistance Issues

Antibiotic resistance is a major issue in infections handled and prevented in the ICU. The emergence of multidrug-resistant organisms (MDROs) poses significant threats to patient outcomes, complicating treatment protocols and lengthening hospital stays. According to recent estimates, approximately 4.95 million deaths were associated with bacterial antimicrobial resistance globally in 2019, highlighting its escalated burden on healthcare systems, particularly in high-stakes environments such as the ICU (Murray *et al.*, 2022). Using broad-spectrum antibiotics for a long time in critically ill patients causes the development of antibiotic-resistant pathogens. Hence, having strong infection control and stewardship programs is necessary to limit resistance and improve how antibiotics are used, which helps critically ill patients live longer. It is important for ICU managers to know the local patterns of antibiotic resistance and the susceptibility of common pathogens. The Surviving Sepsis Campaign guidelines underscore the importance of delivering timely antimicrobials, ideally within one hour of sepsis recognition, while ensuring that such empiric therapy is adapted according to local data (Evans *et al.*, 2021). This way of prescribing helps deal with the rise of resistant organisms, since it requires choosing treatments that are effective but also unlikely to cause more resistance. Moreover, if healthcare teams are educated on the right way to prescribe antibiotics and the dangers of using them too much, they will be more careful when using antibiotics. They help maintain the usefulness of current antibiotics and encourage new progress in the field of antimicrobial drugs. Also, since antibiotic resistance is increasing, we must keep researching and supporting new ways to treat infections. Because of antibiotic resistance around the world, it is important to invent new medicines and treatments to fight severe infections. Highlighting this need, studies indicate that the number of deaths attributable to leading resistant pathogens underscores the urgency of developing new antimicrobial strategies, alongside enhancing existing practices (Murray *et al.*, 2022). Besides antibiotics, using high-dose vitamin C and corticosteroids is being discussed, but their use should be studied carefully. To manage antibiotic resistance in the ICU, one must use accurate diagnostics, customized treatment plans, and continue working on research and development to achieve better results in managing patients and preventing infections.

10.4.3. Importance of Antibiotic Stewardship

Antibiotic stewardship is now seen as a key part of controlling and managing infections in the ICU. AMR is becoming more common, which results in patients spending more time in the hospital, paying more for treatment, and having a higher risk of death. Recent research estimates that in 2019, bacterial AMR was responsible for about 4.95 million deaths, which stresses the importance of proper stewardship measures. They are designed to help us use antibiotics more wisely, so that they continue to work for patients in the future. When antibiotic stewardship is improved in the ICU, it can lead to better patient outcomes and lessen the number of resistant infections, which is especially important for those patients depending on these drugs. Moreover, the implementation of antibiotic stewardship programs (ASPs) directly correlates with decreased rates of AMR and improved patient safety. They rely on different methods like tracking how antibiotics are prescribed, teaching healthcare workers about the right use of antibiotics, and setting rules for treating infections. Recent studies point out that combinations of pathogens and drugs, such as carbapenem-resistant Enterobacteriaceae, are now considered major public health dangers, mainly in places where resources are limited, like sub-Saharan Africa. With strong ASPs, healthcare units can manage the presence of resistant bacteria in their area and modify their actions to fit the local trends, keeping antibiotics working for a longer period.

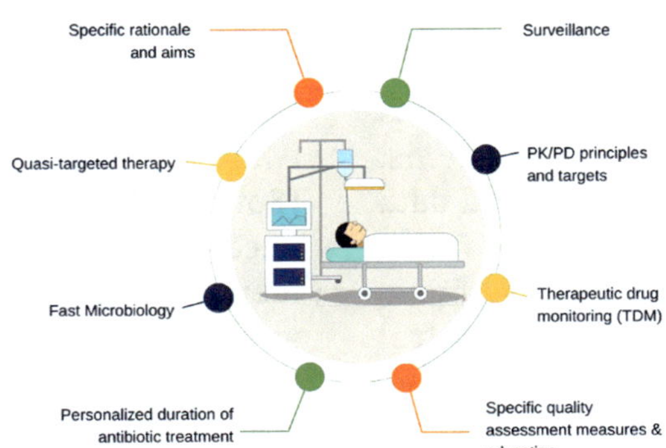

Figure 10.14. The main components and themes related to the clinical application of antimicrobial stewardship principles in the intensive care unit.

Source: https://janesthanalgcritcare.biomedcentral.com/articles/10.1186/s44158-023-00095-6.

Such strategies help patients in the ICU and also support the goals of public health. Antibiotic stewardship efforts are necessary to address antimicrobial resistance, which affects people worldwide. As AMR becomes more serious, mainly for vulnerable people, not managing antibiotics properly can cause significant health emergencies. Many low-income areas lack data on AMR and antibiotic use, which makes it harder to handle infections. When healthcare leaders focus on stewardship, they can improve infection prevention in the ICU while ensuring that important antibiotics are accessible and infection control measures are effective in different healthcare areas. Such endeavors are essential in battling the pervasive threat of AMR and safeguarding the health of future generations as antibiotic-resistant infections continue to challenge global health systems (Figure 10.14).

Test Your Knowledge

1. What are the key principles outlined in guidelines for appropriate antibiotic use in healthcare settings?
2. How does misuse or overuse of antibiotics contribute to the development of antibiotic resistance?

10.5. Monitoring and Surveillance of Infections

Learning Outcome

1. Discuss the infection tracking systems
2. Explain the data collection and analysis
3. Define reporting and feedback mechanisms

It is very important to monitor and closely watch infections in the ICU to maintain patient safety and the best possible outcomes. The purpose of surveillance is to identify, study, and deal with infections, which is necessary since ICU patients usually have weakened immune systems. Healthcare institutions that use organized data collection can spot trends in infections, which allows them to take action promptly. In addition, these systems can assess the infection control measures, such as hand washing, antibiotic use, and staff education programs. By this way, the risk of HAIs is reduced, and better care and use of resources are achieved in the ICU. In addition to traditional methods, hospitals are increasingly utilizing EHRs and real-time data analysis to monitor infections. They enable doctors to quickly monitor new infections, which is crucial in the ICU, where time is of the essence. Machine learning can be used to identify the patterns in large data to predict an infection outbreak. As a result, the country can act swiftly when infections increase, which reduces their impact. Furthermore, integrating surveillance data with antimicrobial resistance profiles can inform treatment decisions and guide appropriate antibiotic use, thereby combating the growing threat of AMR (Murray *et al.*, 2022). It supports the goal of making patients healthier and less likely to get infections in healthcare settings. The importance of continuous monitoring and surveillance cannot be overstated, especially in the context of sepsis-associated complications, which significantly challenge ICU management (Sonneville *et al.*, 2023). Sepsis-associated encephalopathy demands close attention to identify it early so the right treatments can be given. They also go beyond tracking infections; they include careful observation of how patients react to treatment and if some drugs may harm the nervous system. Assessments are done regularly to ensure that oxygen levels, blood pressure, and the body's metabolism are at their best, which is very important for patients with serious infections. Ultimately, a comprehensive surveillance strategy not only addresses immediate infection control needs but also fosters long-term recovery and minimizes the risk of persistent complications for patients transitioning out of the ICU (Figure 10.15).

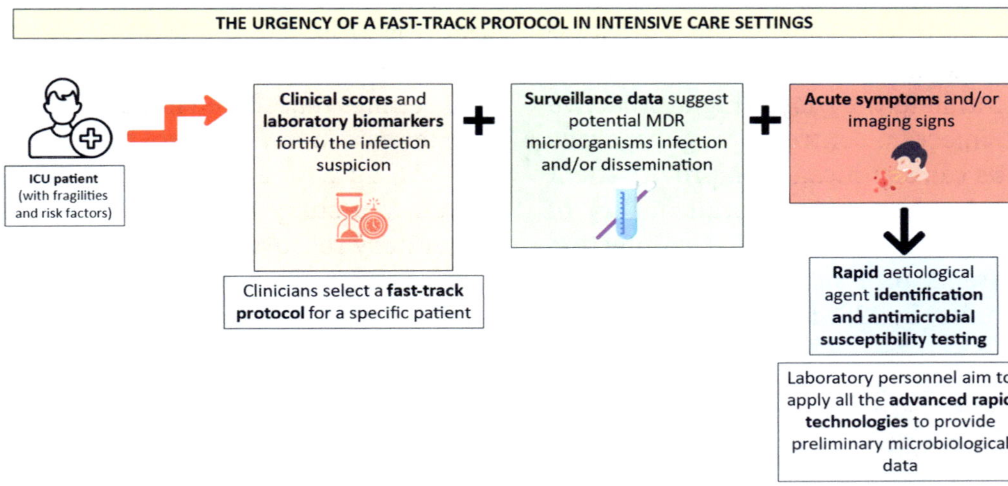

Figure 10.15. Proposal of a diagnostic workflow organization in ICU patients. The ICU patients must hold several risk factors and fragilities to require a fast-track protocol after the suspicion of a severe infection. This suspicion is often fortified by clinical scores and laboratory biomarkers, along with MDR colonization data and acute symptoms.

Source: https://www.mdpi.com/antibiotics/antibiotics-13-00238/article_deploy/html/images/antibiotics-13-00238-g002.png.

10.5.1. Infection Tracking Systems

Infection tracking systems are essential components of infection control and management in ICUs. They help healthcare providers to detect, and deal with HAIs promptly. Using electronic health records and data analytics, infection tracking systems can provide instant updates about infection trends and patterns. Because of this, ICU staff can identify high-risk patients and make necessary changes to their care plans . Besides, monitoring antibiotic resistance trends through these systems helps to plan and execute effective antimicrobial stewardship strategies, which boosts the success of infection control efforts. Once an infection is found, having effective tracking systems helps with both real-time monitoring and thorough reporting, which is very useful for improving quality. If healthcare centers keep infection data in a central database, this helps ensure that all departments use the same approach to reporting trends. By working together, healthcare professionals can share what has worked well in other places and use those practices. By tracking infections, facilities can see how they measure up to national or regional standards, which may encourage them to improve care and safety for patients. Following these systems is in line with the guidelines set by healthcare regulatory bodies, which stress responsibility and openness in managing infections. Assessment and follow-up are essential in infection tracking systems because they give important information about the success of infection management. Systematically reviewing the collected data helps healthcare professionals spot the interventions that reduce infection rates the most. It is also essential for infection tracking to document what happens to patients after they have infections, so we can learn about any issues and how fast they improve. By joining this information with other healthcare systems, the ICU can always learn and adapt. Ultimately, by fostering a proactive approach to infection control through rigorous tracking, ICUs can significantly improve patient outcomes and enhance the overall quality of care, reflecting the crucial role that infection tracking systems play in modern healthcare delivery (Aguilar, 2022; Choi *et al.*, 2021).

10.5.2. Data Collection and Analysis

The process of collecting and reviewing data is essential for handling infections in ICUs. Collecting data correctly is necessary to know about the infections, their rates, and possible outbreaks of HAIs. Having this information allows healthcare professionals to design the best prevention and control strategies for the patients they serve. As an illustration, by using systematic reviews, surveillance, and hospital data, it is possible to find out what risks and trends are linked to infections in critically ill patients. Using data collection effectively allows ICU teams to assess the impact of infection control strategies, which is important for ongoing improvement. In the end, strong data makes it possible to decide on actions that reduce infection risks and keep patients safe. Data analytics advances help ICU teams gain more knowledge about different pathogens and how they become resistant to treatments. Predictive statistical modeling allows researchers to estimate how AMR affects mortality rates, as shown in a study of data from 204 countries. This kind of analysis takes into account both how pathogens react to drugs and the characteristics of the patients, which helps to explain the results of infections in critical care settings. Using large datasets, scientists can identify patients at higher risk of AMR, necessitating targeted strategies to address the problem. Such targeted analysis not only aids in managing infections more effectively but also facilitates the development of best practices for antibiotic stewardship efforts within ICUs (Murray *et al.*, 2022). Besides, there are many difficulties in gathering and analyzing data in ICU settings that should not be ignored. A lack of proper data in low-resource places makes it hard to keep up with and address infections. It was noted in a study that increasing microbiology laboratory resources and better data collection are necessary to handle the problems of AMR and other infections. When these gaps are fixed, healthcare systems can better track infections and act quickly and effectively. Stronger data collection frameworks foster an environment of transparency and accountability in infection management efforts, ultimately leading to improved patient outcomes in ICUs (Chopra *et al.*, 2020). It shows that data is essential for guiding policies and practices in infection control and that a good data analysis approach is necessary for modern critical care.

10.5.3. Reporting and Feedback Mechanisms

Effective reporting and feedback mechanisms are pivotal in managing infection control within the ICU. They are designed to find and resolve problems and also to encourage healthcare professionals to be transparent and responsible. If inconsistencies in practice arise or new infection patterns emerge, real-time data enables prompt adjustments to protocols. Frontline staff often mention when infection control measures are not followed or when they do not have enough personal protective equipment. Furthermore, the integration of these feedback loops encourages team collaboration and adaptability, which are essential in the ever-evolving landscape of healthcare delivery, particularly during unprecedented times like the COVID-19 pandemic, where challenges surrounding hospital-acquired infections are exacerbated (Maben *et al.*, 2020). Using formal feedback systems extensively improves how staff feel and how engaged they are. If healthcare workers believe their ideas are essential, it helps them feel responsible for infection control. People can give feedback at team meetings or through anonymous surveys, so they do not worry about being punished for their opinions. When staff are involved, it leads to better following of infection prevention guidelines since everyone participates in solving issues related to the environment, patient contact, and procedures. Prioritizing clear communication and giving regular feedback in healthcare institutions helps the team follow infection control rules and also strengthens their mental well-being. Increased engagement leads to a more committed workforce that is keen on maintaining high standards of patient safety (Rochwerg *et al.*, 2017). Also, using technology to simplify reporting and feedback supports better infection control in the ICU. With electronic health records, surveillance, and mobile apps, it is easier to collect data about infections and how well control measures are being followed. They not only monitor incidents but also provide valuable insights that can help improve processes. Also, these systems can send timely messages about infection outbreaks to the ICU team, so they are prepared to act accordingly. Because of this approach, healthcare professionals can concentrate more on treating their patients instead of handling paperwork. Thus, fostering an environment that values transparency, active communication, and continuous improvement not only strengthens infection control efforts but ultimately enhances patient outcomes in the ICU (Maben *et al.*, 2020).

Test Your Knowledge

1. How do infection tracking systems help in monitoring and controlling healthcare-associated infections?
2. Why is accurate data collection and analysis essential for effective infection prevention strategies?

10.6. Education and Training for Healthcare Staff

Learning Outcome

1. Explain the importance of ongoing education
2. Define the training programs and workshops
3. Discuss the assessment of staff competency

Effective education and training for healthcare staff are critical components in the realm of infection control and management, especially within ICUs, where the stakes are significantly high. The quick spread of diseases, for example, COVID-19, has highlighted that healthcare professionals require up-to-date knowledge and skills to address new pathogens. It is essential that training covers infection control, using PPE, and the mental strength needed to handle stress at work. Since more patients and tough ethical situations challenge healthcare workers, they must continue their education to improve patient care and safety. The evidence suggests that targeted training can significantly mitigate risks associated with infection transmission in critical care settings (Mokhtari *et al.*, 2020). Nurses are responsible for handling a large part of the infection management in the ICU. Because of the long shifts and emotional stress from patient losses, they require training that covers medical skills and emotional support. Recent studies suggest that better training in mental health can help both patients and healthcare workers. It is clear from reports that nurses are experiencing high levels of burnout and anxiety, which shows that their training and development should be dealt with proactively. By integrating mental health awareness into infection control training, healthcare systems can foster a more resilient workforce equipped to navigate the complexities of critical care during crises, ultimately leading to better management of infectious diseases in ICUs (Maben *et al.*, 2020). Also, training staff with simulation exercises has been found to help them manage infection control situations in ICUs. With these training methods, participants have a chance to practice what they learn in a simulation, which makes them feel more confident and skilled when they see real patients. The simulations ought to address the difficulties of major infectious disease outbreaks, such as fast decision-making and working together as a team under pressure. Providing frequent updates to training programs, which include lessons from past outbreaks, ensures staff are aware of the latest rules and best ways to handle situations. As healthcare continues to evolve, an emphasis on continuous education and adaptive training for ICU staff will be paramount in combating infection risks and improving patient outcomes (Mokhtari *et al.*, 2020) (Figure 10.16).

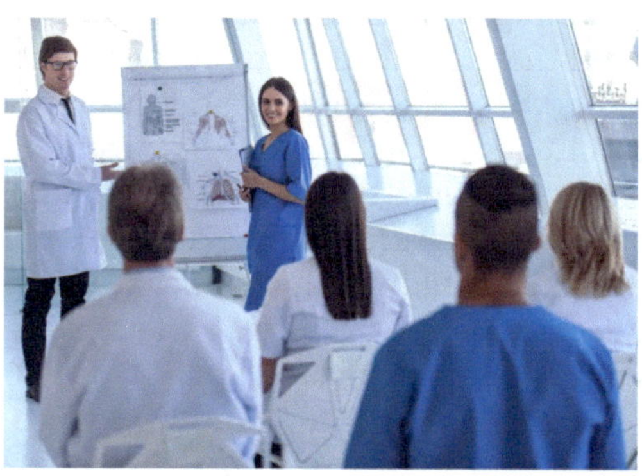

Figure 10.16. Education and training for healthcare staff.

Source: https://careskillstraining.org/wp-content/uploads/2024/03/medical-doctors-at-the-conference-2023-11-27-05-12-44-utc-1024x684.webp.

10.6.1. Importance of Ongoing Education

Because infectious diseases and antimicrobial resistance are constantly changing, ongoing education is very important in ICUs. Because treating infections in vulnerable populations is not easy, healthcare professionals should be aware of the newest research, guidelines for diagnosis, and available therapies. Recent advancements in the study of invasive fungal diseases highlight the importance of continuous learning, as outdated practices may lead to missed diagnoses and poor patient's outcomes. Ongoing education helps to address these challenges and equips healthcare workers with the skills to implement evidence-based practices effectively, ultimately enhancing patient safety and care quality in critical settings (Azim *et al.*, 2024). In addition, the fact that infection control measures are not always followed in the same way in different healthcare facilities shows that more targeted education is necessary. For instance, a study assessing infection control practices in primary healthcare centers revealed significant discrepancies in compliance among healthcare workers, emphasizing the importance of tailored training programs (Mulay *et al.*, 2024). Such variations can negatively influence patient outcomes, mainly in ICU areas where infections are common. When institutions encourage continuous learning, healthcare workers are aware of the latest guidelines and can follow them properly. Because of this approach, the risk of healthcare-associated infections is reduced, which is especially important for ICU patients who often have several health issues . Besides helping staff improve their skills, ongoing education encourages them to work together as a team. Reasonable infection control in an ICU depends on teams working together and communicating well. When healthcare professionals continue their education, they can work together and share what they have learned. Regularly attending training sessions, workshops, and simulation exercises enables

ICU teams to discuss complex cases and develop strategies grounded in the latest evidence. This alignment strengthens the overall infection control efforts and ensures a comprehensive approach to managing infections in critically ill patients, thereby enhancing overall patient care within the ICU (Azim *et al.*, 2024).

10.6.2. Training Programs and Workshops

Infection control and management in the ICU is effective when principles are taught regularly in well-designed training programs and workshops. They are essential for ensuring healthcare professionals are aware of the latest methods to prevent hospital-acquired infections. Because of the problems caused by COVID-19, clinical staff should keep learning and practicing the most effective ways to handle cases. According to current standards, training must reflect not only the emerging evidence but also the organizational strategies that accommodate situations, such as surges in patient volume (Aziz *et al.*, 2020). Workshops that simulate real situations allow participants to practice infection control, which helps them feel more prepared to use these measures in the ICU. How well training programs work depends on their ability to keep up with new clinical practices. Workshops should use approaches that are proven to work and that also show how the theory can be applied in real life. critical function of these meetings is to unite doctors, nurses, and other healthcare workers to improve patient care by working together. Training should include necessary steps, like hand washing and sterilizing equipment, and also focus on dealing with the emotional challenges of working in the ICU. Moreover, integrating pilot studies and feasibility checks, as outlined by guidelines such as the CONSORT extension for studies in this domain, can provide valuable insights into the effectiveness of training interventions (Eldridge *et al.*, 2016). This means that the process is planned to increase the following of infection control rules by reviewing and adjusting them. As well as teaching clinical practices, workshops are places where important news about new and resistant germs is shared. Since there are more complicated infectious diseases, these educational sessions help ICU staff stay prepared and informed. Also, using simulation exercises can significantly help staff in learning how to handle crises, as they can practice in a safe environment before real emergencies happen. After workshops, regular assessments help find out if staff are ready and which areas need more training. By systematically updating training curricula by the latest research and experiences, healthcare facilities can significantly improve their infection control measures, ensuring the safety and well-being of both patients and staff in the ICU (Figure 10.17).

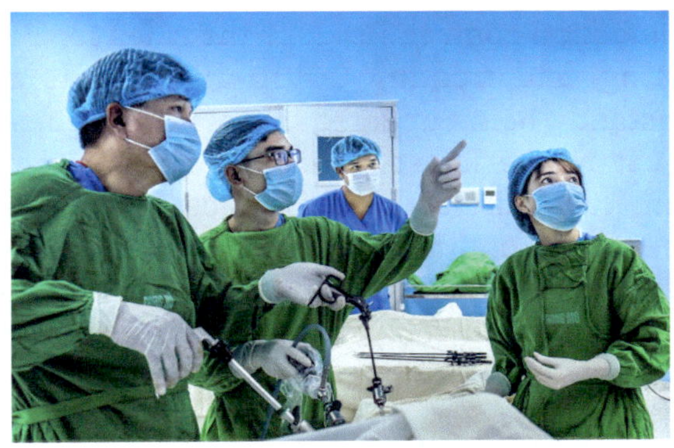

Figure 10.17. Infection control and management in the ICU.

Source: https://www.who.int/images/default-source/wpro/countries/viet-nam/health-topics/hsd/health-workforce/health-workforce-1.tmb-1200v.jpg?Culture=en&sfvrsn=cec3f2bc_4.

10.6.3. Assessment of Staff Competency

Ensuring that staff are competent in the ICU is very important for infection control and management. Since patients in critical care are more likely to get infections due to their treatment and time spent in the hospital, staff members need substantial knowledge and abilities in advanced infection control. By regularly assessing competency, companies can find out where their employees need more training. Working together with professionals from other areas increases competency as everyone can learn from each other's experiences in managing infections. Many studies have shown that creating a learning environment in the ICU encourages staff to follow infection control measures, which helps patients recover. Effective communication, teamwork, and role clarity are fundamental aspects of this assessment process that must be emphasized in competency evaluations (Kleinpell *et al.*, 2021). Because the COVID-19 pandemic caused healthcare challenges to increase, it is now more important than ever to assess staff competency in infection control. Because the rules for PPE, testing, and treating COVID-19 patients are constantly being updated, nurses must quickly adjust to the latest standards. How well the team can handle these changes affects both their safety and the success of patient care in the ICU. Even with more stress and greater workloads, staff competency assessments have allowed healthcare professionals to find and use strategies to manage infection control problems. Assessments carried out during multidisciplinary rounds and team meetings help everyone to be open and work together. This collective approach has been essential in sustaining high standards of care and mitigating the spread of infections within the ICU (Dykes *et al.*, 2020). It is essential to look at both the technical abilities and the mental health of ICU staff, since stress and burnout may lower their performance and risk harm to patients. Making psychological safety a part of regular assessments helps ensure staff feel supported, which can lead to more open talks about managing infections. Organizations in charge should include mental health initiatives in their evaluation of competence, since ICU staff deal with a lot of stress. The link between how well staff can do their jobs and how they feel emotionally shows why an integrated approach to infection control is necessary. By assessing both hard and soft skills comprehensively, healthcare facilities can ensure a workforce well-equipped to tackle the complexities of infection management in the ICU (Kleinpell *et al.*, 2021).

Test Your Knowledge

1. Why is ongoing education important for maintaining high standards of infection control in healthcare settings?
2. How do training programs and workshops enhance staff knowledge and compliance with infection prevention protocols?

SUMMARY

In reflecting on infection control and management within the ICU, it is imperative to acknowledge the evolving landscape of clinical practice guided by rigorous research and evidence-based guidelines. The Campaigns now stress that sepsis must be managed promptly and appropriately, which is very important for patients' recovery. These guidelines recommend a thorough approach that infections, emphasizing the importance of early antibiotic use and fluid resuscitation tailored to the patient's needs. By fostering a deeper understanding of sepsis management, these guidelines aim to mitigate the immediate risks associated with infections in critically ill patients, thereby improving survival rates and reducing long-term morbidity, a goal central to the ethos of ICU care (Evans *et al.*, 2021). In addition, the importance of using various medical specialties within the ICU is very high. When specialists in infectious diseases, nursing, and pharmacy are involved in treatment planning, it helps consider both the medical and the social factors that affect a patient's health. Research indicates that the presence of risk factors such as total parenteral nutrition and acute kidney injury in ICU patients necessitates timely interventions to prevent complications like candidemia (Poissy *et al.*, 2020). Thus, healthcare providers need to keep learning about these risk factors and how to assess risk with the help of scoring systems. Taking these steps can help ensure the hospital is clean and safe, which benefits patients. The treatment of infections in the ICU requires both prompt actions and the cooperation of a team. Because guidelines keep changing with new research, healthcare professionals should be flexible and committed to learning new things all the time. The focus on long-term care in the latest guidelines points out that sepsis survivors need help with physical, mental, and emotional issues after they leave the hospital. Ultimately, achieving excellence in infection control within the ICU hinges on collaboration among clinical teams, adherence to best practices, and a steadfast focus on patient-centered care, ensuring that all efforts translate into meaningful improvements in patient health and quality of life (Evans *et al.*, 2021; Poissy *et al.*, 2020).

Controlling infections in ICUs helps patients survive and reduces the chances of lasting problems caused by infections. Controlling infections depends greatly on understanding AMR, which is a serious risk to health around the world. In 2019, it was found that bacterial AMR caused about 4.95 million deaths, making it one of the main reasons for death globally. It points out that good data collection and effective infection prevention measures for different pathogens are needed, especially in places where there are fewer resources and antimicrobial resistance may be higher. The high mortality rates associated with infections in ICUs, especially those linked to resistant pathogens, demonstrate an urgent need for enhanced diagnosis, surveillance, and treatment protocols to mitigate infection risks and manage the burdens of AMR effectively (Murray *et al.*, 2022). There has been a lot of interest from recent studies in the success of resuscitation efforts for septic shock patients in ICUs. The use of passive leg raises during dynamic assessment was shown to help patients with septic shock by improving their outcomes. Those receiving the intervention had a lower net fluid balance at 72 hours, which went hand in hand with a lower need for renal replacement therapy and mechanical ventilation. The findings advocate for physiologic titration of fluids based on real-time assessments of fluid responsiveness, emphasizing its role in improving patient outcomes and enhancing the overall management of septic patients in an ICU setting (Douglas *et al.*, 2020). In short, dealing with infections in the ICU means using various methods such as addressing antimicrobial resistance, using proven treatment plans, and updating resuscitation techniques for critically ill patients. Using strong data on AMR and constantly monitoring fluid responsiveness in septic patients is the way to improve how infections are managed in critical settings. Collectively, these efforts can enhance recovery rates, decrease ICU lengths of stay, and ultimately save lives while addressing the evolving challenges posed by infections and the persistence of resistant strains in vulnerable patient populations (Douglas *et al.*, 2020; Murray *et al.*, 2022).

KEY TERMS FROM THIS CHAPTER

- Airborne precautions
- Aseptic technique
- Droplet precautions
- Hand hygiene
- Isolation
- Nosocomial infection
- Sepsis
- Ventilator-associated pneumonia (VAP)
- Antimicrobial stewardship
- Contact precautions
- Environmental cleaning
- Infection surveillance
- Multidrug-resistant organisms (MDROs)
- Personal protective equipment (PPE)
- Standard precautions

CRITICAL THINKING QUESTIONS

1. What is the most effective method for preventing healthcare-associated infections (HAIs) in the ICU?
- a. Routine use of prophylactic antibiotics
- b. Daily bathing with chlorhexidine
- c. Strict adherence to hand hygiene protocols
- d. Frequent room disinfection with UV light

2. Which of the following is not a component of the ventilator-associated pneumonia (VAP) prevention bundle?
- a. Elevation of the head of the bed
- b. Daily sedation vacation
- c. Routine bronchoscopy
- d. Peptic ulcer disease prophylaxis

3. Central line-associated bloodstream infections (CLABSIs) can be minimized by:
- a. Replacing lines every three days
- b. Using maximum sterile barrier precautions during insertion
- c. Using antibiotics in all central lines
- d. Using povidone-iodine for skin antisepsis

4. Which organism is most commonly associated with catheter-associated urinary tract infections (CAUTIs) in ICU settings?
- a. *Pseudomonas aeruginosa*
- b. *Escherichia coli*
- c. *Staphylococcus aureus*
- d. Candida albicans

5. In an ICU setting, the use of contact precautions is essential when managing patients with infections caused by:
- a. Influenza virus
- b. *Mycobacterium tuberculosis*
- c. *Clostridioides difficile*
- d. *Plasmodium falciparum*

Short Answer Questions

1. What is the most common source of hospital-acquired infections (HAIs) in the ICU?
2. What are the "4 moments" for hand hygiene in the ICU according to WHO guidelines?
3. What is the primary reason for isolating patients infected with multidrug-resistant organisms (MDROs)?
4. Which diagnostic marker is most commonly used in the ICU to help differentiate between bacterial and non-bacterial infections?
5. Describe two key strategies for preventing catheter-associated urinary tract infections (CAUTIs).
6. What is antimicrobial stewardship, and why is it critical in the ICU setting?

Answer to Critical Thinking Questions

1. (c); 2. (c); 3. (b); 4. (b); 5. (c)

REFERENCES

1. Aguilar, J. (2022). Addressing health concerns interrupted by the COVID-19 pandemic. *Acta Medica Philippina*. https://www.semanticscholar.org/paper/80cb18cbb54d684f5b9448b9d1b01bf1444a7335 (accessed on 22 May 2025).
2. Azim, A., & Ahmed, A. (2024). Diagnosis and management of invasive fungal diseases in non-neutropenic ICU patients, with focus on candidiasis and aspergillosis: A comprehensive review. *Frontiers in Cellular and Infection Microbiology, 14*. https://www.semanticscholar.org/paper/b207db8a8ec2e8727434fde1d053b8ddc3668df9 (accessed on 22 May 2025).
3. Aziz, S., Arabi, Y. M., Alhazzani, W., Evans, L., Citerio, G., Fischkoff, K., Salluh, J. I., *et al.* (2020). Managing ICU surge during the COVID-19 crisis: Rapid guidelines. *Intensive Care Medicine, 46*(7), 1303–1325. https://doi.org/10.1007/s00134-020-06092-5.
4. Buetti, N., Marschall, J., Drees, M., Fakih, M. G., Hadaway, L., Maragakis, L. L., Monsees, E., *et al.* (2022). Strategies to prevent central line-associated bloodstream infections in acute-care hospitals: 2022 update. *Infection Control and Hospital Epidemiology, 43*(5), 553–569. https://doi.org/10.1017/ice.2022.87.
5. Buising, K., Williamson, D. A., Cowie, B. C., MacLachlan, J. H., Orr, E., MacIsaac, C., Williams, E., *et al.* (2020). A hospital-wide response to multiple outbreaks of COVID-19 in health care workers: Lessons learned from the field. *The Medical Journal of Australia, 214*, 101. https://doi.org/10.5694/mja2.50850.
6. Castillo, E., Rojas-Fermín, R., Reyes, Y., Blanco, C., Villegas, A. M., & Mena Lora, A. M. (2025). P-404. A nationwide survey of infection prevention and control and high-level disinfection and sterilization practices in the Dominican Republic. *Open Forum Infectious Diseases, 12*. https://www.semanticscholar.org/paper/80678a15db95f189c7acbb19663312fd4f00bb34 (accessed on 22 May 2025).
7. Choi, J. H., Lee, J., Park, E., Bae, S., Kim, D., Kim, Y. H., & Choi, I. (2021). Nutrition and metabolism research abstracts. *JPEN. Journal of Parenteral and Enteral Nutrition, 45*(S1), 7–240. https://www.semanticscholar.org/paper/02cbd73c3bb6faeac33e59cc28bf6d9f1085eba0 (accessed on 22 May 2025).
8. Chopra, V., Flanders, S. A., O'Malley, M., Malani, A. N., & Prescott, H. C. (2020). Sixty-day outcomes among patients hospitalized with COVID-19. *Annals of Internal Medicine, 174*(4), 576–578. https://doi.org/10.7326/m20-5661.
9. Codjoe, F. S., & Donkor, E. S. (2017). Carbapenem resistance: A review. *Medical Sciences, 6*, 1. https://doi.org/10.3390/medsci6010001.
10. Douglas, I. S., Alapat, P., Corl, K., Exline, M. C., Forni, L. G., Holder, A. L., Kaufman, D. A., *et al.* (2020). Fluid response evaluation in sepsis hypotension and shock. *CHEST Journal, 158*, 1431–1445. https://doi.org/10.1016/j.chest.2020.04.025.
11. Dykes, S., & Chu, C. H. (2020). Now more than ever, nurses need to be involved in technology design: Lessons from the COVID-19 pandemic. *Journal of Clinical Nursing, 30*(1, 2), 1–8. https://doi.org/10.1111/jocn.15581.
12. Eldridge, S., Chan, C., Campbell, M. J., Bond, C., Hopewell, S., Thabane, L., & Lancaster, G. (2016). CONSORT 2010 statement: Extension to randomized pilot and feasibility trials. *BMJ, 355*, i5239. https://doi.org/10.1136/bmj.i5239.

13. Evans, L., Rhodes, A., Alhazzani, W., Antonelli, M., Coopersmith, C. M., French, C., Machado, F. R., *et al.* (2021). Executive summary: Surviving sepsis campaign: International guidelines for the management of sepsis and septic shock 2021. *Critical Care Medicine, 49*, 1974–1982. https://doi.org/10.1097/ccm.0000000000005357.

14. Kang, J., Hang, Y., Liu, Z., Yuan, M., Qiu, X., Ye, Y., Zang, Y., *et al.* (2025). Analysis of pathogenic bacteria and associated risk factors of bloodstream infections in ICU patients undergoing ECMO support using mNGS technology. *International Journal of Clinical Practice*. https://www.semanticscholar.org/paper/42df4cdaa8a40d0a618859a7474a3c3b237ddf12 (accessed on 22 May 2025).

15. Kleinpell, R., Grabenkort, W. R., Boyle, W. A., Vines, D., & Olsen, K. M. (2021). The Society of Critical Care Medicine at 50 years: Interprofessional practice in critical care: Looking back and forging ahead. *Critical Care Medicine, 49*(12), 2017–2032. https://doi.org/10.1097/ccm.0000000000005276.

16. Liu, Y., Wang, Q., Zhao, C., Chen, H., Li, H., *et al.* (2020). Prospective multi-center evaluation on risk factors, clinical characteristics and outcomes due to carbapenem resistance in *Acinetobacter baumannii* complex bacteraemia: Experience from the Chinese Antimicrobial Resistance Surveillance of Nosocomial Infections (CARES) Network. *Journal of Medical Microbiology*. https://www.semanticscholar.org/paper/bb62e6a594cbd3dca9be8bc072514c2197d415b1 (accessed on 22 May 2025).

17. Maben, J., & Bridges, J. (2020). Covid-19: Supporting nurses' psychological and mental health. *Journal of Clinical Nursing, 29*, 2742–2750. https://doi.org/10.1111/jocn.15307.

18. Mokhtari, R., Moayedi, S., & Golitaleb, M. (2020). COVID-19 pandemic and health anxiety among nurses of intensive care units. *International Journal of Mental Health Nursing, 29*(6), 1275–1277. https://doi.org/10.1111/inm.12800.

19. Mulay, M., Naik, S., Wyawahare, A., Mahajan, S. M., & Kulkarni, S. S. (2024). Awareness and monitoring of infection control practices among healthcare workers in three primary health centers in India. *GMS Hygiene and Infection Control, 19*. https://www.semanticscholar.org/paper/c80fd4e91edc4af1bc7724e918de4744c92a8dec (accessed on 22 May 2025).

20. Murhekar, M., & Kumar, C. P. G. (2022). Health-care-associated infection surveillance in India. *The Lancet Global Health, 10*, e1222–e1223. https://doi.org/10.1016/s2214-109x(22)00317-5.

21. Murray, C. J. L., Ikuta, K. S., Sharara, F., Swetschinski, L. R., Robles Aguilar, G., Gray, A. P., Han, C., *et al.* (2022). Global burden of bacterial antimicrobial resistance in 2019: A systematic analysis. *The Lancet, 399*, 629–655. https://doi.org/10.1016/s0140-6736(21)02724-0.

22. Ng, K., Poon, B. H., Puar, T., Quah, J., Loh, W. J., Wong, Y. J., Tan, T. Y., *et al.* (2020). COVID-19 and the risk to health care workers: A case report. *Annals of Internal Medicine, 172*, 766–767. https://doi.org/10.7326/l20-0175.

23. Orishko, A., Imber, J., Roccuzzo, A., Stähli, A., & Salvi, G. (2024). Tooth- and implant-related prognostic factors in treatment planning. *Periodontology 2000, 95*(1), 102–128. https://www.semanticscholar.org/paper/72c5d1cd71aa4181bfe4ed8fe4e5680f4f0e0e9c (accessed on 22 May 2025).

24. Othman, A. A., & Abdelazim, M. S. (2017). Ventilator-associated pneumonia in adult intensive care unit prevalence and complications. *The Egyptian Journal of Critical Care Medicine, 5*, 61–63. https://doi.org/10.1016/j.ejccm.2017.06.001.

25. Park, Y., & Choi, S. (2025). Factors affecting the direct and indirect performance of infection control for centrally inserted central catheters among ICU nurses. *Healthcare*. https://www.semanticscholar.org/paper/97dfb5f084dd77a616001fae792f1e6d7fcdc245 (accessed on 22 May 2025).

26. Patiño-Marín, N., Villa García, L. D., Aguirre López, E. C., Medina-Solís, C., Martínez Zumarán, A., Martínez Rider, R., Márquez Preciado, R., *et al.* (2025). Sterilization and disinfection: Ensuring infection control in dental practices. *Cureus, 17*. https://www.semanticscholar.org/paper/31ef89201b8a30984c236f95f9936408b8e5e9a2 (accessed on 22 May 2025).

27. Poissy, J., Damonti, L., Bignon, A., Khanna, N., von Kietzell, M., Boggian, K., Neofytos, D., *et al.* (2020). Risk factors for candidemia: A prospective matched case-control study. *Critical Care, 24*. https://doi.org/10.1186/s13054-020-2766-1.

28. Pourajam, S., Kalantari, E., Talebzadeh, H., Mellali, H., Sami, R., Soltaninejad, F., Amra, B., *et al.* (2022). Secondary bacterial infection and clinical characteristics in patients with COVID-19 admitted to two intensive care units of an academic hospital in Iran during the first wave of the pandemic. *Frontiers in Cellular and Infection Microbiology, 12*. https://doi.org/10.3389/fcimb.2022.784130.

29. Rajah, K. H. (2025). Contemporary management strategies for appendicular abscess: A narrative review. *Malaysian Journal of Medical Research*. https://www.semanticscholar.org/paper/8808653aa9cde127f63d40f257c358d0958430b2 (accessed on 22 May 2025).

30. Rochwerg, B., Brochard, L., Elliott, M., Hess, D., Hill, N. S., Nava, S., Navalesi, P., *et al.* (2017). Official ERS/ATS clinical practice guidelines: Noninvasive ventilation for acute respiratory failure. *European Respiratory Journal, 50*, 1602426. https://doi.org/10.1183/13993003.02426-2016.

31. Sharma, S. J., Mohler, J. L., Mahajan, S. D., Schwartz, S. A., Bruggemann, L., & Aalinkeel, R. (2023). Microbial biofilm: A review on formation, infection, antibiotic resistance, control measures, and innovative treatment. *Microorganisms, 11*(6), 1614. https://doi.org/10.3390/microorganisms11061614.

32. Sonneville, R., Benghanem, S., Jeantin, L., de Montmollin, É., Doman, M., Gaudemer, A., Thy, M., *et al.* (2023). The spectrum of sepsis-associated encephalopathy: A clinical perspective. *Critical Care, 27*. https://doi.org/10.1186/s13054-023-04655-8.

33. Tabah, A., Lipman, J., Barbier, F., Buetti, N., & Timsit, J. (2022). Use of antimicrobials for bloodstream infections in the intensive care unit, a clinically oriented review. *Antibiotics, 11*. https://www.semanticscholar.org/paper/fe7087a2053efe2ba84fe691c1b51da8e2c8fb0a (accessed on 22 May 2025).

34. Wiersinga, W. J., Rhodes, A., Cheng, A. C., Peacock, S. J., & Prescott, H. C. (2020). Pathophysiology, transmission, diagnosis, and treatment of coronavirus disease 2019 (COVID-19). *JAMA, 324*(8), 782–793. https://doi.org/10.1001/jama.2020.12839.

35. World Health Organization. (2020). Clinical management of severe acute respiratory infection (SARI) when COVID-19 disease is suspected: Interim guidance. *Pediatric I Medycyna Rodzinna, 16*(1), 9–26. https://doi.org/10.15557/pimr.2020.0003.

36. Xie, Y., Cao, S., Dong, H., Li, Q. Y., Chen, E., Zhang, W., Yang, L., *et al.* (2020). Effect of regular intravenous immunoglobulin therapy on prognosis of severe pneumonia in patients with COVID-19. *Journal of Infection, 81*(2), 318–356. https://doi.org/10.1016/j.jinf.2020.03.044.

NUTRITIONAL SUPPORT IN CRITICAL ILLNESS

11

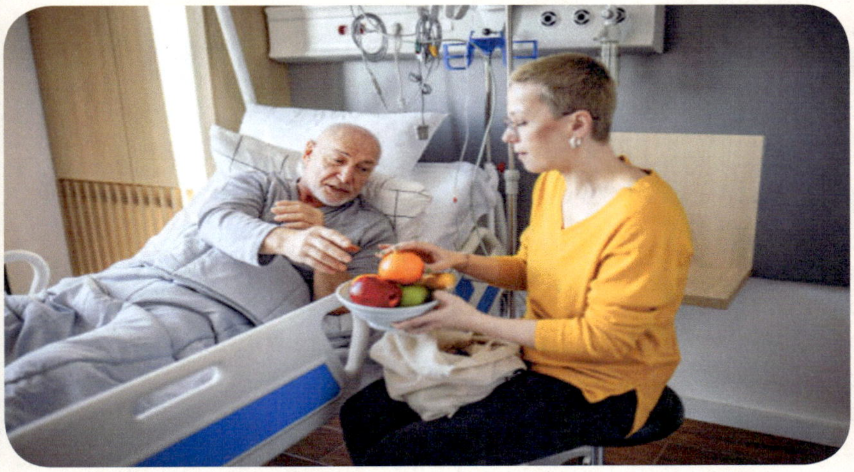

LEARNING OBJECTIVES

After studying this chapter, you will be able to:

1. Explain the types of nutritional support.
2. Define nutritional requirements in critical illness.
3. Discuss outcomes of nutritional support.
4. Understand the challenges and barriers to nutritional support.

Introduction

Nutritional care is important in helping patients recover and achieve better results when they are critically ill. Nutrition and critical care are linked because inadequate nutrition can slow down healing and make catabolic states worse in critically ill patients. For this reason, it is essential to use nutritional plans based on evidence and adapted to each patient, mainly for those with sepsis, since their metabolism can change a lot. As evidenced by guidelines from the Surviving Sepsis Campaign, the integration of nutritional support into the management of septic patients can improve overall care effectiveness and patient survival (Rhodes *et al.*, 2017). Moreover, the role of proper nutritional interventions extends into the realm of cognitive health, emphasizing the need for a robust approach to prevent complications such as delirium, which are prevalent in critically ill populations (Livingston *et al.*, 2020). So, it is essential to know the details of nutritional needs to provide the best care for patients in critical situations.

Definition of Critical Illness

It is essential to understand the meaning of critical illness to provide appropriate nutritional care for patients who are very sick. A critical illness is a wide range of conditions where organs do not function properly and need close observation and special care. This state might happen because of trauma, serious infections, or primary operations, which can cause significant changes in how the body uses nutrients. For example, if a patient is critically ill, their metabolism may be higher, and they may lose more protein than usual. Hence, they need ,exceptional nutritional help to recover and avoid additional problems. In these circumstances, working together across different medical specialties is very important, since managing critical illness often requires teamwork among various healthcare providers. Moreover, recognizing conditions such as Pediatric Feeding Disorder (PFD) helps elucidate the complexities surrounding feeding-related challenges in critically ill populations, emphasizing the need for comprehensive strategies that integrate medical, psychosocial, and nutritional support (Browne *et al.*, 2019; Wilson *et al.*, 2018).

Importance of Nutrition in Critical Care

Nutrition is important in critical care because it greatly helps patients to recover and achieve better results. Nutritional care helps protect metabolism from the adverse effects of stress and disease, and it also helps prevent nutrient shortages in critically ill patients. When patients eat properly, healthcare providers can help the immune system, encourage healing, and cut down on the time spent in the hospital. Research also indicates that individualized nutrition can help reduce health problems associated with prolonged bed rest, a common occurrence in intensive care units. Furthermore, as chronic conditions like dementia can increase the complexity of patient care, appropriate dietary management becomes even more essential in preventing additional health crises, such as delirium and decreased cognitive function (Livingston *et al.*, 2020). Hence, establishing effective nutritional protocols is vital for ensuring holistic patient care during critical illness (Yoshikawa *et al.*, 2020) (Figure 11.1).

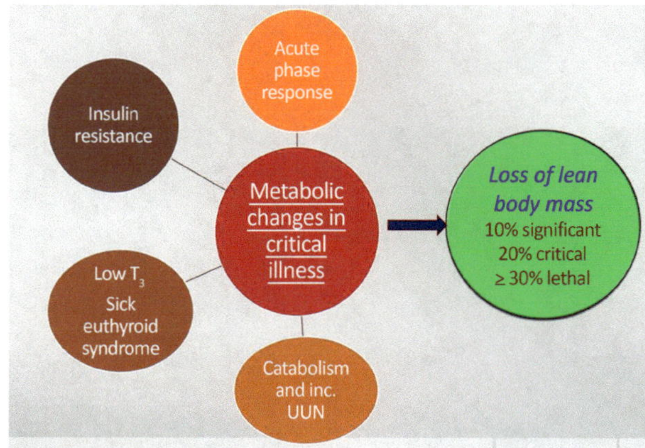

Figure 11.1. Importance of nutrition in critical care.

Source: https://image3.slideserve.com/6524570/importance-of-nutrition-in-critical-care-l.jpg.

Overview of Nutritional Support Methods

Giving proper nutrition is crucial in critical illness to help patients recover and control their metabolism. Because critical illness causes a hypermetabolic state, the primary nutritional interventions are enteral and parenteral nutrition. Most of the time, enteral nutrition is chosen because it uses the gut, which keeps it healthy and reduces the danger of infections that can happen with intravenous nutrition. Trouble with the gastrointestinal tract can stop enteral nutrition from working well, making clinicians turn to parenteral nutrition. Making these decisions even harder is the difficulty in measuring a patient's nutritional status, especially their lean body mass, which is commonly reduced in critically ill people.

Tools like bioelectrical impedance analysis and ultrasound are being explored to enhance assessment accuracy, yet their validation for bedside use remains inconsistent (de Rosa *et al.*, 2023). Ultimately, employing evidence-based strategies for nutritional support can significantly improve recovery times and reduce morbidity rates in critical care settings, as highlighted by recent research (Shetti, 2024).

Impact of Malnutrition on Recovery

Patients who are critically ill and malnourished find it harder to recover, their bodies are weaker, and they stay in the hospital for a more extended period. When a person is critically ill, their body needs more nutrients. However, they often eat less because of the illness, which can result in significant nutritional deficiencies that slow down recovery. Studies indicate that critically ill patients often exhibit increased muscle loss, aggravating their existing health conditions and leading to worse prognostic outcomes, necessitating urgent nutritional interventions in the ICU setting (Smith *et al.*, 2024). Furthermore, the systemic inflammation and immune dysfunction associated with malnutrition can contribute to a cycle of vulnerability, where patients are at risk of infections and complications, thereby delaying their return to baseline health. Nutritional support that is specifically designed for each patient is essential because it helps reduce adverse effects and supports their recovery.

Goals of Nutritional Support in Critical Illness

When someone is critically ill, nutritional support is mainly intended to cover the increased metabolic needs, prevent muscle wasting, and help them recover. As critically ill patients face a hypermetabolic state characterized by increased energy and protein requirements, appropriate nutritional interventions become paramount, cited by Shetti (2024). Effective nutritional strategies enhance recovery processes, reduce the duration of mechanical ventilation, and minimize length of stay in the intensive care unit (ICU). Providing patients with proper nutrients through enteral feeding can help prevent malnutrition-related issues, including weakness and prolonged recovery times. Furthermore, the administration of intermittent enteral feeding has shown advantages in reaching energetic targets more quickly. However, it may be associated with increased gastrointestinal complications such as diarrhea cited by Hrdý *et al.* (2025). So, providing the best nutritional care is important for improving the outcome of critically ill patients.

Role of Healthcare Professionals in Nutritional Care

Healthcare professionals are responsible for providing the proper nutritional support to patients with critical illness to help them recover well. Doctors, dietitians, and nurses in the interdisciplinary team up to analyze a patient's nutrition and design specific plans that address the body's metabolic changes due to illness. It is important to watch these plans, as malnutrition can slow down healing and raise the risk of death. Healthcare staff should be cautious for signs of nutritional shortfalls and respond by making changes as soon as possible, using practices that follow modern guidelines. Furthermore, as the COVID-19 pandemic has shifted healthcare dynamics, the focus on nutrition has become even more pronounced, particularly among vulnerable populations affected by both the virus and pre-existing health disparities, emphasizing the importance of timely nutritional interventions in achieving optimal patient outcomes (Stewart *et al.*, 2020; Yoshikawa *et al.*, 2020).

Current Trends in Nutritional Support

In recent years, the field of nutritional support in critical illness has witnessed significant advancements, aligning with emerging research and clinical practices. Tailoring nutrition therapy based on a person's needs and health issues is now seen as very important by many healthcare providers. Recent research indicates that early enteral feeding is crucial for patients, especially those with severe respiratory issues like COVID-19, as it provides the necessary energy and protein. Such tailored approaches not only optimize nourishment but also mitigate complications like malnutrition and prolonged hospitalization (Livingston *et al.*, 2020). Furthermore, the utilization of immune-modulating nutrients is being explored to bolster immune responses in critically ill patients, reflecting a shift towards a more holistic perspective on nutritional support (Naicker *et al.*, 2020). They demonstrate a strong focus on helping people in vulnerable groups to recover better and live better lives.

Challenges in Providing Nutritional Support

The challenges in providing nutritional support during critical illness are multifaceted and significantly impact patient outcomes. Being malnourished, which is common among critical patients, makes it harder for them to recover and can result in more health complications and deaths. Since metabolism, digestion, and other conditions can be changed, it is necessary to use special nutritional plans that can be hard to carry out. With the COVID-19 pandemic, health systems are overburdened, which has made it harder to provide routine nutritional care. Furthermore, socioeconomic factors and food insecurity can hinder access to adequate nutrition, particularly for vulnerable populations, resulting in disparities in care (Yoshikawa *et al.*, 2020). Emerging evidence emphasizes that a comprehensive approach, integrating nutrition as a core component of critical care, can enhance recovery, underscoring the urgency of addressing these barriers in nutritional support (Sattar *et al.*, 2020).

11.1. Types of Nutritional Support

Learning Outcome

1. Discuss the enteral nutrition: definition and methods
2. Explain the parenteral nutrition: definition and methods
3. Define oral nutritional supplements: types and benefits
4. Understand the timing of nutritional interventions
5. Analyze the assessment of nutritional needs
6. Describe the role of feeding tubes in enteral nutrition
7. Explain the complications associated with parenteral nutrition
8. Discuss the transitioning from parenteral to enteral nutrition
9. Define personalized nutrition plans for patients

During critical illness, the kind of nutrition given to the patient is essential for their recovery and general care. Usually, enteral nutrition is tried first by delivering food directly to the gut so that patients can get enough calories, and gut function is preserved. If enteral nutrition cannot be used, parenteral nutrition is given by injecting nutrients into a vein. Latest studies point out that personalized nutritional plans should be designed according to what each patient needs. For instance, specialized formulas tailored for inflammatory responses can significantly enhance recovery metrics, especially in respiratory conditions like COVID-19, where patient demands fluctuate rapidly (Livingston *et al.*, 2020). Including sufficient micronutrients in nutrition can support the immune system, thereby decreasing the risk of secondary infections and improving outcomes for critically ill patients. Hence, using a combination of nutritional methods is very important for those with critical illness.

11.1.1. Enteral Nutrition: Definition and Methods

Nutrients are given directly into the stomach or intestines through a tube in enteral nutrition, helping patients who cannot eat on their own. This method is important for people who are seriously ill, as their health problems can affect their digestive system. Nasogastric tubes, gastrostomy, and jejunostomy are used to make sure patients get the proper nutrition and avoid malnutrition, which can significantly influence their recovery and chances of survival. Research indicates that adequate enteral feeding can mitigate complications associated with prolonged hospitalization, such as extended mechanical ventilation and poor clinical outcomes (Somani *et al.*, 2025). Moreover, as patients transition from intensive care to general wards, developing structured rehabilitation strategies that incorporate optimized enteral nutrition is crucial for fostering physical independence and improving overall patient outcomes (McWilliams *et al.*, 2025) (Figure 11.2).

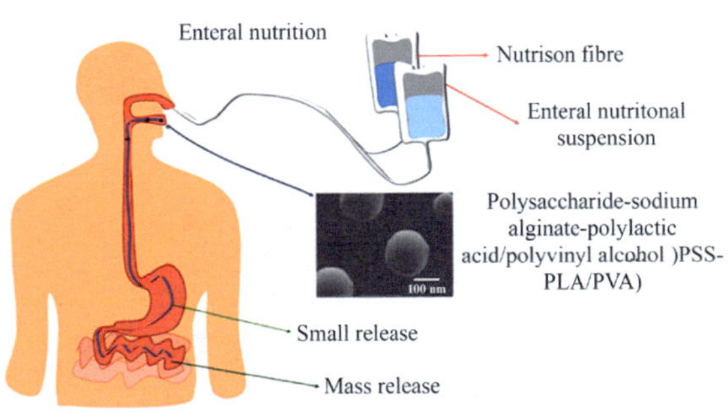

Figure 11.2. Enteral nutrition administration and absorption route.

Source: https://www.researchgate.net/figure/Enteral-nutrition-administration-and-absorption-route_fig1_361667721.

11.1.2. Parenteral Nutrition (PN): Definition and Methods

In the context of critical illness, PN serves as a vital intervention for patients unable to meet their nutritional needs through oral or enteral routes. PN is a way to provide nutrients through the veins, which makes it possible to give patients the specific macronutrients and micronutrients they need to recover. Various methods exist for implementing PN, including the use of total parenteral nutrition (TPN), which provides complete nutritional support, and supplementary parenteral nutrition, often utilized alongside enteral feeding. Recent findings underscore the importance of the composition of intravenous lipid emulsions (ILEs) within PN formulations, particularly for surgical patients, thereby enhancing clinical outcomes and recovery from severe conditions (Martindale *et al.*, 2025). Additionally, establishing a timely initiation of nutritional support, whether through early enteral nutrition or parenteral means, is critical, as malnutrition significantly correlates with increased morbidity and mortality in critically ill patients (Zhang *et al.*, 2024). Collectively, these elements highlight the essential role of PN in optimizing patient care during critical illness (Figure 11.3).

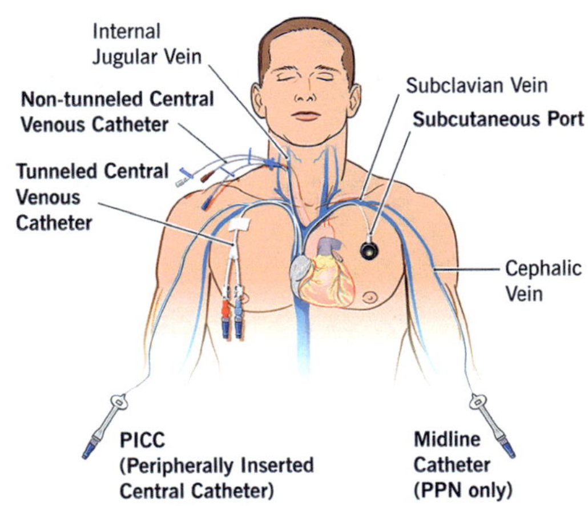

Figure 11.3. Parenteral nutrition (PN).

Source: https://my.clevelandclinic.org/-/scassets/images/org/health/articles/22802-parenteral-nutrition.

11.1.3. Oral Nutritional Supplements (ONS): Types and Benefits

In critical illness, ONS plays a crucial role in improving patient outcomes. Different ONS are available, such as standard, high-protein, fiber-enriched, and immune-modulating, which are meant to help with various nutritional needs. For example, high-protein supplements help patients who are losing muscle or recovering from surgery by giving them the amino acids needed for repair and recovery.

Adding fiber to a patient's diet may help manage digestive problems, and immune-modulating formulas with arginine, glutamine, and omega-3 fatty acids can improve the immune system and reduce inflammation. By offering tailored nutritional support, these supplements can bolster recovery, decrease length of hospital stays, and potentially improve survival rates in critically ill patients, a goal echoed by established guidelines for nutritional care (Rhodes *et al.*, 2017; Taylor *et al.*, 2016) (Figure 11.4).

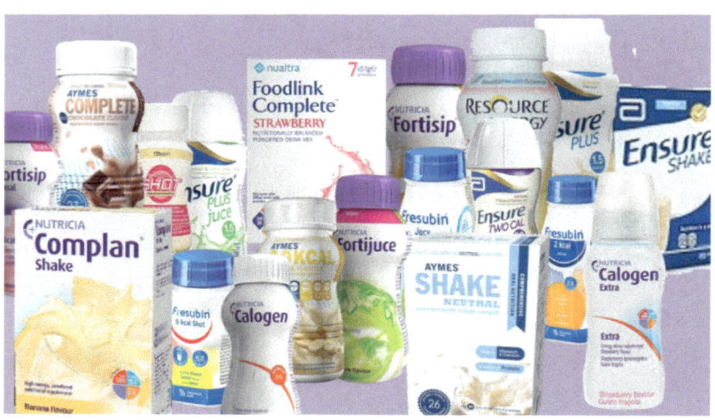

Figure 11.4. Oral nutritional supplement (ONS).

Source: https://media.licdn.com/dms/image/v2/C4E12AQFn-GhSsgJz8g/article-cover_image-shrink_600_2000/article-cover_image-shrink_600_2000/0/1611570044686?e=2147483647&v=beta&t=eych6miR_yuk9iYCfuJSlst9HCYasWTTJFUg6csXfjM.

11.1.4. Timing of Nutritional Interventions

Providing nutritional support is crucial for patients with critical illness, as their bodies require increased energy. Early initiation of enteral nutrition is recommended to mitigate the risk of malnutrition and muscle wasting, which are prevalent in critically ill patients (Shetti, 2024). This way of eating helps the immune system and also helps maintain lean body mass, which is very important for recovery. Moreover, the strategic timing of these interventions, particularly within the first 24–48 hours of ICU admission, can enhance clinical outcomes and reduce the length of mechanical ventilation (Dumitriu *et al.*, 2025). Healthcare providers need to watch the patient's nutrition and adjust their care plan accordingly as the patient's needs evolve during hospitalization. So, giving nutritional strategies that are prompt and tailored to each patient is key to helping critically ill individuals recover and have a better outcome.

11.1.5. Assessment of Nutritional Needs

Assessing nutritional needs is very important in "Nutritional Support in Critical Illness" to help patients recover. When a person has a critical illness, their metabolism can change, and their ability to absorb nutrients may be affected, so each patient needs an individual assessment. Effective assessment strategies include thorough clinical evaluations and methodologies like bioelectrical impedance analysis (BIA), which can elucidate shifts in body composition during illness. By employing BIA, healthcare providers can better understand the intricate physiological changes that accompany critical conditions, thus informing tailored nutritional interventions (Dumitriu *et al.*, 2025). Also, it is important to understand that patients have needs in many areas, such as their physical, emotional, and social well-being. As evidenced by studies on vulnerable populations, such as orphans, addressing comprehensive needs can significantly enhance overall well-being and recovery during critical episodes, further demonstrating the importance of holistic nutritional assessments (Victoria *et al.*, 2024) (Figure 11.5).

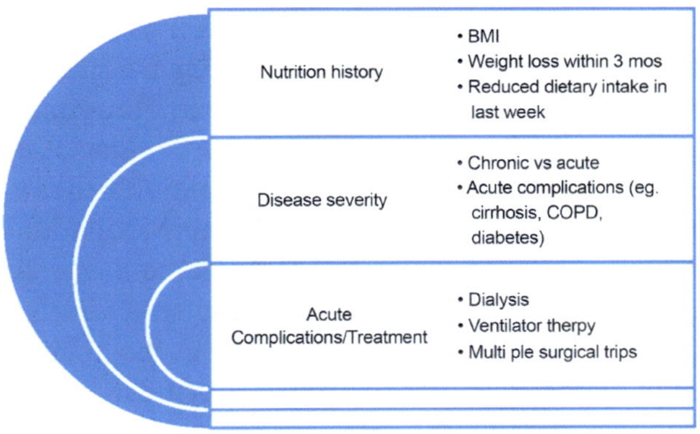

Figure 11.5. Nutrition assessment in the critically ill.

Source: https://www.researchgate.net/figure/Nutrition-assessment-in-the-critically-ill_fig1_313261163.

11.1.6. Role of Feeding Tubes in Enteral Nutrition

In patients who are critically ill, feeding tubes are important for ensuring that enteral nutrition is provided, which helps meet their body's needs and aids in their recovery. Tubes used for enteral feeding are helpful because they support gastrointestinal activity and the strength of the gut, which are usually reduced in these patients. Emerging guidelines suggest that low-volume enteral feeds can stimulate intestinal function without overwhelming the system, thereby mitigating the risks associated with high-volume feeding, such as ischemic bowel necrosis (Weimann *et al.*, 2016). Furthermore, the careful administration of enteral nutrition fosters the preservation of mucosal health.. It contributes to reduced rates of infection, a critical consideration in the management of sepsis and septic shock (Rhodes *et al.*, 2017). By adhering to recommended practices and monitoring biomarkers of gut function, healthcare providers can optimize nutritional support, ultimately enhancing patient outcomes during critical illness (Figure 11.6).

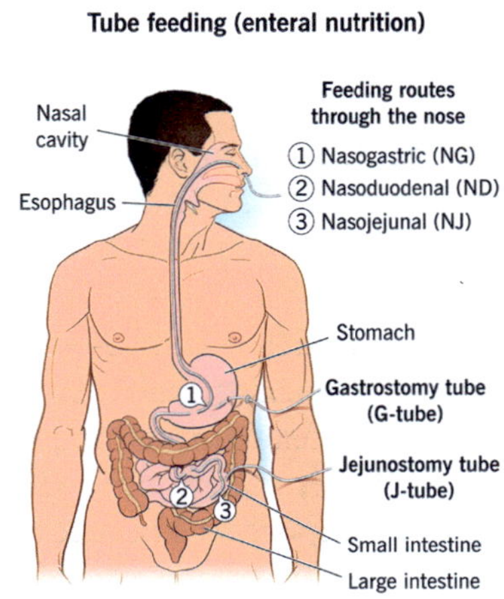

Figure 11.6. Feeding tube placement depends on your condition and how long you willyou will need enteral nutrition.

Source: https://my.clevelandclinic.org/-/scassets/images/org/health/articles/21098-tube-feeding-enteral-nutrition.jpg.

11.1.7. Complications Associated with Parenteral Nutrition (PN)

While PN is needed to give nutrients to critically ill patients, it can still cause some problems. Side effects of PN are metabolic problems, a greater risk of infection, and issues with the digestive system. Studies suggest that patients receiving enteral nutrition (EN) may experience higher rates of digestive complications compared to those on PN, indicating the need for careful selection of nutritional support routes based on individual patient conditions (Shams *et al.*, 2024). Furthermore, the presence of acute kidney injury (AKI), common in critically ill patients, complicates PN, as these individuals often require tailored nutritional assessments to prevent hyperglycemia, fluid imbalances, and electrolyte disturbances (Fiaccadori *et al.*, 2018). Therefore, it is important to watch for these issues and adjust nutritional plans so that the benefits of PN are high and the risks are low, which helps patients recover better from severe illness.

11.1.8. Transitioning from Parenteral to Enteral Nutrition

Moving from parenteral to EN is an important step for critically ill patients, since it helps support their metabolism and lowers the risk of problems linked to long-term parenteral nutrition. Initiating EN within 24–48 hours of admission has been associated with improved gut integrity, decreased infectious morbidity, and shorter intensive care unit (ICU) stays, demonstrating its importance in recovery during critical illness (Vinícius Cruzat *et al.*, 2018). This shift not only conserves the functionality of the gastrointestinal (GI) tract but also mitigates metabolic derangements that arise from prolonged parenteral nutrition (Vinícius Cruzat *et al.*, 2018). However, it is essential to assess individual patient factors, such as GI function and the risk of aspiration, prior to transition (McClave *et al.*, 2016). Regular observation is important to ensure the patient is tolerating the nutrition and feeding plans, and that the plans are updated to improve results and reduce the risks of both methods.

11.1.9. Personalized Nutrition Plans for Patients

In the field of critical illness, giving patients personalized nutrition plans has become very important for their care. When nutritional care is adapted to the needs of each patient, their recovery and quality of life can improve a lot. Research indicates that a well-structured dietary approach, which includes a comprehensive assessment of nutritional status immediately following diagnosis, plays a crucial role in managing conditions like cancer and post-surgical recovery (Caetano *et al.*, 2024). Personalized nutrition plans consider various factors, including age, gender, and lifestyle, enabling healthcare providers to devise strategies that promote optimal macro- and micronutrient intake (Chojnacka *et al.*, 2024). This way of feeding patients helps prevent malnutrition and meets their individual metabolic needs, which strengthens them as they deal with their illnesses. Thus, the shift toward personalized nutrition is essential in the holistic management of patients facing critical health challenges (Figure 11.7).

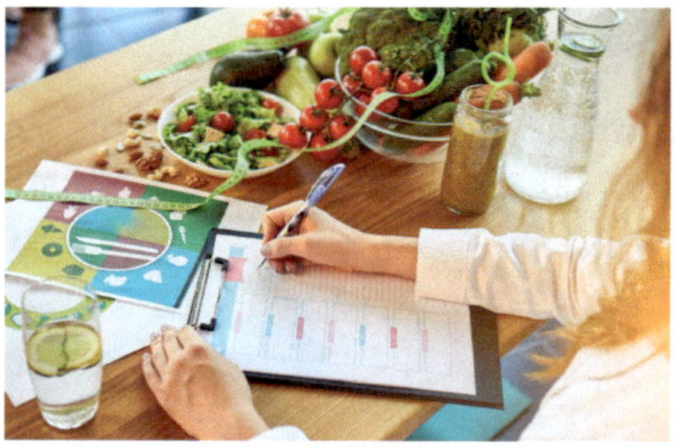

Figure 11.7. Patients personalized nutrition plans.

Source: https://external-content.duckduckgo.com/iu/?u=https%3A%2F%2Fwww.totalhealthandfitness.com%2Fwp-content%2Fuploads%2F2023%2F02%2Fpersonalized-nutrition-Large.jpeg&f=1&nofb=1&ipt=2c732857171866fe54381edab4f641fa7031734614c3160b0ed514a6a417912a.

Test Your Knowledge

1. What are the common methods of delivering enteral nutrition, and when is it indicated?
2. How does parenteral nutrition differ from enteral nutrition in terms of administration and clinical use?
3. What are the benefits of oral nutritional supplements, and why is timely nutritional intervention important in patient care?

11.2. Nutritional Requirements in Critical Illness

Learning Outcome

1. Define macronutrient needs: carbohydrates, proteins, fats
2. Discuss micronutrient needs: vitamins and minerals
3. Explain the energy expenditure in critically ill patients
4. Describe the factors influencing nutritional requirements
5. Identify the role of inflammation in nutritional needs
6. Analyze the assessment tools for determining nutritional needs
7. Discuss the adjustments for specific conditions (e.g., sepsis, trauma)
8. Explain the importance of protein in wound healing
9. Define monitoring and adjusting nutritional support

Because critical illness changes the body's needs and can cause metabolic issues, proper nutrition for patients is essential. Starting nutrition early is important because it helps improve outcomes by reducing the breakdown of the body due to illness, preserving lean muscles, and aiding recovery. The evidence suggests that both enteral and parenteral nutrition strategies must be tailored to the individual's specific metabolic needs, particularly in cases of sepsis or septic shock, where energy and protein requirements may be significantly elevated (Evans *et al.*, 2021). For pediatric populations, particularly critically ill neonates, there remains considerable debate regarding the optimal timing and composition of nutritional interventions; guidelines indicate that a systematic approach is essential for addressing these complexities effectively (Moltu *et al.*, 2021). As a result, carefully assessing what nutrients patients need is very important for the care of critically ill patients to aid in their recovery and lower their risk of complications.

11.2.1. Macronutrient Needs: Carbohydrates, Proteins, and Fats

Good nutrition in critical illness means making sure to provide enough carbohydrates, proteins, and fats. Carbohydrates provide the primary energy for the body, help control blood sugar, and power cells, especially in sick patients with high metabolic rates. Proteins play a vital role in tissue repair and immune function, and their increased needs are often evident in critically ill individuals, necessitating higher protein intake to prevent muscle wasting and support healing (Formenti *et al.*, 2021). Essential fatty acids and energy come from fats, and people may need to adjust their intake based on how their bodies use them. Recent studies underscore the importance of tailored nutritional support, advocating for balanced macronutrient ratios to address the unique demands of critical care patients (Mustafa, 2024). A careful assessment of each patient's macronutrient needs is therefore imperative in improving outcomes and facilitating recovery in critical illness (Figure 11.8).

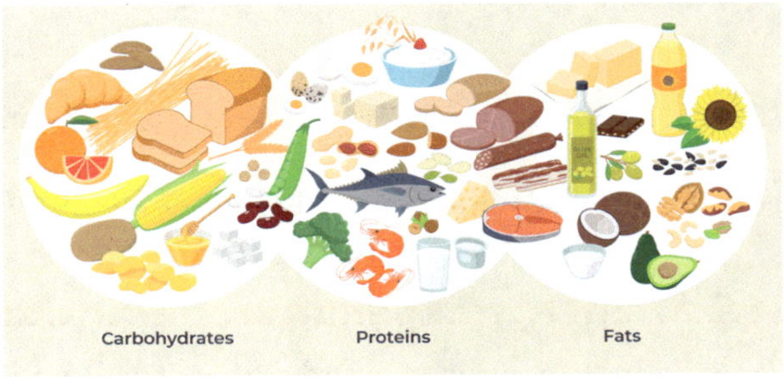

Figure 11.8. Macronutrients.

Source: https://innerbody.imgix.net/macronutrients-nutrition.jpg.

11.2.2. Micronutrient Needs: Vitamins and Minerals

Getting enough vitamins and minerals is very important for the immune system and the overall recovery of a person with a critical illness. Vitamins A, C, D, and E, as well as zinc, iron, and selenium, are important for the immune system and the normal functions of the body. It is clear from their interactions that these nutrients help each other, which means it is important to have enough of them in your diet to prevent problems caused by illness. Research shows that various populations experiencing chronic conditions, such as those impacted by COVID-19, often present with inadequate micronutrient levels, which can exacerbate health risks and hinder recovery processes (Gao *et al.*, 2020). Thus, ensuring that critically ill patients receive appropriate micronutrient supplementation is vital, as even marginal deficiencies can impair immunity and prolong recovery time (Gombart *et al.*, 2020). Addressing these needs can ultimately enhance patient outcomes in critical care settings (Figure 11.9).

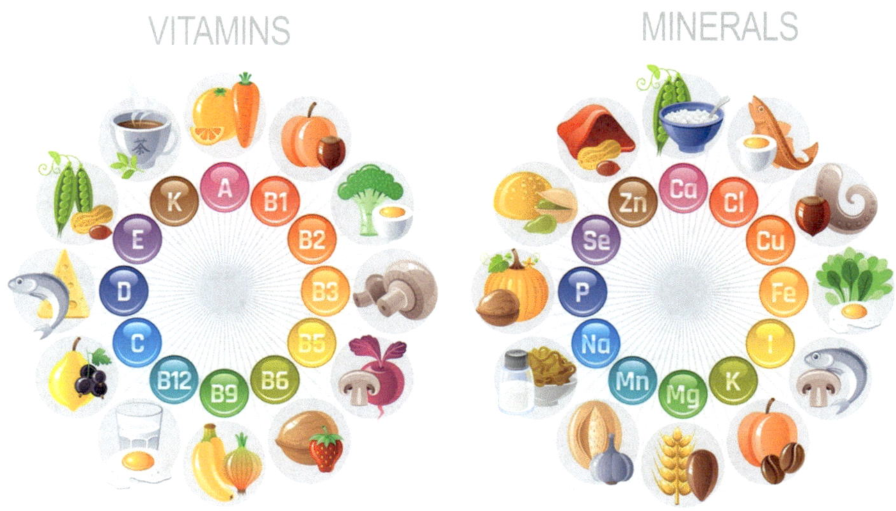

Figure 11.9. Micronutrients specifically vitamins and minerals.

Source: https://blog.nasm.org/hubfs/image-png-1.png.

11.2.3. Energy Expenditure in Critically Ill Patients

Measuring the energy needs of critically ill patients is not easy, but it is essential for good nutrition. Indirect calorimetry (IC) has emerged as the gold standard for determining resting energy expenditure (REE), allowing for a more tailored approach to nutrition that actively addresses individual metabolic needs. Studies indicate that IC-guided nutrition significantly enhances energy delivery, thereby reducing short-term mortality in this vulnerable population, as evidenced by findings that showcase a notable decrease in mortality risk when energy intake aligns with metabolic requirements (Duan *et al.*, 2021). However, because energy use in critical illness can vary, it introduces additional challenges, as the patient's metabolic needs may fluctuate. The initial catabolic phase may lead to potential overfeeding if exogenous nutrition attempts to surpass endogenous energy production, which is often elevated in early stages (Moonen *et al.*, 2021). Therefore, accurately measuring and adjusting nutritional support based on energy expenditure is crucial for optimizing outcomes in critically ill patients (Figure 11.10).

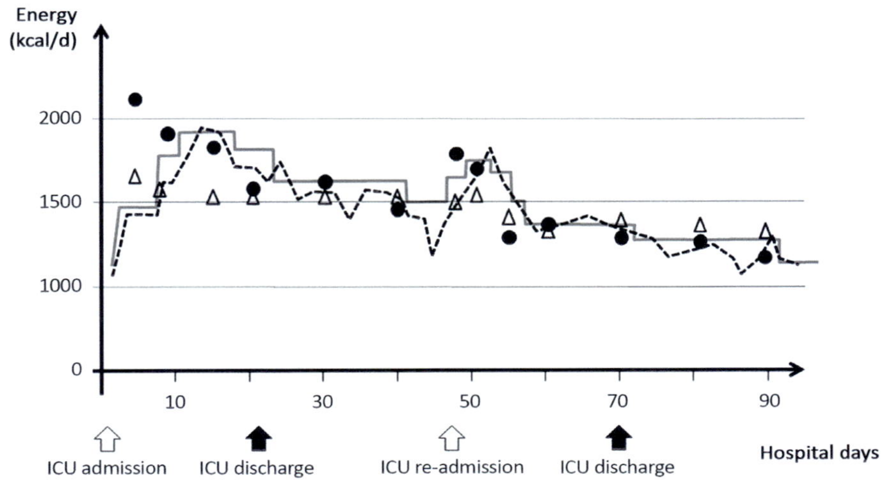

Figure 11.10. Evolution of energy expenditure in critically ill patients.

Source: https://www.researchgate.net/figure/Evolution-of-energy-expenditure-in-critically-ill-patients-The-evolution-of-energy_fig3_304339946.

11.2.4. Factors Influencing Nutritional Requirements

It is important to understand what affects nutritional needs to create good nutritional support for critically ill patients. Different factors, such as a person's metabolic rate, other health problems, and past surgeries, are important in determining what nutrients a person needs. For instance, patients undergoing bariatric surgery often face challenges due to anatomical changes, which can impair gastrointestinal function and alter nutrient absorption, complicating nutritional management (Correia *et al.*, 2024). Additionally, the variability in insulin dosing protocols among hospitals underscores the importance of tailored approaches to nutritional care, particularly in the context of glycemic control, which can directly affect recovery and overall outcomes (Chiang *et al.*, 2024). Since critical illness can cause more metabolic problems and make the body need more nutrients, it is important to do a thorough nutritional assessment for each patient to help them recover.

11.2.5. Role of Inflammation in Nutritional Needs

In critically ill patients, the link between inflammation and nutrition is obvious, because an inflammatory reaction can make it harder for them to get the nutrition they need. Acute inflammation usually causes catabolism, which makes the body require more energy and protein for healing. Moreover, the inflammatory status influences the gut microbiota, which plays a vital role in nutrient absorption and modulation of immune responses, highlighting the need for tailored nutritional interventions (Cryan *et al.*, 2019). Recent guidelines underscore that adequate nutritional support should address these altered requirements while also managing the metabolic disturbances induced by critical illness (Taylor *et al.*, 2016). Proper nutrition can help patients recover and also reduce how severe the inflammation becomes, which highlights the importance of using nutrition in the care of critically ill patients.

11.2.6. Assessment Tools for Determining Nutritional Needs

Correctly assessing nutrition in critical care is important for helping patients recover and avoiding issues. Several ways to assess threats are used, and BIA is seen as especially helpful. BIA allows clinicians to see how a patient's body composition changes in real time, which helps them adjust the patient's nutritional care. Additionally, the use of innovative devices like Glucosafe 2 (GS2) has revolutionized the management of nutritional requirements and glucose control in intensive care. The device helps healthcare professionals give precise directions, so patients can keep their blood glucose within the right range and still receive proper nutrition. This dual approach of employing BIA alongside GS2 highlights the importance of comprehensive assessments in ensuring effective nutritional strategies, ultimately enhancing patient outcomes in critical illness (de Watteville *et al.*, 2025; Dumitriu *et al.*, 2025) (Figure 11.11).

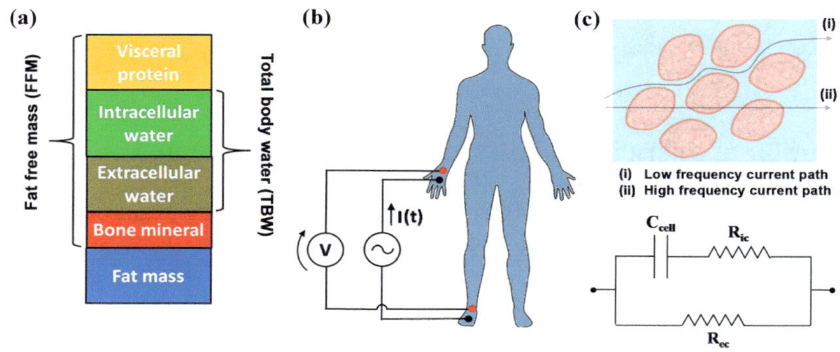

Figure 11.11. Bioelectrical impedance analysis (BIA) principle of work.

Source: https://www.researchgate.net/figure/Bioelectrical-Impedance-Analysis-BIA-principle-of-work_fig5_319317929.

11.2.7. Adjustments for Specific Conditions (e.g., Sepsis, Trauma)

Because critically ill patients with sepsis and trauma need different nutrition, adjustments must be made according to their condition. Such conditions usually result in significant changes in the body's metabolism, which alters how much nutrition is needed. For instance, sepsis is characterized by heightened energy expenditure and altered macronutrient utilization due to the inflammatory response, which may demand increased caloric intake to mitigate muscle wasting and organ failure (Huang *et al.*, 2022).

Similarly, trauma causes the body to react in many ways, which may lead to a quicker metabolism and require particular vitamins and minerals to help the body heal. In the context of COVID-19, the Surviving Sepsis Campaign has emphasized the importance of tailoring nutritional interventions for critically ill patients to enhance immune function and support overall recovery (Alhazzani *et al.*, 2020). So, taking these specific needs into account is important for choosing the best nutritional approach in critical illness.

11.2.8. Importance of Protein in Wound Healing

Protein is important for healing wounds, since it affects many important functions needed for recovery. New tissue is formed with the help of proteins, which also support the production of collagen, which is essential for the strength and integrity of healing tissue. Having enough protein in your diet helps your immune system, which reduces the chance of infections at the wound site. Research indicates that insufficient protein intake can hinder healing and exacerbate complications, particularly for patients undergoing surgery or managing chronic wounds. This points out that it is important to include enough protein in the diet of critically ill patients. Nurses and healthcare providers should assess patients' protein intake and make adjustments to their diet or recommend supplements as needed to support their health. These interventions, highlighted in recent literature, underscore the vital connection between nutritional support and effective wound healing (Alshahrani *et al.*, 2024; Hill *et al.*, 2025).

11.2.9. Monitoring and Adjusting Nutritional Support

It is critical to monitor and modify nutritional care for critically ill patients, since they may easily become malnourished and lose muscle, which can slow their recovery. Since critical illness is constantly changing, the nutrition plan should be adjusted to meet the patient's evolving metabolic needs. Using indirect calorimetry helps doctors precisely measure how many calories the patient needs. Frequently checking patients' nutrient intake using clinical tools can help find any differences between what is prescribed and what they eat so that action can be taken quickly. In light of the challenges presented by prolonged ICU stays, particularly in patients with persistent critical illness, strategies for continuous monitoring and modification of nutritional support can significantly enhance patient outcomes, including reduced morbidity and mortality rates (Shetti, 2024; Smith *et al.*, 2024).

Test Your Knowledge

1. What roles do carbohydrates, proteins, and fats play in meeting the macronutrient needs of critically ill patients?
2. Why are vitamins and minerals essential in critical care, and how are micronutrient needs assessed?
3. What factors influence energy expenditure and nutritional requirements in critically ill patients?

11.3. Outcomes of Nutritional Support

Learning Outcome

1. Identify the impact on length of hospital stay
2. Define influence on recovery rates
3. Describe the role in reducing complications
4. Understand the effects on immune function
5. Explain the relationship between nutrition and mortality
6. Discuss quality of life post-critical illness
7. Understand the cost-effectiveness of nutritional interventions
8. Explain the long-term outcomes of nutritional support

How well nutritional support works in critical illness depends on a patient's initial level of inflammation, which can have a significant impact on outcomes such as survival. For instance, a secondary analysis of the EFFORT trial revealed that patients receiving individualized nutritional support experienced a notable reduction in 30-day mortality, irrespective of their initial inflammatory levels, except those with high inflammation, where support appeared ineffective (Merker *et al.*, 2020). As a result, it is important to use individual nutritional strategies since inflammation can influence metabolism and appetite during sickness. Furthermore, this complexity is echoed in pediatric critical care, where the lack of robust trials often leads to varied nutritional practices across intensive care units (Tume *et al.*, 2020). All in all, these findings suggest that understanding the interplay between inflammation and nutrition is crucial for enhancing outcomes in critical care.

11.3.1. Impact on Length of Hospital Stay

How much time critically ill patients spend in the hospital is strongly affected by their nutritional support, which significantly influences their recovery and the final results. It seems that early and effective nutrition support can help prevent complications and allow patients to leave the hospital sooner. If patients are given enteral feeding within 24–48 hours of admission, they often have better metabolic function and fewer infections, which helps them leave the hospital sooner. Furthermore, inadequate nutrition can exacerbate acute kidney injury, potentially leading to a more extended hospital stay. For example, studies have indicated an association between malnutrition and adverse outcomes, including extended treatment durations for critically ill patients, emphasizing the urgent need for individualized care strategies in these settings (Naicker *et al.*, 2020; Rhodes *et al.*, 2017). Therefore, optimizing nutritional support is critical in enhancing recovery trajectories and minimizing hospital stay lengths for patients facing critical illness (Figure 11.12).

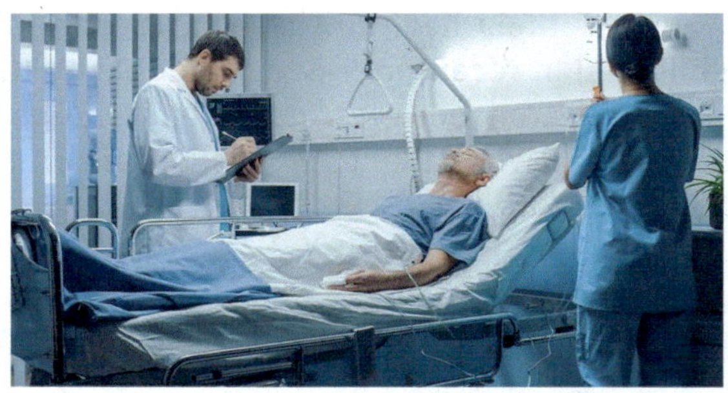

Figure 11.12. The average length of stay for a patient in the U.S. is 4.5 days. Many hospitals are aware that length of stay is an important metric to keep track of, and that it's better to strive for shorter lengths of stay where possible.

Source: https://www.pulsara.com/blog/every-minute-counts-how-increased-length-of-stay-impacts-patients-and-hospitals.

11.3.2. Influence on Recovery Rates

The role of nutritional support in the recovery of critically ill patients is crucial, since it dramatically improves their health and clinical outcomes. Nutritional care helps the body heal well and lowers the chance of developing complications in critical illness. Studies have shown that nutrition tailored to each person's metabolic needs can accelerate recovery by enhancing immunity and reducing inflammation. Nutritional adequacy helps wounds heal faster, speeds up rehabilitation, and lowers the death rate among people who are critically ill. Also, the type of dialysis chosen can alter cardiac biomarkers, and this connection can reveal the way a patient recovers. The presence of elevated cardiac markers, such as cTNT and NT-proBNP, indicates the necessity for comprehensive management strategies that include nutritional support to address underlying health stresses during recovery (Maslach *et al.*, 2016; Rosa *et al.*, 2017) (Figure 11.13).

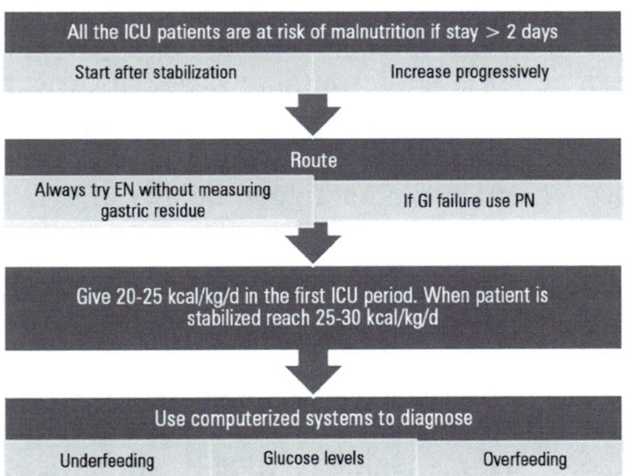

Figure 11.13. Flow chart to achieve nutritional support effectiveness in critically ill patients.

Source: https://www.researchgate.net/figure/Flow-chart-to-achieve-nutritional-support-effectiveness-in-critically-ill-patients_fig1_312519436.

11.3.3. Role in Reducing Complications

Nutritional support is essential in critical illness because it helps to reduce problems and improve patient outcomes. Strong nutritional support at the beginning can significantly decrease the chances of metabolic disorders and support recovery. Evidence suggests that tailored nutritional strategies, such as early enteral nutrition and personalized diet plans, are essential in preventing malnutrition and minimizing muscle wasting among critically ill patients (Shetti, 2024).

Also, dealing with metabolic problems such as starvation ketoacidosis highlights the need for proper nutrition. In particular, patients exhibiting signs of hypoalbuminemia and low body mass index upon ICU admission are at heightened risk for complications like hemodynamic instability and shock (Ottaviani *et al.*, 2024). Supposenutritional status is managed well early in treatment, clinicians can reduce the adverse effects of critical illness, which results in shorter stays in the ICU and a lower risk of complications and death.

11.3.4. Effects on Immune Function

The health of the immune system in critical illness is greatly influenced by nutrition, and this can make the disease more severe and slow down recovery. Malnutrition weakens the immune system, which makes people more likely to get infections, stay in the hospital for longer, and die more often. Shortages of vitamins A, C, D, E, zinc, and selenium may result in a weak immune system that does not mobilize many immune cells and has diminished inflammatory responses. Obesity is also related to a weaker immune system, which can result in extra adipose tissue boosting inflammatory markers and lowering the ability of the immune system to fight off infections, possibly causing more severe outcomes in critical illness. These relationships underscore the critical role of optimal nutrition in supporting immune function, ultimately emphasizing the need for targeted nutritional interventions in managing critically ill patients (Sattar *et al.*, 2020; Yoshikawa *et al.*, 2020).

11.3.5. Relationship Between Nutrition and Mortality

The link between nutrition and mortality in critically ill patients is now recognized as very important for better outcomes. Malnutrition, prevalent among those with chronic critical illnesses, adversely impacts immune function, recovery rates, and overall survival (Chen *et al.*, 2024). It is essential to address the hypermetabolic state driven by critical illness, which exacerbates nutritional needs and contributes to muscle wasting, thereby increasing the risk of complications and mortality (Shetti, 2024). If patients receive proper nutrition early, their recovery in the hospital can improve, they may need less time on a ventilator, and their chances of complications can decrease. Tailoring nutrition to each patient's needs, such as personalized nutrition and immunonutrition, helps address the problems of malnutrition, proving how important nutritional intervention is in critical care. Thus, ensuring appropriate nutritional support not only enhances patient recovery but is also vital in reducing mortality rates among critically ill individuals (Figure 11.14).

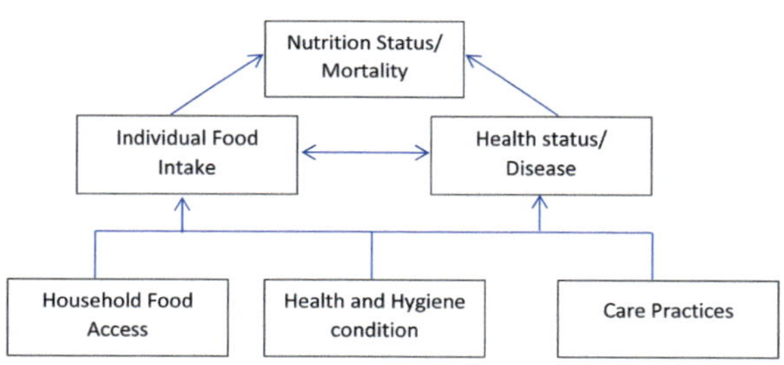

Figure 11.14. Conceptual framework of nutrition and COVID-19 mortality and survival among older persons.

Source: https://journals.sagepub.com/doi/10.1177/00469580211059738?icid=int.sj-abstract.similar-articles.4.

11.3.6. Quality of Life Post-Critical Illness

It is now more important than ever to understand how patients feel after critical illness, since healthcare is focusing on personalized care. In these cases, giving nutritional support is very important, since it helps patients recover better after they leave the hospital. Research indicates that individualized nutritional interventions can significantly reduce complications and enhance functional recovery, ultimately influencing the quality of life in survivors of critical illness (Merker *et al.*, 2019). Having family members involved in nutrition care can help patients recover more easily by giving them more support. The IMPACT trial exemplifies this by showcasing how family involvement in nutritional advocacy can enhance patient outcomes and satisfaction with care (Heyland *et al.*, 2018). While refining post-critical care practices, it is clear that meeting nutritional needs is significant for helping these people recover and maintain a good quality of life.

11.3.7. Cost-Effectiveness of Nutritional Interventions

More attention is being given to how cost-effective nutritional interventions are in critical illness, as managing critically ill patients is very expensive. Using well-structured rehabilitation methods with nutritional support can significantly improve recovery, which helps lower the cost of long-term care. For instance, research indicates that 84% of ICU survivors require ongoing nutritional support, yet many are discharged without a coordinated nutrition plan, leading to persistent malnutrition and complications during recovery (McWilliams *et al.*, 2025). This inadequacy not only hinders physical rehabilitation but may subsequently increase healthcare resource utilization (O'Neill *et al.*, 2025). If healthcare systems provide nutritional and rehabilitation programs in the ICU and general ward in that case, they may be able to lower future expenses by helping patients live better and reducing the number of readmissions. All in all, making nutritional interventions better helps improve patient outcomes and saves money in critical care.

11.3.8. Long-Term Outcomes of Nutritional Support

More and more, it is understood that how critically ill patients are fed affects their long-term recovery and growth. It has been found that the proper nutrition for kids can significantly affect their health now and in the future. For instance, the PEPaNIC randomized controlled trial demonstrated that delaying parenteral nutrition during the first week of PICU admission led to reduced infections and quicker recovery, while subsequent follow-up revealed no adverse effects on growth metrics; in fact, neurocognitive and psychosocial development showed improvement two to four years later (Eveleens *et al.*, 2020). Additionally, early nutritional deficits, particularly in iron, can increase the risk of long-term developmental impairments in infants, thereby underscoring the importance of appropriate dietary interventions during critical phases of growth (N/A, 2020). They show that specialized nutritional programs are needed to help both current health and future development.

Test Your Knowledge

1. How does proper nutritional support impact the length of hospital stay in critically ill patients?
2. In what ways does nutrition influence recovery rates and overall patient outcomes?
3. How does adequate nutrition help reduce complications and support immune function in critical care?

11.4. Challenges and Barriers to Nutritional Support

Learning Outcome

1. Identifying malnutrition in critical care
2. Explain the limitations of current assessment tools
3. Discuss the patient tolerance and gastrointestinal issues
4. Define resource availability and access to nutrition
5. Understand the interdisciplinary communication barriers
6. Analyze the ethical considerations in nutritional support
7. Define cultural and personal preferences in nutrition
8. Discuss the variability in clinical guidelines
9. Explain the future research needs in nutritional support

There are many problems and obstacles when providing nutrition to patients with critical illness, which make it challenging to give the best care. A major problem is that healthcare professionals do not use existing guidelines as much as they should, which is partly because of poor training and limited support for teams that focus on nutrition. Also, delays in getting nutritional products and differences in priorities among healthcare workers make the situation worse. Also, because of complications like changes in metabolism and digestion, it is difficult to ensure proper nutrition in these patients. These barriers are compounded by economic factors, as many healthcare facilities allocate limited budgets to nutritional interventions, impacting the quality of care (Hossain *et al.*, 2019). Furthermore, misunderstanding among caregivers regarding the importance of nutritional support can lead to neglect of these vital interventions, resulting in poorer patient outcomes (Rosa *et al.*, 2017).

Overcoming these problems is important for improving the success of nutritional support in critical care.

11.4.1. Identifying Malnutrition in Critical Care

It is important to identify malnutrition in critical care so that patients receive the best nutritional care. Metabolic changes brought on by critical illnesses usually mean the body uses more energy and breaks down muscle, which may affect a person's nutrition. If malnutrition is recognized at an early stage, it becomes possible to give the right treatments, which can improve patient recovery, shorten time spent in intensive care, and enhance outcomes. To find malnutrition, clinicians depend on clinical assessments, biochemical tests, and measurements of physical features. Moreover, the presence of chronic critical illness complicates the nutritional landscape, as patients may experience prolonged hospitalization and lingering organ dysfunction, which exacerbates the risk of malnutrition (Chen *et al.*, 2024). Addressing malnutrition through individualized nutritional therapy not only supports metabolic demands but also enhances overall clinical management and patient well-being (Shetti, 2024) (Figure 11.15).

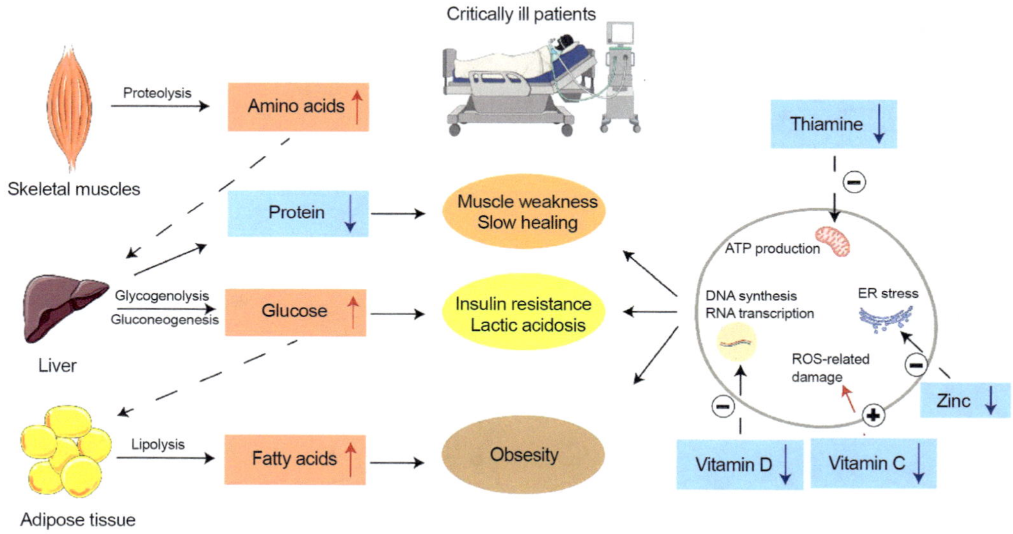

Figure 11.15. Malnutrition caused by metabolic dysregulation in critically ill patients.

Source: https://www.researchgate.net/figure/Malnutrition-caused-by-metabolic-dysregulation-in-critically-ill-patients-downward_fig1_362929809.

11.4.2. Limitations of Current Assessment Tools

Because of the shortcomings of current nutritional assessment methods, nutritional support strategies are not as effective in critical illness. The tools currently available often do not correctly recognize the many changes in the body that happen with critical illness, which can result in the wrong classification of nutrition requirements. For example, usual methods can miss the higher metabolic needs and changes in nutrient uptake that happen with conditions such as delirium or diabetes, which are common in critically ill patients. Not assessing properly can result in feeding patients too much or too little, which can harm both their recovery and the results. Besides, tools that rely mainly on body mass index or body measurements usually neglect the value of lean body mass and metabolism, which are important signs of nutritional risk in patients. Thus, a comprehensive reevaluation of assessment methods is imperative to ensure that nutritional interventions are effectively tailored to the unique needs of this vulnerable population (Davies *et al.*, 2018; Livingston *et al.*, 2020).

11.4.3. Patient Tolerance and Gastrointestinal Issues

Nutritional support, how well the patient handles it, and the state of the GI system are very important for critically ill patients to recover well. Early enteral nutrition (EEN) has been shown to enhance patient tolerance, reducing the incidence of complications such as infections and promoting overall recovery (Blaser *et al.*, 2017). However, patient-specific factors, including obesity, can complicate nutritional delivery. Research indicates that obesity, defined by a body mass index (BMI) that categorizes individuals as having excess body fat, can impair health and increase the risk of long-term medical complications, thus necessitating careful management of nutritional strategies (Wharton *et al.*, 2020). Gastrointestinal problems such as not being able to eat, aspiration, and slow motility are common in critically ill patients; this may require changing the nutritional support plan to improve tolerance and reduce risks. Consequently, a nuanced understanding of patient tolerance and GI status is essential for enhancing nutritional support in critical illness (Figure 11.16).

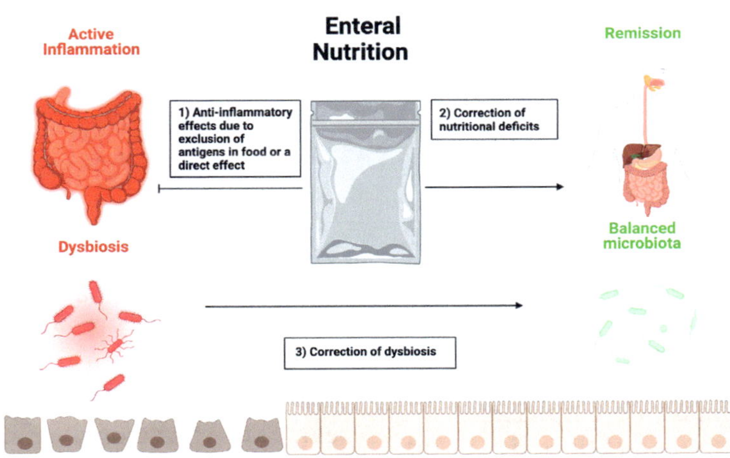

Figure 11.16. Mechanism showing the proposed effects of EEN. EEN improves outcomes in Crohn's disease patients by potentially: (1) reducing antigens in whole foods and/ or direct anti-inflammatory effects, 34-38 (2) improving micronutrient and macronutrient deficiencies 22-28 and (3) correcting gut microbiota disturbances. 29-31 EEN, exclusive enteral nutrition.

Source: https://www.researchgate.net/figure/Mechanism-showing-the-proposed-effects-of-EEN-EEN-improves-outcomes-in-Crohns-disease_fig1_354886097.

11.4.4. Resource Availability and Access to Nutrition

The amount of resources available strongly affects nutrition, which is very important for health, especially in severe illnesses. Not having enough healthy food can make health problems worse, delay recovery, and make a person more vulnerable to infections. Diverse agricultural practices and technological advancements are essential in enhancing food availability and safety, as highlighted the synergies between agriculture and health (Hawkes *et al.*, 2025). Also, some groups, including those living in fishing communities, encounter problems where both nutrition and health are concerned, especially with diseases such as HIV/AIDS. Research indicates that addressing these intertwined issues can significantly improve the well-being of these communities by ensuring both food security and adequate nutritional intake (Lintelo, 2025). So, taking into account both the ecological and socio-economic aspects is necessary for better nutritional care in critical illnesses.

11.4.5. Interdisciplinary Communication Barriers

For nutritional support in critical illness, healthcare providers must communicate well across specialties, though several barriers may prevent this. Typically, healthcare teams are not connected, which results in care that is not coordinated and gaps in understanding what critically ill patients should eat. Not having all the information shared can cause misunderstandings about a patient's nutrition and the care plan. As highlighted by N/A (2010), implementing a four-step approach to reduce hospital readmissions emphasizes the importance of education and care coordination among multidisciplinary teams. Furthermore, Rocca *et al.* (2022) underscore that registered dietitians (RDs) significantly contribute to transitions of care by ensuring that nutrition information is effectively communicated across various healthcare settings. If different medical teams do not work together, the advantages of having RDs involved in care can be missed, which may result in poor health outcomes for critical patients. For this reason, it is essential to overcome these barriers to improve nutritional care in such difficult situations.

11.4.6. Ethical Considerations in Nutritional Support

Ethical issues around nutrition are important and fundamental in critical illness, especially for children, because their nutritional needs can vary widely. There are many ethical issues for clinicians, for example, deciding whether to use enteral or PN for critically ill children with special metabolic needs. Specifically, guidelines indicate the need for careful assessment of macro- and micronutrient requirements, informed by the patient's clinical status and the risks associated with overfeeding, which can lead to adverse outcomes (Marino *et al.*, 2020). There are also crucial ethical aspects related to breastfeeding and the utilization of donor human milk, particularly for vulnerable infants in neonatal intensive care units (Israel-Ballard *et al.*, 2019). Noticing and dealing with these complexities enables healthcare professionals to provide fair access to nutritional support for critically ill patients and decrease risks while improving their outcomes.

11.4.7. Cultural and Personal Preferences in Nutrition

When caring for critically ill patients, considering their cultural and personal likes and dislikes is very important for good nutritional support. A patient's culture, beliefs, and personal preferences usually affect what they want to eat. They can strongly affect how well and how easily nutritional interventions are accepted and used. For example, diets from different cultures can be high in nutrients or flavors that make patients more likely to eat them, which is very important in critical care. Furthermore, considering the implications of obesity, characterized as a complex chronic disease, it becomes essential to tailor nutritional support strategies that respect individual preferences while addressing health concerns, to optimize outcomes and improve quality of life (Wharton *et al.*, 2020). Additionally, addressing cultural factors may mitigate potential risks associated with inadequate nutrition, which can lead to functional decline and increased morbidity in vulnerable populations (Montero-Odasso *et al.*, 2022) (Figure 11.17).

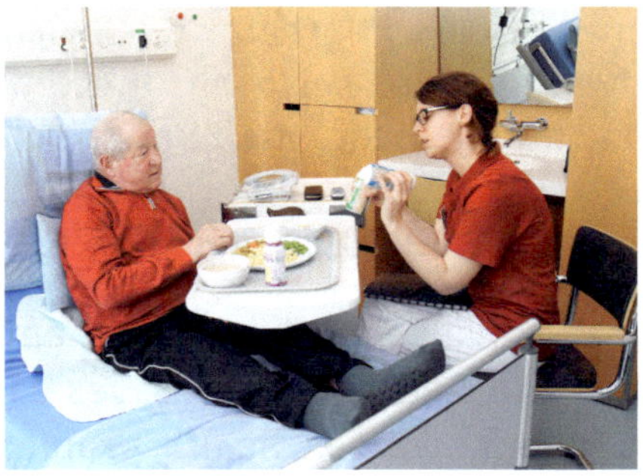

Figure 11.17. Cultural and Personal Preferences in Nutrition.

Source: https://scx2.b-cdn.net/gfx/news/hires/2019/individualnu.jpg.

11.4.8. Variability in Clinical Guidelines

Because clinical guidelines vary, it is difficult to provide the right nutrition to critically ill patients. The fact that experts may have different opinions, evidence is constantly changing, and each patient's situation is different, causes these differences. For instance, organizations like the American Diabetes Association continuously update their recommendations to reflect current best practices, acknowledging the variability in treatment approaches that can arise from differing interpretations of evidence (N/A, 2018). Similarly, the Surviving Sepsis Campaign guidelines illustrate how systematic reviews can yield varied recommendations, with many emerging as either strong or weak based on the quality of available evidence (Rhodes *et al.*, 2017). Because of this inconsistency, healthcare providers may become confused which can complicate the process of providing proper nutrition in critical care. Therefore, clinicians need to recognize these differences to help their patients recover through better nutrition during critical illnesses.

11.4.9. Future Research Needs in Nutritional Support

The discussions about nutrition in critical illness reveal many gaps that should be addressed by more research. While recent randomized controlled trials have demonstrated no benefit and potential harms from early full nutritional support, particularly due to anabolic resistance and exacerbated metabolic conditions, the timing and nature of these interventions remain inadequately explored (Man *et al.*, 2024). Most studies have mainly looked at nutritional care in the first days after admission to the ICU, so there is little information on what is best for patients after leaving the ICU. For this reason, more studies are needed to find out when and how to start nutrition for critical illness patients, depending on their needs. Furthermore, given the variability in micronutrient status and its assessment challenges, future research should aim to clarify effective protocols for micronutrient therapy while considering common comorbidities like dementia, which complicate care in older hospitalized patients (Livingston *et al.*, 2020).

Test Your Knowledge

1. What are the common challenges in identifying malnutrition in critically ill patients, and how can it be addressed?
2. How do gastrointestinal issues and patient tolerance affect the delivery of nutritional support in critical care?
3. What barriers, including resource limitations and poor interdisciplinary communication, can hinder effective nutritional management in the ICU?

SUMMARY

Nutritional care is critical during critical illness because it greatly helps patients recover and achieve better outcomes. It appears that personalized nutrition can significantly reduce the chances of complications, shorten hospital stays, and help people recover faster. Critical illness can change how the body uses nutrients, so a flexible and well-planned nutritional approach is needed to help the patient. It is also essential to focus on the nutrition of people who are at greater risk, such as the elderly and those with pre-existing conditions, since their health can be seriously affected if they do not get proper nutrition. As highlighted by recent studies, timely recognition and intervention can improve not only physical health but also psychological well-being, ultimately benefiting both individuals and the healthcare system as a whole (Livingston *et al.*, 2020; Singhal, 2020).

All in all, providing nutrition to patients in critical illness involves many aspects and has a significant impact on their outcomes. It is important to assess and treat nutrition issues early and according to the needs of each patient, because malnutrition may worsen health problems and keep them in the hospital longer. Also, recent research indicates that specially designed diets can boost the immune system and the rate of recovery, highlighting how important macronutrients and micronutrients are for healing. Mental health plays a big role in recovery, too, as delirium and anxiety are common among critically ill patients, which shows the importance of treating all aspects of a patient's health. Effective management strategies must be implemented to address both nutritional and psychological aspects, ultimately promoting better quality of life for patients and families during challenging times (Livingston *et al.*, 2020; Rogers *et al.*, 2020). For this reason, using an integrated care model is important for improving the recovery of critically ill patients.

KEY TERMS FROM THIS CHAPTER

- Enteral nutrition (EN)
- Gastrostomy
- Hypocaloric feeding
- Indirect calorimetry
- Macronutrients
- Nitrogen balance
- Protein catabolism
- Resting energy expenditure (REE)
- Feeding intolerance
- Glycemic control
- Immunonutrition
- Jejunostomy
- Micronutrients
- Parenteral nutrition (PN)
- Refeeding syndrome
- Trophic feeding

CRITICAL THINKING QUESTIONS

1. **When should enteral nutrition ideally be initiated in a critically ill patient who is hemodynamically stable?**
   a. Within 24–48 hours of ICU admission
   b. After five days of fasting
   c. Only after parenteral nutrition has failed
   d. Immediately after extubation
2. **Which of the following is not a known complication of parenteral nutrition?**
   a. Hyperglycemia
   b. Liver dysfunction
   c. Refeeding syndrome
   d. Improved gut mucosal integrity
3. **What is the most appropriate initial route for nutritional support in a critically ill patient with a functional gastrointestinal tract?**
   a. Total parenteral nutrition (TPN)
   b. Peripheral parenteral nutrition (PPN)
   c. Enteral nutrition
   d. Intravenous glucose and electrolytes only
4. **Which electrolyte abnormality is most characteristic of refeeding syndrome?**
   a. Hyperkalemia
   b. Hypernatremia
   c. Hypophosphatemia
   d. Hypocalcemia
5. **Protein requirements in critically ill patients are generally increased. What is the recommended protein intake for most ICU patients?**
   a. 0.5 g/kg/day
   b. 1.2–2.0 g/kg/day
   c. 2.5–3.0 g/kg/day
   d. >3.5 g/kg/day

Short Answer Questions

1. What are the primary goals of nutritional support in critically ill patients?
2. Why is early nutritional support important in critical illness?
3. What is the difference between enteral and parenteral nutrition, and when should each be used?
4. What are the risks associated with inadequate nutrition in critically ill patients?
5. What factors influence the energy needs of critically ill patients?

Answer to Critical Thinking Questions

1. (a); 2. (d); 3. (c); 4. (c); 5. (b)

REFERENCES

1. Alhazzani, W., Møller, M. H., Arabi, Y. M., Loeb, M., Gong, M. N., Fan, E., Oczkowski, S., *et al.* (2020). Surviving Sepsis Campaign: Guidelines on the management of critically ill adults with coronavirus disease 2019 (COVID-19). *Intensive Care Medicine, 46*, 854–887. https://doi.org/10.1007/s00134-020-06022-5.
2. Alshahrani, F. M., Alzubali, M. A., Alsammak, A. S. H., Al Muteri, M. K., Alabyad, J. A. M., Abutaleb, E. Z., Alanazi, B. M. N., *et al.* (2024). Wound healing in pediatric patients with chronic skin wounds: The critical role of nutrition and nursing interventions. *Journal of Eco Humanism*. https://www.semanticscholar.org/paper/1e8f47b79fac97806bde621ddc4076f0247e2213 (accessed on 22 May 2025).
3. Beyer, A. C. (2017). Holistic healing for hearing voices: Self-care for patients with schizophrenia. https://core.ac.uk/download/151162201.pdf (accessed on 22 May 2025).
4. Browne, J., Cohen, S. S., de Camargo, O. K., Delaney, *et al.* (2019). Pediatric feeding disorder: Consensus definition and conceptual framework. https://core.ac.uk/download/286544045.pdf (accessed on 22 May 2025).
5. Caetano, T., & Rocha, R. R. P. (2024). Major considerations of neurological therapy in cancer patients: A systematic review. https://core.ac.uk/download/622812230.pdf (accessed on 22 May 2025).
6. Chen, W., Song, J., & Gong, S. (2024). Advances in nutritional metabolic therapy to impede the progression of critical illness. *Frontiers in Nutrition, 11*. https://www.semanticscholar.org/paper/55f86763d41c4f8ba22d06a6f8a5f6534ccd9196 (accessed on 22 May 2025).
7. Chiang, H. H., Kahn, S., & Hirsch, I. B. (2024). Starting insulin algorithms for non-critical illness: A survey of 32 academic hospitals in the United States. *Diabetes Technology & Therapeutics*. https://www.semanticscholar.org/paper/b4fe44050103d63f81e184310fa365d248c334e5 (accessed on 22 May 2025).
8. Chojnacka, N., Cymer, R., Jurasz, K., Klarycki, *et al.* (2024). The role of nutritional treatment in postsurgical convalescence process. https://core.ac.uk/download/620863336.pdf (accessed on 22 May 2025).
9. Correia, M., & Rosenfeld, R. (2024). Nutritional management during critical illness in those with previous obesity surgery. *Current Opinion in Clinical Nutrition and Metabolic Care, 27*, 192–199. https://www.semanticscholar.org/paper/6da061fb058e8f83fcda418e03fae42a95def6d5 (accessed on 22 May 2025).
10. Cruzat, V. F., Rogero, M. M., Keane, K. N., Curi, R., & Newsholme, P. (2018). Glutamine: Metabolism and immune function, supplementation and clinical translation. *Nutrients, 10*, 1564. https://doi.org/10.3390/nu10111564.
11. Cryan, J. F., O'Riordan, K. J., Cowan, C. S. M., Sandhu, K. V., Bastiaanssen, T. F. S., Boehme, M., Codagnone, M. G., *et al.* (2019). The microbiota-gut-brain axis. *Physiological Reviews, 99*, 1877–2013. https://doi.org/10.1152/physrev.00018.2018.
12. Davies, M. J., D'Alessio, D. A., Fradkin, J., Kernan, W. N., Mathieu, C., Mingrone, G., Rossing, P., *et al.* (2018). Management of hyperglycemia in type 2 diabetes, 2018: A consensus report by the American Diabetes Association (ADA) and the European Association for the Study of Diabetes (EASD). *Diabetes Care, 41*, 2669–2701. https://doi.org/10.2337/dci18-0033.

13. De Rosa, S., Samoni, S., Villa, G., & Ronco, C. (2017). Management of chronic kidney disease patients in the intensive care unit: Mixing acute and chronic illness. *Blood Purification, 43*, 151–162. https://doi.org/10.1159/000452650.

14. de Rosa, S., Umbrello, M., Pelosi, P., & Battaglini, D. (2023). Update on lean body mass diagnostic assessment in critical illness. *Diagnostics, 13*. https://www.semanticscholar.org/paper/d5af603d7ac07eb90cd64365c14ccb4755137708 (accessed on 22 May 2025).

15. de Watteville, A., Pielmeier, U., Di Marco, M., Gayet-Ageron, A., Siegenthaler, N., Parel, N., Wozniak, H., *et al.* (2025). Glucosafe 2—A new tool for nutritional management and insulin-therapy in the intensive care unit: Randomized controlled study (the Glucosafe 2 protocol). *PLOS One, 20*. https://www.semanticscholar.org/paper/4ea8f8a684451a139d6c4a3d340886de07a96d50 (accessed on 22 May 2025).

16. Duan, J., Zheng, W. H., Zhou, H., Xu, Y., & Huang, H. B. (2021). Energy delivery guided by indirect calorimetry in critically ill patients: A systematic review and meta-analysis. *Critical Care, 25*. https://doi.org/10.1186/s13054-021-03508-6.

17. Dumitriu, A., Cobilinschi, C., Dumitriu, B., Vâlcea, S., Ungureanu, R., Popa, A., Ene, R., *et al.* (2025). Advancing nutritional care through bioelectrical impedance analysis in critical patients. *Nutrients, 17*. https://www.semanticscholar.org/paper/d056b88f2584aa26b200a564c6d54af43b3e07b8 (accessed on 22 May 2025).

18. Evans, L., Rhodes, A., Alhazzani, W., Antonelli, M., Coopersmith, C. M., French, C., Machado, F. R., *et al.* (2021). Surviving Sepsis Campaign: International guidelines for management of sepsis and septic shock 2021. *Critical Care Medicine, 49*, e1063–e1143. https://doi.org/10.1097/ccm.0000000000005337.

19. Eveleens, R. D., Joosten, K. F. M., & Verbruggen, S. C. A. T. (2020). The role of parenteral nutrition in pediatric critical care, and its consequences on recovery. https://core.ac.uk/download/566894246.pdf (accessed on 22 May 2025).

20. Fiaccadori, E., Parenti, E., & Maggiore, U. (2018). Nutritional support in acute kidney injury. *Journal of Nephrology, 21*(5), 645–656. https://www.semanticscholar.org/paper/9b4342fb196182dc23225ca6804489e849fb671d (accessed on 22 May 2025).

21. Formenti, P., Bichi, F., Castagna, V., Pozzi, T., & Chiumello, D. (2021). Nutrition support in patients with acute respiratory distress syndrome COVID-19. *Nutrition in Clinical Practice, 36*, 500–501. https://www.semanticscholar.org/paper/426622404c79b326a182fd723b7be47303ec0740 (accessed on 22 May 2025).

22. Gao, Y., Ding, M., Dong, X., Zhang, J., Azkur, A. K., Azkur, D., Gan, H., *et al.* (2020). Risk factors for severe and critically ill COVID-19 patients: A review. *Allergy, 76*, 428–455. https://doi.org/10.1111/all.14657.

23. Gombart, A. F., Pierre, A., & Maggini, S. (2020). A review of micronutrients and the immune system–working in harmony to reduce the risk of infection. *Nutrients, 12*(1), 236. https://doi.org/10.3390/nu12010236.

24. Hawkes, C., & Ruel, M. T. (2025). *Understanding the Links Between Agriculture and Health*. https://core.ac.uk/download/pdf/6288827.pdf (accessed on 22 May 2025).

25. Health Care Leader Action Guide to Reduce Avoidable Readmissions. (2010). https://core.ac.uk/download/71351784.pdf (accessed on 22 May 2025).

26. Heyland, D. K., Davidson, J. E., Skrobik, Y., Roze des Ordons, A., Van Scoy, L. J., Day, A. G., Vandall-Walker, V., *et al.* (2018). Improving partnerships with family members of ICU patients: Study protocol for a randomized controlled trial. *Trials, 19*, Article 119. https://doi.org/10.1186/s13063-017-2379-4.

27. Hill, B., Mitchell, A., Szydlowska, A., Sparks, C., Dunn, H., & Berry, H. (2025). The role of nutrition in wound healing and implications for nursing practice. *British Journal of Nursing, 34*(4), S39–S42. https://www.semanticscholar.org/paper/a491f49aba5aa6990024702d77fb49abd2331ae8 (accessed on 22 May 2025).

28. Hossain, M., & Purohit, N. (2019). Improving child and adolescent mental health in India: Status, services, policies, and way forward. *Indian Journal of Psychiatry, 61*, 415. https://doi.org/10.4103/psychiatry.indianjpsychiatry_217_18.

29. Hrdý, O., Vrbica, K., Duba, J., Slezak, M., Straževská, E., Agalarev, V., Duba, M., *et al.* (2025). Intermittent enteral nutrition shortens the time to achieve nutritional goals in critically ill patients. *Scientific Reports, 15*. https://www.semanticscholar.org/paper/f8ba220c6f0a45d98e92c3cd9a767108972186dd (accessed on 22 May 2025).

30. Huang, W., Liu, D., Zhang, H., Ding, X., & Wang, X. (2022). Focus on host/organ unregulated response: A common cause of critical illness. *Chinese Medical Journal*. https://doi.org/10.1097/cm9.0000000000002374.

31. Israel-Ballard, K., Cohen, J., Mansen, K., Parker, M., Engmann, C., Kelley, M., Brooks, E., *et al.* (2019). Call to action for equitable access to human milk for vulnerable infants. *The Lancet Global Health, 7*, e1484–e1486. https://doi.org/10.1016/s2214-109x(19)30402-4.

32. Livingston, G., Huntley, J., Sommerlad, A., Ames, D., Ballard, C., Banerjee, S., Brayne, C., *et al.* (2020). Dementia prevention, intervention, and care: 2020 report of the Lancet Commission. *The Lancet, 396*, 413–446. https://doi.org/10.1016/s0140-6736(20)30367-6.

33. Mahmud, I., & Mbuya, N. (2016). Water, sanitation, hygiene, and nutrition in Bangladesh: Can building toilets affect children's growth? https://core.ac.uk/download/75783689.pdf (accessed on 22 May 2025).

34. Man, A., Gunst, J., & Reintam Blaser, A. (2024). Nutrition in the intensive care unit: From the acute phase to beyond. *Intensive Care Medicine, 50*(9), 1035–1048. https://doi.org/10.1007/s00134-024-07458-9.

35. Marino, L. V., Moullet, C., & Jotterand Chaparro, C. (2020). The impact of nutrition on clinical outcomes in the critically ill child. *Pediatric Medicine, 3*, 21. https://doi.org/10.21037/pm-20-73.

36. Maslach, C., & Leiter, M. P. (2016). Understanding the burnout experience: Recent research and its implications for psychiatry. *World Psychiatry, 15*(2), 103–111. https://doi.org/10.1002/wps.20311.

37. McClave, S. A., Taylor, B., Martindale, R. G., Warren, M., Johnson, D. R., Braunschweig, C., McCarthy, M. S., *et al.* (2016). Guidelines for the provision and assessment of nutrition support therapy in the adult critically ill patient. *Journal of Parenteral and Enteral Nutrition, 40*, 159–211. https://doi.org/10.1177/0148607115621863.

38. McWilliams, D., Gustafson, O., Wyer, N., Couper, K., Kimani, P., Kandiyali, R., Barghouthy, D., *et al.* (2025). Physiotherapy and optimized enteral nutrition in the post-acute phase of critical

illness (PHOENIX): Protocol for a mixed methods feasibility randomized controlled trial. *BMJ Open, 15*. https://www.semanticscholar.org/paper/0014d7a49ddc7073ab54742adf2b7d479ef0ced9 (accessed on 22 May 2025).

39. Merker, M., Felder, M., Gueissaz, L., Bolliger, R., Tribolet, P., Kaegi-Braun, N., Gomes, F., *et al.* (2020). Association of baseline inflammation with effectiveness of nutritional support among patients with disease-related malnutrition. *JAMA Network Open, 3*, e200663. https://doi.org/10.1001/jamanetworkopen.2020.0663.

40. Merker, M., Gomes, F., Stanga, Z., & Schüetz, P. (2019). Evidence-based nutrition for the malnourished, hospitalized patient: One bite at a time. *Schweizerische Medizinische Wochenschrift*. https://doi.org/10.4414/smw.2019.20112.

41. Moltu, S. J., Bronský, J., Embleton, N. D., Gerasimidis, K., Indrio, F., Köglmeier, J., de Koning, B., *et al.* (2021). Nutritional management of the critically ill neonate. *Journal of Pediatric Gastroenterology and Nutrition, 73*, 274–289. https://doi.org/10.1097/mpg.0000000000003076.

42. Montero-Odasso, M., van der Velde, N., Martin, F. C., Petrović, M., Tan, M. P., Ryg, J., Aguilar-Navarro, S. G., *et al.* (2022). World guidelines for falls prevention and management for older adults: A global initiative. *Age and Ageing, 51*. https://doi.org/10.1093/ageing/afac205.

43. Moonen, H. P. F. X., Beckers, K. J. H., & van Zanten, A. R. H. (2021). Energy expenditure and indirect calorimetry in critical illness and convalescence: Current evidence and practical considerations. *Journal of Intensive Care, 9*. https://doi.org/10.1186/s40560-021-00524-0.

44. Mustafa, N. (2024). Clinical nutrition and health. *Albus Scientia*. https://www.semanticscholar.org/paper/279dd0b9e5ad9323980830a1a1bfa31a2ae18ec5 (accessed on 22 May 2025).

45. Naicker, S., Yang, C. W., Hwang, S. J., Liu, B. C., Chen, J., & Jha, V. (2020). The novel coronavirus 2019 epidemic and kidneys. *Kidney International, 97*, 824–828. https://doi.org/10.1016/j.kint.2020.03.001.

46. O'Neill, B., Bradley, J., Connolly, B. A., Bruce, J., Underwood, M., Lall, R., Ji, C., *et al.* (2025). Remote multicomponent rehabilitation compared to standard care for survivors of critical illness after hospital discharge (iRehab): A protocol for a randomized controlled assessor-blind clinical and cost-effectiveness trial. *NIHR Open Research*. https://www.semanticscholar.org/paper/266c46e225b5c8cde730c1b62d474eec7f0b6092 (accessed on 22 May 2025).

47. Ottaviani, I., Tantillo, S., Miggiano, L., Guarnera, M., Menghini, M., Talarico, F., Mazzanti, F., *et al.* (2024). Fasting in critical illness: The role of ketonuria–A retrospective observational study. *Journal of Anesthesia, Analgesia and Critical Care, 4*. https://www.semanticscholar.org/paper/578d9c904932b6b1572e28e049fc784a2ef05ca3 (accessed on 22 May 2025).

48. Rhodes, A., Evans, L., Alhazzani, W., Levy, M. M., Antonelli, M., Ferrer, R., Kumar, A., *et al.* (2017). Surviving sepsis campaign: International guidelines for management of sepsis and septic shock: 2016. *Critical Care Medicine, 45*(3), 486–552. https://doi.org/10.1097/ccm.0000000000002255.

49. Rocca, N. (2022). Implementation of a transitions of care nutrition intervention for malnourished patients. https://core.ac.uk/download/541293064.pdf (accessed on 22 May 2025).

50. Rogers, J., Chesney, E., Oliver, D., Pollak, T. A., McGuire, P., Fusar-Poli, P., Zandi, M. S., *et al.* (2020). Psychiatric and neuropsychiatric presentations associated with severe coronavirus

infections: A systematic review and meta-analysis with comparison to the COVID-19 pandemic. *The Lancet Psychiatry, 7*, 611–627. https://doi.org/10.1016/s2215-0366(20)30203-0.

51. Sattar, N., McInnes, I. B., & McMurray, J. J. V. (2020). Obesity is a risk factor for severe COVID-19 infection. *Circulation, 142*, 4–6. https://doi.org/10.1161/circulationaha.120.047659.
52. Shams, M. M. K., Alawady, D. E. S., Abd Elaziz, F. K. E., & Hassan, M. M. E. (2024). Impact of enteral and parenteral nutrition on mortality and morbidity of mechanically ventilated severely septic critically ill patients. *QJM: An International Journal of Medicine*. https://www.semanticscholar.org/paper/ef5da1b25368ecb6cf884964829a78414ee69950 (accessed on 22 May 2025).
53. Shetti, A. (2024). Nutritional support in critical care patients: Challenges, strategies, and recent advances. *IP Journal of Nutrition, Metabolism and Health Science*. https://www.semanticscholar.org/paper/3f4e9b7244d9713b8b7a737b47b84a0a7f97722b (accessed on 22 May 2025).
54. Singhal, T. (2020). A review of coronavirus disease-2019 (COVID-19). *The Indian Journal of Pediatrics, 87*, 281–286. https://doi.org/10.1007/s12098-020-03263-6.
55. Somani, N., Batth, N. K., Beri, N., Jindal, P., & Kansal, M. (2025). Evaluating the impact of enteral nutrition on pediatric outcomes in PICU patients: A study of morbidity and mortality effects. *National Board of Examinations Journal of Medical Sciences*. https://www.semanticscholar.org/paper/06891e16a9b1f62267e161116a93c836020e8878 (accessed on 22 May 2025).
56. Stewart, D. E., & Appelbaum, P. S. (2020). COVID-19 and psychiatrists' responsibilities: A WPA position paper. *World Psychiatry, 19*(3), 406–407. https://doi.org/10.1002/wps.20803.
57. Taylor, B., McClave, S. A., Martindale, R. G., Warren, M., Johnson, D. R., Braunschweig, C., McCarthy, M. S., *et al.* (2016). Guidelines for the provision and assessment of nutrition support therapy in the adult critically ill patient. *Critical Care Medicine, 44*(2), 390–438. https://doi.org/10.1097/ccm.0000000000001525.
58. Te Lintelo, D. (2025). Food security, nutrition and HIV/AIDS in African fisheries: Emerging evidence and research directions: A literature review. https://core.ac.uk/download/pdf/6515119.pdf (accessed on 22 May 2025).
59. Tume, L. N., Valla, F. V., Joosten, K. F. M., Jotterand Chaparro, C., Latten, L., Marino, L. V., Macleod, I., *et al.* (2020). Nutritional support for children during critical illness: European Society of Pediatric and Neonatal Intensive Care (ESPNIC) metabolism, endocrine and nutrition section position statement and clinical recommendations. *Intensive Care Medicine, 46*, 411–425. https://doi.org/10.1007/s00134-019-05922-5.
60. Viner Smith, E., Lambell, K., Tatucu-Babet, O. A., Ridley, E., & Chapple, L. (2024). Nutrition considerations for patients with persistent critical illness: A narrative review. *JPEN. Journal of Parenteral and Enteral Nutrition, 48*(4), 658–666. https://doi.org/10.1002/jpen.2623.
61. Wei, P. F. (2020). Diagnosis and treatment protocol for novel coronavirus pneumonia (Trial version 7). *Chinese Medical Journal, 133*, 1087–1095. https://doi.org/10.1097/cm9.0000000000000819.
62. Weimann, A., & Felbinger, T. W. (2016). Gastrointestinal dysmotility in the critically ill. *Current Opinion in Clinical Nutrition & Metabolic Care, 19*(4), 353–359. https://doi.org/10.1097/mco.0000000000000300.

63. Wharton, S., Lau, D. C. W., Vallis, M., Sharma, A. M., Biertho, L., Campbell-Scherer, D., Adamo, K. B., *et al.* (2020). Obesity in adults: A clinical practice guideline. *Canadian Medical Association Journal, 192*, E875–E891. https://doi.org/10.1503/cmaj.191707.

64. Wilson, C. (2018). Breastfeeding as a mechanism to reduce postpartum depression with weight as a major contributing factor in Hispanic women. https://core.ac.uk/download/215485163.pdf (accessed on 22 May 2025).

65. Yewande, S. V., Oberhiri, O. K., Peter, S. O., Jesse, O., Gabriel, A., Bewaji, A. O., & Reginald, A. U. (2024). Psychosocial wellbeing of orphans in Kaduna state: A comprehensive assessment. *The American Journal of Social Science and Education Innovations*. https://www.semanticscholar.org/paper/b5828e5114c237c4cfc306725b1ef84625368f2a (accessed on 22 May 2025).

66. Yoshikawa, H., Wuermli, A. J., Britto, P. R., Dreyer, B. P., Leckman, J. F., Lye, S. J., Ponguta, L. A., *et al.* (2020). Effects of the global coronavirus disease-2019 pandemic on early childhood development: Short- and long-term risks and mitigating program and policy actions. *The Journal of Pediatrics, 223*, 188–193. https://doi.org/10.1016/j.jpeds.2020.05.020.

67. Zhang, H., Zhao, L., & Jia, B. (2024). Research progress on nutritional support in the neonatal and pediatric populations receiving extracorporeal membrane oxygenation. *Frontiers in Nutrition, 11*. https://www.semanticscholar.org/paper/e30da9b251223cdac8ccf871906daa46adba8e1d (accessed on 22 May 2025).

END-OF-LIFE CARE AND PALLIATIVE MEDICINE IN THE ICU

12

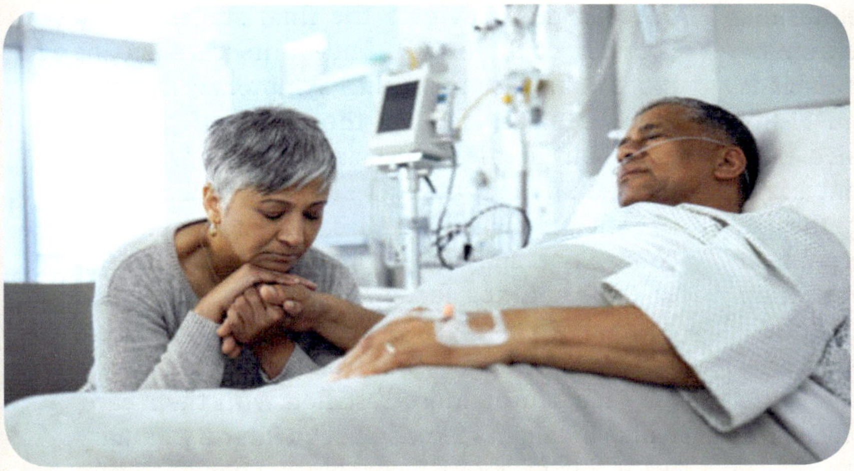

LEARNING OBJECTIVES

After studying this chapter, you will be able to:

1. After studying this chapter, you will be able to.
2. Define the role of the ICU in end-of-life care.
3. Explain the principles of palliative medicine.
4. Explore communication with patients and families.
5. Discuss pain management in end-of-life care.
6. Illustrate advanced directives and patient autonomy.

Introduction

The concept of end-of-life care (EOLC) has emerged as a critical component of patient management within the Intensive Care Unit (ICU). Because medical advances allow people to live longer, the ethical issues related to terminal illnesses and critical health situations are more noticeable. EOLC includes actions that make sure patients are comfortable, treated with dignity, and that their wishes and those of their families are respected in the final stages of life. Good communication is essential, since misunderstandings between patients and their loved ones can cause distress. For this reason, including structured EOLC communication protocols in critical care can significantly improve the quality of care given in the ICU. When these communication problems are resolved, healthcare providers can create a setting that is both patient-focused and caring, which helps both patients and their families. Training in palliative care remains a vital yet often inconsistent aspect of fellowship programs in Pulmonary and Critical Care Medicine (PCCM). Although palliative care is recognized as important, there is considerable variation in the quality and depth of teaching about it among fellows. Research indicates that a mere 61% of PCCM fellows reported receiving one or two forms of EOLC training, with nearly half expressing that their training was inadequate (Yuan *et al.*, 2025). Because of this gap, it is clear that school curricula should include more lessons and activities on EOLC principles, such as active discussions and conflict management. Having more confidence in leading EOLC talks can significantly affect both patients' results and the satisfaction of ICU staff. Making sure training is standardized can help critical care clinicians handle the emotional aspects of end-of-life care. The European Society of Intensive Care Medicine (ESICM) has taken significant steps toward optimizing end-of-life and palliative care practices by developing evidence-based recommendations. This initiative involves an international panel of experts focusing on key areas such as communication, family-centered care, and the integration of palliative care within the ICU framework (Kesecioglu *et al.*, 2024). The guidelines point out that access to healthcare resources affects EOLC, and they urge respect for patients' wishes, use of decision-making structures, and help for families with communication. It is suggested that palliative care be introduced early and that standardized ways be used to check for symptoms in patients who could die soon. By dealing with both the emotional and administrative parts of EOLC, such efforts aim to enhance the experience for patients, their families, and the medical team, showing the importance of proper training and following set procedures in critical care.

Definition of End-of-Life Care (EOLC)

End-of-life care is focused on helping patients feel comfortable and respected, rather than focusing on medical treatments that could cure them. This care is made to help patients with terminal illnesses who have many physical, emotional, and psychological needs. A team involving different specialists is needed to make sure the patient's wishes and values are respected during the management of pain, anxiety, and distress. Good communication, talking about advanced directives, and matching treatment to what the patient wants are all important in end-of-life care. This holistic approach not only enhances the quality of life for patients but also offers critical support to families during an exceptionally challenging time, allowing them to share meaningful moments with their loved ones as they navigate the final stages of life (Cowfer *et al.*, 2020). End-of-life care means more than just managing symptoms; it offers many services that fit the needs of patients and their families. A crucial aspect is providing emotional and mental support to both the patient and their loved ones. This means offering counseling, spiritual support, and information to help families face what is happening and deal with their grief. According to research, patients who get comprehensive end-of-life care tend to be more satisfied with their care, which highlights the value of an interdisciplinary team. Furthermore, incorporating palliative care principles in the ICU setting can meaningfully alter decision-making processes, transitioning focus from life-sustaining treatments to quality of life considerations (Baumgartner *et al.*, 2020). So, seeing end-of-life care as a complex subject helps improve the outcomes for patients and their families. Making care decisions is important at the end of life, and patients are included in the process. It means that healthcare providers should have sensitive talks about what to expect in terms of prognosis, available treatments, and what care will be like as the end approaches. If healthcare teams prioritize transparency and patient autonomy, patients feel more comfortable sharing their thoughts. Teaching healthcare workers how to communicate well in pediatric palliative care has helped them feel more confident about having these necessary talks. In addition, encouraging collaborative goal-setting between patients, families, and healthcare professionals helps create personalized care plans that honor the patient's values while addressing their needs effectively (Cowfer *et al.*, 2020). Ultimately, a robust understanding of end-of-life care facilitates a supportive framework for managing the complexities of dying, both for patients and the families that care for them (Figure 12.1).

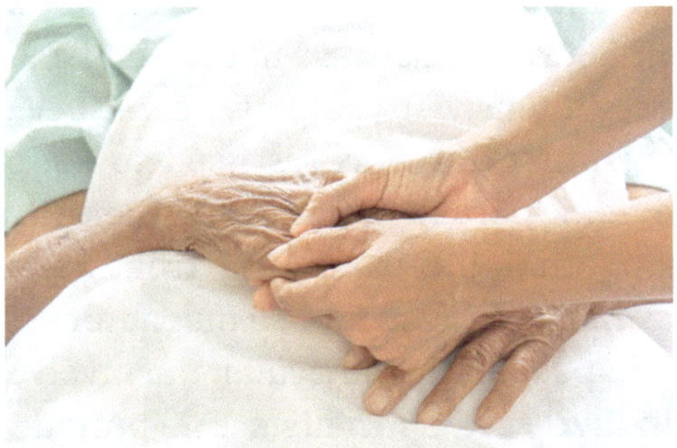

Figure 12.1. End-of-Life Care (EOLC).

Source: https://medicine.nus.edu.sg/nursing/wp-content/uploads/sites/2/2022/06/Geriatric-Care-Level-2-2jpg.jpg.

Importance of Palliative Medicine in the Intensive Care Unit (ICU)

More people now see that palliative medicine in the ICU is essential for improving how end-of-life care is provided. As stated by the European Society of Intensive Care Medicine, palliative care can optimize patient-centered care, significantly improving outcomes for both patients and their families while supporting ICU staff in delivering compassionate care (Alampi *et al.*, 2024). This is particularly pertinent as one in five hospital deaths now occurs in the ICU, a trend projected to double by 2030, increasing the necessity for effective end-of-life interventions (Ghabeljoo *et al.*, 2017). Taking care of the physical, emotional, and spiritual needs of patients close to the end of life is what palliative care does to improve their well-being and respect their dignity. Also, using standard palliative care processes in the ICU can help balance medical treatment with compassionate care. With evidence indicating inadequate management of end-of-life discomforts, the integration of standardized tools for symptom assessment and early palliative care involvement is vital (Ghabeljoo *et al.*, 2017). This way of working helps dying patients and also supports important communication among healthcare staff, patients, and their families. Effective communication strategies, including structured family conferences and culturally sensitive interventions, allow for more precise understanding and alignment of care goals, thereby reducing family distress and conflicting decisions during a pivotal time (Alampi *et al.*, 2024). Focusing on the happiness and mental health of staff is just as important as other topics in palliative medicine in the ICU. The provision of support systems that mitigate feelings of burnout among healthcare providers is essential in maintaining a compassionate caregiving environment (Alampi *et al.*, 2024). When ICU staff deal with end-of-life care, having access to conflict management resources and communication training can make their jobs more satisfying and less stressful. Thanks to these strategies, palliative medicine supports patients and their families as well as the medical staff which helps create a culture of respect and empathy in the ICU.

12.1. The Role of the Intensive Care Unit (ICU) in End-of-Life Care (EOLC)

Learning Outcome

1. Understanding the ICU environment
2. Discuss the common conditions leading to end-of-life scenarios
3. Define ethical considerations in the ICU

The ICU plays a critical role in guiding end-of-life care, as it handles challenging medical decisions that can impact on patients. Because the situation is so severe, healthcare providers must decide how to weigh the importance of keeping patients alive against the quality of their lives. A study indicated that a significant proportion of ICU practitioners reported making decisions regarding life support without sufficient time for comprehensive discussions with families or patients, underscoring the urgency often inherent in critical care settings (Seale *et al.*, 2009). Because decisions must be made quickly, there is a risk that patients' wishes and dignity will not be honored, which can cause problems for patients and their families. In addition, nurses in the ICU are very important because they provide comfort and care to patients at the end of their lives. They are the primary caregivers who usually get close to dying patients and their families and support their wishes. Research has revealed several factors that influence nurses' caring behaviors, which are essential for delivering high-quality end-of-life care (Nilmanat *et al.*, 2011). Personal traits, technology, and the environment in which care is given are some of these factors, and they can have a significant effect on patients at the end of life. Improving these variables helps ICUs to provide better care for patients, supporting their physical, emotional, and mental health. In addition, since ethics plays a significant role in ICU decisions, it is important to involve many different specialists for complete care. Because of the many needs at this time, intensivists, palliative care specialists, nurses, and social workers need to cooperate on providing care to patients and their families. Realizing that life-extending treatments are more complicated than those meant for comfort is very important. In particular, the involvement of palliative care specialists can provide vital support in navigating family discussions and care planning, helping mitigate the emotional burden on ICU staff and enhancing the overall quality of end-of-life experiences for patients and their loved ones (Seale *et al.*, 2009). This multidisciplinary framework is essential to honoring patients' values while striving to meet the ethical mandates of care in the ICU setting (Figure 12.2).

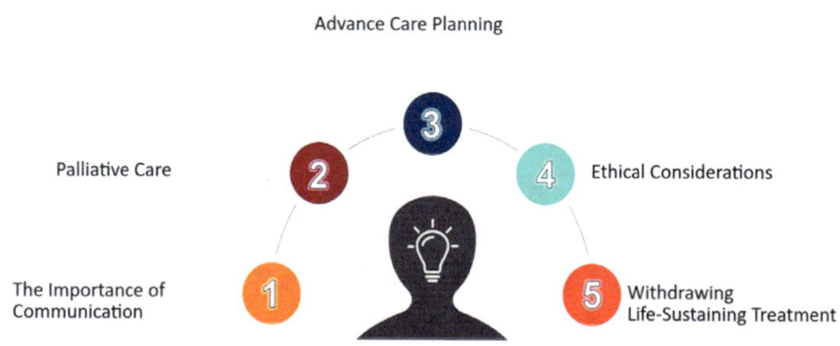

Figure 12.2. The importance of end-of-life care in the intensive care unit (ICU).

Source: https://fastercapital.co/i/End-of-life-care--Honoring-Life--End-of-Life-Care-in-the-ICU--Understanding-the-Importance-of-End-of-Life-Care-in-the-ICU.webp.

12.1.1. Understanding the Intensive Care Unit (ICU) Environment

The ICU is designed for patients who are very ill and need extra medical care and close observation. Knowing about the many parts of the ICU is vital for providing good end-of-life care and palliative medicine. Having advanced medical tools, many kinds of healthcare workers, and the issues faced by patients' families make the situation complex. Because the ICU is usually stressful and full of uncertainties, it requires nurses to be both medically and emotionally supportive. In this setting, healthcare providers must be adept at navigating the intricate dynamics among clinicians, patients, and families, ensuring that communication is clear and compassionate during a time when decisions regarding patient care are paramount (Pamplin *et al.*, 2021). Also, the ICU requires staff to make quick choices under much pressure. These clinicians should weigh the benefits of intense medical treatment against what the patient wants and their quality of life. The ongoing challenges of resource allocation become even more poignant during crises, as highlighted by the strains observed during the COVID-19 pandemic (Anderson *et al.*, 2020).

Because of the crisis, healthcare providers had to update their care methods and saw how valuable telemedicine and remote support were for patients. Knowing these dynamics helps healthcare providers follow palliative care principles by aiming to ease suffering and make the days ahead of terminally ill patients as comfortable as possible. Involving family is very important in the ICU, especially when making decisions about end-of-life care. Because of the stress, families may struggle to understand medical terms and deal with strong emotions, which can make it hard for them to participate in care decisions. Providers need to connect with family members, talk openly, and provide help and advice as the family decides. As healthcare systems evolve to meet growing demands, integrating palliative care principles within the ICU becomes vital to honor patients' values and preferences while providing comprehensive end-of-life care (Anderson *et al.*, 2020). By fostering a collaborative environment that includes family input, clinicians can better tailor interventions and ultimately improve patient experiences in this challenging healthcare setting (Figure 12.3).

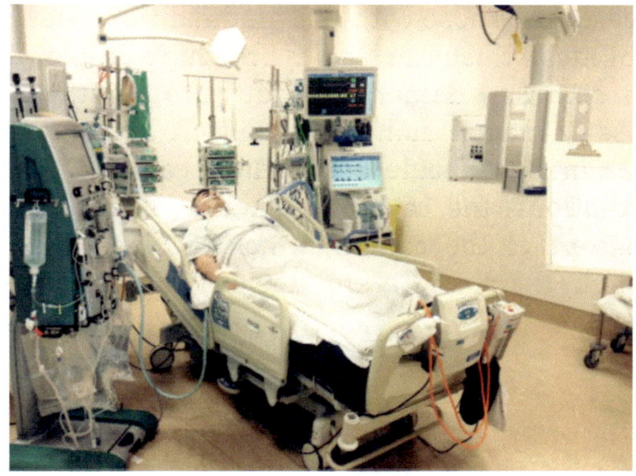

Figure 12.3. The intensive care unit (ICU)'s multifaceted aspects is crucial for delivering effective end-of-life care and palliative medicine.

Source: https://www.slideshare.net/slideshow/end-of-life-care-in-the-intensive-care-unit-icu-presentation-from-acute-hospital-network-march-2015-ahn34/73344707.

12.1.2. Common Conditions Leading to End-of-Life Scenarios

Many conditions that result in end-of-life situations are chronic illnesses and sudden medical events that seriously affect a patient's quality of life. Respiratory diseases, such as chronic obstructive pulmonary disease (COPD) and advanced lung cancer, frequently result in significant breathing difficulties that can culminate in acute respiratory failure. Besides, some heart conditions, such as congestive heart failure and end-stage coronary artery disease, can cause a steady decline, leading patients to have ongoing discomfort and less ability to function. To manage such conditions, it is important to use comprehensive strategies that often rely on palliative care as patients change, and this means using both drugs and non-drug methods to help patients feel better and live more comfortably in the ICU. Neurological disorders, including amyotrophic lateral sclerosis (ALS) and advanced dementia, also rank among the prominent conditions contributing to end-of-life scenarios. Those with ALS gradually lose motor abilities, which can lead to breathing problems. In contrast, dementia leads to a significant loss of mental abilities, making it difficult for patients to decide about their care. In both situations, the care plan should reflect what matters to the patient, which can be difficult when their ability to decide changes. The ethical complexities surrounding advanced care planning and the potential for rapid terminal sedation reflect the critical role of clinicians in navigating these sensitive discussions, paving the way for tailored, compassionate end-of-life options that prioritize the dignity and comfort of these patients (Wilkinson *et al.*, 2023) (Figure 12.4).

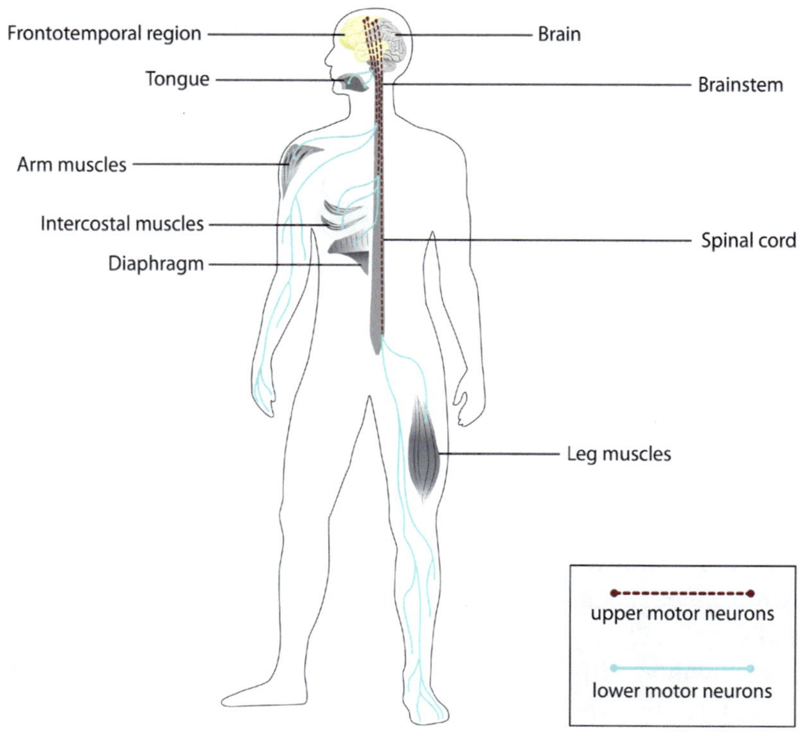

Figure 12.4. Parts of the nervous system affected by amyotrophic lateral sclerosis (ALS).

Source: https://upload.wikimedia.org/wikipedia/commons/1/16/ALS_Affected_neurons_and_muscles.png.

Cancer is still one of the main reasons people face end-of-life situations, especially if it is diagnosed late. Patients with cancer regularly have severe and lasting pain, which is made worse by the side effects of their treatments and the illness. When someone has a terminal illness, the mental and emotional stress often makes their pain worse, so a care plan should include both pain relief and therapy. Having oncologists, palliative care specialists, and social workers work together is important for handling all the challenges patients face. Clarity around treatment goals and patient preferences is crucial, especially when contemplating surgery or other life-extending interventions that may not align with the patient's desire for quality over quantity of life, thus enriching the discourse surrounding end-of-life options and reinforcing the need for ethical deliberation in clinical settings (Anstey *et al.*, 2023).

12.1.3. Ethical Considerations in the Intensive Care Unit (ICU)

While treating patients in the ICU at the end of life, decisions are strongly influenced by ethical issues. An important ethical idea is medical futility, which describes treatments that have little or no chance of helping the patient. Healthcare professionals in critical care should not use treatments that are against what the patient wants and believes. Clinicians need to handle the challenges of medical futility, since recognizing useless interventions depends on open communication with patients and their families. Discussing possible outcomes and what is important to the patient ensures that the care aligns with their wishes for life quality. Establishing a framework for understanding futility, as outlined, provides a basis for ethically sound decision-making that respects the patient's autonomy while maintaining professional integrity (Kopar *et al.*, 2022). Because of the ethical issues in the ICU, it is often necessary to use advanced ways of communicating and resolving conflicts. Making decisions at the end of life often includes families who find it difficult to understand the medical details or what their loved one's condition means. In these emotional situations, healthcare teams should be caring and provide patients with correct, , andprecise information about their condition and treatment. Being ethical in the ICU means that healthcare workers always involve families in the decision-making process.

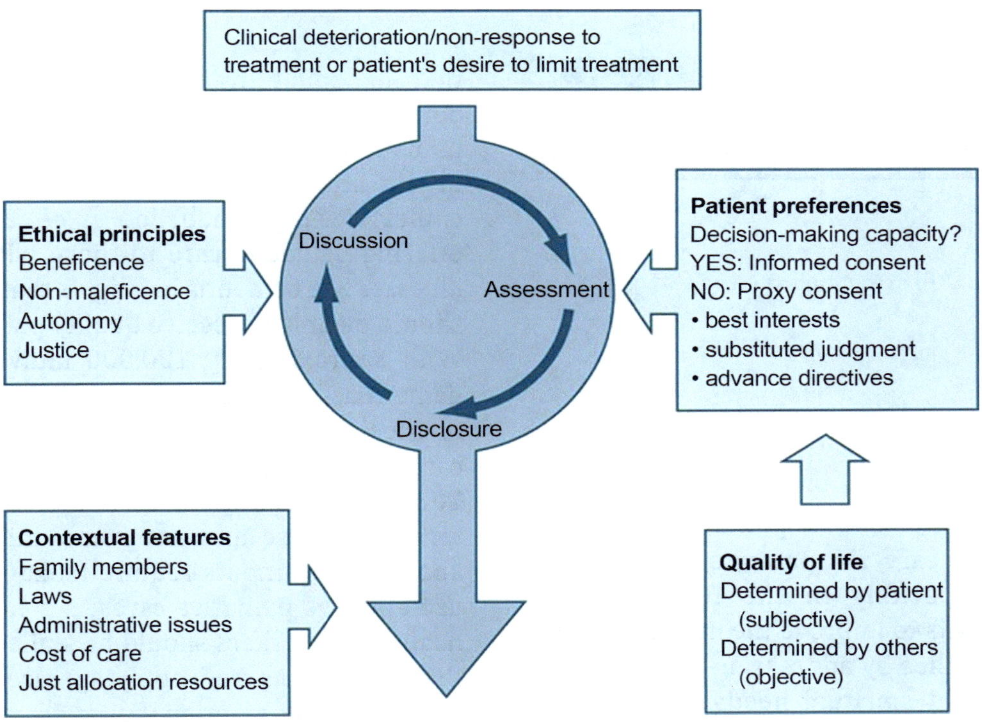

Figure 12.5. The decision-making process.

Source: https://nursekey.com/ethical-issues-in-critical-care/.

Discussions about end-of-life care can be guided by interdisciplinary teams, which also ensure that ethical issues are handled well. In practice, addressing what constitutes reasonable care involves framing palliative measures positively and emphasizing the importance of aligning interventions with the patient's values and goals (Anderson *et al.*, 2020). Furthermore, there is a big concern in the ICU about moral distress, which occurs when healthcare providers are required to act against their ethics, mainly when dealing with end-of-life care. The stress of handling critical care, especially during a crisis like COVID-19, can make medical staff feel more morally distressed when they cannot give the compassionate care they think their patients need. Institutions should create a caring environment for their staff to help alleviate moral distress. It means creating an environment where providers are encouraged to talk about their worries and get support. Having structured support systems, such as mental health resources, can assist in lowering the risks caused by moral distress. As we navigate complex ethical landscapes in the ICU, cultivating resilience among providers becomes vital for sustaining high-quality care and preserving the ethical integrity of end-of-life practices (Kopar *et al.*, 2022) (Figure 12.5).

Test Your Knowledge

1. What are the key features of the ICU environment that influence patient care and decision-making?
2. What are some common medical conditions that may lead to end-of-life situations in the ICU?

12.2. Principles of Palliative Medicine (PM)

Learning Outcome

1. Understand the definition and goals of palliative care
2. Distinction between curative and palliative approaches
3. Explain the importance of interdisciplinary teams in palliative care

It is important to use palliative medicine principles to care for patients with serious illnesses, especially in the ICU. Palliative medicine works to improve the lives of patients and their families by addressing their physical, emotional, and spiritual needs. Because this model covers physical, emotional, social, and spiritual health, healthcare professionals must cooperate to provide care. Given the rise in ICU admissions and the proportion of hospital deaths occurring in these settings, there is an urgent need for effective end-of-life (EOL) care strategies that honor patients' preferences and values. Specifically, research has shown that inadequate treatment of EOL discomforts persists among ICU patients, highlighting a gap in palliative care practices that necessitates urgent attention and improvement within the clinical setting (Ghabeljoo *et al.*, 2017). Also, offering palliative care to those with terminal illnesses like dementia highlights that all patients should be able to receive quality palliative care. With approximately 100,000 individuals with dementia succumbing to the disease annually in the UK, the need for accessible palliative care becomes even more crucial (Birch *et al.*, 2008). Problems such as not recognizing the terminal phase and not communicating well about what patients require make it harder to use effective palliative care. As a consequence, healthcare workers should be skilled in finding these problems and applying care plans that focus on pain, emotional support, and include the family. Using palliative interventions at an early stage can significantly improve a patient's comfort and quality of life, which is in line with the main principles of palliative medicine. Early planning and teamwork among different healthcare professionals are essential for palliative medicine to work well in the ICU.

Team members, patients, and families need to communicate well to handle the many aspects of end-of-life care. Research indicates a lack of standardization in EOL care practices, often resulting in inadequate access to palliative care services and preventable suffering for patients (Ghabeljoo *et al.*, 2017). Talking about what care should involve and what patients hope to achieve can support patients and their families during this challenging period. In addition, teaching healthcare staff about palliative care can help create an atmosphere that supports giving quality EOL care to critically ill patients. When palliative medicine is valued in the ICU, healthcare systems can meet the many needs of patients and their families who are dealing with serious illnesses.

12.2.1. Definition and Goals of Palliative Care

Palliative care is a comprehensive approach that seeks to enhance the quality of life for patients facing serious, often terminal, illnesses. It focuses primarily on alleviating symptoms such as pain, anxiety, and distress, rather than solely on curative treatment. Palliative care's philosophy stresses that illness affects people in many ways and that people's psychological, social, and spiritual needs should be considered as well as their physical health. By using a team from several areas, palliative care tries to support both patients and their families with the proper guidance and resources at every stage of the illness. Since the ICU can involve tough decisions about care and treatment, this approach is essential there. Ultimately, the goal of palliative care is to foster dignity, comfort, and peace for individuals at the end of life (Lyon *et al.*, 2022). Because ICU patients often experience much distress and do not know what to expect, palliative care's goals become especially important. The primary purpose here is to help patients and their families participate in deciding on their care. It helps respect what each person wants and tries to ease the emotional stress that comes with serious illness. Palliative care teams collaborate with other medical staff to ensure that treating symptoms is a primary concern, even as other medical treatments are used. Moreover, families are helped through counseling and bereavement services, which recognize how important they are in the patient's care. In this way, palliative care provides a vital framework for enhancing the overall quality of life for patients in the ICU (Schönhofer *et al.*, 2020).

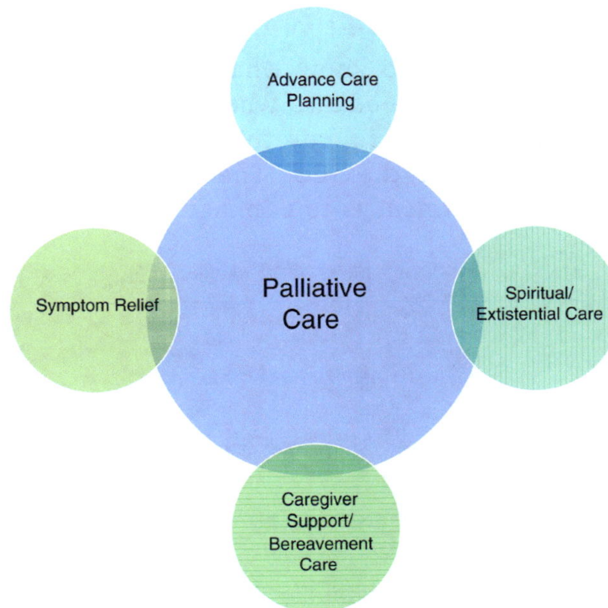

Figure 12.6. Model of palliative care.

Source: https://onlinelibrary.wiley.com/cms/asset/6d9edaa2-b70f-4a90-89da-1cd5ca02936c/clc23307-fig-0001-m.jpg.

Ethical questions about end-of-life care are a major part of palliative care in the ICU. When patients face conditions that could be life-threatening, talking about continuing aggressive treatment becomes more important. In this situation, palliative care guides both healthcare workers and families in understanding the different treatment choices and what patients prefer. Because palliative care teams involve many fields, they can take into account medical, emotional, and ethical concerns. Training ICU staff in palliative care can help them improve their communication skills, which are important for sharing difficult news and handling family issues. By fostering a compassionate and patient-centered atmosphere, palliative care not only addresses immediate needs but also prepares all involved for the emotional implications of end-of-life care (Lyon *et al.*, 2022) (Figure 12.6).

12.2.2. Distinction Between Curative and Palliative Approaches

It is important to know what the main aims are for each type of care when looking at the difference between curative and palliative approaches in the ICU. The main goal of curative treatment is to eliminate the disease and extend life, often through the use of potent treatments that may suppress symptoms but do not constantly improve quality of life. In contrast, palliative care tries to ease pain and improve how people feel by offering comprehensive and helpful support. It is crucial because when patients and families choose treatments that may not succeed, it can cause disagreements. Physicians must recognize these dynamics to avoid treatment inertia, which can exacerbate distress for both patients and their families (Avati *et al.*, 2018). Being aware of these differences helps families and healthcare providers talk about what the patient wants and the best care options as they come closer to death. A growing problem is making sure that patients who might benefit from palliative care are recognized and involved as quickly as possible.

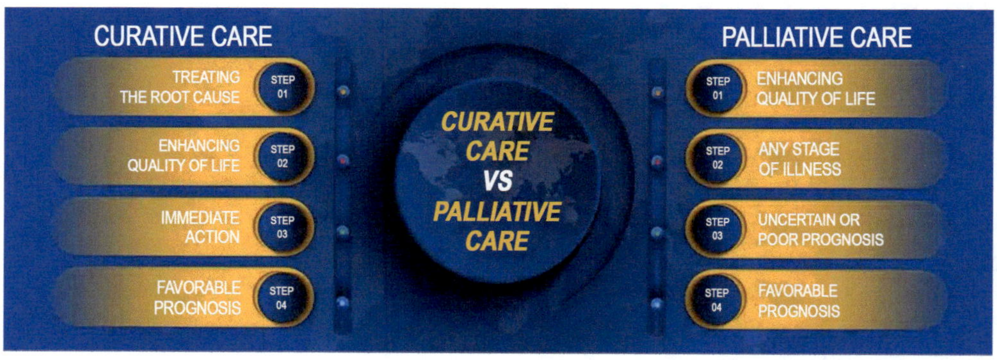

Figure 12.7. Curative care versus palliative care.

Source: https://safehandshhc.com/wp-content/uploads/2023/08/abc-1024x355.webp.

Even though most decisions in medicine are focused on curing, they may not be what the patient wants or needs when facing the end of life. Advanced predictive models, such as those that utilize Electronic Health Records (EHRs), have been employed to identify patients eligible for palliative interventions proactively. By focusing on mortality predictions, healthcare professionals can streamline the palliative referral process and reduce the burden of time-consuming chart reviews, enabling a more responsive approach to patient care (Avati *et al.*, 2018). Identifying these conditions early on makes it more likely for patients to get palliative care, together with or instead of curative care, according to what they prefer. Also, the way care addresses a person's mind and spirit is essential for telling curative medicine apart from palliative medicine. Although curative treatments focus only on physical symptoms, palliative care supports patients emotionally, spiritually, and in all other ways, regardless of their religious beliefs. Since many patients with serious illnesses say they are spiritual but not religious, it is necessary to provide integrative and non-religious care in palliative care.

Looking into these feelings helps patients better understand themselves and achieve inner peace when things are hard. Having interdisciplinary teams lead these discussions protects patients' dignity and helps them make sense of their health issues. Through thoughtful integration of both medical and spiritual support, palliative care can transform the end-of-life experience from one of suffering to one of acceptance and solace (Figure 12.7).

12.2.3. Importance of Interdisciplinary Teams in Palliative Care

In the ICU, where patients often have many severe symptoms and medical issues, working in teams from different specialties is very important. When physicians, nurses, social workers, and chaplains team up, they can manage patients by treating their physical, emotional, and spiritual issues. Studies suggest that teamwork greatly improves the quality of care in these important places.

For example, initiatives like RWJFs Interdisciplinary Nursing Quality Research emphasize how diverse nursing-led quality improvement projects can lead to significant enhancements in patient care outcomes, showcasing the critical role interdisciplinary collaboration plays in effective palliative strategies (N/A, 2012). Interdisciplinary teams in ICUs also help by making sure that palliative care is tailored to each patient and their family members. Studies show that ICU-based palliative care helps, but the practice of such care is not always consistent and sometimes overlooks important factors. Successful practices often involve creating symbiotic relationships between palliative care specialists and ICU teams, which allow for smoother operational dynamics (Meddick-Dyson & Stephanie, 2023).

When team members can work together and use their different skills, it leads to better symptom control and better communication with families during important choices. Using interdisciplinary teams in palliative care helps the ICU develop a holistic approach to health. Working together in this way helps create a learning environment and allows everyone to find solutions to the challenges of end-of-life care. When different opinions are shared, the palliative care team gains access to a broader range of knowledge and experience, which helps them find new and better ways to help patients. Both the obstacles and supports in these collaborative efforts are emphasized in the context of palliative care implementation strategies. Thus, enhancing the effectiveness of interdisciplinary teams not only contributes to better patient outcomes but also fosters an invaluable resource for future care practices in ICUs (Meddick-Dyson & Stephanie, 2023).

Test Your Knowledge

1. What is the definition of palliative care, and what are its primary goals in patient management?
2. How does a palliative care approach differ from a curative approach in terms of treatment objectives?

12.3. Communication with Patients and Families

Learning Outcome

1. Discuss the strategies for effective communication.
2. Define addressing emotional and psychological needs.
3. Explain the involving families in decision-making processes.

Good communication with patients and their families is critical in end-of-life care and palliative medicine, especially in the ICU. Healthcare professionals must handle emotional challenges while ensuring that medical information is communicated clearly. It means discussing what is likely to happen and the available treatments, as well as learning about what matters to patients and their families. If families participate in making decisions, they usually feel more supported and involved, which can help reduce their anxiety and strengthen their trust in the healthcare team. If there is not enough clear communication, it can cause misunderstandings, more stress, and less satisfaction with care, which affects both patients and their families. So, open and understanding communication should be a primary focus in the ICU. Along with managing medical issues, doctors should be aware of the emotional and psychological needs of patients and their families at the end of life. It is challenging in the ICU, since time is usually limited and things can change very fast. Healthcare providers must handle the demanding side of critical care and still comfort families dealing with loss. Listening to what families have to say, using gestures to communicate, and making sure families have plenty of opportunities to speak up can support them. Furthermore, healthcare teams ought to have resources and mental health support ready to help families get through this experience. In the end, well-planned communication helps both by sharing information and by comforting patients, which supports a fuller approach to patient care. We should understand that effective communication is something that we keep working on, not just in one conversation. Checking how well patients and their families understand the care plan and how they feel helps in adapting the care and making sure it matches their wishes. Because of telemedicine and other new technologies, healthcare providers can still stay in contact and give updates, even if they cannot meet patients physically during the pandemic. Working together, physicians, nurses, social workers, and chaplains can improve the way patients and their families are supported by using different skills. As the paradigm of end-of-life care continues to evolve, prioritizing communication remains a cornerstone of delivering compassionate and effective palliative care within the ICU setting (Lambertini *et al.*, 2020; Weissman *et al.*, 2018).

12.3.1. Strategies for Effective Communication

Effective communication is a cornerstone in enhancing the quality of end-of-life care in the ICU. It requires not only disseminating information about medical conditions and treatment options but also addressing the emotional and psychological needs of patients and their families. Training programs designed for healthcare professionals, particularly those in Pulmonary and Critical Care Medicine (PCCM) fellowship, play a crucial role in fostering such communication skills. It is shown that fellows who have more end-of-life conversations feel much more confident in handling them, underlining the role of practical experience in improving their skills. Moreover, factors like strong mentorship and favorable ICU environments contribute positively to fellows' capabilities in facilitating effective communication, underscoring the necessity for structured training integrated into fellowship curricula (Yuan *et al.*, 2025). Also, international guidelines stress the use of evidence-based methods to improve communication in the ICU, especially when patients are approaching the end of their lives.

The European Society of Intensive Care Medicine (ESICM) has developed recommendations advocating for structured decision-making strategies, which aid healthcare providers in navigating complex conversations surrounding palliative care. They highlight the need to use family-focused care and give families simple printed materials to help them understand medical terms, which can lower their anxiety. In family conferences, families can openly discuss their needs and wishes, and their independence is continually respected. Implementing these strategies demonstrates a commitment to compassionate care, effectively addressing the emotional needs of both patients and families during critical times (Kesecioglu *et al.*, 2024).

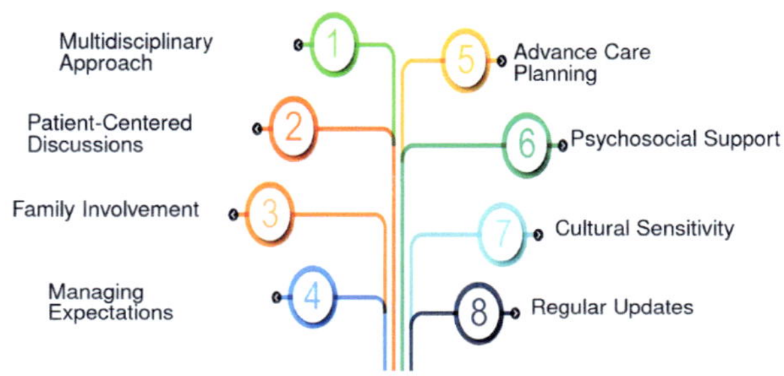

Figure 12.8. The importance of communication in palliative care in the intensive care unit (ICU).

Source: https://fastercapital.co/i/Palliative-care--Providing-Comfort--Palliative-Care-in-the-ICU--The-Importance-of-Communication-in-Palliative-Care.webp.

It is also important to handle conflicts and prevent clinician burnout to maintain good communication in the ICU. Healthcare providers can encounter situations that make patients or families upset, which might result in arguments about how care should be handled. Having conflict-management rules in place supports families and staff in solving problems positively. Supporting healthcare providers and promoting their mental health can prevent burnout, so they stay caring and effective in their work. When these strategies are part of ICU practice, they can help improve how end-of-life communication is handled. Ultimately, prioritizing effective communication strategies is essential for improving patient care, family satisfaction, and staff well-being in the challenging setting of end-of-life and palliative medicine in the ICU (Kesecioglu *et al.*, 2024) (Figure 12.8).

12.3.2. Addressing Emotional and Psychological Needs

In the context of end-of-life care and palliative medicine in the ICU, addressing emotional and psychological needs is crucial for both patients and their families. Critical illness can make people feel many things, such as fear, anxiety, and despair. Intensive care can be very stressful for patients, so healthcare providers must understand that stress can come from both the seriousness of the condition and the unknown outcomes.

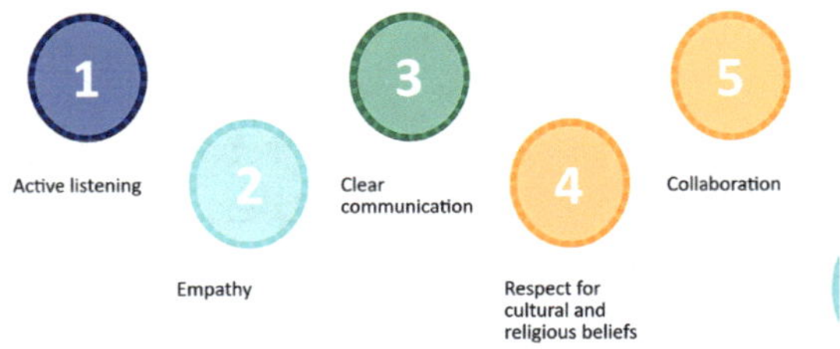
1
Active listening
2
Empathy
3
Clear communication
4
Respect for cultural and religious beliefs
5
Collaboration

Figure 12.9. Essential skills for end-of-life (EoL) care.

Source: https://fastercapital.co/i/End-of-life-care--Honoring-Life--End-of-Life-Care-in-the-ICU--Essential-Skills-for-End-of-Life-Care.webp.

At this point, being able to communicate effectively is very important because it supports trust and allows feelings to be expressed. If caregivers explain things clearly, treat patients with care, and make sure everyone feels understood, they can help individuals face their fears and decide on the best treatment and end-of-life plans. Also, the mental effects reach families who may lose a loved one, so healthcare teams should use supportive strategies that address all aspects of care. Family members often experience anticipatory grief, a process marked by sorrow and distress as they witness their loved ones face impending death (Figure 12.9).

Offering psychological support and resources like counseling and palliative care consultations is important for ICU teams to handle these emotional needs. They can assist family members in dealing with their emotions, which makes it easier to talk about values, hopes, and fears. According to research, when relatives get enough emotional support, they are better able to cope both during and after the loss, which can greatly improve their experience of the end-of-life process.

Thus, it is important to use multidisciplinary methods that combine emotional and psychological care to help families become more resilient during this hard time. Also, patients with specific diseases, such as hematologic malignancies, require unique psychological support from palliative services. People with these cancers usually experience severe physical discomfort as well as emotional distress because they are unsure about their treatment and outcome. When these factors interact, patients may feel more hopeless and anxious, which makes palliative care more complicated.

Many patients with hematologic malignancies have incorrect views about their illness, which can make their emotional problems worse and lower their quality of life. So, to meet the psychological needs of these patients, specialized palliative care is needed to inform and help them cope with their complex emotions. Ultimately, such a focus on emotional care not only aids patients but also enhances the overall efficacy of end-of-life care initiatives within the ICU setting, ensuring that individuals receive comprehensive support during their most vulnerable moments (El-Jawahri *et al.*, 2020; René Robert *et al.*, 2020).

12.3.3. Involving Families in Decision-Making Processes

The involvement of families in decision-making processes within the ICU is essential for ensuring that the care provided aligns with the values and preferences of critically ill patients. Families may feel much emotional distress at this point, and being involved in talks about treatment can make them feel less helpless.

When family members are involved in decisions, healthcare providers can make sure the environment respects the importance of family. In addition, families often know what the patient wants and how they feel, which may not be evident to the medical team. This collaborative approach fosters a sense of shared responsibility. It can ultimately lead to more personalized and satisfactory care plans, particularly in palliative contexts where the objectives may focus on comfort and dignity rather than curative measures (Davidson *et al.*, 2016). Talking effectively with families is very important in the process of including them in decisions.

Talking openly and kindly about the patient's illness, the outlook, and treatment choices helps families feel confident and better informed. Allowing families to share their views helps everyone learn more about what the patient needs. Families are involved in decision-making about care when the ethical principle of patient autonomy is respected, especially when a person is dying. Also, having family members involved in making decisions can strengthen their emotional strength, as they know the reasons for the decisions and feel appreciated by the healthcare team. This structured communication strategy, therefore, not only improves relational dynamics but also enhances the overall quality of end-of-life care (Davidson *et al.*, 2016).

Although family involvement is recognized as valuable, there are still many things that can make it difficult for families to be involved in ICU decisions. Because of their training, healthcare professionals may give more weight to their own decisions than to what the family wants, which might leave family members feeling excluded and irritated. Also, stress and grief can make it difficult for families to be involved in important healthcare talks. Addressing these hurdles with counseling and clear resources is very important. Following the current guidelines, healthcare teams can be trained to use family-centered care, which can help them have more meaningful talks with patients. The importance of establishing a collaborative atmosphere cannot be overstated; as evidenced in recent literature, such an approach is instrumental for driving effective engagement and enhancing the overall quality of end-of-life care decisions (Davidson *et al.*, 2016) (Figure 12.10).

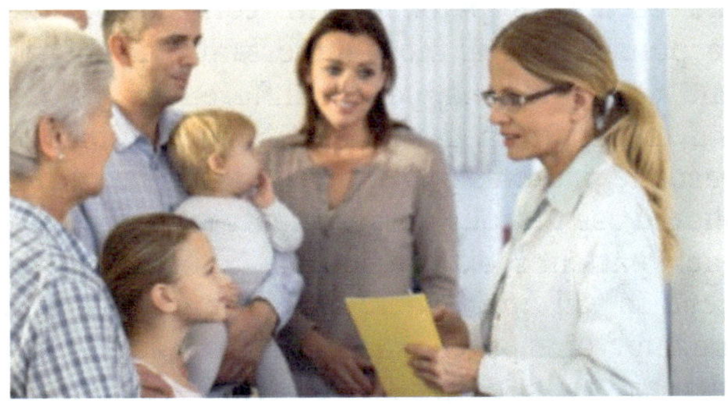

Figure 12.10. Decision-making processes within the ICU.

Source: https://www.healthychildren.org/English/health-issues/conditions/developmental-disabilities/Pages/Involving-Your-Child-in-the-Decision-Making-Process.aspx.

Test Your Knowledge

1. What strategies can healthcare providers use to ensure effective communication with critically ill patients and their families?
2. How can the emotional and psychological needs of patients and families be addressed in critical care settings?

12.4. Pain Management in End-of-Life Care

Learning Outcome

1. Analyze the assessment of pain in critically ill patients
2. Define pharmacological interventions for pain relief
3. Discuss the non-pharmacological approaches to pain management

Managing pain well is very important for end-of-life care, especially in the ICU. At the end of life, caring for patients with compassion and responsiveness is most important. Pain at the end of life can happen in different ways and may result from the illness or from efforts to ease the patient's pain. So, healthcare providers should use thorough assessments to understand each patient's experience of pain. Caregivers need to tell apart acute and chronic pain and look for any psychological factors that might increase the patient's distress. Addressing these complexities requires a thorough understanding of treatment options and an awareness of how these choices impact not just the patient, but also their families and the broader healthcare team (Lyon *et al.*, 2022). It is essential in palliative medicine to use a methodical approach to managing pain. Strategies may vary widely, incorporating pharmacological methods such as opioids, nonsteroidal anti-inflammatory drugs (NSAIDs), and adjuvant therapies based on the patient's specific needs and responses. Non-medicine therapies, for example, cognitive-behavioral therapy, acupuncture, or massage therapy, may help to manage pain symptoms. For patients in the ICU, where technology is advanced and can cause stress, using both methods at once is very important. Effective communication among the interdisciplinary team members is crucial to ensure that pain management plans are tailored to each patient, fostering an environment where both comfort and dignity are prioritized (Price *et al.*, 2018). In addition, the emotional and mental aspects of pain should not be ignored in caring for someone at the end of their life. Those with terminal illness usually face profound questions about life, which can add to their physical pain. So, to give comprehensive palliative care, one must know how emotional distress can influence pain management. Providing counseling or spiritual care can significantly improve how patients feel and allow them to talk about their pain and discomfort. Also, including family in care discussions helps ensure that the patient's goals are followed, making the process more team-based and valuable. Ensuring that nurses and other staff members are adequately trained in both pain management techniques and the emotional aspects of care is crucial for delivering compassionate end-of-life care in the ICU (Lyon *et al.*, 2022) (Figure 12.11).

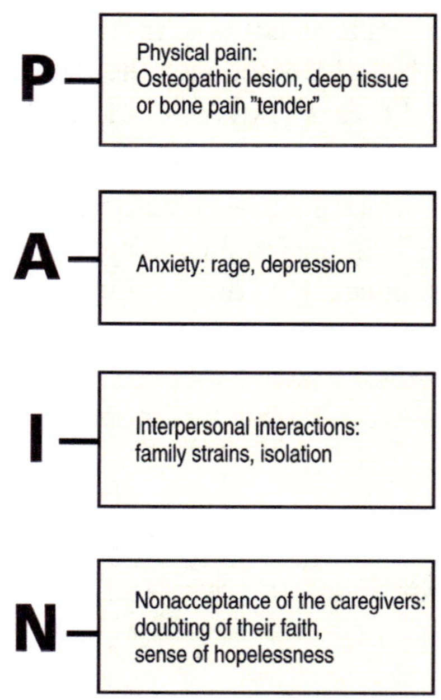

Figure 12.11. Patient's perception of "total pain."

Source: https://www.degruyterbrill.com/document/doi/10.7556/jaoa.2005.20003/html.

12.4.1. Assessment of Pain in Critically Ill Patients

The assessment of pain in critically ill patients is a crucial component of end-of-life care and palliative medicine in the ICU. It can be tough to assess pain in these patients because they may be unconscious, on a ventilator, and have many other health problems. In this situation, healthcare providers should use pain assessment tools that are reliable and fit the needs of this group. Using observational pain scales to look at non-verbal signs of pain is very important. Furthermore, the incorporation of the Clinical Frailty Scale (CFS) can help identify patients' functional status and customize pain management strategies accordingly, enhancing the quality of palliative care provided in the ICU (Rockwood *et al.*, 2020). A proper and organized assessment of pain helps manage symptoms better and makes end-of-life care more satisfying for everyone. Therefore, because it is so difficult to assess pain in critically ill patients, a team effort involving various healthcare workers is required. Physicians, nurses, social workers, and palliative care specialists to join efforts to assess and communicate about the patient's pain. Because critically ill patients can behave differently due to their medical situation, working in a team helps us notice the differences in their pain expression. As noted, older adults with frailty and cognitive impairment face heightened risks associated with surgical procedures and post-operative pain management (Lee *et al.*, 2018). If healthcare providers are aware of these complexities, they can provide pain management that aligns with patients' desires and expectations. Pain management that fits the patient's needs leads to more comfort and a decent end-of-life journey. Pain management strategies should not stop at the immediate care given in the hospital. It is crucial in the ICU to encourage patients and their families to talk openly about pain management and treatment goals. Talking to patients and their families about pain relief options helps them feel more in control and respected, which can be lost in critical care. Also, providing detailed training to healthcare staff on the need to assess and manage pain in seriously ill patients can help improve care standards. Palliative care interventions have shown promise in significantly improving outcomes such as quality of life and symptom control in surgical patients, emphasizing the importance of integrating pain management within the broader framework of critical care (Lee *et al.*, 2018). In summation, an approach that emphasizes thorough assessment, interdisciplinary collaboration, and preemptive communication can fundamentally transform the end-of-life care experience for critically ill patients (Figure 12.12).

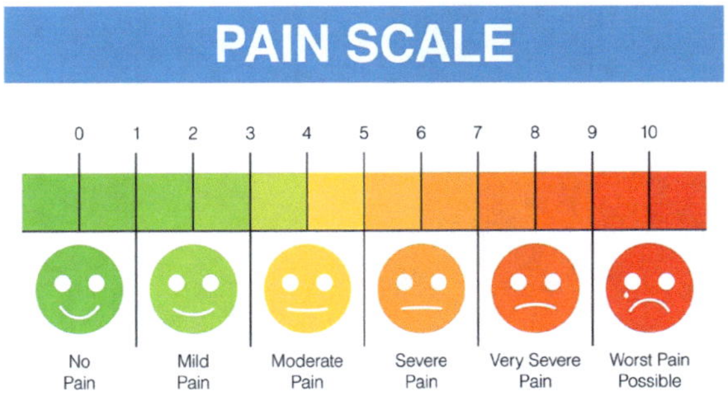

Figure 12.12. Pain assessment in the critically ill patient.

Source: https://cdn.ausmed.com/ausmed-blog-images/2018/05/20180509_body.jpg.

12.4.2. Pharmacological Interventions for Pain Relief

When caring for patients at the end of life in the ICU, drugs for pain relief are essential for their dignity and comfort. Opioids are the main drugs used in pain management to provide important relief from pain. Pain medications can be given by mouth, through a vein, or by applying them to the skin, which makes it easier to control pain. In the ICU, where patients can have different physiological needs, such methods are important and fundamental.

As Chowdhury (2024) outlines, proper management of opioid administration involves not only dose adjustments to mitigate side effects like sedation and respiratory depression but also continuous monitoring to optimize the therapeutic outcome while ensuring the patient's quality of life is preserved. Treating pain in critically ill people requires using both drugs and non-drug strategies. Doctors and nurses may also give other medications, such as NSAIDs and adjuvant analgesics, to help patients feel less pain and depend less on opioids. This multimodal approach not only addresses complex pain syndromes but also minimizes the adverse effects associated with high-dose opioid therapy (Figure 12.13).

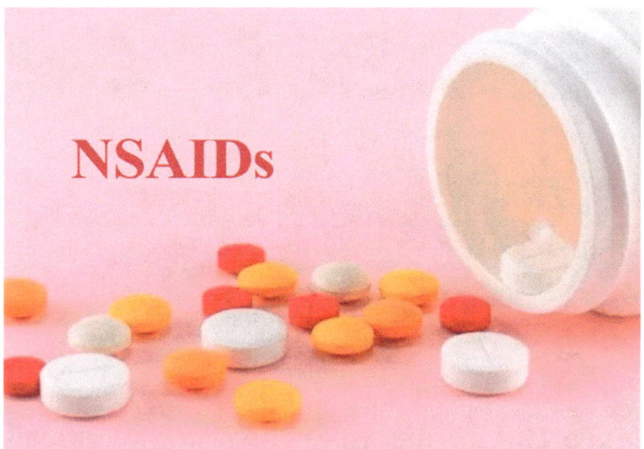

Figure 12.13. Pharmacological Interventions for Pain Relief.

Source: https://samarpanphysioclinic.com/wp-content/uploads/2021/11/NSAIDs-%E2%80%93-Non-Steroidal-Anti-Inflammatory-Drugs-1200x900.webp.

According to findings from a recent audit, while pharmacological management of symptoms is prevalent, it is equally essential to document assessments meticulously to ensure an adequate understanding of pain management efficacy (Loh *et al.*, 2023). With this documentation, personalized care plans can be made, and it is easier to remember to reassess symptoms regularly in the ICU to ensure proper end-of-life care. It is essential to include pharmacological treatments along with a complete approach to symptom management to provide the best care for patients at the end of life in the ICU. In this situation, the palliative care team is critical because they help manage difficult symptoms and support the emotional and social needs of patients and their families. When healthcare providers and patients/families work together, it leads to a more helpful environment for pain management. Since palliative care is now seen as important in ICUs, it is still necessary for healthcare workers to know the details of pain relief medications.

12.4.3. Non-Pharmacological Approaches to Pain Management

In the context of end-of-life care and palliative medicine within the ICU, non-pharmacological approaches to pain management are increasingly recognized for their significance in improving patient quality of life. They cover many types of treatments that help both the body and the mind. Mindfulness, guided imagery, and relaxation therapy are proven to reduce anxiety and encourage a calm state, which is very important for patients who are aware of their approaching death. Incorporating non-pharmacological measures alongside pharmacologic treatments can lead to a more holistic approach in palliative care, ultimately contributing to an enhanced patient experience in critical care settings, as evidenced by the multidisciplinary efforts underway in supportive care frameworks like Integrative Obstetric programs (Ben-Arye *et al.*, 2025). Also, studies have found that non-pharmacological strategies play an important role in managing pain when used together with other treatments, especially in patients who have major procedures or chronic pain. Combining physical therapy, acupuncture, and psychotherapy in healthcare allows doctors to control pain without needing to give patients dangerous drugs. Since patients in the ICU may experience complex pain from their diseases and the procedures they receive, this approach is critical. Studies today suggest that using a variety of these techniques can both ease pain and offer better emotional support and ways to cope for patients and their families. By establishing effective communication between healthcare teams about available non-pharmacological resources, the ICU can better address the multifaceted nature of pain management (de Souza *et al.*, 2024). Incorporating non-pharmacological approaches in palliative care emphasizes the patient's needs and preferences in the ICU. It respects that every person's pain is different and encourages healthcare providers to work together with patients. When healthcare providers talk to patients and their families about pain management, they can adjust treatments that fit patients' values, preferences, and emotions. For these strategies to be successful, healthcare organizations must back them up, train their staff, and keep researching to see if they are effective. With the progress of palliative medicine, it is necessary to include and standardize non-pharmacological methods, so that all patients are cared for with respect and their pain is handled in a kind and appropriate way.

Test Your Knowledge

1. What methods are commonly used to assess pain in critically ill patients who may be unable to communicate?
2. What pharmacological options are available for managing pain in the ICU, and how are they selected?

12.5. Advanced Directives and Patient Autonomy

Learning Outcome

1. Understanding advanced directives and living wills
2. Describe the role of patient autonomy in decision-making
3. Understand the challenges in honoring patient wishes in the ICU

In the context of end-of-life care within the ICU, advanced directives play a pivotal role in safeguarding patient autonomy. They allow people to state their health care wishes, especially when they are too sick to speak for themselves. Advanced directives help patients take part in deciding their care, and they are important for healthcare professionals to guide treatment that fits the patient's wishes. In Argentina, laws have been put in place to ensure these rights are respected, which strengthens the ethical duty of clinicians to respect patients' decisions about their end-of-life care. By prioritizing advanced directives, healthcare systems can foster an environment where dignity and respect for individual autonomy are upheld, providing patients and families with a more straightforward path through the complexities of decision-making in critical care settings (Guzmán, 2025). Even though advanced directives are very useful, there are many difficulties in using them in the ICU. A study conducted in the context of chronic kidney disease (CKD) patients revealed alarming statistics regarding the lack of palliative care involvement, even as mortality rates escalated during critical health crises, such as the COVID-19 pandemic (Correa *et al.*, 2025). Many patients with CKD who were admitted to the ICU passed away without proper palliative care, which suggests healthcare providers may not always follow advanced directives when a patient is in an emergency. A lack of training in how to communicate, not knowing the rules, and cultural issues usually stop people from using advanced directives effectively. Handling these issues helps patients make their own choices and get care that matches what they want. Being able to make healthcare decisions for oneself is tied to acknowledging a person's values and rights. Respecting autonomy is especially important in end-of-life care in the ICU, since patients have to make challenging medical decisions. If healthcare providers discuss advanced directives before a crisis, patients are more likely to feel in control and understood during their care. Encouraging compassion among medical teams allows providers to manage these delicate talks more smoothly. Ultimately, integrating advanced directives into ICU protocols not only respects patient autonomy but also promotes a humane approach to end-of-life care that aligns with ethical practices (Guzmán, 2025).

12.5.1. Understanding Advanced Directives and Living Wills

Advanced directives and living wills are essential in end-of-life care in the ICU. Advance directives let individuals state what medical care they want if they are unable to express their wishes themselves. By using this strategy, patients can make their own choices, which helps medical staff and family members decide what to do in serious situations. Advanced directives work well when both the patient and the healthcare provider understand what they say. In discussing advanced care planning, it is essential to recognize that misinterpretation or lack of knowledge about these directives can lead to conflicts between patient preferences and the medical interventions that occur, underscoring the necessity for ongoing education in this area as part of end-of-life discussions (Guzmán, 2025). Living wills, which are advance directives, are vital in ICU situations where quick medical decisions are needed. They detail situations where patients want to refuse specific treatments, such as those to prolong life, if they are diagnosed with a terminal or irreversible illness. Thus, healthcare providers must know the finer points of living wills to support patient autonomy. Because the ICU is so intense and offers many advanced treatments, it can be difficult to tell what patients want and what the medical team can do. If healthcare workers wanted.

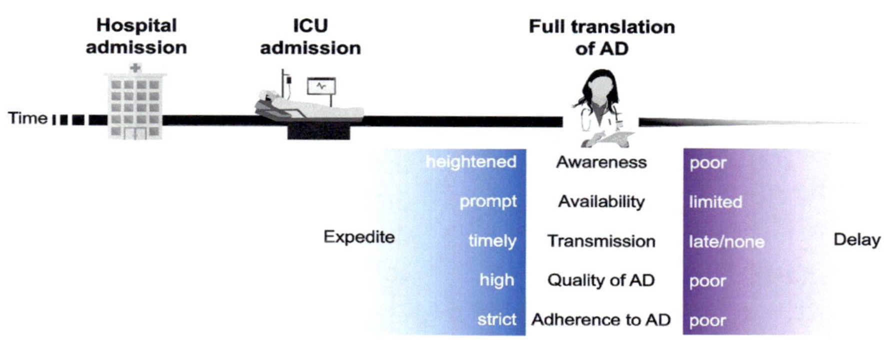

Figure 12.14. Challenges regarding the identification, transmission, and implementation of patients' advance directives during critical care.

Source: https://jintensivecare.biomedcentral.com/articles/10.1186/s40560-023-00705-z.

They may also be unaware of a patient's living will and provide treatment that contradicts the patient's wishes. Hence, fostering an environment where living wills are regularly discussed and respected is crucial in delivering compassionate end-of-life care (Wheless *et al.*, 2025). Although advanced directives and living wills seem worthwhile, many obstacles prevent their proper use in ICUs. Many healthcare workers say they do not feel prepared to talk about these delicate subjects with patients and their families. Sometimes, cultural and ethical issues can make it harder to discuss end-of-life wishes, which can cause patients' preferences to be poorly documented or communicated. Such problems point to the need for healthcare organizations to improve their training and educational programs on advanced care planning. Also, using protocols that encourage healthcare teams to talk with patients and families about advance directives can make end-of-life care more effective. By addressing these barriers, healthcare professionals can better uphold the principles of informed consent and patient autonomy, ultimately providing dignified care to those transitioning through critical illnesses (Guzmán, 2025) (Figure 12.14).

12.5.2. The Role of Patient Autonomy in Decision-Making

Navigating the intricacies of end-of-life care within the ICU setting necessitates a profound respect for patient autonomy, particularly as it pertains to decision-making. Patient autonomy is the ethical idea that individuals should be able to decide about their healthcare. At the end of life, this principle matters a lot because patients may need to make difficult medical choices that can greatly influence their health and quality of life. Allowing patients to express their choices helps make the care more about them, which can lead to more satisfaction with the services they receive. When medical care is guided by autonomy, it reflects the patient's wishes and values, which makes the decision-making process more complete and important. Even so, making decisions about care at the end of life can be very hard for patients and those providing care. Many people who are patients may feel emotional distress, experience a decline in mental abilities, or have trouble understanding their health problems, which can make it hard for them to decide what is best for them.

This example underlines the importance of healthcare professionals in helping people discuss their options, what might happen, and what they want. Since providers have to share difficult medical information and deal with patients' emotions, effective communication becomes essential. Additionally, issues regarding advanced directives and surrogate decision-makers must be addressed to ensure that patients' wishes align with subsequent medical decisions, thus reinforcing the crucial nature of autonomy in palliative care frameworks (Lyon *et al.*, 2022). Allowing patients to make their own decisions can help them live better in the ICU. Based on research, those who are involved in making decisions about their care report being more satisfied and having less anxiety about the unknown aspects of their illness and treatment. Because of the growing number of older people and those with chronic diseases, it is crucial to stress the role of autonomy in planning health care. It is expected that by 2050, the need for end-of-life care will rise sharply, which means healthcare providers must pay more attention to what patients want. This emphasis on autonomy not only empowers patients but also enhances the quality and appropriateness of care, ultimately fostering a more compassionate and responsive healthcare environment (Figure 12.15).

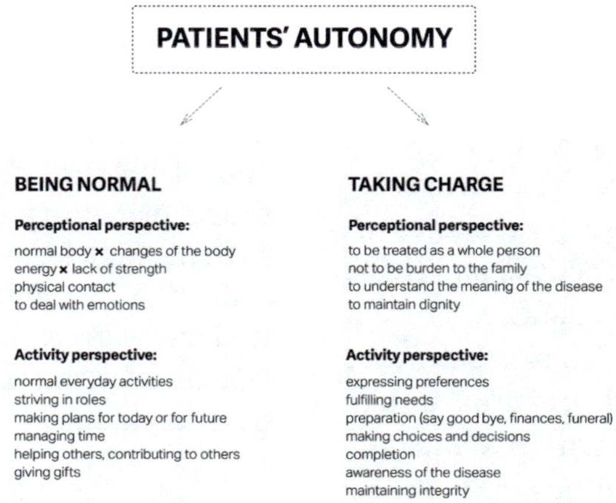

Figure 12.15. Structural model of autonomy for patients at the end of life (EoL).

Source: https://www.sciencedirect.com/science/article/pii/S0885392418314878.

12.5.3. Challenges in Honoring Patient Wishes in the Intensive Care Unit (ICU)

In the ICU, healthcare providers frequently encounter significant challenges when attempting to honor patient wishes, particularly regarding end-of-life care. Many ethical problems occur when beneficence, which supports actions that help patients, and autonomy, which supports a patient's decision-making, conflict. Families and medical teams may have to make decisions that go against what the patient said they wanted. Suppose a patient has previously stated they want little treatment. In that case, the team's decision to pursue aggressive care might cause both the family and the healthcare providers to feel uneasy and distressed. Recognizing the complexity involved in such situations is vital for ensuring that patient wishes are respected and upheld in accordance with ethical guidelines (Varkey, 2020) (Figure 12.16).

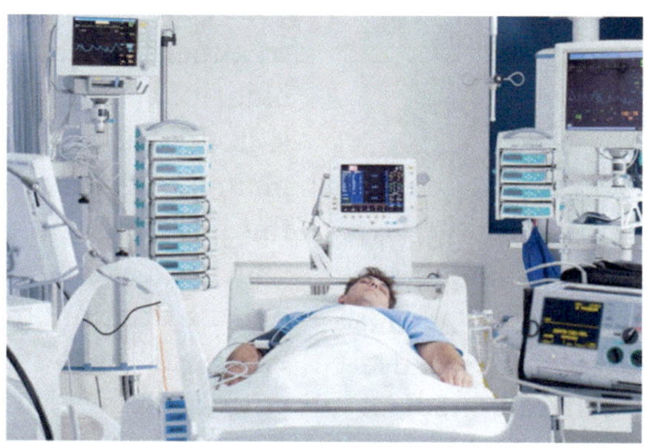

Figure 12.16. Honoring Patient Wishes in the Intensive Care Unit (ICU).

Source: https://www.usnews.com/dims4/USNEWS/71985c6/2147483647/thumbnail/970x647/quality/85/?url=https%3A%2F%2Fwww.usnews.com%2Fcmsmedia%2Fd3%2F23%2Fdfb649b847439f73d4c8c72739e1%2F141024-eicupatient-stock.jpg.

Another challenge in honoring patient wishes is the variability in the advance care planning process. Many patients do not engage in discussions about their preferences prior to entering the ICU, leaving families to make decisions under extreme stress and uncertainty. If advance directives are not detailed enough, there may be disagreements about what the patient wanted in particular circumstances. Families may also struggle with making important decisions, feeling unsure about how to navigate the vast amount of medical information and choices available. Sufficient education and support for families during this process are critical to bridging the gap between patient wishes and actionable choices, ultimately leading to a more compassionate approach to end-of-life care and palliative medicine in the ICU (Lapid *et al.*, 2020). Also, having several healthcare providers involved can make it more difficult to honor what the patient wants in the ICU. Having different specialties can cause team members to have varying views on a patient's condition, which may lead to mixed messages. Because of this dissonance, family members may struggle to speak up for their loved ones and might end up confused. Because of time pressure, doctors and patients may not have the time to discuss preferences in detail. Making sure that there is open communication among the medical team, the patient, and the family is important for respecting what matters to the patient. By adopting an integrative and communicative approach, it becomes possible to navigate the ethical complexities inherent in critical care while honoring patient autonomy (Varkey, 2020).

Test Your Knowledge

1. What are advanced directives and living wills, and how do they guide care in critical situations?
2. How does the principle of patient autonomy influence medical decision-making in the ICU?

SUMMARY

In the discussion on end-of-life care and palliative medicine within the ICU, it is imperative to recognize the critical need for a paradigm shift toward comprehensive palliative care for all patients, particularly those with terminal illnesses, such as dementia. Although palliative care is now seen as important for patient well-being, many people are still not given the proper support when they most need it. According to the literature, especially for dementia patients, difficulties in determining a prognosis and in communication continue to prevent many from receiving palliative care. Handling these challenges is necessary to improve how care is given and to ensure that patients are adequately supported as they approach the end of their lives. Integrating palliative care into the ICU setting can bridge gaps in service accessibility and ultimately uplift the standard of care for critically ill patients (Birch *et al.*, 2008). Economically, the importance of strong palliative care services cannot be ignored. It seems that palliative care can help lower costs compared to standard care by managing symptoms well and improving the coordination between different healthcare providers. It has been found that palliative care can improve the patient and family experience, and at the same time reduce healthcare expenses by reducing unnecessary treatments and hospital stays. This shows that using cost-effective palliative care in the ICU is important and helps overcome the belief that it is always more expensive. A well-structured palliative care framework can therefore enhance the quality of life for patients while simultaneously representing a sensible financial investment for healthcare systems (Brick *et al.*, 2013). End-of-life care in the ICU requires an approach that centers on the patient's needs and uses palliative care. This way, the healthcare system should actively remove barriers and encourage different medical experts to communicate, so that patients and families are given the best care for their needs. In addition, new research helps discover the best approaches and the unique needs of people with conditions such as dementia. These initiatives will help people learn how to use resources well and improve training for healthcare workers in giving quality palliative care. Ultimately, embracing this holistic vision not only honors the dignity of patients navigating life's final chapter but also redefines the objectives of ICU care in a manner that prioritizes comfort, compassion, and holistic health (Birch *et al.*, 2008; Brick *et al.*, 2013).

It is important to focus on the educational gaps that still exist among healthcare workers when looking at EOL care and palliative medicine in the ICU. Lack of proper knowledge and training may make it challenging to communicate with patients and their families about decisions at the end of life. While it is acknowledged that these discussions have been important since the late 1960s, most medical schools still do not prepare students well for EOL care. The TRIPLE curriculum at Johns Hopkins School of Medicine actively helps students develop the skills needed to handle end-of-life situations by using standardized patients and simulations. Having providers ready for these sensitive talks improves the care given in the ICU. The curriculum also gives a clear structure for using different teaching methods, helping students grasp EOL care principles well. The use of didactic lessons, hands-on activities, and simulations with standardized patients makes sure the curriculum highlights the importance of emotional and communication skills needed for discussing EOL options with families. The strong positive feedback from participants, with an average satisfaction rating of 4.6 out of 5, underlines the effectiveness of this educational approach in fostering confidence among healthcare providers addressing complex EOL issues (Lyon *et al.*, 2022). As a result, such training will likely be included in future updates to medical education, demonstrating a dedication to preparing professionals who can compassionately help patients and their families in critical care situations. In addition, better EOL and palliative care training affects many areas of medical care, not just the ICU. A well-equipped doctor can guide patients in planning for the future, including organ donation and creating living wills, and can also effectively manage patients in various medical settings. The integration of EOL learning underscores the relevance of these skills in an era where a growing aging population presents a pressing need for compassionate care (Lyon *et al.*, 2022). Paying attention to the emotional and ethical aspects of death and dying helps medical professionals and students build a supportive environment, which can improve how patients feel and recover. Giving healthcare providers the skills for these responsibilities is a moral duty that improves the quality of care in the ICU and other areas.

KEY TERMS FROM THIS CHAPTER

- Advanced care planning
- Bereavement support
- Do not intubate (DNI)
- End-of-life care
- Euthanasia
- Hospice care
- Life-sustaining treatment
- Pain management
- Advanced directives
- Comfort measures
- Do not resuscitate (DNR)
- Ethical dilemmas
- Family-centered care
- ICU (intensive care unit)
- Organ donation
- Palliative care

CRITICAL THINKING QUESTIONS

1. **Which of the following is a primary goal of palliative care in the ICU?**
   a. Cure the underlying disease
   b. Prevent all possible complications
   c. Provide comfort and relieve suffering
   d. Achieve the longest possible survival
2. **Which of the following medications is most commonly used for managing pain in terminally ill patients in the ICU?**
   a. Acetaminophen
   b. Morphine
   c. Ibuprofen
   d. Methotrexate
3. **In the context of end-of-life care, which of the following interventions is most commonly used to manage dyspnea in critically ill patients?**
   a. High-flow oxygen therapy
   b. Diuretics
   c. Benzodiazepines
   d. Opioids
4. **The decision to withdraw life-sustaining treatment in an ICU patient is best made by:**
   a. The primary care physician only
   b. A multidisciplinary team, including the patient's family
   c. The ICU nursing staff
   d. The hospital administrator
5. **What is the role of sedation in end-of-life care in the ICU?**
   a. To induce a state of unconsciousness until death occurs
   b. To relieve pain and distress in terminally ill patients, ensuring comfort
   c. To hasten death by stopping the patient's respiratory function
   d. To maintain patients in an awake, alert state

Short Answer Questions

1. What are the main goals of palliative care in the ICU?
2. How does palliative care differ from curative or life-prolonging treatments in the ICU?
3. What are the key components of end-of-life care in the ICU?
4. Why is it important to initiate palliative care early in the ICU for patients with life-limiting conditions?
5. What is the role of comfort measures in end-of-life care in the ICU?

Answer to Critical Thinking Questions

1. (c); 2. (b); 3. (d); 4. (b); 5. (b)

REFERENCES

1. Alampi, D., Arabi, Y. M., Azoulay, E., Benbenishty, J., Benoit, D., Boulanger, C., Cecconi, M., *et al.* (2024). European Society of Intensive Care Medicine guidelines on end of life and palliative care in the intensive care unit. https://core.ac.uk/download/638812564.pdf (accessed on 22 May 2025).
2. Anderson, B. R., Ivascu, N. S., Brodie, D., Weingarten, J. A., Manoach, S., Smith, A., Millerman, K., *et al.* (2020). Breaking silos: The team-based approach to coronavirus disease 2019 pandemic staffing. *Critical Care Explorations, 2*, e0265. https://doi.org/10.1097/cce.0000000000000265.
3. Anstey, M., & Senthuran, S. (2023). The what-if approach to perioperative planning. *Anesthesia and Intensive Care, 51*, 168–169. https://www.semanticscholar.org/paper/2610979e5b8c05533ba222292f0b1db189ba4a1c (accessed on 22 May 2025).
4. Avati, A., Jung, K., Harman, S., Downing, N. L., Ng, A. Y., & Shah, N. H. (2018). Improving palliative care with deep learning. *BMC Medical Informatics and Decision Making, 18*. https://doi.org/10.1186/s12911-018-0677-8.
5. Baumgartner, H., De Backer, J., Babu-Narayan, S. V., Budts, W., Chessa, M., Diller, G. P., Lung, B., *et al.* (2020). 2020 ESC guidelines for the management of adult congenital heart disease. *European Heart Journal, 42*, 563–645. https://doi.org/10.1093/eurheartj/ehaa554.
6. Ben-Arye, E., Biron-Shental, T., Rosa, W. E., Samuels, N., Levy, O., Keshet, Y., Armon, S., *et al.* (2025). Acupuncture in obstetrics: Delivery room integrative medicine for anxiety and pain. *BMJ Supportive & Palliative Care*. https://www.semanticscholar.org/paper/1d23ef47b5d7e5c7564a0cf1718ea2db82cdea03 (accessed on 22 May 2025).
7. Birch, D., & Draper, J. (2008). A critical literature review exploring the challenges of delivering effective palliative care to older people with dementia in the acute hospital setting. https://core.ac.uk/download/82906952.pdf (accessed on 22 May 2025).
8. Brick, A., Normand, C., Smith, S., & O'Hara, S. (2013). Evidence on the cost and cost-effectiveness of palliative care: A literature review. https://core.ac.uk/download/75777777.pdf (accessed on 22 May 2025).
9. Chowdhury, M. K. (2024). Opioid analgesics in palliative care. *Bangladesh Journal of Medicine*. https://www.semanticscholar.org/paper/535b51766a6e79a28c0b1040795d233cb5c43576 (accessed on 22 May 2025).
10. Correa, T. L., Guelli, M., & Tavares de Carvalho, R. (2025). Palliative care for patients with chronic kidney disease and severe COVID-19 in Brazil: A retrospective study in a quaternary hospital. *Annals of Palliative Medicine, 14*(1), 4–12. https://www.semanticscholar.org/paper/891b7ceb88915d2553d73d9d54876457f67dd25b (accessed on 22 May 2025).
11. Cowfer, B., McGrath, C., & Trowbridge, A. (2020). Teaching pediatric palliative care communication skills to fourth-year medical students through role-play. *MedEdPORTAL*. https://doi.org/10.15766/mep_2374-8265.10991.
12. Davidson, J. E., Aslakson, R. A., Long, A. C., Puntillo, K., Kross, E. K., Hart, J. L., Cox, C. E., *et al.* (2016). Guidelines for family-centered care in the neonatal, pediatric, and adult ICU. *Critical Care Medicine, 45*, 103–128. https://doi.org/10.1097/ccm.0000000000002169.
13. de Souza, D. N., Lorentz, N. A., Charalambous, L. T., Galetta, M., Petrilli, C. A., & Rozell, J. (2024). Comprehensive pain management in total joint arthroplasty: A review of contemporary

approaches. *Journal of Clinical Medicine, 13*. https://www.semanticscholar.org/paper/e23d3d2c9fac9a9aa1ac32c3f525ecda60c914d0 (accessed on 22 May 2025).

14. El-Jawahri, A., Nelson, A. M., Gray, T. F., Lee, S. J., & LeBlanc, T. W. (2020). Palliative and end-of-life care for patients with hematologic malignancies. *Journal of Clinical Oncology, 38*, 944–953. https://doi.org/10.1200/jco.18.02386.

15. Ghabeljoo, J. (2017). End of life care practices for patients who die in intensive care units (ICU). https://core.ac.uk/download/70419827.pdf (accessed on 22 May 2025).

16. Guzmán, C. (2025). Intensive care and death with dignity: Ethical, clinical and regulatory aspects at the end of life. *SCT Proceedings in Interdisciplinary Insights and Innovations*. https://www.semanticscholar.org/paper/6c1ce2c6c2cdbf1ca852ebc0138e2dbdde130798 (accessed on 22 May 2025).

17. Jeffers, J., Bord, S., Hooper, J. E., Fleishman, C., Cayea, D., & Garibaldi, B. T. (2021). End-of-life care: A multimodal and comprehensive curriculum for graduating medical students utilizing experiential learning opportunities. *MedEdPORTAL*. https://doi.org/10.15766/mep_2374-8265.11149.

18. Kesecioglu, J., Rusinova, K., Alampi, D., Arabi, Y., Benbenishty, J., Benoît, D., Boulanger, C., *et al.* (2024). European Society of Intensive Care Medicine guidelines on end of life and palliative care in the intensive care unit. *Intensive Care Medicine, 50*, 1740–1766. https://www.semanticscholar.org/paper/d534f87b0dde6a97ecf50a3e5fc175a4aac8008e (accessed on 22 May 2025).

19. Kopar, P. K., Visani, A., Squirrell, K., & Brown, D. (2022). Addressing futility: A practical approach. *Critical Care Explorations, 4*, e0706. https://doi.org/10.1097/cce.0000000000000706.

20. Lambertini, M., Toss, A., Passaro, A., Criscitiello, C., Cremolini, C., Cardone, C., Loupakis, F., *et al.* (2020). Cancer care during the spread of coronavirus disease 2019 (COVID-19) in Italy: Young oncologists' perspective. *ESMO Open, 5*, e000759. https://doi.org/10.1136/esmoopen-2020-000759.

21. Lapid, M. I., Koopmans, R. T. C. M., Sampson, E. L., Van den Block, L., & Peisah, C. (2020). Providing quality end-of-life care to older people in the era of COVID-19: Perspectives from five countries. *International Psychogeriatrics, 32*, 1345–1352. https://doi.org/10.1017/s1041610220000836.

22. Lee, K. C., Senglaub, S. S., Walling, A. M., Mosenthal, A. C., & Cooper, Z. (2018). Quality measures in surgical palliative care. *Annals of Surgery, 269*, 607–609. https://doi.org/10.1097/sla.0000000000003136.

23. Loh, C. S., Watkins, M., & Ashok, S. (2023). 48 End-of-life care in the intensive care unit. *Poster Presentations*. https://www.semanticscholar.org/paper/2e234863436e0583679c816a888f3391d73dec53 (accessed on 22 May 2025).

24. Lyon, A. R., López-Fernández, T., Couch, L. S., Asteggiano, R., Aznar, M. C., Bergler-Klein, J., Boriani, G., *et al.* (2022). 2022 ESC guidelines on cardio-oncology developed in collaboration with the European Hematology Association (EHA), the European Society for Therapeutic Radiology and Oncology (ESTRO) and the International Cardio-Oncology Society (IC-OS). *European Heart Journal, 43*, 4229–4361. https://doi.org/10.1093/eurheartj/ehac244.

25. Meddick-Dyson, S. (2023). Implementation lessons learnt when evaluating palliative care interventions in the intensive care unit: Relationships between implementation determinants, strategies, and models of delivery. https://core.ac.uk/download/603272487.pdf (accessed on 22 May 2025).

26. Nilmanat, K., & Prompahakul, C. (2011). Review: Factors relating to nurses' caring behaviors for dying patients. https://media.neliti.com/media/publications/154583-EN-review-factors-relating-to-nurses-caring.pdf (accessed on 22 May 2025).

27. Pamplin, J., Scott, B., Quinn, M. T., Little, J. R., Goede, M. R., Pappas, P. A., Jolly, B., *et al.* (2021). Technology and disasters: The evolution of the National Emergency Tele-Critical Care Network. *Critical Care Medicine, 49*, 1007–1014. https://doi.org/10.1097/ccm.0000000000005001.

28. Price, D., & Kocan, M. J. (2018). Clinical nurse specialists fostering palliative care skills. *AACN Advanced Critical Care, 29*, 84–90. https://doi.org/10.4037/aacnacc2018286.

29. Robert, R., Kentish-Barnes, N., Boyer, A., Laurent, A., Azoulay, É., & Reignier, J. (2020). Ethical dilemmas due to the Covid-19 pandemic. *Annals of Intensive Care, 10*. https://doi.org/10.1186/s13613-020-00702-7.

30. Rochwerg, B., Brochard, L., Elliott, M., Hess, D., Hill, N. S., Nava, S., Navalesi, P., *et al.* (2017). Official ERS/ATS clinical practice guidelines: Non-invasive ventilation for acute respiratory failure. *European Respiratory Journal, 50*, 1602426. https://doi.org/10.1183/13993003.02426-2016.

31. Rockwood, K., & Theou, O. (2020). Using the Clinical Frailty Scale in allocating scarce health care resources. *Canadian Geriatrics Journal, 23*, 254–259. https://doi.org/10.5770/cgj.23.463.

32. Schönhofer, B., Geiseler, J., Dellweg, D., Fuchs, H., Moerer, O., Weber-Carstens, S., Westhoff, M., *et al.* (2020). Prolonged weaning: S2k guideline published by the German Respiratory Society. *Respiration, 99*, 982–1084. https://doi.org/10.1159/000510085.

33. Seale, C. (2009). Hastening death in end-of-life care: A survey of doctors. https://core.ac.uk/download/20572783.pdf (accessed on 22 May 2025).

34. Steinhorn, D. M., Din, J., & Johnson, A. (2017). Healing, spirituality and integrative medicine. *Annals of Palliative Medicine, 6*, 237–247. https://doi.org/10.21037/apm.2017.05.01.

35. Varkey, B. (2020). Principles of clinical ethics and their application to practice. *Medical Principles and Practice, 30*, 17–28. https://doi.org/10.1159/000509119.

36. Weissman, G. E., Kerlin, M. P., Yuan, Y., Gabler, N. B., Groeneveld, P. W., Werner, R. M., & Halpern, S. D. (2018). Population trends in intensive care unit admissions in the United States among Medicare beneficiaries, 2006–2015. *Annals of Internal Medicine, 170*, 213. https://doi.org/10.7326/m18-1425.

37. Wheless, M., Uhelski, A. R., Cimino, S., Domenico, H., Martin, S. F., Karlekar, M., Heumann, T., *et al.* (2025). End-of-life (EOL) outcomes and healthcare utilization for patients with hepatocellular carcinoma (HCC) who received immune checkpoint inhibition (ICI). *Journal of Clinical Oncology*. https://www.semanticscholar.org/paper/88b8c2a32f559ee9e167b15e97960586bd1120c0 (accessed on 22 May 2025).

38. Wilkinson, D., Gilbertson, L., Oakley, J., & Savulescu, J. (2023). Expanding choice at the end of life. *Journal of Medical Ethics, 49*, 269–270. https://www.semanticscholar.org/paper/9aa084ea1ad072deb8e267e1aa51318b244e9d36 (accessed on 22 May 2025).

TRAUMA AND BURN MANAGEMENT IN THE ICU

13

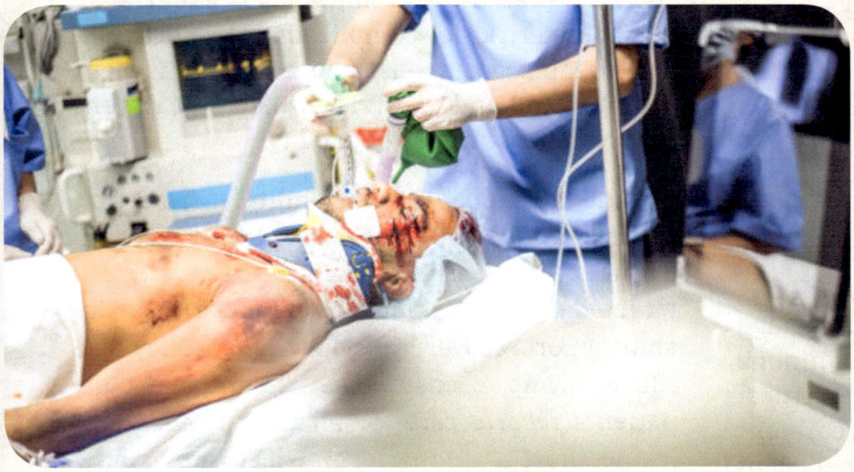

LEARNING OBJECTIVES

After studying this chapter, you will be able to:

1. Understanding trauma and burns.
2. Discuss about initial assessment and stabilization.
3. Describe advanced management strategies.
4. List the outcomes and long-term care.

Introduction

The intensive care unit (ICU) serves as a critical environment for the management of trauma and burn patients, necessitating a multidisciplinary approach to optimize recovery and minimize complications. Because there are more trauma and severe burn cases, it is very important to know how to treat patients in the ICU. Injuries sustained in traumatic events often lead to systemic complications such as venous thromboembolism (VTE), which underscores the necessity of timely pharmacologic prophylaxis to mitigate associated risks. Evidence-based algorithms, like those developed by the Western Trauma Association, provide guidance on pharmacologic prophylaxis tailored to trauma patients, indicating that early intervention significantly reduces VTE rates and enhances overall patient outcomes (Ley *et al.*, 2020). Moreover, the ongoing pandemic has further strained surgical capacities, revealing the need for robust contingency planning to maintain essential surgical services in the ICU environment (Kjetil Søreide *et al.*, 2020). Addressing all these problems together is required to improve trauma and burn care in critical care units.

Definition of Trauma and Burns

Trauma and burns represent significant medical challenges, often requiring intensive management in critical care settings, such as the ICU. Trauma happens when someone experiences a physical injury because of something happening from outside, such as accidents, falls, or violence. Because of this, people may suffer from hemorrhagic shock or organ failure, and urgent and thorough medical care is required. Burns are divided by their depth and size, and they are caused by heat, electricity or chemicals, which can damage cells and lead to inflammation that puts survival at risk. Significantly, trauma and burns often go together, since this leads to more complications for the patient and makes it harder to manage them in the ICU. Understanding the definitions and implications of trauma and burns is critical for the development of effective treatment protocols that address the unique needs of these patients (Donohue *et al.*, 2019; Levey *et al.*, 2017) (Figure 13.1).

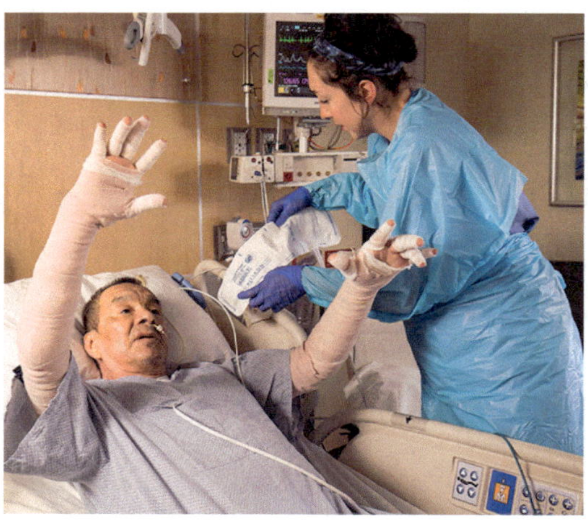

Figure 13.1. Trauma and burns.

Source: https://healthcare.utah.edu/sites/g/files/zrelqx136/files/files/migration/inpatient-unit-patient.jpg.

Importance of Intensive Care Unit (ICU) for Trauma and Burn Patients

ICU care is very important for trauma and burn patients because these patients usually have serious medical problems that need specialized care. Since trauma and burns can lead to significant stress on the body and organ damage, it is crucial to use special ICU treatments to help patients recover. For instance, trauma patients with concurrent substance abuse, such as methamphetamine use, experience heightened risks for complications like delirium and pulmonary embolism, necessitating vigilant monitoring and individualized treatment protocols (Stanton *et al.*, 2024).

Furthermore, the variability in infection control and antibiotic susceptibility across different ICU settings highlights the necessity for targeted treatment strategies to reduce mortality and support recovery (Blackley *et al.*, 2024). The ICU is set up to ensure that trauma and burn patients receive care for all their needs, both in the short and long term, which shows how important it is for these conditions.

Statistics on Trauma and Burn Incidents

Trauma and burn cases cause significant problems in critical care, directly affecting the outcomes of patients and the resources used by healthcare teams. Statistics indicate that falls account for a substantial portion of trauma-related injuries, especially among the elderly, with frailty being a critical factor that heightens the risk of readmission due to falls after initial trauma incidents (Hatcher *et al.*, 2019). Furthermore, military contexts highlight the prevalence of trauma in children during conflicts, with a considerable percentage of pediatric admissions derived from surgical and trauma-related issues (Idenburg *et al.*, 2015). It is obvious from these high numbers that better trauma and burn management plans are necessary in ICUs. Because the number of trauma cases is growing, healthcare providers need to adjust to the new needs of these patients and make sure their care plans cover both emergency treatment and recovery over time. This way of treatment is necessary to support the survival and recovery of people with trauma and burns.

The Role of the Intensive Care Unit (ICU) In Patient Outcomes

For people with traumatic injuries and severe burns, the ICU is essential in shaping their outcomes. Since these situations are crucial, various professionals need to cooperate because studies have found that teamwork helps reduce errors and aids in faster patient recovery. For example, protocols developed through collaborative efforts, such as those facilitated by the Burn Padlet, have been shown to improve the standardization of care and optimize resources, ultimately enhancing patient outcomes in burn management (Palacio *et al.*, 2025).

Additionally, research highlights that patients with stimulant use during the treatment of burns faced worse outcomes, emphasizing the critical need for specialized interventions like addiction medicine (Stanton *et al.*, 2025). Taking care of both the physical and mental needs of patients, the ICU helps them recover well in the long run. For this reason, the ICU plays a key role in trauma and burn management, affecting important patient outcomes.

Key Challenges in Trauma and Burn Management

Managing trauma and burn patients in the ICU requires handling several important challenges that affect patient outcomes. A serious problem is preventing VTE, since trauma patients are more likely to develop it because of being immobile and the coagulation changes caused by their injuries. Current guidelines emphasize the need for timely pharmacologic prophylaxis, yet many patients experience delays or interruptions in treatment, heightening the risk of complications (Ley *et al.*, 2020). Moreover, the integration of noninvasive mechanical ventilation (NIV) plays a crucial role in managing acute respiratory failure among these patients. However, its application requires careful consideration of clinical conditions and protocols (Rochwerg *et al.*, 2017). Thus, ICU staff have to develop and update special protocols for each trauma and burn patient, since it is hard to start proper interventions and monitor side effects.

Relevance to Current Medical Practices

The importance of current medical practices for trauma and burns in the ICU is very high, mainly because guidelines and antimicrobial resistance are constantly changing. Updated guidelines, such as the 2023 guideline for the management of patients with aneurysmal subarachnoid hemorrhage, underscore the need for evidence-based approaches that prioritize patient-centric care, aligning treatment protocols with the latest research and clinical data (Hoh *et al.*, 2023). At the same time, more cases of multidrug-resistant infections make it hard for trauma and burn patients to receive effective antibiotic treatment. The challenges presented by antibiotic-resistant organisms, as highlighted by recent studies, necessitate innovative treatment strategies and alternative antimicrobial therapies to enhance patient outcomes in the ICU (Frieri *et al.*, 2016). Consequently, using the latest guidelines and dealing with antimicrobial resistance are very important for improving trauma and burn management in critical care.

13.1. Understanding Trauma and Burns

Learning Outcome

1. Discuss the types of trauma: blunt versus penetrating
2. Explain the classification of burns: first, second, third, and fourth degree
3. Define mechanisms of injury in trauma cases
4. Understand the pathophysiology of burn injuries
5. Identify the common causes of trauma and burns
6. Understand the psychological impact of trauma and burns
7. Identify the risk factors associated with severe injuries
8. Define the assessment tools for trauma and burn severity
9. Explain the importance of early recognition and intervention

Knowing about trauma and burns is necessary in ICU management to help patients recover well and avoid complications. A lot of tissue damage can occur as a result of trauma, so it requires a medical approach that handles both the initial effects and the long-term recovery process. Burns are often followed by a rush of inflammation, which can result in infections and sepsis, and make the chance of death much greater if not handled well. Effective interprofessional collaboration is crucial in these cases, as the ICU team—comprising physicians, nurses, pharmacists, and other specialists—must work together to deliver comprehensive care plans tailored to each patient's unique needs (Kleinpell *et al.*, 2021). Moreover, research has indicated that impaired immune responses following sepsis, often a consequence of severe trauma or burns, complicate recovery and increase the risk of recurrent infections, underscoring the necessity of vigilant monitoring and proactive therapeutic interventions in the ICU (Delano *et al.*, 2016).

13.1.1. Types of Trauma: Blunt Versus Penetrating

Being able to distinguish between blunt and penetrating trauma is important in handling trauma and burn cases in the ICU. Forces that hit the body without breaking the skin, such as a direct impact, usually cause internal injuries like organ lacerations and contusions, and have higher severity scores than penetrating trauma. Penetrating trauma means that an object goes inside the body, resulting in wounds both on the surface and inside, such as those caused by a knife or gunshot injuries. Although penetrating trauma happens more often, blunt trauma usually results in worse injuries and more problems. In a recent evaluation of breast trauma cases, for instance, the incidence of blunt injuries demonstrated higher injury severity scores than penetrating types, underscoring significant variations in management decisions and outcomes based on trauma type (Sargent *et al.*, 2022). Understanding these mechanisms is critical for optimizing patient care in the ICU setting (Elkbuli *et al.*, 2020) (Figure 13.2).

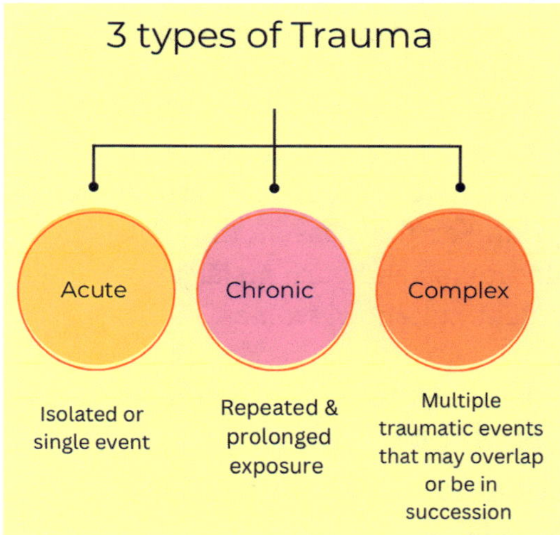

Figure 13.2. Types of trauma.

Source: https://blog.psychmoments.com/wp-content/uploads/2023/02/3typesoftrauma-1024x1024.png.

13.1.2. Classification of Burns: First, Second, Third, and Fourth Degree

Proper management of trauma and burn cases in the ICU depends on knowing how to classify burns. Burns are given a degree depending on how much tissue is damaged. In a first-degree burn, only the outer layer is damaged, which causes redness and some pain, without blisters. Second-degree burns go deeper into the skin, resulting in blisters and more intense pain.

Classification	Characteristics
First degree	Partial thickness burns. * Characterized by erythema (localized redness). * Appear sunburn-like. * Are not included when calculating burn size. * Usually heal by themselves.
Second degree	Partial thickness burns. * Part of skin has been damaged or destroyed. * Have blisters containing clear fluid. * Pink underlying tissue. * Often heal by themselves.
Third degree	Full thickness burns. * Full skin has been destroyed. * Deep red tissue underlying blister. * Presence of bloody blister fluid. * Muscle and bone may be destroyed. * Require professional treatment.
Fourth degree	Full thickness burns. * Penetrate deep tissue to fat, muscle, bone. * Require immediate professional treatment.

Figure 13.3. Classification of burns.

Source: https://www.researchgate.net/profile/Allison-Jackson-2/publication/265860345/figure/tbl1/AS:601771277836319@1520484861591/Classification-of-Burns.png.

Third-degree burns damage the deeper tissues, and these burns may appear white or charred; they usually need grafting and special treatment. Fourth-degree burns, which are the most severe, reach the muscles, tendons, and bones, so they usually require a lot of surgery and rehabilitation. Clinicians can provide patients with the proper treatment and better results when they fully understand these classifications. Recent advancements, such as Bromelain-based Enzymatic Debridement for mid- to deep dermal burns, demonstrate the evolving approaches to burn management in critical care settings (Apfelbaum *et al.*, 2021; Hirche *et al.*, 2020) (Figure 13.3).

13.1.3. Mechanisms of Injury in Trauma Cases

Trauma cases exhibit a complex interplay of mechanisms that contribute significantly to patient outcomes in the intensive care unit (ICU). Knowing about these mechanisms is very important for effective care and treatment. Blunt trauma, penetrating trauma, and thermal injuries are some of the sources of injuries, all of which need different care methods. For example, patients suffering from chest trauma may experience compromised respiratory function due to noninvasive mechanical ventilation (NIV) needs, highlighting the importance of prompt intervention to prevent acute respiratory failure (Rochwerg *et al.*, 2017).

Additionally, the consequences of sepsis in trauma patients can complicate recovery, leading to alterations in hemodynamics and oxygenation that undermine healing processes (Bateman *et al.*, 2016). Ultimately, a thorough grasp of these injury mechanisms helps clinicians tailor treatment strategies, thereby improving outcomes for critically injured patients and enhancing their overall management within the ICU setting (Figure 13.4).

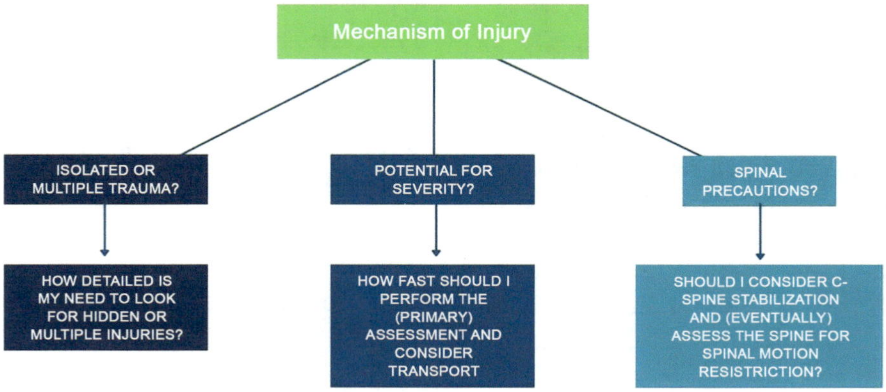

Figure 13.4. Mechanism of injury.

Source: https://limmereducation.com/storage/media/trauma-assessment_mechanism-of-inury_flowchart.jpg.

13.1.4. Pathophysiology of Burn Injuries

Burn injuries cause many changes in the body, both locally and systemically, which have a major impact on outcomes in intensive care. The initial effect of a burn is to break the skin's barrier, which injures the tissue and starts an inflammatory process. Because of this, pro-inflammatory cytokines are released, and they make the capillaries more permeable, which can lead to fluid shifts in burn patients.

Much energy is needed to treat severe burns, which can make it harder for the body to recover since it is already tired. The presence of sepsis further exacerbates these processes, as illustrated by its association with dysregulated immune responses that pose additional risks for burn victims (Delano *et al.*, 2016). Moreover, impaired immune responses can lead to secondary infections, complicating management strategies in the ICU (Rochwerg *et al.*, 2017). Having a good knowledge of these mechanisms is helpful in managing trauma and burns.

13.1.5. Common Causes of Trauma and Burns

Knowing the typical reasons behind trauma and burns is necessary for treating patients in the ICU properly. accidents. Things like car accidents cause many cases of trauma, falls, and violence, which often result in serious injuries that must be treated with intensive care. The primary sources of burns are flames, hot liquids, and electric currents. Managing trauma and burns is more challenging in the ICU because patients there can develop infections and problems with several organs. It is critical to address underlying issues such as fluid balance in trauma patients and the strategic administration of pharmacologic prophylaxis to prevent venous thromboembolism, as highlighted by recent studies of Ley *et al.* (2020) and the ongoing debate regarding vasopressor management in septic shock (Douglas *et al.*, 2020). Understanding these causes not only informs clinical practice but also shapes preventive measures within healthcare settings (Figure 13.5).

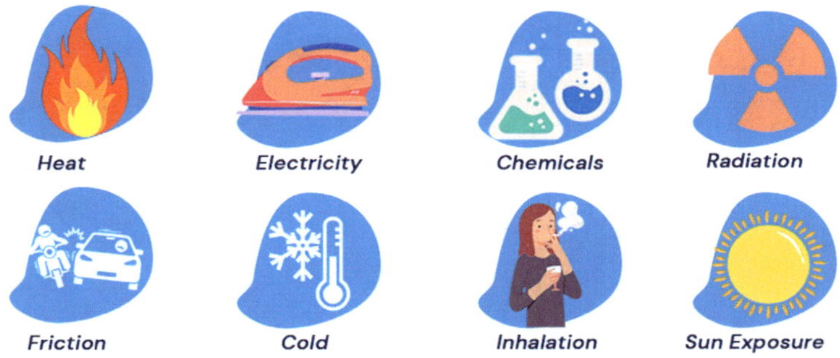

Figure 13.5. Causes of burns.

Source: https://ongocare.com/wp-content/uploads/2023/05/Causes-of-Burns.jpg.

13.1.6. Psychological Impact of Trauma and Burns

Patients in the ICU who have experienced trauma and burns often deal with strong psychological effects, which are usually made worse by the seriousness of their injuries and the emergency care setting. Patients may experience a range of psychological responses, including anxiety, depression, post-traumatic stress disorder (PTSD), and feelings of isolation, particularly when separated from their families during treatment. Burns can cause much physical rehabilitation, which is both difficult and emotionally straining for patients as they deal with body image problems and the possibility of long-term mental health issues. Thus, trauma and burn management should always include psychological support as a key part of care. Interprofessional teams, as highlighted by recent research, play a vital role in addressing these psychological needs by integrating mental health professionals into the ICU setting, ensuring a holistic approach to patient recovery (Kleinpell *et al.*, 2021; Perkins *et al.*, 2021) (Figure 13.6).

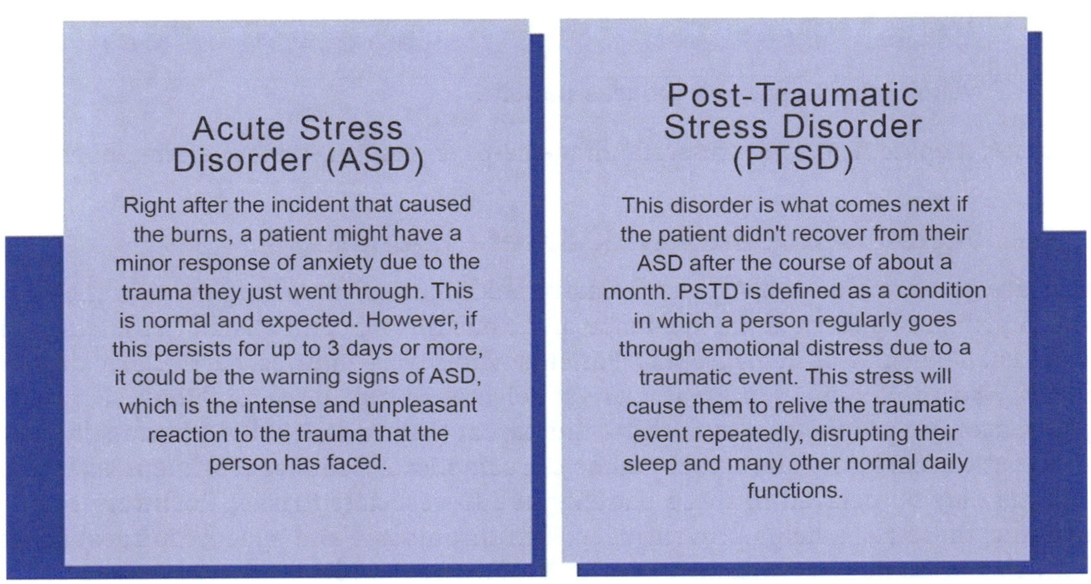

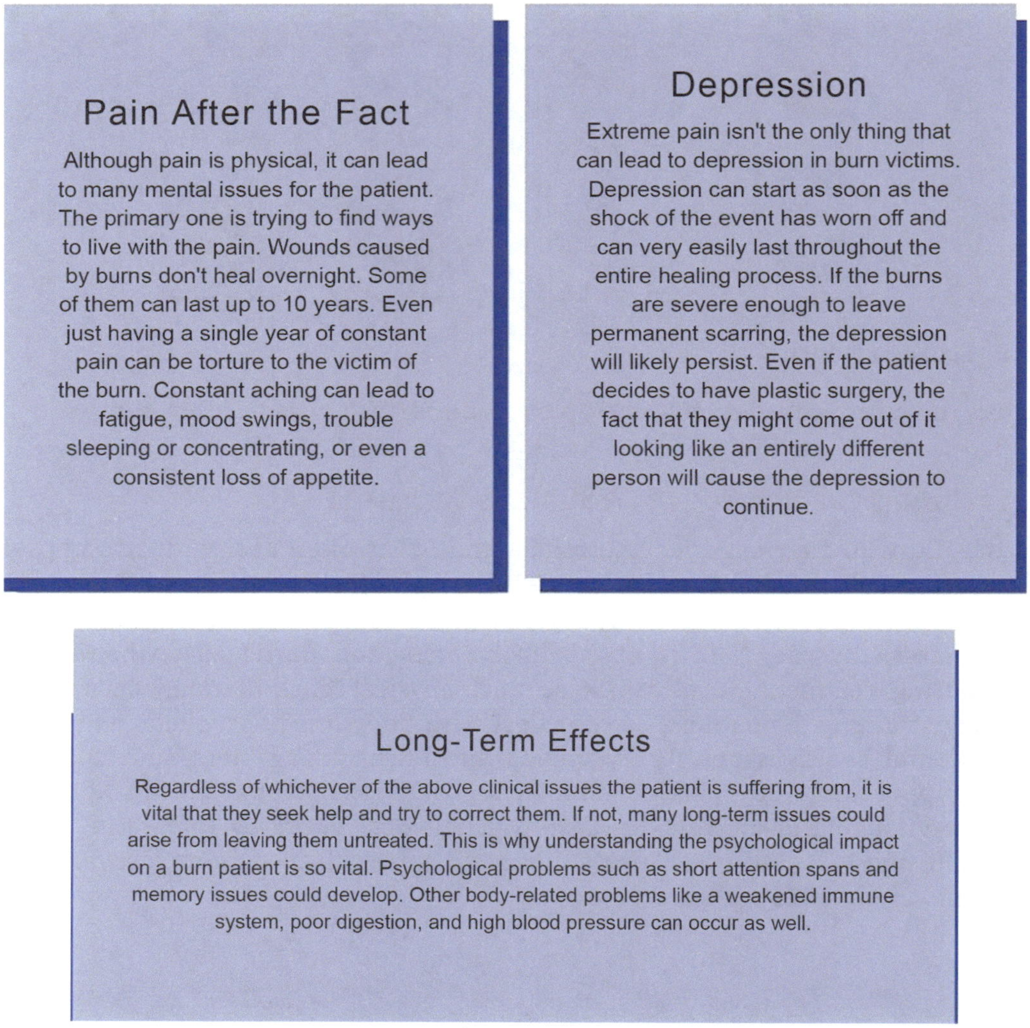

Figure 13.6. Psychological impact on a burns patient.

Source: https://thepatelfirm.com/understanding-the-psychological-impact-after-a-burn-injury/.

13.1.7. Risk Factors Associated with Severe Injuries

Since there are severe risks involved in trauma-related injuries, managing them in the ICU is very important. A primary concern is the incidence of venous thromboembolism (VTE), which presents a significant challenge in this demographic. Patients with severe injuries, particularly those with an Injury Severity Score (ISS) of 10 or greater, are at heightened risk for developing VTE, necessitating timely pharmacologic prophylaxis to mitigate this threat (Ley *et al.*, 2020). Additionally, conditions such as traumatic brain injury and spinal trauma can complicate treatment regimens, as the initiation of prophylaxis may be delayed in these patients due to associated risks (Rochwerg *et al.*, 2017). Knowing about these risks helps prevent deep vein thrombosis and speeds up recovery for each patient, which proves how important it is to tailor care in the ICU.

13.1.8. Assessment Tools for Trauma and Burn Severity

The evaluation of the degree of trauma and burn helps choose the best treatment and ensures the best results for patients in the ICU. Various tools and scoring systems, such as the Abbreviated Injury Scale (AIS) and the Total Body Burn Surface Area (TBSA), serve as fundamental frameworks for quantifying injuries and stratifying patients according to the severity of their conditions. Correct assessment helps with triage and the use of specific interventions, which are important for managing sepsis and breathing problems. For instance, understanding the extent of burn injuries directly impacts fluid resuscitation strategies that mitigate the risk of further complications, including organ dysfunction (Gotts *et al.*, 2016). Furthermore, assessments utilizing criteria for mechanical ventilation can guide individualized treatment plans, particularly in cases of severe respiratory distress associated with trauma or burn injuries (Rochwerg *et al.*, 2017). Thus, robust assessment tools are vital for effective trauma and burn management in the ICU (Figure 13.7).

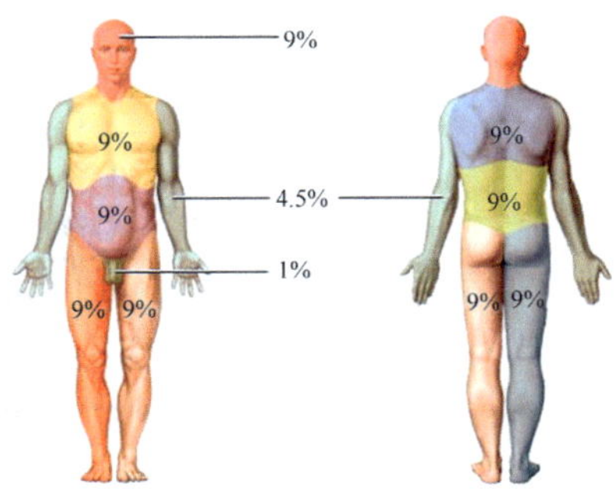

Figure 13.7. Total body surface area.

Source: https://www.health.state.mn.us/communities/ep/surge/burn/tbsa.html.

13.1.9. Importance of Early Recognition and Intervention

In critical care, early detection and treatment of trauma and burns increase the chances of a good outcome and decrease the risk of death for patients. Taking quick action allows healthcare teams to deal with the complications of sepsis and organ failure, stopping them from worsening into septic shock, which can be fatal. As evidenced by multiple studies, efficient interprofessional collaboration in the ICU, where each team member's expertise is leveraged, is crucial for implementing evidence-based practices rapidly (Kleinpell *et al.*, 2021). Furthermore, recognizing the long-term implications of sepsis, including immune dysfunctions that can continue post-recovery, emphasizes the necessity of ongoing assessment and intervention following the initial trauma (Delano *et al.*, 2016). Therefore, promptly finding and treating problems in critically ill patients helps them in the short and long term.

Test Your Knowledge

1. How do blunt and penetrating traumas differ in terms of mechanisms and clinical presentation?
2. What are the key features distinguishing first, second, third, and fourth-degree burns?
3. What are the common causes and underlying pathophysiological changes associated with trauma and burn injuries?

13.2. Initial Assessment and Stabilization

Learning Outcome

1. Discuss the primary survey in trauma management
2. Explain the secondary survey for comprehensive evaluation
3. Discuss the burn assessment: the rule of nines
4. Understand the airway management in trauma patients
5. Define fluid resuscitation protocols for burn victims
6. Discuss the pain management strategies in the ICU
7. Identify the monitoring vital signs and hemodynamic stability
8. Discuss the use of imaging studies in trauma assessment
9. Define multidisciplinary approach to initial care

Critical care staff must first assess and stabilize trauma and burn patients to achieve the best results. The first step is to quickly check the patient's airway, breathing, circulation, and neurological status, which is known as the ABCs of trauma care. Recognizing life-threatening injuries like respiratory distress or hemorrhagic shock early on helps clinicians take action quickly, which reduces the chances of complications and death. Furthermore, effective stabilization often necessitates the initiation of enteral nutrition within 24–48 hours following admission, as this can support gut integrity and prevent complications associated with prolonged immobility and malnutrition (McClave *et al.*, 2016). Collaboratively, multidisciplinary teams guided by A.S.P.E.N. and SCCM clinical guidelines enhance the assessment protocols, allowing for tailored nutrition therapy to be established early in a patient's ICU stay (McClave *et al.*, 2016). It meets the patient's current needs and also supports a lasting recovery.

13.2.1. Primary Survey in Trauma Management

The first thing to do in trauma management is the primary survey, which tells you what should be done first and what is most urgent. This systematic evaluation adheres to the principles of the Advanced Trauma Life Support (ATLS) protocols, allowing clinicians to quickly identify and address critical injuries in patients, such as compromised airway, breathing difficulties, and circulatory inadequacies.

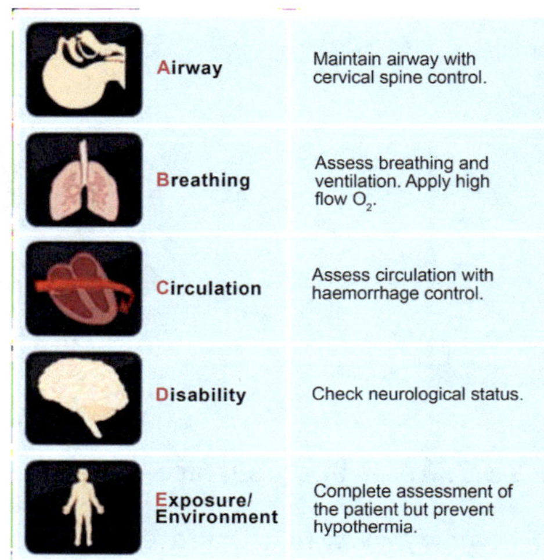

Figure 13.8. Primary survey in trauma management.

Source: https://www.rcemlearning.co.uk/modules/abdominal-trauma/lessons/clinical-assessment-and-risk-stratification-37/topic/primary-survey/.

It is especially clear why a primary survey matters in complicated cases, for example, those involving patients with both traumatic and burn injuries, as knowing all the details about the patient is crucial for successful treatment. For instance, stimulant use in burn patients has been shown to prolong hospital stays and intensify complications, thereby emphasizing the need for immediate and precise assessment of airway and circulatory status to mitigate risks associated with their underlying substance use (Stanton *et al.*, 2025). Additionally, in rare cases involving multisystem trauma, such as lightning strikes, a well-executed primary survey can facilitate a multidisciplinary approach to comprehensive care and optimal patient outcomes (Shauly *et al.*, 2025) (Figure 13.8).

13.2.2. Secondary Survey for Comprehensive Evaluation

After the initial assessment in ICU trauma and burn management, the secondary survey is very important for further evaluating the patient. By doing a thorough check, the team aims to spot injuries that might have been missed and measure the seriousness of any existing ones, which helps decide the next steps for treatment. In the secondary survey, the patient's medical history is reviewed, a physical exam is done, and key tests are ordered. The guidelines established by authoritative bodies emphasize the need for careful airway management, especially in cases where the airway may be compromised due to trauma or burns (Apfelbaum *et al.*, 2021). Additionally, NIV has emerged as a vital intervention in managing acute respiratory failure in these patients, underscoring the necessity of incorporating respiratory assessments into the secondary survey (Rochwerg *et al.*, 2017). By carefully evaluating patients, healthcare providers can closely monitor them and provide the best treatments, which greatly benefits ICU patients.

13.2.3. Burn Assessment: The Rule of Nines

In emergency medicine, especially when dealing with trauma and burns in the ICU, it is very important to assess how severe the burn is. A common technique is the Rule of Nines, which helps quickly determine the area of the body burned.

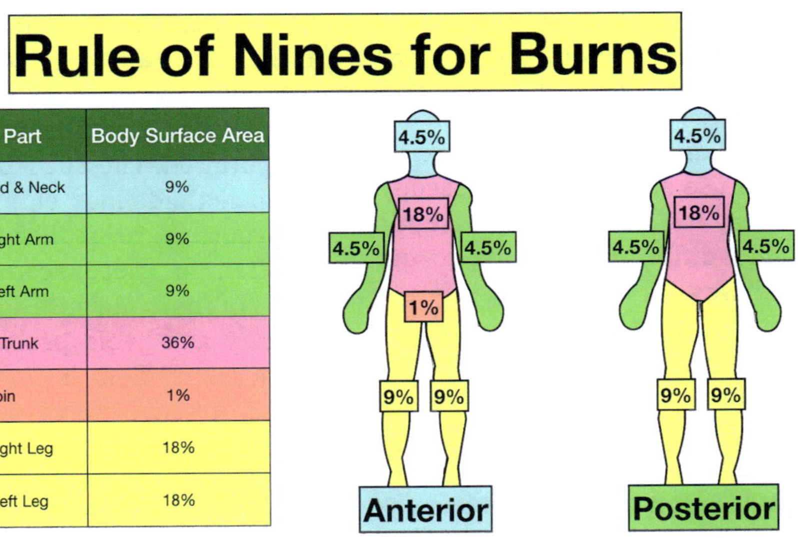

Body Part	Body Surface Area
Entire Head & Neck	9%
Entire Right Arm	9%
Entire Left Arm	9%
Entire Trunk	36%
Groin	1%
Entire Right Leg	18%
Entire Left Leg	18%

Figure 13.9. Rule of nines for burns.

Source: https://images.squarespace-cdn.com/content/v1/5e48489da899cd09424943db/26aef1cb-d80b-4be9-99e6-0e650529bc95/rule-of-nines-chart-diagram.png.

For adults, the body is divided into sections, with each section accounting for about 9% of the total TBSA, which helps doctors make quick choices about fluid therapy and where to transfer the patient. Accurate assessment is paramount, as burn injuries are a leading cause of mortality worldwide, with significant implications for patient outcomes and resource allocation in emergency care (Dalamagka, 2024). Furthermore, the evolution of treatment protocols, particularly for populations vulnerable to severe burns, emphasizes the need for an integrated approach to both pain management and rehabilitation (Elsadek, 2024). This underscores the importance of utilizing the Rule of Nines in conjunction with comprehensive patient care strategies in the ICU (Figure 13.9).

13.2.4. Airway Management in Trauma Patients

Managing the airway in trauma patients with burns is difficult since it involves thinking about the changes to their body and breathing caused by the trauma. It is important to check for laryngeal and supraglottic edema and any changes in the airway that may make standard intubation methods difficult. In several cases, it is not enough to use standard laryngoscopy, so practitioners may have to rely on fiberoptic bronchoscopy and different methods to get access to the airway. Tracheostomy should be performed for patients with severe upper airway burns or breathing problems, since early airway support can prevent more issues from developing. Studies highlight that patients with methamphetamine intoxication often face prolonged hospitalization and specific airway-related challenges, underscoring the need for tailored interventions and a multidisciplinary approach to achieve optimal outcomes in trauma management, particularly in the critical care setting (Mittal *et al.*, 2024; Stanton *et al.*, 2024) (Figure 13.10).

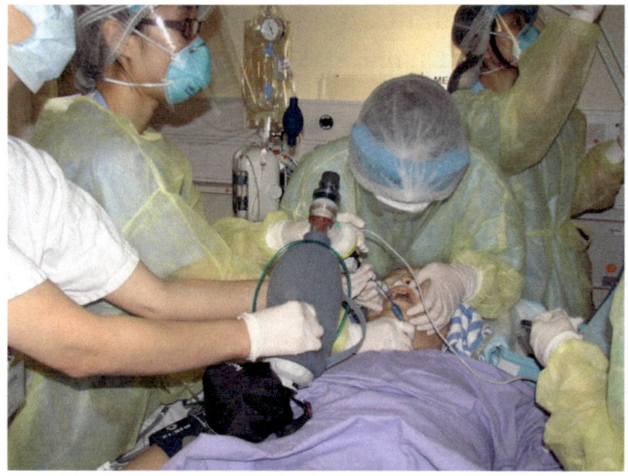

Figure 13.10. Airway management and initial resuscitation of the trauma patient.

Source: https://www.hksccm.org/images/stories/JournalNewsUpdate/IMG_4073.JPG.

13.2.5. Fluid Resuscitation Protocols for Burn Victims

Fluid resuscitation is vital for managing burn victims, especially when they are in the ICU. It is important to replace fluids in time to deal with hypovolemia, which is common in severe burn cases because of skin injury and evaporation. The 2021 European Resuscitation Council Guidelines emphasize evidence-based approaches to resuscitation that could be applied in these scenarios (Perkins *et al.*, 2021). Their purpose is to replace lost fluids quickly and avoid problems that may happen if too much fluid is given, such as abdominal compartment syndrome. Despite advancements in understanding the cellular responses to burn injuries, many clinical practices remain rooted in long-standing protocols that are continually refined through observation and research (Nielson *et al.*, 2016). So, it is important to keep updating the way fluids are given to burn patients to help improve their outcomes, which highlights the need to use new guidelines along with experience.

13.2.6. Pain Management Strategies in the Intensive Care Unit (ICU)

Pain management in the ICU is very important, especially for those with trauma or burns, since not treating pain well can cause a longer recovery and emotional issues. Multimodal analgesia means using both drugs and non-drug therapies such as physical therapy and cognitive behavioral techniques, together. This system aims to relieve pain and lower the use of opioids which helps reduce the chance of side effects and addiction. An interprofessional team must collaborate to tailor pain management strategies to the specific needs of the patient, ensuring that both physical and emotional aspects of pain are addressed (Kleinpell *et al.*, 2021). Furthermore, adherence to recommended guidelines and algorithms, effective communication, and ongoing assessment of pain levels contribute to improved outcomes for trauma and burn patients in the ICU (Ley *et al.*, 2020).

13.2.7. Monitoring Vital Signs and Hemodynamic Stability

Careful monitoring of vital signs and blood pressure is crucial for trauma and burn patients in the ICU, since sudden changes may indicate serious problems. Healthcare teams can act promptly if they regularly check blood pressure, heart rate, and oxygen saturation. For instance, in cases involving significant blood loss, as demonstrated in a pediatric burn study, whole blood transfusions have been shown to maintain hemodynamic stability during surgical procedures, providing crucial components like red blood cells and plasma to enhance oxygen delivery and support recovery (Decker *et al.*, 2025). Similarly, in instances of severe abdominal trauma, meticulous monitoring and timely interventions, including damage control surgery and appropriately timed transfusions, are essential to stabilize patients post-operation and avert complications like volume overload (Nur *et al.*, 2023). Being so careful about oversight helps a business stay alive now and recover in the long run.

13.2.8. Use of Imaging Studies in Trauma Assessment

Regular imaging studies are important in the intensive care unit to check for trauma, especially lightning injuries. Imaging modalities, including computed tomography (CT) and magnetic resonance imaging (MRI), provide critical insights into the extent of injuries, facilitating the identification of craniofacial fractures and other life-threatening conditions. For instance, a case study involving a 70-year-old male patient revealed that imaging studies were pivotal in diagnosing bilateral Le Fort II and III-like fractures, which guided a conservative management approach that obviated the need for surgical intervention (Shauly *et al.*, 2025).

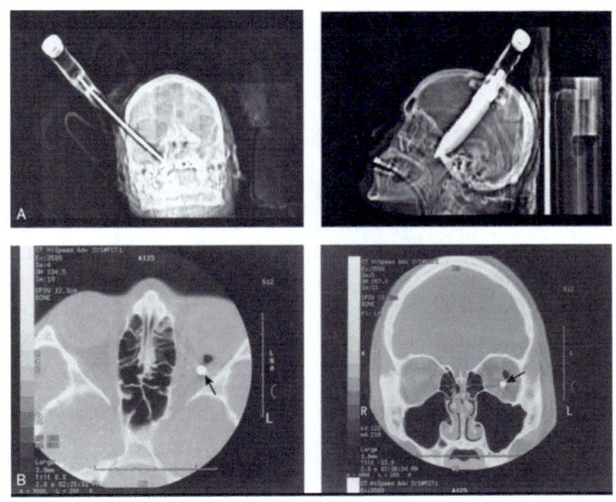

Figure 13.11. Trauma radiography.

Source: https://radiologykey.com/wp-content/uploads/2016/03/B9780323073226500125_f13-054-9780323073226.jpg.

Additionally, the use of imaging is crucial in evaluating burn injuries, wherein techniques like ultrasound can assess tissue viability, ultimately informing treatment options such as the application of autologous skin cell suspensions

(Olaveson, 2025). Therefore, imaging studies are integral to tailoring interdisciplinary care strategies for trauma patients in the ICU (Figure 13.11).

13.2.9. Multidisciplinary Approach to Initial Care

Using a multidisciplinary team greatly improves the results of trauma and burn management in the ICU. It allows surgeons, critical care doctors, nurses, physiotherapists, and nutritionists to cooperate, using their different skills to benefit the patient. Experts can make better decisions about care when they collaborate closely, which can significantly affect the outcomes of critically injured patients. For instance, Kjetil Søreide *et al.* (2020) highlight that the ongoing pandemic has underscored the importance of adaptive surge planning and interdisciplinary protocols, particularly concerning infection control and resource allocation. Additionally, Griffin *et al.* (2020) illustrate that effective communication and education among team members can lead to improved patient engagement and streamlined care processes. As a result, this integrated approach improves the first care given and also helps trauma and burn patients recover better in the ICU.

Test Your Knowledge

1. What are the key components of the primary and secondary surveys in trauma management, and how do they differ?
2. How is the Rule of Nines used to assess the extent of burn injuries in patients?
3. What are the essential principles of airway management and fluid resuscitation in trauma and burn patients?

13.3. Advanced Management Strategies

Learning Outcome

1. Define surgical interventions for trauma patients
2. Understand the burn wound care and dressing techniques
3. Discuss the infection prevention and control measures
4. Explain the nutritional support for critically ill patients
5. Define rehabilitation and physical therapy considerations
6. Describe the psychological support and counseling services
7. Explain the use of advanced technologies in monitoring
8. Identify the role of pharmacological agents in management
9. Define ethical considerations in trauma and burn care

Using advanced management approaches in trauma and burn care within the ICU is very important for achieving the best results for patients. The complexities of burn injuries are exacerbated by factors such as substance use, as evidenced by the findings that stimulant-positive burn patients experience more extended hospital stays, increased complications, and more severe injuries (Stanton *et al.*, 2025). For better care of these patients, it is important to combine addiction medicine with usual burn management practices. Furthermore, engaging frontline staff through initiatives like Quality Conversations fosters a culture of continuous improvement, where root causes of issues such as hospital-acquired pressure injuries (HAPIs) are identified collaboratively (Smith, 2025). Using the knowledge of inter-professional teams, healthcare facilities can plan effective prevention measures that help trauma and burn patients recover quickly and also rehabilitate them for the long term. When staff are involved in care strategies, patients often do better, and the ICU handles important challenges more efficiently.

13.3.1. Surgical Interventions for Trauma Patients

When treating trauma patients, surgeons are especially needed for complex injuries such as those caused by high-voltage electricity and burns. Many trauma patients have severe wounds that must be treated quickly with surgery to stop complications and help them heal. For instance, those suffering from train-surfing injuries exhibit extensive burns and may necessitate numerous surgical procedures, as evidenced by a study showing an average of 5.3 surgeries per patient, significantly higher than in other injury types (Koenig *et al.*, 2025). Additionally, patients who are stimulant-positive demonstrate more extended hospital stays and increased surgical demands, highlighting the need for tailored surgical strategies to address the complications arising from their condition (Stanton *et al.*, 2025). Effective surgical management not only shortens recovery time but also enhances overall patient outcomes in the ICU, making it a vital component of trauma and burn care protocols (Figure 13.12).

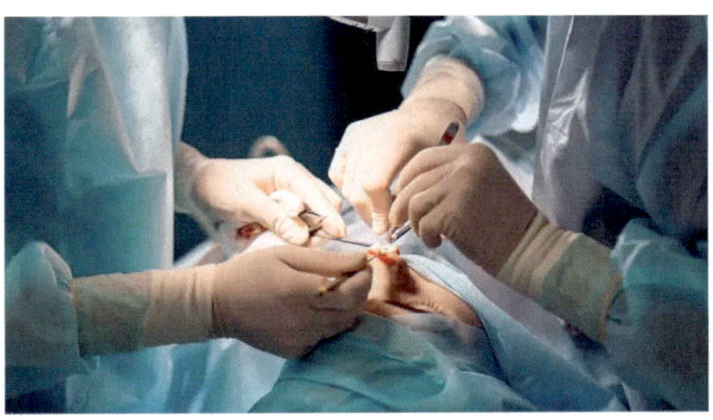

Figure 13.12. Trauma surgery.

Source: https://www.apex-hospital.co.in/wp-content/uploads/2024/11/Trauma-Surgery-Types-Preparation-Procedure-Risks-and-Complications.jpg.

13.3.2. Burn Wound Care and Dressing Techniques

Caring for burn wounds and changing dressings properly is important in the ICU to help wounds heal and avoid infections. Selecting a dressing calls for attention to the burn severity, health of the patient, and the risk of complications in those with weakened immune systems. With these new dressings, the risk of infection can be lowered, and the wound remains moist, which is necessary for a good recovery. Infections, such as those caused by *Pseudomonas aeruginosa*, pose significant risks in burn patients and can complicate the healing process and increase mortality rates, highlighting the necessity for careful monitoring and appropriate antimicrobial strategies (Bassetti *et al.*, 2018). Furthermore, the systemic effects of burns, including sepsis and immune dysregulation, call for a holistic approach to patient care, as these factors can lead to sustained alterations in immune function post-recovery (Delano *et al.*, 2016). Proper dressing techniques ultimately play a crucial role in enhancing patient outcomes (Figure 13.13).

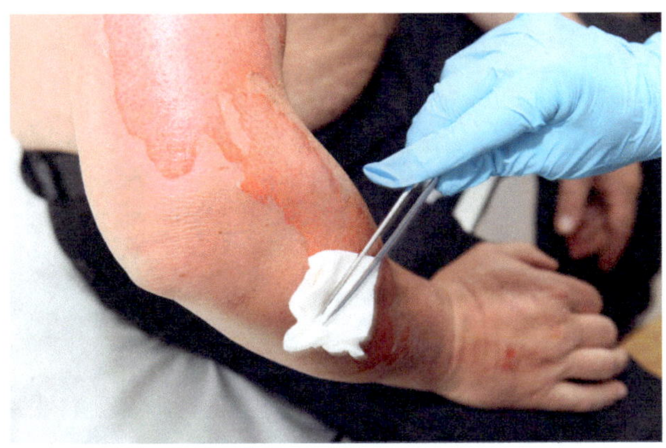

Figure 13.13. Manage wound care directly after a burn injury.

Source: https://wp02-media.cdn.ihealthspot.com/wp-content/uploads/sites/522/2023/04/iStock-171137633.jpg.

13.3.3. Infection Prevention and Control Measures

In the ICU, especially for those with trauma or burns, preventing infections is very important for a better outcome and fewer complications. Central line-associated bloodstream infections (CLABSI) pose significant risks, with studies identifying risk factors such as the duration of central venous catheter (CVC) use and administration of certain sedatives, which can lead to increased infection rates despite existing prevention protocols (Marks *et al.*, 2024). Similarly, ventilator-associated pneumonia (VAP) remains a serious concern, significantly affecting recovery times and healthcare costs. Implementing evidence-based VAP prevention bundles has been shown to reduce both incidence rates and patient ventilator days, underscoring the necessity of continuous nursing education on infection control practices (Alfano *et al.*, 2024). Thus, carefully following these rules improves patient safety and helps save resources in the ICU.

13.3.4. Nutritional Support for Critically Ill Patients

Nutrition is essential in the ICU for critically ill patients, mainly those who have suffered trauma and burns. With hypermetabolism and catabolism being common in these patients, their dietary needs go up, so they require specialnutritional support. Enteral nutrition is usually chosen because it maintains the health of the digestive tract and lowers the chance of infections. Multidisciplinary teams, including registered dietitians, are essential in assessing each patient's unique nutritional status and formulating appropriate feeding plans that align with their metabolic demands and clinical conditions (Kleinpell *et al.*, 2021). Furthermore, evidence suggests that timely nutritional support positively influences recovery and can lead to improved outcomes, especially in sepsis management, a common complication in critically ill patients (Gotts *et al.*, 2016). Thus, effective nutritional strategies must be integral to trauma and burn management protocols in the ICU setting (Figure 13.14).

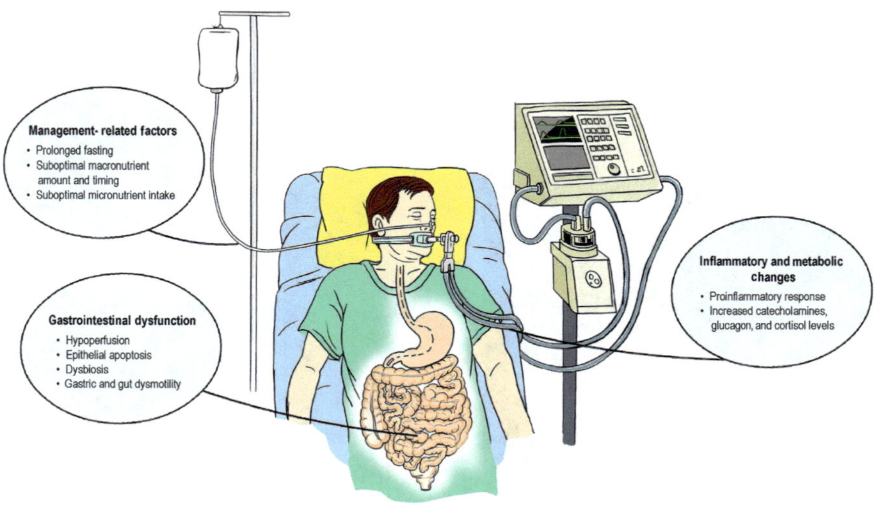

Figure 13.14. Nutrition support for critically ill patients.

Source: https://external-content.duckduckgo.com/iu/?u=https%3A%2F%2Faspenjournals.onlinelibrary.wiley.com%2Fcms%2Fasset%2F8b3339cb-2e38-4c1e-931a-686ca9775a6f%2Fjpen2228-fig-0001-m.jpg&f=1&nofb=1&ipt=2399ccc10633b7b03a88d88294d8093597ecfa30ff4684cd913eb3dd2ac3c8fd.

13.3.5. Rehabilitation and Physical Therapy Considerations

Rehabilitation and physical therapy are important for critically ill patients in the ICU, mainly after trauma and burn injuries. Early mobilization has been accepted as a helpful approach, supporting better function, less need for ventilators, and shorter stays in intensive care and the hospital. Evidence suggests that implementing physical therapy interventions such as passive and active mobilizations can be safely initiated even in unstable patients, thereby promoting physical recovery (Abdulsatar *et al.*, 2015).

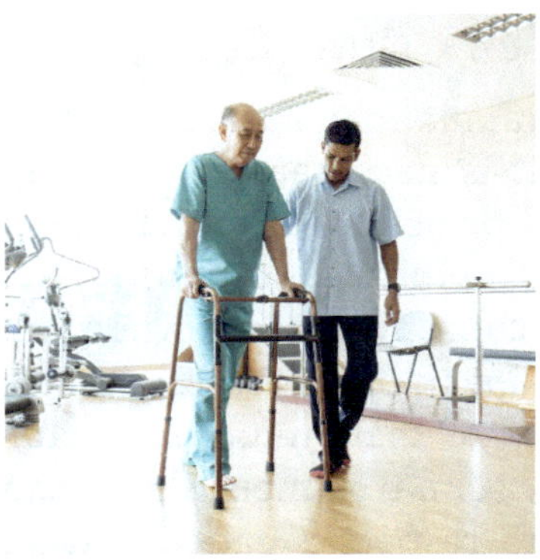

Figure 13.15. The initial phase of cardiac rehabilitation occurs soon after your cardiac event.

Source: https://www.verywellhealth.com/thmb/MkKqCkDzeBwkJE50plDyTLYoL_w=/1500x0/filters:no_upscale():max_bytes(150000):strip_icc()/GettyImages-1091940910-a4e6ab8a96a44a7eac6320a271fc0b15.jpg.

Furthermore, the Chelsea Critical Care Physical Assessment tool (CPAx) has emerged as a valuable measure for assessing the physical function and morbidity of critically ill patients. The use of the CPAx tool not only assists in evaluating patient progress but also fosters a better understanding of the relationship between physical therapy interventions and overall recovery trajectories (Whelan *et al.*, 2017). Ultimately, these considerations underscore the necessity for integrated rehabilitation strategies in the management of trauma and burn patients in critical care environments (Figure 13.15).

13.3.6. Psychological Support and Counseling Services

Having psychological support and counseling services in trauma and burn management in the ICU is very important for patient care. After severe trauma or burns, patients often feel a lot of psychological distress, including PTSD and anxiety, which may slow down their physical recovery. Providing trauma counseling centers can give patients the psychological help they need to cope with the emotions caused by their injuries. These centers are designed not only to facilitate recovery but also to enhance the quality of life for individuals by providing tailored psychological interventions at various recovery stages (Kim *et al.*, 2025). Moreover, research underscores the importance of a supportive environment in reducing the psychological impacts associated with traumatic incidents, emphasizing that psychological support must be integrated with other therapeutic approaches to foster resilience and recovery (Souza, 2024). Care strategies that cover many aspects can greatly improve the outcomes of ICU patients who have suffered trauma and burns.

13.3.7. Use of Advanced Technologies in Monitoring

The use of advanced technology in monitoring has greatly changed trauma and burn management in the ICU, helping patients by providing more precise and instant data. Nowadays, advanced algorithms and wearable devices are used in monitoring, which makes it possible to check vital signs and body functions regularly. Because of these advancements, healthcare professionals can respond quickly, which is very important for handling the changing conditions that come with severe trauma and major burns. Evidence suggests that the collaborative efforts of the interprofessional ICU team, as emphasized by

Dr. Max Harry Weil, contribute to the successful implementation of these technologies in clinical practice, ensuring that each patient receives comprehensive care tailored to their unique needs (Kleinpell *et al.*, 2021). As a result, the combination of cutting-edge monitoring tools and dedicated healthcare teams fosters a safer, more effective environment for critically ill patients undergoing trauma and burn treatment (Hoh *et al.*, 2023) (Figure 13.16).

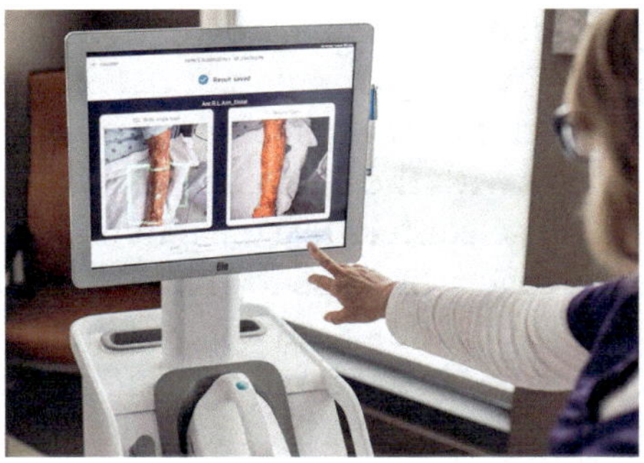

Figure 13.16. The use of advanced technology in monitoring trauma and burn management.

Source: https://www.spectral-ai.com/wp-content/uploads/2024/08/burns-assessment.jpg.

13.3.8. Role of Pharmacological Agents in Management

In the ICU, drugs are very important for handling both trauma and burn patients, since their conditions are often very complex. They are important for controlling pain, sedating patients, and preventing blood clots, mainly in critically injured people. For instance, low molecular weight heparin, such as enoxaparin, has been established as a standard for VTE prophylaxis, significantly reducing incidence rates when administered early and continuously post-injury (Ley *et al.*, 2020). Analgesics and sedatives are given to patients to help them feel more comfortable, which is important for their recovery and to manage their stress responses. The integration of a multidisciplinary approach in pharmacotherapy allows ICU teams to tailor medication regimens that consider individual patient factors, thereby improving outcomes and fostering safety in critically ill patients (Kleinpell *et al.*, 2021). By working together, doctors and pharmacists highlight the role of drugs in caring for patients with trauma and burns in the ICU.

13.3.9. Ethical Considerations in Trauma and Burn Care

Because trauma and burn care in the ICU are complex, it is necessary to carefully consider the ethical principles involved in patient care. Many times, ethical questions come up about informed consent, mainly when patients are unable to speak or understand because of the seriousness of their injuries. Doctors have to weigh how soon treatment should start against the need to respect a patient's wishes, which can be made harder when family members disagree on what is best. Moreover, the risk of HAPIs in critically ill patients raises significant ethical concerns about the standard of care and resource allocation in the ICU environment (Wyatt *et al.*, 2021). Additionally, the rise of antibiotic-resistant infections, such as those caused by *Pseudomonas aeruginosa*, underscores the importance of ethical stewardship in antibiotic use to avoid compromising patient outcomes and public health (Alghamdi *et al.*, 2022). So, dealing with these ethical issues is essential for the best possible care of trauma and burn patients.

Test Your Knowledge

1. What types of surgical interventions are commonly performed in the management of trauma patients?
2. What are the key principles of burn wound care and the techniques used for dressing burn injuries?
3. Why are infection prevention measures and adequate nutritional support critical in the care of critically ill trauma and burn patients?

13.4. Outcomes and Long-term Care

Learning Outcome

1. Describe the factors influencing recovery in trauma and burn patients
2. Discuss the complications associated with severe injuries
3. Explain long-term rehabilitation needs
4. Identify the quality of life assessments post-discharge
5. Understand the follow-up care and outpatient services
6. Discuss the community resources for trauma and burn survivors
7. Focus on research on improving patient outcomes
8. Identify the role of support groups and peer networks
9. Explain the future trends in trauma and burn management.

Outcomes in trauma and burn management extend far beyond the immediate physical recovery achieved in the ICU. Evidence suggests that effective pain management strategies significantly influence long-term outcomes, especially concerning opioid use, which can present both benefits and risks. For instance, while opioids may alleviate pain in patients with extensive burns, their administration is intricately linked to a potential increase in adverse events, including higher mortality rates in lower TBSA cases, as noted in Kleinhapl *et al.* (2025). Additionally, the focus on holistic long-term care is crucial, where interdisciplinary approaches, such as orthoclastic care in managing complex fractures, have shown low infection rates and high union success, showcasing effective outcomes in trauma patients (Madhvani *et al.*, 2024). Thus, understanding and implementing comprehensive long-term care strategies is vital for enhancing the quality of life and overall prognosis for patients recovering from severe trauma and burns (Figure 13.17).

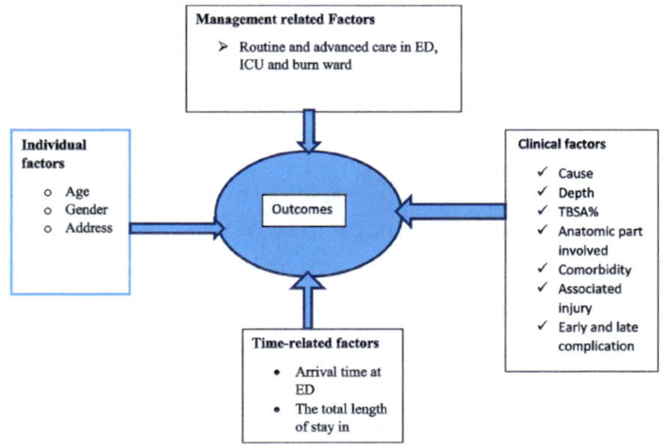

Figure 13.17. Conceptual framework showing the outcome of burn injury and associated factors.

Source: https://bmcemergmed.biomedcentral.com/articles/10.1186/s12873-022-00758-7.

13.4.1. Factors Influencing Recovery in Trauma and Burn Patients

A variety of factors that are connected play a role in the recovery of trauma and burn patients, not just the initial injury. A patient's age and ethnic background are very important factors in how well they respond to treatment. For instance, older individuals and those of African-American ethnicity have been shown to exhibit higher incidences of complications, such as heterotopic ossification (HO), which adversely affect recovery trajectories and functional outcomes (Chaij *et al.*, 2025). Furthermore, the severity of injury significantly correlates with hospitalization duration and overall recovery; patients with complex or penetrating injuries typically experience longer lengths of stay and increased complications (Gupta *et al.*, 2025). The existence of depression and ongoing pain can make it harder for someone to recover. Therefore, knowing about both physical and mental factors is important for designing interventions that help trauma and burn patients recover in the ICU.

13.4.2. Complications Associated with Severe Injuries

Severe injuries can cause many complications that can seriously affect how patients do in the ICU. One of the primary concerns is the risk of VTE, which includes deep vein thrombosis (DVT) and pulmonary embolism (PE). Trauma patients are particularly susceptible, with studies showing DVT rates as high as 58% in the absence of pharmacologic prophylaxis, underscoring the need for preventive measures in the ICU setting (Ley *et al.*, 2020).

Additional complications can arise from the management strategies employed, such as fluid overload due to aggressive resuscitation protocols, which may exacerbate conditions like acute respiratory distress syndrome (ARDS) and lead to prolonged mechanical ventilation (Douglas *et al.*, 2020). Therefore, a comprehensive approach that includes vigilant monitoring and appropriate prophylactic interventions is essential to mitigate these complications and improve the overall prognosis for patients suffering from severe injuries in the ICU (Figure 13.18).

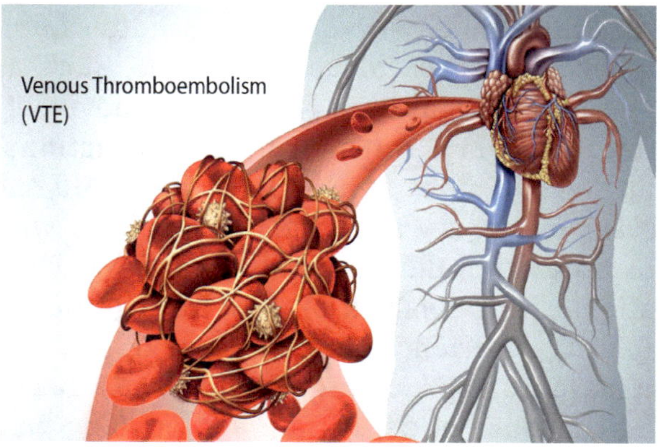

Figure 13.18. Complications Associated with Severe Injuries.

Source: https://vegasvascular.com/venous-thromboembolism-vte/.

13.4.3. Long-Term Rehabilitation Needs

Their recovery from trauma and burns often requires much more time than just their first hospital stay in the ICU. They usually have to manage a range of physical, mental, and social problems during their recovery. Having rehabilitation programs is important since they help patients recover function and support their mental and social health. It appears that personalized rehabilitation, which includes both physical therapy and psychological help, greatly enhances the long-term results of these patients, proving that an interdisciplinary approach is necessary. For instance, the incorporation of evidence-based guidelines, such as those outlined in the 2023 Guideline for the Management of Patients with Aneurysmal Subarachnoid Hemorrhage, emphasizes the need for ongoing assessment and modification of treatment plans to meet evolving patient needs (Hoh *et al.*, 2023). Additionally, the 2021 European Resuscitation Council Guidelines reinforce the significance of long-term support systems in enhancing patient outcomes post-trauma (Perkins *et al.*, 2021).

13.4.4. Quality of life (QoL) Assessments Post-Discharge

Checking on QoL after patients are discharged from the ICU is necessary in trauma and burn management because it indicates how effective the care was. After a patient is discharged, healthcare professionals assess their QoL to see how critical injuries have affected their physical, mental, and social health. Evidence suggests that integrating interprofessional collaboration in the ICU, as highlighted by Kleinpell *et al.* (2021), can optimize care transitions and enhance recovery outcomes. Furthermore, various studies underline the necessity for personalized QoL evaluations, particularly for trauma patients at risk of complications like VTE, which underscores the importance of postoperative management strategies outlined in Ley *et al.* (2020). When healthcare providers pay attention to QoL, they can design rehabilitation programs to fit each patient, address their particular needs, and help them recover better, emphasizing the need for teamwork in post-ICU care.

13.4.5. Follow-Up Care and Outpatient Services

Both physical and psychological recovery are supported by effective follow-up care and outpatient services in trauma and burn management. Many patients continue to recover for a long time after trauma, and they need close outpatient care to supervise their recovery, address complications, and assist in rehabilitation. The incidence of postoperative complications remains significant, with reports indicating that up to 31.5% of surgical trauma patients experience issues that necessitate additional care (Khan *et al.*, 2013). Traumatic injuries can also lead to mental health problems that greatly influence how patients recover, which is why mental health care is so important for follow-up. Current studies advocate for the integration of trauma psychology within outpatient services, as they can enhance patient outcomes significantly—around 8.7% of trauma patients at a Level I center were referred for psychological intervention, which emphasizes the necessity of tailored follow-up services (Mladen *et al.*, 2023). In general, a whole-person approach to outpatient care is necessary to help trauma and burn patients recover well.

13.4.6. Community Resources for Trauma and Burn Survivors

Community resources are important for the recovery of people affected by trauma and burns in the ICU. They provide support groups, rehabilitation, and counseling, which help people heal and reconnect with their community. Many survivors deal with mental and emotional problems after an injury, so they require services that focus on these areas. Also, community organizations provide social assistance, helping those affected by traumatic events manage their recovery. As seen in evidence-based recommendations for various traumatic conditions, such as those outlined in the 2023 guidelines for managing aneurysmal subarachnoid hemorrhage, a collaborative approach can significantly enhance patient outcomes (Hoh *et al.*, 2023). Similarly, the comprehensive guidelines provided by the European Resuscitation Council emphasize the importance of continued care and resource access for optimal recovery following life-threatening events (Perkins *et al.*, 2021).

13.4.7. Research on Improving Patient Outcomes

Trauma and burn care for patients in the ICU is now guided more by evidence-based guidelines and protocols. Research has illustrated that implementing structured algorithms for interventions, such as the Western Trauma Association's recommendations for pharmacologic prophylaxis against VTE, significantly reduces complication rates among trauma patients by ensuring timely and appropriate care (Ley *et al.*, 2020). Similarly, advancements in the use of NIV for acute respiratory failure have demonstrated marked improvements in patient recovery, facilitating better oxygenation and reducing the need for invasive procedures (Rochwerg *et al.*, 2017). This research points out that clinical practice should use scientific findings to improve treatment and encourage teamwork among different specialists. As a result, regularly improving these protocols helps achieve better patient results and reduces the complications faced by critically injured people.

13.4.8. Role of Support Groups and Peer Networks

Support groups and peer networks are now seen as an important part of care for patients with trauma and burns in the ICU. These networks help patients emotionally and give them advice that helps them cope with the hardships of recovery. Talking with people who have gone through the same thing can help ICU patients feel less alone and anxious. Studies reveal that being part of a structured group helps people improve their mental health and learn better ways to cope, which allows them to adjust more easily to rehabilitation and daily living. Furthermore, as outlined in the "2023 Guideline for the Management of Patients With Aneurysmal Subarachnoid Hemorrhage," patient-centric support mechanisms align medical interventions with the psychosocial needs of patients and their families, highlighting the importance of emotional support in clinical practice (Hoh *et al.*, 2023). Peer networks thus contribute to a holistic approach, effectively bridging the emotional and physical aspects of recovery (Apfelbaum *et al.*, 2021) (Figure 13.1).

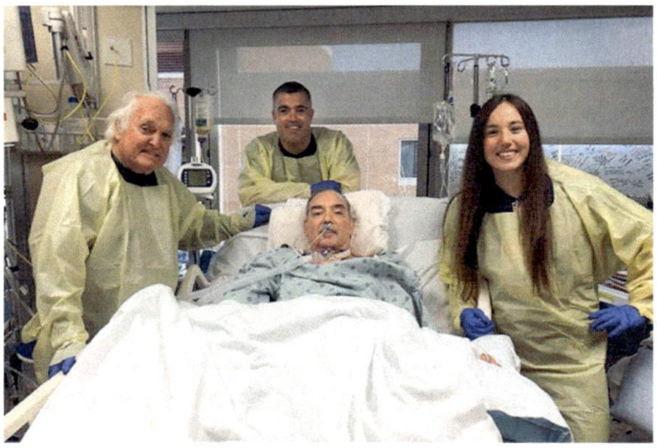

Figure 13.19. Support groups and peer networks.

Source: https://www.hopkinsmedicine.org/-/media/burn/images/burn-patient.jpg?h=440&iar=0&w=640&hash=8A7A2A3424EFADED3F0D0A6D53656A57.

13.4.9. Future Trends in Trauma and Burn Management

Moving forward, the main trends in trauma and burn management will probably involve better teamwork between various professionals and more research-based methods. The collaboration among general and emergency surgeons, intensivists, and infectious disease specialists is crucial for addressing the complexities of skin and soft-tissue infections, which frequently occur in trauma cases, and demonstrating the value of teamwork in developing effective treatment protocols (Sartelli *et al.*, 2018). Furthermore, advancements in enteral nutrition (EN) will play a pivotal role in supporting recovery during the ICU stay, emphasizing the need for systematic approaches to minimize complications associated with nutritional support (Boullata *et al.*, 2016). If medical professionals follow these changes, they can help patients recover and manage care more efficiently, so that trauma and burn management in the ICU continues to adapt to new demands and medical science.

Test Your Knowledge

1. What types of surgical interventions are commonly performed in the management of trauma patients?
2. What are the key principles of burn wound care and the techniques used for dressing burn injuries?
3. Why are infection prevention measures and adequate nutritional support critical in the care of critically ill trauma and burn patients?

SUMMARY

In short, proper management of trauma and burns in the ICU helps patients recover well and prevents complications. The implementation of clear protocols, such as the pharmacologic prophylaxis guidelines to prevent VTE, demonstrates the importance of evidence-based practice in trauma care (Ley *et al.*, 2020). Furthermore, strategies such as NIV have been established as essential interventions for patients experiencing acute respiratory failure, showcasing the multifaceted approach required for critically ill individuals (Rochwerg *et al.*, 2017). Following the guidelines and seeing how different clinical factors interact can help healthcare providers support patients' recovery and reduce the dangers linked to trauma and burn injuries. Following these practices and always seeking to improve will result in improved health outcomes for patients in the ICU.

Care for trauma and burn patients in the ICU involves stressing the need for proper fluid resuscitation and it's careful monitoring to help patients recover. Recent studies illustrate that dynamic measures, such as assessing stroke volume changes during passive leg raises, can effectively guide fluid and vasopressor management in patients experiencing septic shock, ultimately leading to a lower net fluid balance and reduced requirements for renal replacement therapy and mechanical ventilation (Douglas *et al.*, 2020). Additionally, the integration of noninvasive mechanical ventilation is highlighted as a valuable intervention for patients with acute respiratory failure, addressing diverse etiologies and contributing to improved care standards (Rochwerg *et al.*, 2017). Because of these factors, using evidence-based methods is essential for supporting recovery and keeping critically ill patients stable in the ICU. Treating patients using individualized plans matches the latest guidelines in managing trauma and burns.

KEY TERMS FROM THIS CHAPTER

- Airway management
- Burns
- Debridement
- Fluid resuscitation
- Hypermetabolic state
- Infection control
- Inotropes
- Shock
- Burn shock
- Carbon monoxide poisoning
- Escharotomy
- Hemodynamic monitoring
- ICU (intensive care unit)
- Inhalation injury
- Pain management
- Tissue perfusion

CRITICAL THINKING QUESTIONS

1. **What is the first priority in the management of a trauma patient upon arrival at the ICU?**
   a. Pain management
   b. Fluid resuscitation
   c. Nutritional support
   d. Wound debridement
2. **Which of the following is the most important factor in determining the severity of a burn injury?**
   a. The age of the patient
   b. The depth of the burn
   c. The presence of infection
   d. The size of the burn in relation to the total body surface area (TBSA)
3. **In burn management, what is the recommended initial fluid resuscitation guideline for adults with burns covering more than 20% TBSA?**
   a. 2 mL/kg of Lactated Ringer's solution per % TBSA burned over the first 24 hours
   b. 4 mL/kg of Lactated Ringer's solution per % TBSA burned over the first 24 hours
   c. 6 mL/kg of Normal Saline per % TBSA burned over the first 24 hours
   d. 8 mL/kg of D5W per % TBSA burned over the first 24 hours
4. **Which of the following is the most common cause of death in critically ill burn patients?**
   a. Acute renal failure
   b. Septic shock
   c. Hypovolemic shock
   d. Respiratory failure
5. **In trauma patients with suspected spinal cord injury, the first intervention should be:**
   a. Intubation and ventilation
   b. Immobilization of the spine
   c. Fluid resuscitation
   d. Immediate surgery for decompression

Short Answer Questions

1. What are the primary goals of trauma and burn management in the ICU?
2. How do the initial management principles differ between trauma patients and burn patients in the ICU?
3. What is the importance of rapid assessment and stabilization in trauma patients upon ICU admission?
4. What is the role of the ABCDE approach (Airway, Breathing, Circulation, Disability, Exposure) in the initial management of trauma patients in the ICU?
5. What are the key differences in managing burn patients compared to other critically ill patients in the ICU?

Answer to Critical Thinking Questions

1. (b); 2. (d); 3. (b); 4. (b); 5. (b)

REFERENCES

1. Abdulsatar, A., Adler, A., Amidei, C., Bailey, S., Balas, M., Baldwin, M., Banwell, B., *et al.* (2015). Early mobilization in the critical care unit: A review of adult and pediatric literature. https://core.ac.uk/download/61659404.pdf.
2. Alfano, A., Riddle, K., Nordstrom, K., Buterakos, R., & Keiser, M. (2024). The impact of nursing education on ventilator-associated pneumonia prevention bundle to reduce incidence of infection: A quality improvement project. *Dimensions of Critical Care Nursing, 43*(1), 40–46. https://www.semanticscholar.org/paper/abc00b6b60376bd6449ae34bb6567fae888b5a2c (accessed on 22 May 2025).
3. Alghamdi, S., Ateeq, M., Atwah, B., Bantun, B., *et al.* (2022). Presence of BlaPER-1 and BlaVEB-1 beta-lactamase genes among isolates of *Pseudomonas aeruginosa* from Burn and Trauma Hospital Peshawar, Pakistan. https://core.ac.uk/download/541142003.pdf (accessed on 22 May 2025).
4. Apfelbaum, J. L., Hagberg, C. A., Connis, R. T., Abdelmalak, B., Agarkar, M., Dutton, R. P., Fiadjoe, J. E., *et al.* (2021). 2022 American Society of Anesthesiologists practice guidelines for management of the difficult airway. *Anesthesiology, 136*(1), 31–81. https://doi.org/10.1097/aln.0000000000004002.
5. Bassetti, M., Vena, A., Croxatto, A., Righi, E., & Guéry, B. (2018). How to manage *Pseudomonas aeruginosa* infections. *Drugs in Context, 7*, 212527. https://doi.org/10.7573/dic.212527.
6. Bateman, R. M., Sharpe, M. D., Jagger, J. E., Ellis, C., Solé-Violán, J., López Rodríguez, M., Herrera-Ramos, E., *et al.* (2016). 36th International Symposium on Intensive Care and Emergency Medicine. *Critical Care, 20*(Suppl. 2). https://doi.org/10.1186/s13054-016-1208-6.
7. Blackley, S. K., Lawrence, J., Blevins, A. C., Howell, C. W., Butts, C., Polite, N. M., Capasso, T. J., *et al.* (2024). A single hospital-wide antibiogram is insufficient to account for differences in antibiotic resistance patterns across multiple ICUs. *The American Surgeon*. https://www.semanticscholar.org/paper/2803c3b9779b10a0426e5639ca926a8c824b0293 (accessed on 22 May 2025).
8. Boullata, J. I., Carrera, A. L., Harvey, L. P., Escuro, A. A., Hudson, L., Mays, A., McGinnis, C., *et al.* (2016). ASPEN safe practices for enteral nutrition therapy. *Journal of Parenteral and Enteral Nutrition, 41*(1), 15–103. https://doi.org/10.1177/0148607116673053.
9. Chaij, J. M., Ghogomu, M., Marzook, F., Golovko, G., Song, J., Wolf, S. E., & El Ayadi, A. (2025). 885 heterotopic ossifications after burn injury results in worse outcomes. *Journal of Burn Care & Research, 46*(S1), S317–S318. https://www.semanticscholar.org/paper/2c32e2aeb68b292ccd4ed1ac027fb517751c2634 (accessed on 22 May 2025).
10. Dalamagka, M. I. (2024). Emergency medicine. *World Journal of Advanced Research and Reviews, 23*(2), 394–401. https://doi.org/10.30574/wjarr.2024.23.2.2389.
11. Decker, P., Jeng, J., Tran, M., Zaky, K., Chen, S. Y., & Urgun, K. (2025). 839 Intraoperative whole blood transfusion improves outcomes in pediatric burn: 1st reported case. *Journal of Burn Care & Research, 46*(Suppl. 1), S283. https://www.semanticscholar.org/paper/e568cdd7c5b6c5725cc6f8dab44e16063e749fb7 (accessed on 22 May 2025).
12. Delano, M. J., & Ward, P. A. (2016). The immune system's role in sepsis progression, resolution, and long-term outcome. *Immunological Reviews, 274*(1), 330–353. https://doi.org/10.1111/imr.12499.

13. Donohue, J., Kennedy, J., Seymour, C., Girard, T., Lo-Ciganic, W., Kim, C., Marroquin, O., *et al.* (2019). Patterns of opioid administration among opioid-naive inpatients and associations with post discharge opioid use. *Annals of Internal Medicine, 171*(2), 81–90. https://www.semanticscholar.org/paper/2f6e53ed932ab9a87dbe619d90419790b339cd81 (accessed on 22 May 2025).

14. Douglas, I. S., Alapat, P., Corl, K., Exline, M. C., Forni, L. G., Holder, A. L., Kaufman, D. A., *et al.* (2020). Fluid response evaluation in sepsis hypotension and shock. *CHEST Journal, 158*(4), 1431–1445. https://doi.org/10.1016/j.chest.2020.04.025.

15. Elkbuli, A., Narvel, R., Boneva, D., & Mckenney, M. (2020). The impact of chronic opioid use on trauma outcomes. *The American Surgeon, 86*(1), 35–37. https://www.semanticscholar.org/paper/f699aee3eb082a23b2927443d7cfb85ba4d5cb3a (accessed on 22 May 2025).

16. Elsadek, H. E. (2024). Management of procedural pain in pediatric burnt patients: A review. *Deleted Journal, 3*(1), 51–61. https://doi.org/10.54536/ajmsi.v3i1.2567.

17. Frieri, M., Kumar, K., & Boutin, A. (2016). Antibiotic resistance. *Journal of Infection and Public Health, 10*(4), 369–378. https://doi.org/10.1016/j.jiph.2016.08.007.

18. Gotts, J. E., & Matthay, M. A. (2016). Sepsis: Pathophysiology and clinical management. *BMJ*. https://doi.org/10.1136/bmj.i1585.

19. Griffin, K., Karas, M., Ivascu, N. S., & Lief, L. (2020). Hospital preparedness for COVID-19: A practical guide from a critical care perspective. *American Journal of Respiratory and Critical Care Medicine, 201*(11), 1337–1344. https://doi.org/10.1164/rccm.202004-1037cp.

20. Gupta, A., Purushothaman, V., & James, J. D. (2025). Optimizing trauma laparotomy outcomes: The role of Enhanced Recovery After Surgery protocols in reducing hospital length of stay. *Trauma Surgery & Acute Care Open, 10*. https://www.semanticscholar.org/paper/d07bd72bced458bed300da635ce1f06386ff8b81 (accessed on 22 May 2025).

21. Hatcher, V. H., Galet, C., Lilienthal, M., Skeete, D. A., & Romanowski, K. S. (2019). Association of clinical frailty scores with hospital readmission for falls after index admission for trauma-related injury. *JAMA Network Open, 2*(11), e1912409. https://doi.org/10.1001/jamanetworkopen.2019.12409.

22. Hirche, C., Almeland, S. K., Dheansa, B., Fuchs, P. C., Governa, M., Hoeksema, H., Korzeniowski, T., *et al.* (2020). Eschar removal by bromelain-based enzymatic debridement (Nexobrid®) in burns: European consensus guidelines update. *Burns, 46*(4), 782–796. https://doi.org/10.1016/j.burns.2020.03.002.

23. Hoh, B. L., Ko, N., Amin-Hanjani, S., Chou, S., Cruz-Flores, S., Dangayach, N., Derdeyn, C. P., *et al.* (2023). 2023 guideline for the management of patients with aneurysmal subarachnoid hemorrhage: A guideline from the American Heart Association/American Stroke Association. *Stroke, 54*. https://doi.org/10.1161/str.0000000000000436.

24. Idenburg, F. J., van Dongen, T. T. C. F., Tan, E., Hamming, J. H., Leenen, L. P. H., & Hoencamp, R. (2015). Pediatric surgical care in a Dutch military hospital in Afghanistan. *World Journal of Surgery, 39*(10), 2413–2421. https://doi.org/10.1007/s00268-015-3136-z.

25. Khan, A., Kuzuku, A., Chandika, A. B., Solagberu, B. A., Mutasingwa, D. R., Norberg, E., Twagirayezu, E., *et al.* (2013). Citywide trauma experience in Mwanza, Tanzania: A need for urgent intervention. https://core.ac.uk/download/pdf/19726063.pdf (accessed on 22 May 2025).

26. Kim, C. S., Kong, J. O., & Koo, J. W. (2025). Trauma counseling centers for psychological support to manage trauma from workplace injuries in Korea: A narrative review. *The Ewha Medical Journal*. https://www.semanticscholar.org/paper/585b012912dd73a6b326227c52bbc7bd527aa63e (accessed on 22 May 2025).

27. Kleinhapl, J., Dempsey, J., Song, J., Suman, O. E., Branski, L., & Wolf, S. E. (2025). 591 the use of opioids in adult burn patients: Long-term dependency risk and outcomes. *Journal of Burn Care & Research, 46*(S1), S172. https://www.semanticscholar.org/paper/5538d616d49e36b00c29a619f9daeb6247df1f4d (accessed on 22 May 2025).

28. Kleinpell, R., Grabenkort, W. R., Boyle, W. A., Vines, D., & Olsen, K. M. (2021). The Society of Critical Care Medicine at 50 years: Interprofessional practice in critical care: Looking back and forging ahead. *Critical Care Medicine, 49*(12), 2017–2032. https://doi.org/10.1097/ccm.0000000000005276.

29. Koenig, V., Lumenta, D., Joestl, J., Ihra, G., Windpassinger, M., Monai, M., & Fochtmann, A. (2025). High-voltage injuries and train surfing: A 30-year review of epidemiology, treatment, and outcomes. *Journal of Clinical Medicine*. https://www.semanticscholar.org/paper/08f7bc10dd573d85c8d1258bb2ea177b7c228d47 (accessed on 22 May 2025).

30. Levey, A., & James, M. (2017). Acute kidney injury. *Annals of Internal Medicine, 167*, ITC66–ITC80. https://www.semanticscholar.org/paper/2478ae2dce4d2223b7be8e55e7acc798625bb1be (accessed on 22 May 2025).

31. Ley, E. J., Brown, C. V. R., Moore, E. E., Sava, J., Peck, K. A., Ciesla, D. J., Sperry, J. L., *et al.* (2020). Updated guidelines to reduce venous thromboembolism in trauma patients: A Western Trauma Association critical decisions algorithm. *Journal of Trauma and Acute Care Surgery, 89*(6), 971–981. https://doi.org/10.1097/ta.0000000000002830.

32. Madhvani, K. R., Fong, A., Clark, T., Eng, K., Condurache, C., McGregor-Riley, J., & Shields, D. (2024). Mid to long-term outcomes of grade III-B open tibial fractures definitively managed with a circular frame: A 13-year prospective database study at a major trauma center. *Journal of Orthopedic Trauma, 38*(8), 447–451. https://www.semanticscholar.org/paper/307cfd95f2b04ae57c5eca3610106c8df29a9fa1 (accessed on 22 May 2025).

33. Marks, K. T., Rosengard, K. D., Franks, J. D., Staffa, S. J., Chan Yuen, J., Burns, J. P., Priebe, G. P., *et al.* (2024). Risk factors for central line-associated bloodstream infection in the pediatric intensive care setting despite standard prevention measures. *Infection Control and Hospital Epidemiology*. https://www.semanticscholar.org/paper/d3f6fd222923e48c2787702aed16c127813981dd (accessed on 22 May 2025).

34. McClave, S. A., DiBaise, J. K., Mullin, G. E., & Martindale, R. G. (2016). ACG clinical guideline: Nutrition therapy in the adult hospitalized patient. *The American Journal of Gastroenterology, 111*(3), 315–334. https://doi.org/10.1038/ajg.2016.28.

35. McClave, S. A., Taylor, B., Martindale, R. G., Warren, M., Johnson, D. R., Braunschweig, C., McCarthy, M. S., *et al.* (2016). Guidelines for the provision and assessment of nutrition support therapy in the adult critically ill patient. *Journal of Parenteral and Enteral Nutrition, 40*(2), 159–211. https://doi.org/10.1177/0148607115621863.

36. Mittal, B. M., McQuitty, R. A., Talon, M., & McQuitty, A. L. (2024). Airway management for acute and reconstructive burns: Our 30-year experience. *Seminars in Plastic Surgery*. https://www.semanticscholar.org/paper/110d920e34ee1c3ce01402bd4c16537b9f37f380 (accessed on 22 May 2025).

37. Mladen, S. (2023). *Analysis of Referrals to Trauma Psychology and Subsequent Development and Proof-Of-Concept Study of Provider Mental Health Training at a Level I Trauma Center*. https://core.ac.uk/download/596339099.pdf (accessed on 22 May 2025).

38. Nielson, C. B., Duethman, N. C., Howard, J. M., Moncure, M., & Wood, J. G. (2016). Burns. *Journal of Burn Care & Research, 38*(4), e469–e481. https://doi.org/10.1097/bcr.0000000000000355.

39. Nur, M. I., & Rismawan, B. (2023). Management of critically ill patient following multiple abdominal traumas with massive hemorrhage: Case report. *Journal of Advanced Research in Medical and Health Science, 6*(1). https://www.semanticscholar.org/paper/58bab835c41f2b49fe881a458816265c5e47b56d (accessed on 22 May 2025).

40. Olaveson, T. (2025). 829 Biosynthetic wound matrixes applied to autologous skin cell suspension-treated burns supports good outcomes. *Journal of Burn Care & Research, 46*(Suppl. 1), S277. https://www.semanticscholar.org/paper/15e5f2a3ceb2b61df2efe8e0dc2a8f0add07fb22 (accessed on 22 May 2025).

41. Palacio, R. M., & Iacobelli, O. (2025). 625 Implementing Burn Padlet to improve interprofessional collaboration within the BTSD interdisciplinary team. *Journal of Burn Care & Research, 46*(Suppl. 1), S196. https://www.semanticscholar.org/paper/2621d8b489379dd75c8a817ae93a5ebc4f017429 (accessed on 22 May 2025).

42. Perkins, G. D., Gräsner, J. T., Semeraro, F., Olasveengen, T. M., Soar, J., Lott, C., Van de Voorde, P., *et al.* (2021). European Resuscitation Council guidelines 2021: Executive summary. *Resuscitation, 161*, 1–60. https://doi.org/10.1016/j.resuscitation.2021.02.003.

43. Rochwerg, B., Brochard, L., Elliott, M., Hess, D., Hill, N. S., Nava, S., Navalesi, P., *et al.* (2017). Official ERS/ATS clinical practice guidelines: Noninvasive ventilation for acute respiratory failure. *European Respiratory Journal, 50*, 1602426. https://doi.org/10.1183/13993003.02426-2016.

44. Sargent, R., Schellenberg, M., Cheng, V., Emigh, B., Matsushima, K., & Inaba, K. (2022). Breast trauma: A decade of surgical interventions and outcomes from US trauma centers. *The American Surgeon, 89*(11), 2321–2324. https://www.semanticscholar.org/paper/a9f19610219122d36f230f271c881a83b79c598b (accessed on 22 May 2025).

45. Sartelli, M., Guirao, X., Hardcastle, T. C., Kluger, Y., Boermeester, M. A., Rașa, K., Ansaloni, L., *et al.* (2018). 2018 WSES/SIS-E consensus conference: Recommendations for the management of skin and soft-tissue infections. *World Journal of Emergency Surgery, 13*(1). https://doi.org/10.1186/s13017-018-0219-9.

46. Shauly, O., Kong, B. H., Brant, N., Marxen, T., Johnson, L., Liu, Y., & Nosanov, L. (2025). 857 The Lightning Le Fort: Contemporary management of lightning strike injuries including craniofacial fractures. *Journal of Burn Care & Research, 46*(Suppl. 1), S296–S297. https://www.semanticscholar.org/paper/1fce4445052107b9772fe1a38f90a742d0d3854b (accessed on 22 May 2025).

47. Smith, C. (2025). 982 quality conversations: Addressing the problem of pressure injuries in burn ICU. *Journal of Burn Care & Research, 46*(S1), S384. https://www.semanticscholar.org/paper/3e111659980f6db67ac5f1e22be8304f9322aea4 (accessed on 22 May 2025).

48. Søreide, K., Hallet, J., Matthews, J. B., Schnitzbauer, A. A., Line, P. D., Lai, P. B. S., Gestal Otero, J. J., *et al.* (2020). Immediate and long-term impact of the COVID-19 pandemic on delivery of surgical services. *British Journal of Surgery, 107*(10), 1250–1261. https://doi.org/10.1002/bjs.11670.

49. Souza, R. P. P. (2024). Enhancing school safety through psychological support: Key findings and strategies. *Revita Systematical*. https://www.semanticscholar.org/paper/0c4012b79931f8dd5c518904a3e31906632e4760 (accessed on 22 May 2025).

50. Stanton, E., Karanas, Y. L., Gillenwater, J., Pham, T. N., & Sheckter, C. (2024). 506 methamphetamine intoxication and inpatient outcomes for burn patients. *Journal of Burn Care & Research, 45*(1), 115. https://www.semanticscholar.org/paper/b06b8561c7a06a624b515441f820cf88e9475b27 (accessed on 22 May 2025).

51. Stanton, E., Manasyan, A., Wong, S., Johnson, M. B., & Gillenwater, J. (2025). 104 integrating addiction medicine into burn care: Optimizing pain management in stimulant-positive patients. *Journal of Burn Care & Research, 46*(S1), S83. https://www.semanticscholar.org/paper/7e9a33c231943d39896be19f23713d742f037446 (accessed on 22 May 2025).

52. Whelan, M. (2017). *The Use of the CPAX Tool in a South African Intensive Care Unit: Clinical Outcomes and Physiotherapists' Perceptions* [Master's thesis, Stellenbosch University]. https://core.ac.uk/download/188772766.pdf (accessed on 22 May 2025).

53. Wyatt, R. L. (2021). *Successfully Spreading Improvement Work Using a Proven Framework* [Doctoral dissertation, University of Alabama at Birmingham]. https://core.ac.uk/download/489537045.pdf (accessed on 22 May 2025).

CARDIOVASCULAR EMERGENCIES IN CRITICAL CARE

14

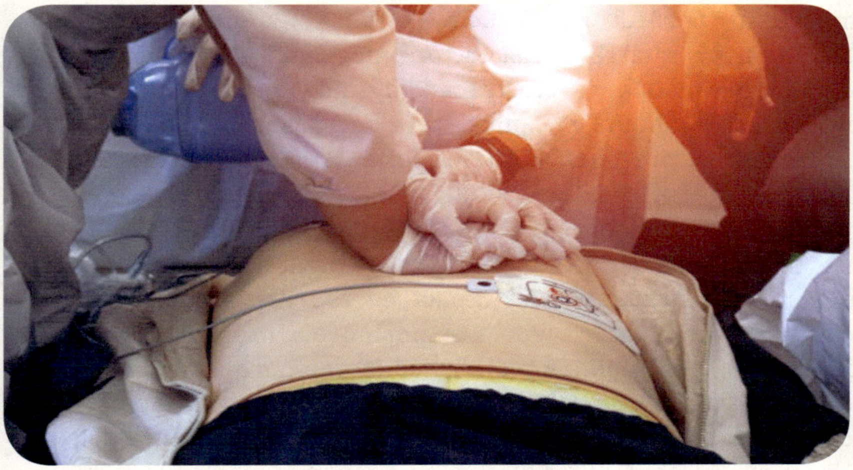

LEARNING OBJECTIVES

After studying this chapter, you will be able to:

1. List the types of cardiovascular emergencies.
2. Focus on the risk factors and prevalence.
3. Discuss the pathophysiology of cardiovascular emergencies.
4. Elaborate on the diagnostic approaches.
5. Describe treatment protocols.

Introduction

Critical care frequently deals with many problems, and cardiovascular emergencies are critical because they can be very complex and progress rapidly. Such emergencies involve many dangerous conditions, for example, myocardial infarction, cardiac arrest, and severe arrhythmias, which must be managed right away. Because cardiovascular diseases are complicated, critical care professionals must know a lot and be able to decide quickly in emergencies. Since these diseases are hazardous and lead to many deaths, it is crucial to use management techniques supported by the latest scientific research and best practices. These strategies will help patients recover better and could save lives as healthcare professionals deal with the rising number of people dealing with cardiovascular diseases. The economic consequences of cardiovascular emergencies in critical care are serious, which makes dealing with these problems more urgent. Stays in the hospital after heart problems are often long and expensive, which may put pressure on healthcare resources. For instance, the costs associated with hypertension care in regions like sub-Saharan Africa reveal a broader trend that challenges health systems worldwide; medications often represent the most substantial expense in treatment plans (Steinert *et al.*, 2023). Healthcare policymakers and providers need to know the economic effects of emergencies, as this knowledge can guide where and how resources are used. Since both financial stability and high-quality care are important today, finding ways to lower costs without harming patient care is an important subject for research and implementation in critical care medicine. Also, it is important to understand the full range of cardiovascular emergencies and the factors that increase the risk of them for proper management. Many studies point out that various factors, including lifestyle and genes can cause these conditions. Factors such as age, pre-existing health conditions, and socioeconomic status can significantly influence the incidence and severity of cardiovascular emergencies (Pleșca *et al.*, 2017). Noticing these variables helps healthcare professionals create plans that handle the crisis and also improve a person's overall health in the future. Because cardiovascular health is tied to public health in many ways, promoting awareness and prevention locally can help lessen the risk of such emergencies. For this reason, it is essential to keep learning about cardiovascular risks and to manage patients in critical care emergencies actively.

Definition of Cardiovascular Emergencies

Cardiovascular emergencies are a serious group of medical problems that happen suddenly and can be life-threatening for the patient. Various emergencies can happen, such as acute myocardial infarction, worsening congestive heart failure, severe arrhythmias, and pulmonary embolism. Because these situations are urgent, a quick and accurate diagnosis is required, along with quick treatment to avoid serious health problems or death. Dealing with these critical events requires emergency care providers, cardiologists, and critical care specialists to join forces and address the problem together. Since cardiovascular disease is constantly evolving, it is necessary to know and define the important features of these emergencies to provide good treatment and better patient outcomes. You need to identify specific symptoms and signs to tell cardiovascular emergencies apart from other medical problems. If a patient has acute chest pain, which is often a sign of myocardial infarction, risk factors, medical history, and tests such as electrocardiograms and biomarkers should be quickly evaluated. Also, if someone presents with syncope or severe shortness of breath, it could mean there are both heart and other systemic issues involved. Noticing and differentiating these signs early can have a significant impact on the way critical care is managed. Furthermore, integrating the guidelines established by the European Society of Cardiology (ESC) and the European Society of Hypertension (ESH) provides a framework that informs clinical practice and aligns with evidence-based medicine, impacting treatment decisions for patients facing these emergencies (Williams *et al.*, 2018). If cardiovascular emergencies are not handled right away, they can result in major complications or even death. It is important to pay close attention to patients who are at high risk, such as the elderly or those with heart problems, when dealing with these crises. Having a clear emergency plan with quick assessment, successful resuscitation, and advanced options is important for good results. In addition, keeping healthcare professionals informed about the latest changes in cardiovascular emergencies improves the care given. As we move forward in demanding healthcare environments, recognizing and understanding the definition of cardiovascular emergencies will play a pivotal role in refining treatment protocols and optimizing patient-centric care (Livingston *et al.*, 2020) (Figure 14.1).

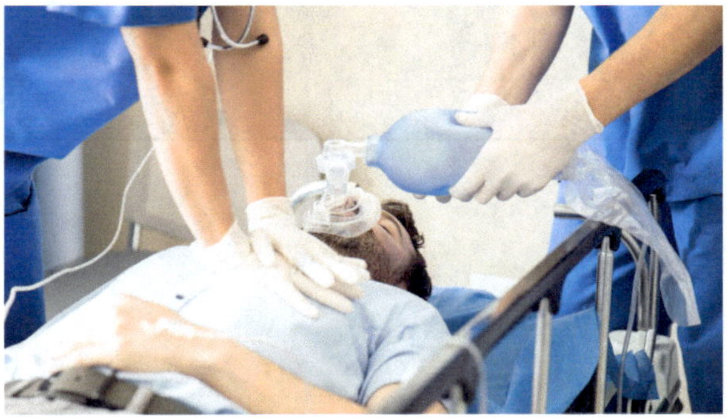

Figure 14.1. Cardiovascular emergencies.

Source: https://d35oenyzp35321.cloudfront.net/cardiac_emergency_cpr_1c299779b8.jpg.

Importance of Timely Intervention

In the realm of cardiovascular emergencies, the significance of timely intervention cannot be overstated. If acute coronary syndrome or severe arrhythmias are recognized and managed quickly, it helps protect the heart and prevents permanent damage. If treatment is delayed, patients may experience more health problems, higher death rates, and take longer to recover, which is why healthcare systems should focus on quick action in such situations. In addition, the education of healthcare professionals matters a lot, since their quick decisions in the clinic can greatly affect patient outcomes. Incorporating innovative teaching methods, such as gamified scenario-writing, has been shown to enhance clinical reasoning skills in nursing students, equipping them for effective intervention during emergencies like those described in Antikchi *et al.* (2025). So, encouraging quick and effective action in cardiovascular emergencies is still very important for better patient care. It is very important to use a multidisciplinary approach when considering how to act quickly in cardiovascular emergencies. It makes sure that cardiologists, nurses and emergency responders can all work together to give complete care. Good communication and strict adherence to protocols enable doctors to quickly identify and treat congenital heart diseases in newborns, which is crucial. It has been demonstrated that using advanced imaging and coordinating teams quickly helps find critical conditions early, which improves patient outcomes. Insights from literature, particularly regarding the urgency of prenatal screening for potential cardiac anomalies, highlight the necessity of integrated efforts across specialties to facilitate decisive interventions noted in Moisa *et al.* (2024). A unified and team-oriented approach helps the team be more active in handling cardiovascular emergencies. In short, acting quickly is very important for treating cardiovascular emergencies effectively. Delays can be very harmful, because each second can affect the chances of a patient surviving and recovering well. Training healthcare professionals to recognize signs of distress and act swiftly is essential, bolstered by research that indicates improved clinical reasoning through innovative educational methods, such as those shown in Antikchi *et al.* (2025). Strong teamwork and open communication among healthcare staff make it easier to make good decisions quickly. The literature points out that quick and coordinated actions are necessary, so timely intervention should always be a primary concern in critical care. To address the difficulties of cardiovascular emergencies and help patients survive, healthcare systems must be very diligent.

Overview of Critical Care Settings

Critical care units are set up to give close attention and care to patients with severe medical conditions, mainly related to the heart and blood vessels. These environments, including intensive care units (ICUs) and emergency departments (EDs), are equipped with advanced technology and staffed by a multidisciplinary team of healthcare professionals, including physicians, nurses, and respiratory therapists. All members are important in making sure that cardiovascular emergencies like acute myocardial infarctions, arrhythmias, and cardiac arrest are handled quickly and effectively. Since urgent care is needed, making decisions and acting promptly is crucial because it can affect the patient's condition. When team members cooperate, they can ensure a planned and efficient response to emergencies in the heart, which may result in higher survival rates. Cardiovascular emergencies in critical care are managed best when healthcare providers have medical knowledge and also collaborate and communicate effectively. Because critical care is constantly changing, frontline doctors need to be ready to respond right away to new developments. A structured induction program focusing on emergency cardiac care has been shown to enhance the competencies of resident doctors, equipping them with the skills needed to adhere to emergency protocols and make quick, informed decisions in high-pressure environments (Sooltan *et al.*, 2025). They are designed to make sure healthcare providers understand critical care and advanced cardiac life support, so that care is given consistently and effectively. Such training and education are necessary because they influence how well patients with heart emergencies are cared for. Also, critical care teams must manage the challenges of somatic symptom disorders that are often expressed as cardiovascular complaints, which can make treatment more difficult. Patients with somatization disorders frequently visit emergency departments with nonspecific symptoms that can mimic cardiac events, posing challenges for healthcare providers in making accurate diagnoses (Garde *et al.*, 2025). For this reason, members of critical care teams should be skilled in managing cardiac emergencies and also in handling the mental and emotional aspects of treating patients. Paying attention to mental health in the protocol for cardiovascular emergencies can result in better and more complete care. Creating an environment that cares for both physical and mental health in critical care allows patients to get better treatment and leads to better overall results.

14.1. Types of Cardiovascular Emergencies

Learning Outcome

1. Discuss the myocardial infarction
2. Explain the cardiac arrest
3. Discuss pulmonary embolism

Many different life-threatening cardiovascular emergencies exist, and all of them require urgent medical treatment. Among these types, myocardial infarction (MI) stands out as a common and critical emergency. If blood flow to a heart area is blocked, MI happens, and this can result in tissue damage and cardiac failure. The clinical presentation of MI often includes chest pain, shortness of breath, and diaphoresis, demanding urgent treatment through interventions such as thrombolysis or percutaneous coronary intervention (PCI). It is dangerous for both adults and young people, mainly those who have predisposing factors such as smoking and high blood pressure. Quickly noticing and handling an MI is crucial for protecting the heart and improving the patient's condition. Therefore, healthcare providers should be knowledgeable about the symptoms and appropriate treatments for this emergency. Another critical type of cardiovascular emergency is congestive heart failure (CHF) exacerbation, often triggered by various factors, including infection, non-compliance with medications, or sudden dietary indiscretions. When the heart does not pump blood well, CHF can result, and this causes fluid to build up in the lungs and leads to symptoms like edema and tiredness. When patients are examined, signs of distress may appear, such as a fast heartbeat, raised blood pressure, and trouble breathing, especially when they are lying down. When a patient with CHF is in critical care, the main approach is to use diuretics to reduce extra fluid and nitrates or inotropes to make the heart work more efficiently. Since CHF is common among older people, it is crucial for healthcare workers in emergency and critical care to understand its various aspects, enabling them to provide prompt and effective treatment. Cardiovascular emergencies can also appear as arrhythmias, which can happen due to ischemic heart disease, changes in electrolytes, or as a medication side effect. Life-threatening arrhythmias, such as ventricular tachycardia (VT) and ventricular fibrillation (VF), require immediate defibrillation and advanced cardiovascular life support (ACLS) protocols to restore normal heart rhythm. A quick response and treatment can stop a heart attack from happening and increase the chances of survival. It is also necessary to know the causes of arrhythmias, as a patient with an MI can develop them without noticing, which can make their condition worse and require prompt attention. The diverse manifestations of cardiovascular emergencies underscore the necessity for comprehensive training and preparedness among healthcare providers in critical care settings to effectively address these complexities (Montgomery *et al.*, 2024; Nadikudhiti *et al.*, 2025).

14.1.1. Myocardial Infarction (MI)

When MI or heart attack develops, it is a serious emergency that must be managed right away in the critical care setting. Atherosclerotic plaques are usually disrupted in MI, which causes blood flow to the heart to be blocked and leads to damage to the heart muscle. It is essential to diagnose and treat this condition as quickly as possible, since myocardial ischemia can turn into permanent myocardial damage in a short time. A quick diagnosis of chest pain, shortness of breath, and pain in the arm is very important for proper medical care. A doctor or nurse will use clinical assessment and tests such as electrocardiograms and biomarkers to confirm the diagnosis and then provide the proper treatment, which could be antiplatelets, thrombolytics, or PCI to restore blood flow and reduce myocardial damage. More women are dying from heart disease during pregnancy, which stresses the need to identify myocardial infarction among pregnant women. In the past three decades, more pregnant women have died from cardiovascular emergencies, which include MI, pointing to the increased risk for this group. Because of the changes in pregnant women, cardiovascular emergencies usually appear differently and require special treatment. It is clear that heart disease, including myocardial infarction, can happen to women, which shows that traditional views about heart disease being mostly a male problem are incorrect and highlights how healthcare systems must respond. The critical care offered in cardiac intensive care units (CICUs) plays a pivotal role in managing these cases, allowing for specialized care and a multidisciplinary approach tailored to the complex physiological changes associated with pregnancy (Kharawala *et al.*, 2025) (Figure 14.2).

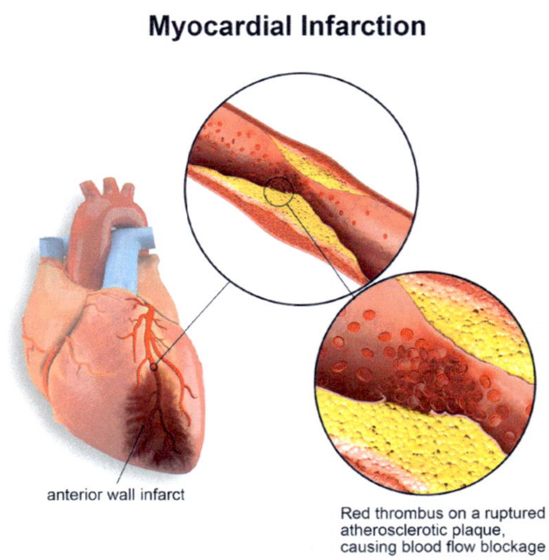

Figure 14.2. Myocardial infarction (MI).

Source: https://upload.medbullets.com/topic/120011/images/e4d2094c_3f91f376.79508c5a.jpg.

High mortality rates linked to myocardial infarction point to the importance of intensive care, since patients in general wards have a much higher risk of dying than those treated in intensive care units.

A review of MI patients in the hospital found that those admitted to general wards were more likely to die, which points to the need to give ICU care to these patients as a matter of urgency. Defibrillation and CPR in an ICU led to much lower death rates than when provided in general wards. The results show that quick action and specialized care are crucial, which is why immediate ICU admission is necessary after an MI diagnosis. Consequently, healthcare institutions must enhance triage protocols to ensure that patients experiencing MI receive the appropriate level of care to optimize treatment outcomes and reduce mortality (Kuwabara *et al.*, 2025).

14.1.2. Cardiac Arrest

A cardiac arrest requires fast medical attention to keep organs from being permanently damaged and to save the patient's life. The heart suddenly stops working properly, which leads to a loss of blood circulation and causes the person to become unconscious in seconds. Arrhythmias, myocardial infarction, and mainly underlying cardiovascular diseases are some of the reasons for cardiac arrest.

Because cardiac arrest is common, healthcare systems are very concerned, especially in CICUs, where being ready and acting fast can make a big difference for patients. As Kharawala *et al.* (2025) highlight, the rise in prevalence of cardiovascular disease complicates its management and warrants ongoing research to develop standardized protocols that can guide the treatment of patients experiencing cardiac emergencies, particularly in vulnerable populations such as pregnant women (Figure 14.3).

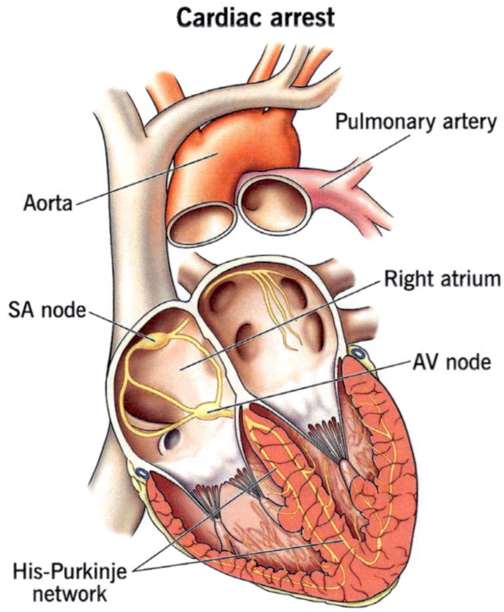

Figure 14.3. Cardiac arrest, your heart stops beating regularly because of a problem with the system that controls your heartbeats.

Source: https://my.clevelandclinic.org/health/diseases/21736-cardiac-arrest.

In the setting of out-of-hospital cardiac arrest (OHCA), prompt initiation of cardiopulmonary resuscitation (CPR) and subsequent advanced cardiac life support (ACLS) are essential. Usually, the first step is for bystanders to notice cardiac arrest and start CPR, which can double or even triple the chances of survival. According to Riba *et al.* (2024), OHCA accounts for nearly 50% of all cardiovascular deaths, illustrating the critical importance of community education on CPR techniques and the use of automated external defibrillators (AEDs). Even with improvements in resuscitation science, it remains challenging to implement these guidelines effectively. Because of this gap, it is clear that better approaches are needed to enhance post-resuscitation care, especially for neurological outcomes, which are often as crucial as restoring blood pressure. The care given after resuscitation in cardiac arrest is not limited to restoring the heart; it also covers ways to improve brain function and prevent further problems. Following the stabilization of the patient, targeted temperature management (TTM) and careful neuroprognostication play pivotal roles. Research has shown that TTM can mitigate neurological injury resulting from hypoxic-ischemic episodes during cardiac arrest (Riba *et al.*, 2024). Even though there are well-established guidelines for using different methods in neuroprognosis, how they are used in healthcare settings is not always the same, which can influence how patients are managed. Furthermore, understanding the intricate relationship between cardiac function and neurological outcomes is paramount, as findings from Kharawala *et al.* (2025) suggest a significant prevalence of cardiac-related pathologies in critically ill populations, underscoring the broader implications of effective management for patients who experience cardiac arrest in various contexts.

14.1.3. Pulmonary Embolism (PE)

PE represents a significant cardiovascular emergency that arises from the obstruction of pulmonary arteries due to blood clots, typically originating from deep vein thrombosis. Acute cases may be without symptoms or may end in sudden death, which is why doctors must act quickly. Common signs in patients are dyspnea, chest pain, and hemoptysis, and these can change in how severe they are. It is very important to notice these symptoms quickly, mainly in people at high risk, to improve patient outcomes. Advanced imaging modalities, particularly computed tomography pulmonary angiography (CTPA), play a critical role in confirming the diagnosis. Furthermore, PE ranks as a leading cause of morbidity and mortality in hospitalized patients, as highlighted by findings that emphasize the necessity of intensive care management for effective treatment and improved survival rates in individuals who experience this life-threatening event (Kuwabara *et al.*, 2025). Treatment for pulmonary embolism often involves anticoagulants, and the usual first-line options are unfractionated heparin and direct oral anticoagulants to stop more clots from forming. If the obstruction is not cleared by usual methods, advanced steps such as catheter-directed thrombolysis or surgical embolectomy may be necessary to remove the blockage and let blood flow through the lungs. Recent advancements in extracorporeal membrane oxygenation (ECMO) reflect the ongoing evolution of treatment methodologies, providing critical support for patients in cardiac arrest secondary to PE (Xie *et al.*, 2024).

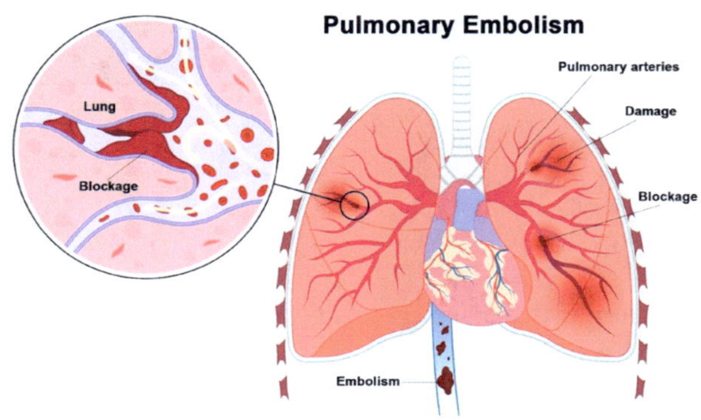

Figure 14.4. Pulmonary embolism (PE).

Source: https://cdn.myhealthteams.com/graphic/652fe70a02ac643b7a2c8274/woriginal/AdobeStock_558730161_copy-7783d25d7de04446ea5685b73e7d1755.webp?1697638153.

Because ECMO can maintain blood flow and oxygen levels, it makes it possible for doctors to perform other important procedures, which is why it matters a lot in treating this life-threatening condition. The role of intensive care units (ICUs) is particularly pertinent in the management of patients with severe pulmonary embolism. Research indicates that mortality rates are markedly lower among patients admitted to ICUs compared to those treated in general wards, highlighting the need for specialized care in acute situations (Kuwabara *et al.*, 2025). Applying early detection guidelines and strong management plans across healthcare facilities such as risk assessment, can help improve the outcomes of people who are at risk for PE. It is very important to keep a close eye on the patient and act quickly, because the situation can get worse very fast if not supervised. Overall, enhancing education and training for healthcare providers on the recognition and management of pulmonary embolism can significantly impact patient survival and recovery in critical care environments (Figure 14.4).

Test Your Knowledge

1. What are the common signs and symptoms of a myocardial infarction, and how is it diagnosed?
2. What are the immediate steps in the management of a patient experiencing cardiac arrest?

14.2. Risk Factors and Prevalence

Learning Outcome

1. Identify the common risk factors (e.g., hypertension, diabetes)
2. Discuss the demographic trends in cardiovascular emergencies
3. Understand the impact of lifestyle choices on prevalence

Having knowledge of the factors that increase the risk of cardiovascular emergencies is necessary to make good prevention and intervention plans in critical care. Age, being obese, hypertension, and diabetes increase the risk of cardiovascular conditions that may become emergencies. Cardiovascular complications are more common in the elderly because of their age and the presence of other health problems. In addition, things like smoking and not being active enough increase these risks, so healthcare providers should take a multi-layered approach to management and education. Because of this wide-ranging knowledge, clinicians are better able to handle cardiovascular emergencies, directing their efforts and resources to the most at-risk people, which reduces the strain on emergency departments. Because cardiovascular emergencies are common in critical care, it is clear that better monitoring and preventive actions are needed. Recent studies have documented alarming rates of preventable medication harm across medical settings, indicating that nearly 3% of patients experience such incidents, with higher rates observed in specific care environments like emergency medicine and intensive care (Hodkinson *et al.*, 2020). It shows that healthcare providers have to deal with both the rising cases of cardiovascular emergencies and the issues that come with managing medications, which can result in adverse outcomes. Because of how often these mistakes occur, it is important to review medication plans and care procedures, mainly for those with heart problems, as even small errors can be dangerous. In addition, delirium and cognitive changes, which are more common in older people, play a major role in increasing the risk of cardiovascular events. Delirium, often exacerbated by factors like dehydration and infection, can lead to an escalation in cognitive impairment and complicate existing cardiovascular ailments (Livingston *et al.*, 2020). It is important to control any existing health problems and use special strategies to stop delirium in order to prevent cardiovascular emergencies in this group. If these risk factors are acknowledged and managed, critical care services can improve patient safety and outcomes, which may result in fewer hospitalizations because of cardiovascular emergencies. Taking mental health and cognitive function into account when assessing patients will play a major role in managing the growing number of cardiovascular emergencies in critical care.

14.2.1. Common Risk Factors (e.g., Hypertension, Diabetes)

When patients in critical care have identifiable risk factors, cardiovascular emergencies can be very difficult to manage. Hypertension is common in these conditions, affecting many people from different groups. When blood pressure is too high, the heart has to work harder and this can cause heart failure, myocardial infarction or stroke. The interplay between hypertension and other comorbidities exacerbates these risks, as individuals with multiple health issues often experience a more severe clinical trajectory (Figure 14.5).

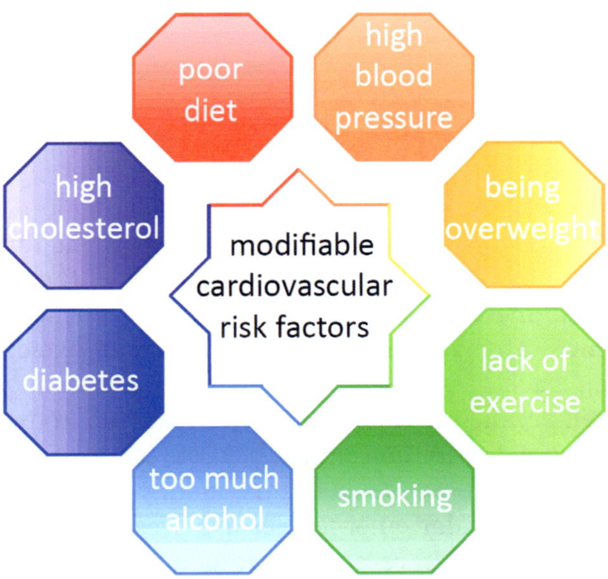
poor diet
high blood pressure
high cholesterol
modifiable cardiovascular risk factors
being overweight
diabetes
lack of exercise
too much alcohol
smoking

Figure 14.5. Some cardiovascular risk factors.

Source: https://www.drholdright.co.uk/coronary-heart-disease-and-angina/.

When chronic hypertension is acutely severe, critical care teams must act quickly, so it is important for cardiovascular emergency specialists to know how to handle this risk factor. If someone has diabetes mellitus, they are at greater risk of experiencing cardiovascular emergencies. Having diabetes makes it more likely for someone to develop coronary artery disease, hypertension, and other heart problems. Insulin resistance and dyslipidemia, which are part of the disease, put patients at a greater risk of acute coronary syndromes and other sudden heart problems.

As shown in recent research on hospitalized COVID-19 patients, diabetes was a common finding, so careful monitoring of blood sugar and its effects on the heart is needed during acute care. Taking care of diabetes in critical care settings can help prevent serious problems and improve patient outcomes. Also, when diabetes and hypertension occur together, it can increase the chance of heart problems. Those with both conditions are commonly at a greater risk for systemic problems that call for urgent and intense treatment in the hospital.

Many studies find that hypertension and diabetes greatly impact the outcomes of patients with cardiovascular emergencies who are hospitalized. For example, a significant number of hospitalized COVID-19 patients exhibited hypertension alongside diabetes, indicating that these common risk factors often co-occur and complicate critical care management (Richardson *et al.*, 2020). As healthcare systems continue to encounter these challenges, it is imperative to prioritize the identification and treatment of these factors, thereby enhancing the efficacy of interventions and improving prognosis for critically ill patients (Livingston *et al.*, 2020) (Figure 14.6).

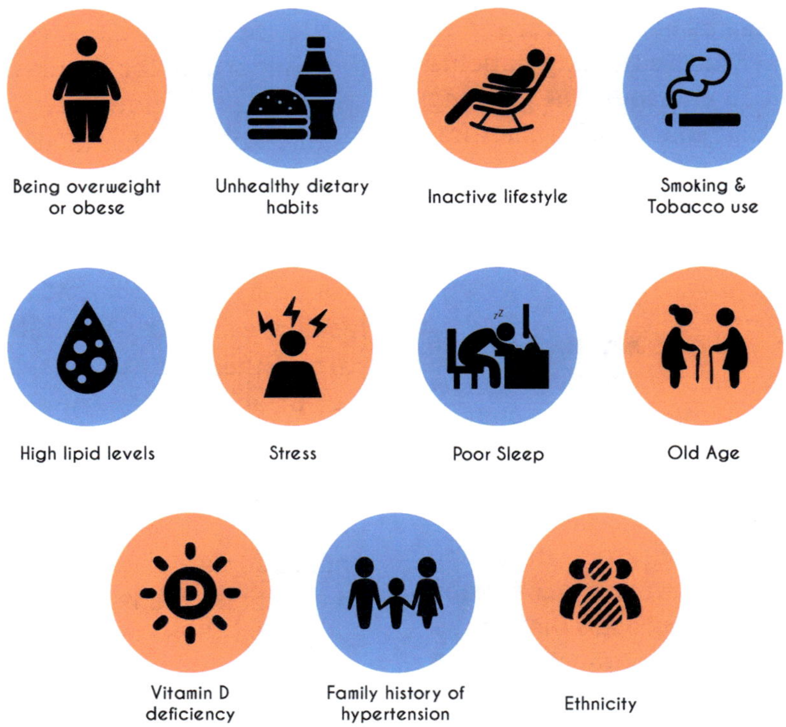
Being overweight or obese
Unhealthy dietary habits
Inactive lifestyle
Smoking & Tobacco use
High lipid levels
Stress
Poor Sleep
Old Age
Vitamin D deficiency
Family history of hypertension
Ethnicity

Figure 14.6. Common risk factors of hypertension and diabetes.

Source: https://d1zxene68j3keg.cloudfront.net/sites/default/files/styles/large/public/Diabetes%20Risk%20Factor%20Revision%20Final.png?itok=BVLW2NV2.

14.2.2. Demographic Trends in Cardiovascular Emergencies

Being aware of changes in the demographics of cardiovascular emergencies is important for developing strategies in critical care. There have been more cases of cardiovascular emergencies among older people, which is related to the worldwide increase in age. Older patients are more likely to have hypertension, diabetes, and obesity, which can make their heart-related emergencies worse. Also, the rise in cities and new ways of living, such as sitting for long periods and eating unhealthy foods, are adding to the problem of these emergencies. This agrees with research in the field, which suggests that special interventions and resource distribution should be used, taking these demographic realities into account, to help patients with cardiovascular events, mainly in critical care settings where quick action is necessary. How cardiovascular emergencies are presented and the outcomes they have can be influenced by gender. It is found in research that men tend to have heart-related issues at a younger age, but women usually have more severe consequences after such an event. Gender and cardiovascular health are linked in many ways, and these links depend on biological, social, and behavioral factors, so the subject needs to be understood in various ways. Men are more likely to have heart attacks because they smoke more and experience more stress, and women might delay getting treatment because they believe heart disease is mainly a problem for men. Paying attention to these demographic details allows healthcare providers to design targeted ways to educate and intervene early, which can lower the risks of death and serious illness from cardiovascular emergencies. Besides age and gender, the social and economic background of people has a major impact on cardiovascular emergencies. Many people from lower socioeconomic groups have difficulties getting healthcare, which can make cardiovascular emergencies more severe. Because not all people can get preventative healthcare and lifestyle help, it is clear that public health programs should focus on those who are most at risk. Moreover, comorbidities such as rheumatoid arthritis and Sjögren's disease, which exhibit unique demographic trends, can complicate cardiovascular presentations and critical care admissions in certain patient cohorts, as illustrated in recent studies highlighting increased ICU admissions associated with these conditions (Domańska-Poboża *et al.*, 2025a; Domańska-Poboża *et al.*, 2025b). Recognizing these demographic trends is crucial for devising effective healthcare policies and targeted interventions that ensure equitable access to care and improved outcomes for all demographic groups facing cardiovascular emergencies (Figure 14.7).

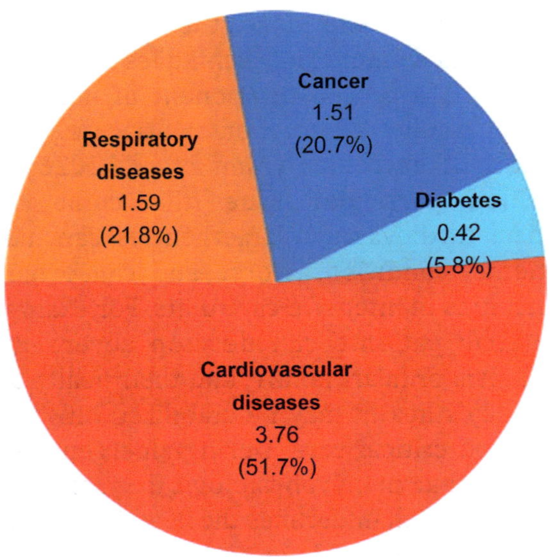

Figure 14.7. The worldwide environment of cardiovascular disease.

Source: https://ars.els-cdn.com/content/image/1-s2.0-S0735109712053715-gr2.jpg.

14.2.3. Impact of Lifestyle Choices on Prevalence

The number of cardiovascular emergencies is highly affected by the way people live, especially among those who are more likely to develop obesity or heart failure. Being overweight can make existing heart problems worse and also change the heart's structure, which makes people more likely to be hospitalized for heart failure. Weight loss efforts, whether from changing one's lifestyle, taking medicine, or having surgery, have a strong chance of improving some heart-related issues. As outlined in recent research, these changes can improve overall cardiac function and may indeed reduce hospital admissions stemming from heart-related complications, underscoring the critical need to address lifestyle factors in managing cardiovascular emergencies effectively (Alansari *et al.*, 2025). Besides helping with weight, living healthily involves changes in diet, exercise, and substance use. A diet rich in processed foods and high in sugars contributes significantly to the rising incidence of cardiovascular diseases, including atrial fibrillation (AF). Lifestyle choices are very important in AF, as research has found that being overweight and not being active are major risk factors for it. If people eat healthier and exercise more, they may reduce their chance of AF, which can help lessen the number of cardiovascular emergencies in critical care. Research confirms that lifestyle changes not only help manage existing conditions but also play a pivotal role in preventing the onset of new cardiovascular issues, highlighting the importance of a holistic approach to cardiovascular health (Fahimi, 2024). Because of the rising number of cardiovascular emergencies, it is important to reconsider how clinical settings address lifestyle-related risks. More and more, medical professionals see that treating cardiovascular diseases requires both medications and lifestyle advice. Taking action in this way can reduce the number of cardiovascular emergencies by focusing on unhealthy eating, lack of exercise, and smoking. Helping patients understand how their choices affect their health can encourage them to look after themselves, which can lessen the need for healthcare for preventable heart conditions. Taking lifestyle factors into account at the beginning of cardiovascular care is important for better patient outcomes and fewer emergencies in critical care.

Test Your Knowledge

1. How do common risk factors like hypertension and diabetes contribute to cardiovascular emergencies?
2. What demographic trends are observed in the incidence of cardiovascular emergencies such as heart attacks and strokes?

14.3. Pathophysiology of Cardiovascular Emergencies

Learning Outcome

1. Define mechanisms of myocardial ischemia
2. Identify the role of the autonomic nervous system
3. Discuss consequences of prolonged hypoxia

Many physiological changes happen in cardiovascular emergencies, which interfere with the heart's normal activities and blood circulation. Such emergencies are usually caused by problems like ischemic heart disease or heart failure, which can result in acute myocardial infarction or make it hard for the heart to pump blood. If the heart's function is reduced, several things happen in the body, such as widening of blood vessels, increased resistance in the blood vessels, and activation of the sympathetic nervous system, all of which can lead to arrhythmias, cardiogenic shock, or sudden cardiac arrest. It is essential to understand these mechanisms in critical care, since quick action can make a big difference for patients going through these dangerous episodes. Hemodynamic monitoring is crucial for dealing with cardiovascular emergencies because it helps medical staff monitor and address the changing condition of the patient's blood flow. Traditional indicators, like mean arterial pressure, provide essential information; however, advanced methods such as reservoir-excess pressure analysis (REPA) offer nuanced insights that are critical in critical care settings. Examining reservoir pressure and diastolic rate constant, practitioners can find out about peripheral vasotonus and the overall condition of the heart. With improved monitoring, medical teams can notice small changes in a patient's blood pressure and heart function, which helps them give more targeted care. Therefore, the integration of sophisticated monitoring techniques into clinical practice is a crucial component of managing cardiovascular emergencies intricately tied to patient outcomes (Alan *et al.*, 2025). In addition, particular issues that come with critical cardiovascular emergencies can make patients' conditions worse and cause many difficulties in intensive care units. For example, obstetric patients can develop severe pre-eclampsia or heart failure, and their health and the baby's health may be stabilized only with advanced critical care. During emergencies, it is clear that many physiological systems are involved, which underlines the need for different medical professionals to be involved. Knowing the reasons behind these emergencies helps healthcare providers work better together and give fast and appropriate care. As the frequency and complexity of cardiovascular emergencies increase, ongoing education and research remain paramount to equip healthcare professionals with the knowledge necessary for effective treatment strategies (Nadikudhiti *et al.*, 2025).

14.3.1. Mechanisms of Myocardial Ischemia (MI)

There are many different and complicated factors involved in MI, which can occur in many different clinical and disease situations. A major reason for ischemia is when there is not enough oxygen for the heart muscle. A disease like coronary artery disease causes the arteries to narrow, and this blockage of blood flow prevents oxygen from reaching the heart muscle. The presence of atherosclerotic plaques can make things worse by narrowing the vessel and sometimes bursting, which can lead to clot formation and a complete blockage. During times of hard work or high emotion, the heart needs more oxygen, which may intensify ischemic events and lead to significant problems and possible heart damage.

Besides changes in the structure of the coronary arteries, myocardial ischemia is marked by trouble with the endothelium and changes in the microcirculation. When endothelial cells are not working properly, they cannot control blood vessel tension and proper blood flow, which worsens ischemic conditions. Inflammation is important, since inflammatory cytokines can cause the blood vessels to change, which leads to more atherosclerosis and a greater chance of myocardial infarction. It has been noted that the COVID-19 pandemic has made it clear that viral infections and cardiovascular conditions are connected, as studies suggest that SARS-CoV-2 may cause myocardial injury through disrupting the endothelium and causing hypercoagulability. This highlights the importance of understanding ischemic mechanisms in the context of emergent clinical scenarios, especially amid global health challenges (Guzik *et al.*, 2020). To manage myocardial ischemia well, it is important to understand how it happens, mainly in the acute phase.

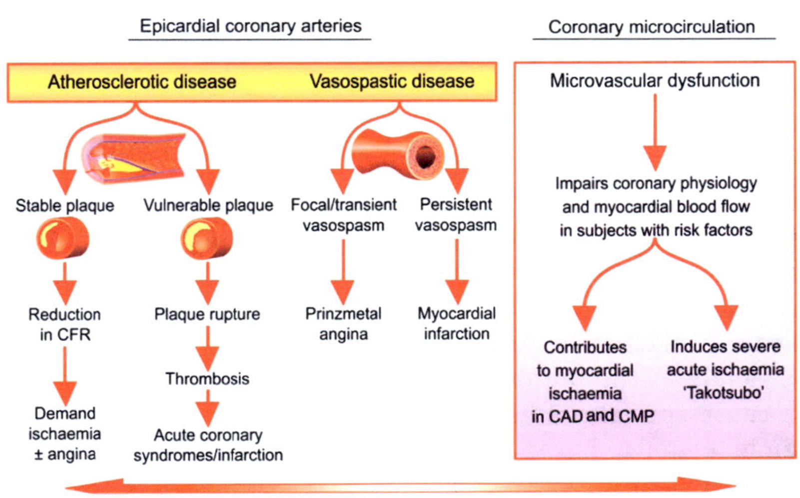

Figure 14.8. Mechanisms of myocardial ischemia (MI).

Source: https://www.researchgate.net/figure/Mechanisms-of-myocardial-ischemia-modified-from-9-with-a-permission-license_fig1_375081344.

The urgent symptoms of myocardial infarction usually mean doctors must decide quickly on antithrombotic drugs and revascularization methods to improve blood flow to the affected part of the heart. Recent recommendations stress that early treatment should be given after ischemic symptoms such as chest pain and increased signs of heart injury are identified. Choosing the right management approach is very important since waiting to treat can result in permanent damage to the heart and a rise in both the morbidity and mortality rates. Therefore, an integrated approach that includes assessment of risk factors, timely diagnosis, and swift therapeutic action is essential for improving outcomes in patients experiencing myocardial ischemia (Anderson *et al.*, 2017) (Figure 14.8).

14.3.2. Role of the Autonomic Nervous System (ANS)

In critical care, the ANS plays a crucial role in managing cardiovascular functions during emergencies. The ANS consists of the sympathetic and parasympathetic branches, which cooperate to keep the body's functions stable when facing stress. When an emergency happens, the sympathetic nervous system is turned on, which makes the heart beat faster, raises blood pressure, and increases the blood pumped by the heart to cope with the situation. It is crucial for shock management, since fast changes in the heart's function are needed to keep organs supplied with blood and oxygen. It is very important for healthcare professionals in critical care to understand these mechanisms because improper control of the ANS can worsen heart problems in patients experiencing emergencies. The autonomic nervous system can cause special problems in critical illnesses, mainly related to how patients respond to infusion therapy. In situations where keeping blood pressure and circulation stable is very important, fluid management is very important. The use of non-invasive methods to measure vital signs allows for monitoring of the autonomic response to fluids, and this helps determine the patient's cardiovascular state and directs additional care. Changes in the stress index may show if therapeutic treatments are working and reveal what is happening in the body's neurohumoral system. It is important to know how age affects the ANS response to infusion treatments in children since this can impact recovery and how doctors manage their care. Recognition of these responses can lead to more effective management strategies in critical care settings, ultimately improving patient outcomes (Budarova *et al.*, 2022) (Figure 14.9).

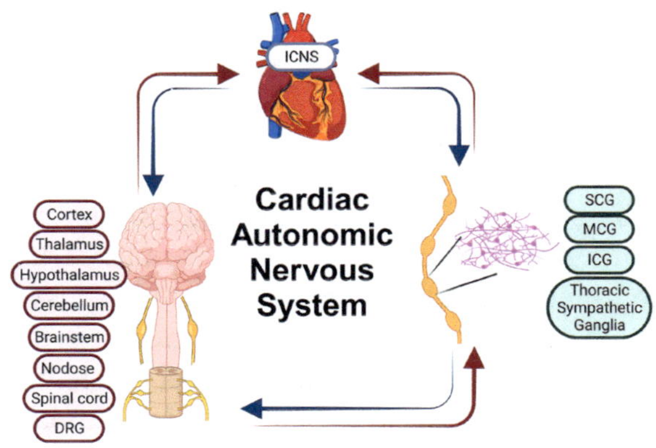

Figure 14.9. Cardiac autonomic nervous system (ANS).

Source: https://www.frontiersin.org/files/Articles/1377171/fnins-18-1377171-HTML-r1/image_m/fnins-18-1377171-g001.jpg.

Also, stress and pain are external factors that can greatly change how the autonomic nervous system affects the heart. When we are stressed in serious situations, catecholamines are released, which activate the sympathetic nervous system and may have either good or bad effects. Managing stress is very important for people with diabetes mellitus, since too much stress hormone can make their blood sugar levels rise and increase their risk of heart problems. Also, yoga and similar practices have been studied for their role in restoring autonomic balance, which might help in critical care settings. By enhancing parasympathetic activity and reducing sympathetic overdrive, such practices may provide adjunctive benefits for patients experiencing cardiovascular emergencies (Sharma *et al.*, 2025). Paying attention to the link between the ANS and cardiovascular health can improve our understanding of managing critical care patients.

14.3.3. Consequences of Prolonged Hypoxia

Long-lasting hypoxia leads to major difficulties for the heart and blood vessels, altering both their form and function. When there is not enough oxygen in the body, the heart rate can increase, and the heart pumps more blood to ensure the body gets enough oxygen. But if hypoxia continues, these changes are not enough and cause adverse outcomes. Long-term hypoxia causes changes in the heart, such as thickening and scarring, which can lower the heart's ability to work properly and increase the risk of heart failure. Also, if hypoxia continues, it can decrease the ability of peripheral tissues to take in and use oxygen, which adds more stress to the heart. It is clear from these cases that vulnerable groups, such as pregnant women and those with heart problems, are more severely affected by long-term hypoxia, so it is critical to have effective treatments in critical care settings. Besides affecting the heart's structure, hypoxia for a long time can also bring about major changes in the electrical activity of the heart. Hypoxia may result in arrhythmias, and these are commonly affected by how much the atria and ventricles stretch and by increased activity of the sympathetic nervous system. It is at these times, when the body needs more oxygen, that arrhythmias can be very dangerous. Long-lasting hypoxia can lead to various heart rhythm problems, which might result in fainting or sudden death. The management of these arrhythmic conditions requires a comprehensive approach that considers the intricate interactions of prolonged hypoxia and underlying cardiovascular pathologies, particularly in critical care environments where rapid interventions may be necessary to stabilize patients (Conti *et al.*, 2024). Studies on the effects of long-term hypoxia on vertebrates have shown that it is very harmful to both adults and those that lay eggs, which has broader implications for cardiovascular emergencies in critical care. It has been found that chronic hypoxia can seriously affect the development of the heart, mainly when the heart is growing rapidly. It becomes essential to examine species-specific responses and the thresholds at which hypoxia manifests physiological consequences (Lock *et al.*, 2024). Spotting these thresholds can help doctors give better predictions and develop new treatments for patients suffering from cardiovascular emergencies due to prolonged hypoxia. Filling these knowledge gaps is important for learning more about hypoxia's many effects on the heart and finding ways to manage them in people at risk.

Test Your Knowledge

1. What are the underlying mechanisms that lead to myocardial ischemia?
2. How does the autonomic nervous system influence cardiovascular function during acute cardiac events?

14.4. Diagnostic Approaches

Learning Outcome

1. Discuss the clinical assessment and history taking
2. Explain the use of imaging techniques (e.g., ECG, echocardiography)
3. Define laboratory tests and biomarkers

In critical care situations involving heart emergencies, accurate diagnosis is very important for quick and effective action. Healthcare professionals rely on clinical reasoning to handle the difficulties of acute heart problems. Advanced imaging methods, including echocardiography and coronary angiography, are vital for fast patient assessments. They supply doctors with important information about the heart's structure and function, which helps identify serious heart problems. Moreover, incorporating tools like electrocardiograms (ECGs) allows for immediate evaluation of arrhythmias or ischemic changes, enabling prompt stabilization of the patient's condition. Using various diagnostic tools together improves medical decision-making and directly affects how patients fare, which is why medical practitioners should receive thorough training in these areas. Improvements in teaching methods are as important as improvements in diagnostics for critical care. In one example, a study with nursing students showed that using a gamified scenario writing method greatly enhanced their ability to deal with urgent cases related to heart care. The findings show that engaging and interactive learning activities help healthcare professionals get ready for situations they will face in real life. Since nurses are key in assessing patients and deciding on care during heart emergencies, improving their clinical reasoning with targeted education is very important. When we make these programs important in nursing education, we prepare future nurses to face cardiovascular emergencies, which helps ensure patients are safe. Additionally, understanding congenital heart diseases (CHDs) in neonates underscores the importance of timely diagnosis and management. Neonatologists and pediatricians working together are necessary to overcome the diagnostic difficulties faced by these patients. Using advanced imaging, such as fetal echocardiography, allows doctors to find cardiac issues early in the pregnancy. This action helps medical teams be ready for postnatal problems and take quick action. Improving communication and teamwork among healthcare staff supports better diagnosis and leads to better outcomes for newborns with severe heart problems. As emerging research continues to refine these diagnostic strategies, a holistic approach to caring for vulnerable populations will remain essential in the realm of cardiovascular emergencies in critical care (Antikchi *et al.*, 2025; Moisa *et al.*, 2024) (Figure 14.10).

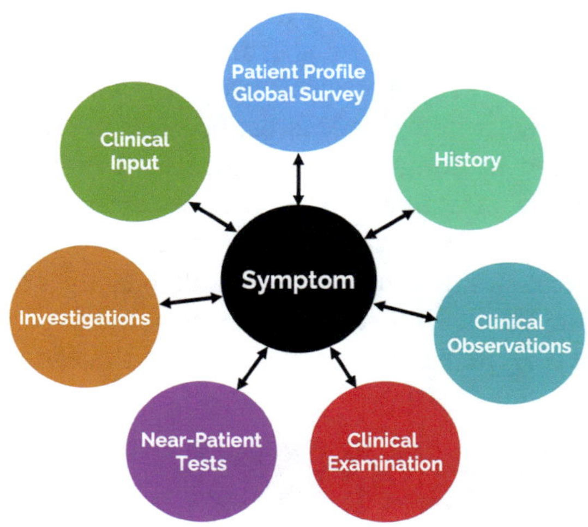

Figure 14.10. Clinical assessment wagon wheel.

Source: https://geekymedics.com/wp-content/uploads/2023/03/Clinical-assessment-wagon-wheel.png.

14.4.1. Clinical Assessment and History Taking

When it comes to cardiovascular emergencies, understanding the patient's condition and history is very important for treatment and diagnosis. When history taking is accurate and organized, healthcare providers can discover a patient's symptoms, past health issues, and risk factors, which are important for making the right decisions. A thorough cardiac history helps identify the causes of chest pain, difficulty breathing, and palpitations, which allows for quick treatment. Also, learning about the patient's age, medical history, and family's cardiovascular history improves the way risks are assessed and decisions are made in emergency rooms.

By using this approach, both the symptoms and a reference point for comparison are found, which supports continuous updates to the management plan as the condition develops. A physical examination is also done during the clinical assessment to look for symptoms of acute cardiac problems in patients with cardiovascular emergencies. Vital signs should be checked, the heart should be listened to, and any signs of peripheral edema should be noted since they may indicate heart failure or too much fluid in the body. Clinicians should also check the patient's mental state and blood flow, since these can significantly affect how urgent the interventions need to be. The potential for life-threatening conditions such as non-ST elevation myocardial infarctions (NSTEMI) or acute heart failure necessitates a thorough examination. By correlating clinical findings from both history and physical examination, healthcare professionals can prioritize immediate diagnostic tests, including electrocardiograms and biomarker assessments, thereby enhancing the efficacy of the treatment provided in critical care situations (Byrne, 2021) (Figure 14.11).

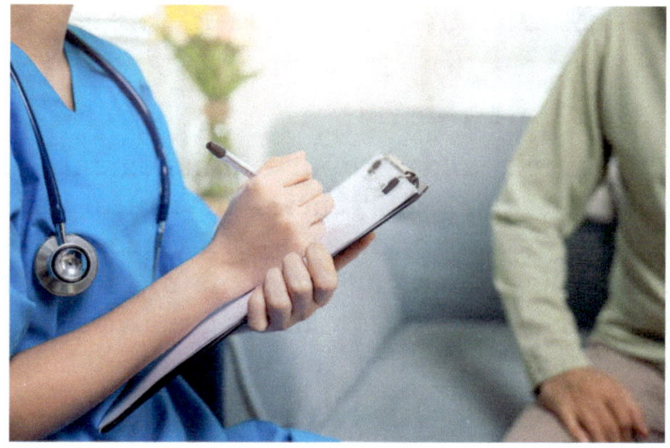

Figure 14.11. Patient history taking.

Source: https://external-content.duckduckgo.com/iu/?u=https%3A%2F%2Fsimplenursing.com%2Fwp-content%2Fuploads%2F2023%2F08%2FiStock-1434595001-scaled.jpg&f=1&nofb=1&ipt=d7c15d1913a7c72cab4b89ea5eba3960f4918738efc8f076445576341b62b1b4.

The integration of clinical assessment findings with established risk models for acute myocardial infarction (AMI) can further refine the evaluation of patients in critical care. It is now widely accepted that clinical risk scores which use several clinical factors, should be used to help predict in-hospital mortality and decide on treatment. For example, a recent study highlighted specific differences between patients who experienced mortality versus those who did not, focusing on factors such as creatinine levels and blood pressure variations, which are crucial in managing AMI (Mohamed *et al.*, 2021). Because of this approach, healthcare teams can handle high-risk patients better and design management strategies that fit each person. Good cardiovascular care in emergencies relies on thorough clinical assessment and a complete medical history, which helps patients with acute heart problems achieve better results and live longer.

14.4.2. Use of Imaging Techniques (Electrocardiograms (ECGs), Echocardiography)

The quick and proper management of cardiovascular emergencies in critical care depends greatly on imaging techniques. ECGs and echocardiography are some of the most often used methods for checking the electrical and structural health of the heart. An ECG helps clinicians detect arrhythmias, signs of ischemia, and signs of myocardial infarction. Such insights are necessary for quick decisions, since early actions can greatly affect how a patient does. Also, because ECGs can be taken anywhere, they are perfect for emergencies that require quick evaluation. ECG is used first to diagnose and also to keep an eye on patients with serious heart problems, making it necessary for acute cardiac care. Echocardiography is a type of imaging that allows doctors to watch the heart in real time. It is important to understand heart failure, abnormalities of heart valves, and congenital heart defects. Because echocardiography is non-invasive and can be used in many ways, including transthoracic and transesophageal methods, it is very useful in emergency situations. When there are suspicions of pericardial effusion or cardiac tamponade, echocardiography can show if there is fluid around the heart and how much, which helps plan further steps. Also, the use of Doppler imaging in echocardiography makes it easier to check hemodynamics and cardiac output, which is very helpful when treating serious heart conditions. Using advanced imaging methods supports the combined effort needed to handle complex cardiovascular emergencies. For example, in instances of CHDs, the timely utilization of fetal echocardiography during pregnancy has shown significant promise for early diagnosis and intervention, enabling healthcare teams to prepare effectively for neonatal care upon delivery (Moisa *et al.*, 2024). Similarly, coronary cameral fistulas and related anomalies benefit from multimodal imaging, as seen in cases where echocardiography and computed tomography angiography work synergistically to confirm diagnoses (Mortezaeian *et al.*, 2024). Using imaging in this way allows doctors to diagnose accurately and plan the best treatment, which helps patients recover from critical heart events. This collaborative framework underscores the necessity of ongoing research and clinical innovation to enhance imaging methods, ultimately improving the management of cardiovascular emergencies in critical care settings (Figure 14.12).

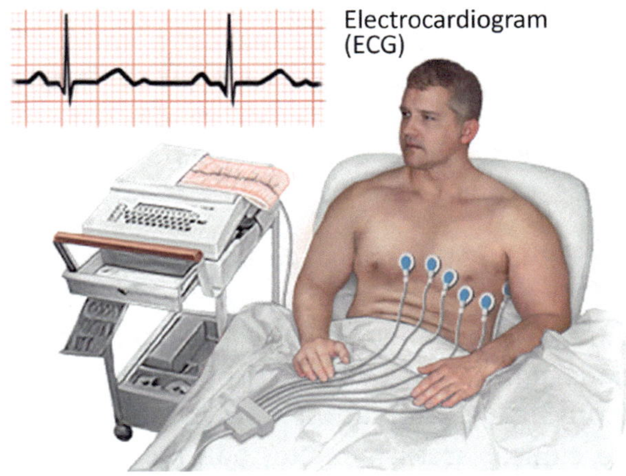

Figure 14.12. An EKG shows the frequency and duration of your heartbeat.

Source: https://ssl.adam.com/graphics/images/en/1135.jpg.

14.4.3. Laboratory Tests and Biomarkers

When a cardiovascular emergency happens in critical care, laboratory tests and biomarkers help quickly identify the problem and direct treatment. They help doctors understand the condition of a patient's heart, find out if there is any damage, and detect heart failure or blood clots. Among the commonly utilized biomarkers are troponins, B-type natriuretic peptide (BNP), and d-dimer, each providing specific insights into underlying pathologies. Elevated troponin levels usually point to myocardial necrosis, which is why they are very useful for diagnosing acute coronary syndromes. Therefore, by combining results from the laboratory with clinical observations, healthcare professionals can assess risk and start proper treatment quickly, which improves patient outcomes. In addition, laboratory tests are helpful in following the course of the disease and how well the treatment is working. Some studies have found that C-reactive protein and lactate dehydrogenase can show signs of inflammation and tissue damage that often happen with serious cardiovascular events. Higher levels of these biomarkers are linked to worse outcomes in people having cardiovascular emergencies. Clinicians can use laboratory data to help decide on intensive care or specialized therapy, which supports better patient management. So, knowing how well biomarkers can predict outcomes helps doctors manage challenging cases with more accuracy. Finally, laboratory tests are important, but they work best when combined with clinical exams and imaging studies. Therefore, a complete assessment approach is needed since no single biomarker can tell us what the underlying disorder is. Laboratory tests, when used together with clinical findings, help to make a correct diagnosis. For instance, in the presence of suspected cardiovascular compromise, timely microbiological sampling in critical care settings can identify underlying infections that may complicate the clinical picture, particularly in the presence of sepsis (Pervaiz *et al.*, 2024). Therefore, the collaboration between laboratory diagnostics and clinical acumen is essential for optimizing care in cardiovascular emergencies, leading to informed, timely interventions that can significantly alter patient trajectories and outcomes (Rop *et al.*, 2024) (Figure 14.13).

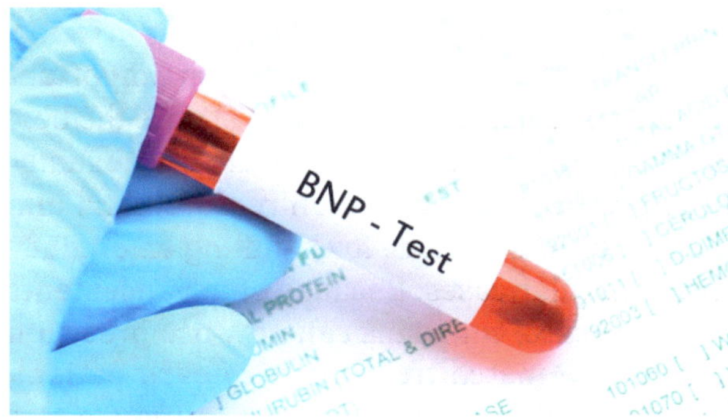

Figure 14.13. Laboratory tests and biomarkers.

Source: https://stgaccinwbsdevlrs01.blob.core.windows.net/newcorporatewbsite/blogs/october2023/detail-main-B-Type-Natriuretic-Peptide-BNP-Test-1.jpeg.

Test Your Knowledge

1. What key information should be gathered during clinical assessment and history taking in suspected cardiac cases?
2. How are imaging techniques like ECG and echocardiography used to diagnose cardiovascular conditions?

14.5. Treatment Protocols

Learning Outcome

1. Define immediate interventions (e.g., Cardiopulmonary Resuscitation (CPR), defibrillation)
2. Discuss the pharmacological management (e.g., anticoagulants, thrombolytics)
3. Focus on surgical options (e.g., angioplasty, bypass surgery)

Developing treatment protocols is very important in cardiovascular emergencies to ensure the best outcomes for patients in critical care. Usually, these protocols are based on research and aim to give a clear structure for handling emergency cardiovascular cases. Because of advancements in critical care, clinicians can now use precision medicine to match treatments to each patient, which makes therapies more effective. As an example, using biomarkers and genomics can help doctors choose treatments that are better suited to each patient. As cardiovascular emergencies are often time-sensitive, such improvements underline the significance of rapidly implementing established protocols that incorporate innovative approaches to patient care (Padte *et al.*, 2024). Moreover, the role of point-of-care ultrasound (POCUS) in treatment protocols for cardiovascular emergencies has emerged as a critical component in modern practice. Clinicians can use POCUS to quickly assess patients, which helps them make decisions faster in emergencies like shock, chest pain, and shortness of breath. The incorporation of multiorgan POCUS (MOPOCUS) into treatment protocols can significantly enhance clinical evaluation processes, providing insights that guide therapeutic interventions. Using these imaging techniques in a planned way helps doctors quickly find conditions that need urgent care, which may lead to better outcomes for patients in critical care. As healthcare continuously evolves, the adaptation of treatment protocols to include advanced diagnostic tools like POCUS is essential in addressing the complexities associated with cardiovascular emergencies (Cheng *et al.*, 2023). The integration of artificial intelligence (AI) into treatment protocols marks another frontier in the management of cardiovascular emergencies. AI helps predict outcomes and detect diseases early, giving doctors the ability to use data quickly for their decisions. In situations where seconds matter, such as in critical care, AI can help by constantly monitoring vital signs and warning of possible complications. AI-based applications in healthcare reduce the time needed for data processing and assessment, which helps improve treatment plans and fits with the trend toward personalized care. AI can play a role in shaping treatment options, which helps raise the standard of care in critical situations. As such, the continuous refinement of treatment protocols to incorporate technological advancements reinforces their relevance and efficacy in addressing the challenges posed by cardiovascular emergencies in critical care (Padte *et al.*, 2024).

14.5.1. Immediate Interventions (e.g., Cardiopulmonary Resuscitation (CPR), Defibrillation)

When someone is having a cardiovascular emergency, CPR and defibrillation must be used quickly to prevent serious harm and death. A lack of heartbeat and breathing in cardiac arrest means blood doesn't reach vital organs, which leads to quick unconsciousness and death unless treated. Giving CPR right away allows healthcare providers to support some blood flow and oxygen supply until more advanced care is provided. The effectiveness of these life-saving measures is significantly influenced by the timeliness of their initiation, which can directly alter outcomes for patients experiencing events such as acute myocardial infarction or arrhythmias (Giuvara *et al.*, 2025) (Figure 14.14).

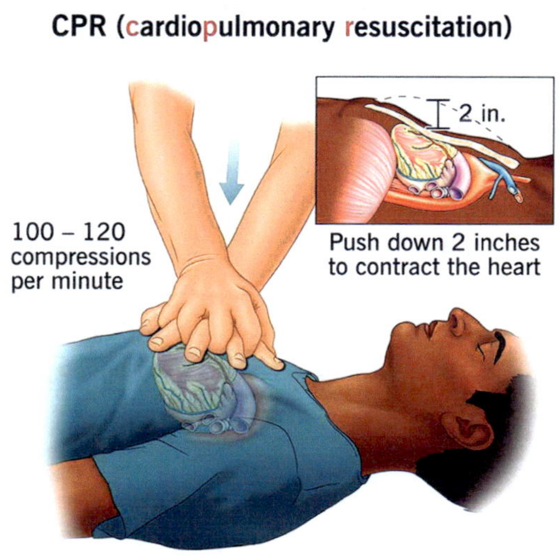

Figure 14.14. Cardiopulmonary resuscitation (CPR) keeps blood moving after cardiac arrest.

Source: https://my.clevelandclinic.org/health/treatments/17680-cardiopulmonary-resuscitation-cpr.

Defibrillation emerges as another essential component of immediate intervention. In situations of ventricular fibrillation or pulseless ventricular tachycardia, fast electric shocks are needed to restore the heart's normal rhythm. Studies highlight the varying rates of defibrillation across different patient care settings, revealing stark disparities in mortality outcomes (Kuwabara *et al.*, 2025). People in intensive care units tend to have much lower death rates than those in general wards, which highlights the need for quick defibrillation in critical situations. The success of defibrillation is greatly influenced by having skilled people and the necessary equipment nearby when someone is having a cardiac emergency. Building a strong infrastructure for fast emergency care is important for lowering deaths from heart problems. Using a variety of medical specialties improves the outcomes of immediate care after a heart event. A successful resuscitation usually depends on using advanced cardiac life support and having teams of emergency responders and critical care professionals work together. For example, after resuscitation from cardiac arrest, ongoing care in the intensive care unit, which may include pharmacological treatment, ventilatory support, and rehabilitation services, plays a vital role in patient recovery (Giuvara *et al.*, 2025). Analysis of patient data suggests that timely and coordinated interventions lead to improved outcomes, with increased rates of survival and functional recovery following hospitalization (Kuwabara *et al.*, 2025). So, having clear steps for responding quickly that involve different specialists can greatly help people with cardiovascular emergencies.

14.5.2. Pharmacological Management (e.g., Anticoagulants, Thrombolytics)

In cardiovascular emergencies, fast and proper medication for pulmonary embolism is important for better patient outcomes. In the first stage of treating thromboembolic events, anticoagulants such as heparin and warfarin are very important. When heparin is given in its low molecular weight form, it quickly stops blood clotting, which is very important in emergencies. Giving heparin can help stop additional clots from forming and lower the immediate threat of pulmonary embolism. Even so, anticoagulants are important for handling these emergencies, but their results can be improved by using updated protocols that evaluate a patient's risks and depend on advanced tools to help decide on treatment, making care in critical situations safer and more effective. Besides anticoagulants, thrombolytics are commonly used to treat serious cases of pulmonary embolism, as fast removal of the clot is necessary. Thrombolytic therapy, such as the use of tissue plasminogen activator (tPA), may facilitate the immediate restoration of blood flow, significantly reducing mortality rates associated with massive pulmonary embolism. Evidence from > critical care reports underscores the importance of timely intervention, as the factor of time can be a decisive element in patient survival. Giving thrombolytics to patients should be done with careful consideration of when they are not appropriate and the risks involved, so strong clinical judgment is necessary. This approach becomes even more compelling in peripheral healthcare settings, where professionals must often navigate resource limitations while striving to implement effective thrombolytic strategies as part of a broader emergency response plan (Chhaperwal *et al.*, 2025).

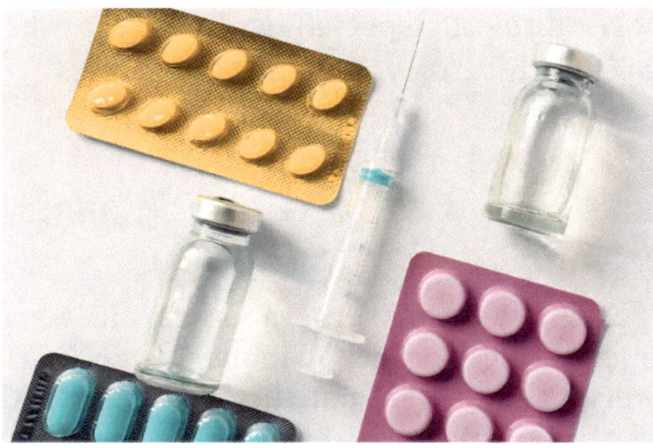

Figure 14.15. Pharmacological Management in cardiovascular emergencies.

Source: https://media.post.rvohealth.io/wp-content/uploads/2023/12/various-colorful-pill-packs-vials-tablets-syringe-1200x628-facebook.jpg.

Also, treating patients with pulmonary embolism or other critical cardiovascular emergencies requires more than just using drugs. It calls for using both medicine and non-medicine approaches. For example, when thrombolysis is not safe because of the risk of bleeding, catheter-directed therapies or embolectomy can be used. They show that it is important for critical care teams to team up and adjust their approaches to suit each patient. Also, knowing the differences between common anticoagulants and newer direct oral anticoagulants allows clinicians to improve treatment plans. Therefore, integrating evidence from systematic reviews and clinical guidelines can ensure that healthcare professionals make informed decisions that prioritize patient safety and therapeutic effectiveness in the management of life-threatening cardiovascular conditions (Huilcarema *et al.*, 2024) (Figure 14.15).

14.5.3. Surgical Options (e.g., Angioplasty, Bypass Surgery)

Among the surgical options available for managing cardiovascular emergencies, angioplasty and coronary artery bypass grafting (CABG) stand out as pivotal interventions. A balloon catheter is inserted during angioplasty to open up narrowed or blocked arteries, which helps restore blood flow. It is used to treat acute coronary syndromes right away, which lowers the risk of heart attack and improves the outcome for patients. If angioplasty is done promptly, people may recover faster than they would with surgery. Still, how well it works over time can depend on how much the patients follow the recommended lifestyle and medicine after surgery, which shows the value of ongoing care. CABG is more often advised for people with severe coronary artery disease or when several arteries are blocked. The surgeon takes a blood vessel from elsewhere in the body and uses it to create a bypass around blocked arteries, making sure the heart muscle gets enough blood. Recent studies suggest that surgery may be more risky initially, but it can significantly benefit certain patient groups. For instance, research has shown that surgeons' experience plays a significant role in clinical outcomes, impacting mortality, morbidity, and complication rates associated with CABG (Sağlam *et al.*, 2025) (Figure 14.16).

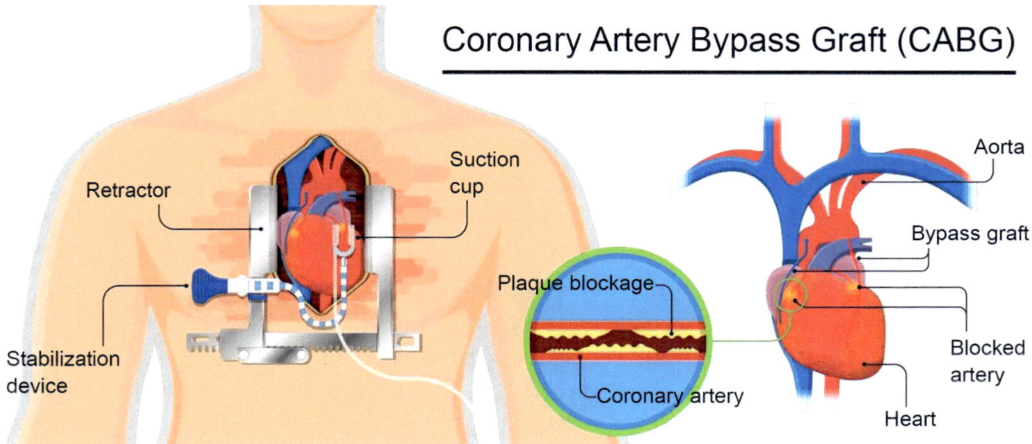

Figure 14.16. Coronary artery bypass grafting (CABG).

Source: https://cdn-assets-eu.frontify.com/s3/frontify-enterprise-files-eu/eyJvYXV0aCI6eyJjbGllbnRfaWQiOiJmcm9udGlmeS1leHBsb3JlciJ9LCJwYXRoIjoiaWhoLWhlYWx0aGNhcmUtYmVy aGFkXC9hY2NvdW50c1wvYz NcLzQwMDA2MjRc L3Byb2plY3RzXC8yMDlcL2Fzc2V0c1wvMzFcLzMzOTU3XC8yNDA0NDUzYzFlYzEyM2Q3ZGY3Mzc 4ZTNiYjE5Y2UyNy0xNjQ3MjY0MDA1LmpwZyJ9:ihh-healthcare-berhad:MMSAakHslcZN81Q3hViCRO7VApeziSUsQjzaGot7yzA?format=webp.

This highlights why it is important for surgeons to have expertise in handling high-risk patients, and it encourages more discussions about improving surgical approaches in critical care. The choice between angioplasty and CABG depends on many things about the patient, for example, their age, health, and the severity of their coronary artery disease. For many people, especially those with diabetes or additional conditions, CABG is more likely to offer lasting results for normal heart function than angioplasty. Additionally, as indicated in the research by Pan *et al.*, metabolic considerations, such as achieving diabetes remission or improved metabolic profiles, are vital in selecting appropriate surgical interventions (Hung *et al.*, 2025). In the end, angioplasty and CABG are key parts of treating cardiovascular emergencies. Knowing the details of each option allows healthcare providers to provide the best care for each patient which improves their long-term heart health.

Test Your Knowledge

1. What are the critical steps involved in immediate interventions like CPR and defibrillation during cardiac emergencies?
2. How are pharmacological agents such as anticoagulants and thrombolytics used in the management of acute cardiac events?

SUMMARY

Managing cardiovascular emergencies is very important in critical care to help patients survive and recover well. Many problems can arise during tracheal intubation, which points to the many difficulties healthcare professionals face in the ICU. Many patients experience changes in their heart rate or blood pressure during intubation, which is a vital action taken in emergencies. It was recently found that 42.6% of patients experienced cardiovascular instability, which emphasizes the importance for healthcare providers to be skilled in handling these situations. Addressing these complications through rigorous training and protocol adherence is essential for improving patient safety during critical interventions (Russotto *et al.*, 2021). Also, knowing what cardiovascular emergencies mean is not limited to a single procedure. The information shows that if these events are not handled well, ICU mortality rates can be very high, reaching 32.8% for those who need emergency intubation. Because of this statistic, it is clear that current emergency protocols are not working well and that a review of strategies is needed, highlighting the importance of using proven practices. Pre-intubation assessments should be improved, and the conditions during intubation should be better managed, especially for people at high risk. By proactively addressing these elements, critical care professionals can significantly mitigate adverse outcomes and enhance overall patient care (Livingston *et al.*, 2020). From studying cardiovascular emergencies in critical care, it is clear that more research and better clinical practices are needed. All stakeholders should focus on teamwork across fields to make sure best practices are always followed and checked. Also, making sure critical care staff receive thorough training can help them handle cardiovascular emergencies more efficiently. Using new strategies and advanced technology in healthcare can greatly help improve patient outcomes. In summary, addressing the intricate realities of cardiovascular emergencies is vital not only for improving immediate response strategies but also for fostering a robust framework for ongoing quality improvement in critical care settings (Russotto *et al.*, 2021).

It is important to see that cardiovascular emergencies in critical care are complex and usually result in a fast decline in a patient's condition. It is necessary to understand acute myocardial infarction, cardiogenic shock, and cardiac arrest to handle these emergencies well. Every one of these conditions brings its own set of problems, which usually need quick and effective medical care. Guidelines extrapolated from existing literature, such as the latest recommendations on treatment protocols and diagnostic criteria, aid healthcare providers in their decision-making process, ensuring timely responses that can significantly impact patient outcomes (Vahanian *et al.*, 2021). Also, thanks to telemedicine and remote monitoring, care can now be given promptly in critical situations, which helps stabilize patients before they need advanced care. Having interdisciplinary teams is very important in dealing with cardiovascular emergencies. It is crucial for cardiologists, critical care nurses, and emergency medical technicians to communicate and cooperate well to handle these emergencies. Research indicates that early identification and intervention by specialized teams can markedly improve survival rates and reduce morbidity associated with cardiac events (Livingston *et al.*, 2020). Because of this, more attention is being given to teamwork and rule following in the educational programs for healthcare workers. Building a teamwork culture and encouraging staff to keep learning allows healthcare facilities to ensure that their team is ready for both the challenges and the detailed care needed in cardiovascular crises. Cardiovascular emergencies can also have major effects on healthcare systems and the people they serve. Because cardiovascular disease is becoming more common worldwide, critical care units have to adapt to handle the higher number of emergencies. So, we must work on solutions for urgent care and also focus on preventing the risk factors that cause these conditions. Strategies such as public health awareness campaigns and community-based interventions are instrumental in promoting cardiovascular health and reducing the incidence of emergencies (Vahanian *et al.*, 2021). Also, recognizing the social and economic factors behind health differences in cardiovascular disease can direct policies that promote equal access to quality care for allTaking care of all these points as a whole is important for improving the way critical care is provided and the health results for patients with cardiovascular emergencies.

KEY TERMS FROM THIS CHAPTER

- Acute coronary syndrome (ACS)
- Angina
- Atrial flutter
- Cardiogenic shock
- Cardiovascular emergencies
- Diastolic dysfunction
- Heart failure (HF)
- Hypotension
- Acute pulmonary edema
- Atrial fibrillation (AF)
- Cardiac arrest
- Cardiopulmonary resuscitation (CPR)
- Defibrillation
- Distributive shock
- Hemodynamic monitoring
- Inotropic support

CRITICAL THINKING QUESTIONS

1. In a patient with acute myocardial infarction (MI), what is the first-line treatment for pain relief and to reduce myocardial oxygen demand?

a. Intravenous morphine

b. Oral aspirin

c. Beta-blockers

d. Nitroglycerin

2. What is the primary treatment for a patient in shock with a systolic blood pressure <90 mmHg and suspected septic shock?

a. Blood transfusion

b. Administration of vasopressors and intravenous fluids

c. Intubation and mechanical ventilation

d. Immediate coronary angiography

3. In the case of acute decompensated heart failure, what is the most appropriate initial intervention?

a. Diuretics and nitrates

b. Anticoagulation therapy

c. Coronary artery bypass graft surgery

d. Beta-blockers and calcium channel blockers

4. Which of the following is a contraindication to thrombolytic therapy in a patient with acute pulmonary embolism (PE)?

a. Age over 70 years

b. Severe hypertension (SBP >180 mmHg)

c. Positive D-dimer test

d. Unilateral leg swelling

5. In a patient with ventricular fibrillation (VF), what is the recommended first step in management?

a. Administer epinephrine

b. Defibrillation (shock)

c. Start chest compressions

d. Perform endotracheal intubation

Short Answer Questions

1. What are the primary causes of acute myocardial infarction (MI), and how do they differ between STEMI and NSTEMI?
2. How are thrombolytics used in treating STEMI and how is it decided if a patient can have thrombolytic therapy?
3. State the differences between compensated and decompensated shock and how they are seen in patients experiencing cardiovascular emergencies.
4. How is the Frank-Starling law relevant to shock and the way fluids are managed in critical care?
5. Which are the main treatment approaches for a patient who has acute heart failure?
6. When should vasopressors be given in shock management?

Answer to Critical Thinking Questions

1. (a); 2. (b); 3. (a); 4. (b); 5. (b)

REFERENCES

1. Alan, Y., Tas, A., Bayhan, M. I., Haj Mohammad, A. I., Umman, S., Parker, K., & Sezer, M. (2025). Reservoir-excess pressure analysis, aiding critical care management by revealing subtle changes in vasomotor status, is closely linked to dicrotic notch morphology. *European Heart Journal: Acute Cardiovascular Care*. https://www.semanticscholar.org/paper/0880d852ef270ffb60636c84b07cc9e47916fab6 (accessed on 22 May 2025).
2. Alansari, H., Lazzara, G., Taha, M. B., & Gorthi, J. (2025). The impact of obesity on cardiovascular diseases: Heart failure. *Methodist DeBakey Cardiovascular Journal, 21*, 44–52. https://www.semanticscholar.org/paper/467ddc7fea81253976b52ee5e927119031e65f79 (accessed on 22 May 2025).
3. Anderson, J. L., & Morrow, D. A. (2017). Acute myocardial infarction. *New England Journal of Medicine, 376*, 2053–2064. https://doi.org/10.1056/nejmra1606915.
4. Antikchi, M., Heydari, S., & Bakhshi, F. (2025). The effect of game-based scenario writing on the clinical reasoning of internship nursing students in cardiovascular emergencies and critical care units. *BMC Medical Education, 25*. https://www.semanticscholar.org/paper/448cb5bffcd72934a61ed4a1079a3ae82f5bf7f0 (accessed on 22 May 2025).
5. Budarova, K. V., Shmakov, A. N., Elizar'eva, N. L., & Kokhno, V. N. (2022). Reaction pattern of the autonomic nervous system to the infusion load in the intensive care in children: A prospective comparative study. *Annals of Critical Care*. https://www.semanticscholar.org/paper/4c90cfe9dd861e7fca30769c7abed897f64e3ad7 (accessed on 22 May 2025).
6. Byrne, J. (2021). Consultation and clinical assessment of the heart and cardiovascular system. *British Journal of Nursing, 30*(18), 1066–1072. https://www.semanticscholar.org/paper/b0c6648f3de0f00a8fe9ce1bc77c569c3046b51d (accessed on 22 May 2025).
7. Cheng, P. J., & Hsu, N. C. (2023). Incorporating multiorgan point-of-care ultrasound into obstetric emergency treatment protocols. *Journal of Medical Ultrasound, 31*, 83–85. https://www.semanticscholar.org/paper/087b32438ab5dee0d7bb822a396962e318170341 (accessed on 22 May 2025).
8. Chhaperwal, P., Kumar, S., Suri, G., Garg, U., Kapoor, S., & Devarakonda, B. V. (2025). A comprehensive clinical acumen enhanced by point-of-care ultrasonography in managing acute life-threatening massive pulmonary thromboembolism in a peripheral setting: A case report. *Annals of Cardiac Anaesthesia, 28*, 61–64. https://www.semanticscholar.org/paper/f40e8f99517d785195071981f71073894b91ac6e (accessed on 22 May 2025).
9. Conti, E., Cascio, N. D., Paluan, P., Racca, G., Longhitano, Y., Savioli, G., Tesauro, M., *et al.* (2024). Pregnancy arrhythmias: Management in the emergency department and critical care. *Journal of Clinical Medicine, 13*. https://www.semanticscholar.org/paper/16a68d14fe944336489b28d0dcc0d9d8cc3b6f1d (accessed on 22 May 2025).
10. De Rop, L., Bos, D. A. G., Stegeman, I., Holtman, G., Ochodo, E. A., Spijker, R., Otieno, J. A., *et al.* (2024). Accuracy of routine laboratory tests to predict mortality and deterioration to severe or critical COVID-19 in people with SARS-CoV-2. *The Cochrane Database of Systematic Reviews, 2024*. https://www.semanticscholar.org/paper/0bbf071dc0684987d9601359186773b3928e092d (accessed on 22 May 2025).

11. Domańska-Poboża, J., Kapica, Ł., Kanecki, K., Lewtak, K., Goryński, P., & Wisłowska, M. (2025). Trends in initial hospitalizations of patients with newly diagnosed Sjogren's disease in Poland between 2012 and 2023: A retrospective data analysis. *Journal of Clinical Medicine, 14*. https://www.semanticscholar.org/paper/b2f16f872a26b9136c97beaf861e2e243bef9962 (accessed on 22 May 2025).

12. Domańska-Poboża, J., Kapica, Ł., Kanecki, K., Nitsch-Osuch, A., Gorycki, P., & Wisłowska, M. (2025). Hospitalizations of patients with rheumatoid arthritis in Polish intensive care units or cardiac intensive care units in 2011–2021: Population study. *Polish Archives of Internal Medicine*. https://www.semanticscholar.org/paper/67c76162162b6e3622f4233f7e8ea1106a7b0be7 (accessed on 22 May 2025).

13. Fahimi, B. (2024). Atrial fibrillation and lifestyle modification: Charting new courses for cardiovascular health. *Clinical Research and Clinical Trials*. https://www.semanticscholar.org/paper/6f7f6e6b2db31e658e5103bdba8b6720ba878f01 (accessed on 22 May 2025).

14. Garde, V., Churchill, M., Greenslade, J., Watt, K., Mallett, A. J., & Morel, D. (2025). Review article: Somatization disorders in emergency department: A critical overview of current challenges and future directions. *Emergency Medicine Australasia, 37*. https://www.semanticscholar.org/paper/7f18744ff0a918672db96afb5aa4eb3efe63b7ff (accessed on 22 May 2025).

15. Giuvara, S., Suciu, A. V., Postoiu, R., Aurelian, S., Daia, C., Băilă, M., Andone, I., *et al.* (2025). Rehabilitation challenges in a case of a female patient with cardio-respiratory arrest resuscitated in an intra-hospital environment, associating multiple cardiovascular comorbidities and metabolic pathology–Case report. *Romanian Journal of Medical Rehabilitation Physical Medicine and Paleoclimatology*. https://www.semanticscholar.org/paper/9b9d2c8a35642d0da1540ae8eaca8e6fc4bff520 (accessed on 22 May 2025).

16. Guaraca Huilcarema, D. P., Yánez Tobar, J. C., Moya Pilay, R. D., Pagalo Tacuri, S. A., Tulcanaza Ochoa, G. F., Garcés López, M. E., & Albán Galarza, M. D. (2024). Pharmacological and nonpharmacological interventions for prevention and management of pulmonary embolism in patients with cardiac comorbidities: A literature review. *International Journal of Medical Science and Clinical Research Studies*. https://www.semanticscholar.org/paper/76197c8f860c01bab6943a59439ebf6f60fcd1fe (accessed on 22 May 2025).

17. Guzik, T. J., Mohiddin, S., Dimarco, A., Patel, V., Savvatis, K., Marelli-Berg, F. M., Madhur, M. S., *et al.* (2020). COVID-19 and the cardiovascular system: Implications for risk assessment, diagnosis, and treatment options. *Cardiovascular Research, 116*, 1666–1687. https://doi.org/10.1093/cvr/cvaa106.

18. Hodkinson, A., Tyler, N., Ashcroft, D. M., Keers, R. N., Khan, K., Phipps, D. L., Abuzour, A. S., *et al.* (2020). Preventable medication harm across health care settings: A systematic review and meta-analysis. *BMC Medicine, 18*. https://doi.org/10.1186/s12916-020-01774-9.

19. Hung, C. M., Lee, H. M., & Chiu, C. C. (2025). The role of metabolic bariatric surgery in improving outcomes for major adverse cardiovascular events. *Annals of Medicine and Surgery, 87*, 1773–1774. https://www.semanticscholar.org/paper/3bebcd662750cd463a5434ca82fa5810ea506943 (accessed on 22 May 2025).

20. Kharawala, A., Nagraj, S., Setia, G., Reynolds, D., & Thachil, R. (2025). Cardiac critical care of the cardio-obstetric patient. *Journal of Intensive Care Medicine*. https://www.semanticscholar.org/paper/61121e2dbcc8580173c519cc94da613e4d6ea5f5 (accessed on 22 May 2025).

21. Kuwabara, M., Yamamoto, T., Tahara, Y., Kikuchi, M., Imamura, H., Takeuchi, I., Sato, N., *et al.* (2025). Utilization of intensive care units and outcomes based on admission wards in cardiovascular emergencies. *Circulation Journal: Official Journal of the Japanese Circulation Society*. https://www.semanticscholar.org/paper/a7308e34e3f098f3d886e36fce642d368178f57e (accessed on 22 May 2025).

22. Livingston, G., Huntley, J., Sommerlad, A., Ames, D., Ballard, C., Banerjee, S., Brayne, C., *et al.* (2020). Dementia prevention, intervention, and care: 2020 report of the Lancet Commission. *The Lancet, 396*, 413–446. https://doi.org/10.1016/S0140-6736(20)30367-6.

23. Lock, M. C., Ripley, D. M., Smith, K. L. M., Mueller, C. A., Shiels, H. A., Crossley, D., & Galli, G. (2024). Developmental plasticity of the cardiovascular system in oviparous vertebrates: Effects of chronic hypoxia and interactive stressors in the context of climate change. *The Journal of Experimental Biology, 227*. https://www.semanticscholar.org/paper/86ac0d3c90f8f534207e350976763dbb6f0b8326 (accessed on 22 May 2025).

24. Mohamed, A. A., Atia, A., El-Barbary, A., & Elian. (2021). Validity of new risk model (McNamara *et al.*, 2016) in predicting in-hospital mortality in patients with acute myocardial infarction. *Benha Journal of Applied Sciences*. https://www.semanticscholar.org/paper/43d647be48dbf4f03f2ee6456eba929200846169 (accessed on 22 May 2025).

25. Moisa, Ş., Brinza, C., Floria, M., & Burlacu, A. (2024). Navigating neonatal cardiovascular emergencies: A comprehensive narrative review on assessment and intervention strategies. *Journal of Cardiovascular Emergencies, 10*, 1–6. https://www.semanticscholar.org/paper/c1f1d04fae84c44b66e8398876447f8502f9ce02 (accessed on 22 May 2025).

26. Montgomery, J. P., Marquez, J. L., Nord, J., Stamper, A. R., Edwards, E. A., Valentini, N., Frank, C. J., *et al.* (2024). Detection of a human adenovirus outbreak, including some critical infections, using multipathing testing at a large university, September 2022–January 2023. *Open Forum Infectious Diseases, 11*(5), ofae192. https://www.semanticscholar.org/paper/a81ccb4ac94ae9922e7440bd977152956bacd53d (accessed on 22 May 2025).

27. Mortezaeian, H., Taheri, M., Anafje, M., Esmaeili, Z., Hassanzadeh, G., & Ebrahimi, P. (2024). Pediatric coronary cameral fistula in a structurally normal heart: A case report and review of the literature. *Journal of Medical Case Reports, 18*. https://www.semanticscholar.org/paper/d9741a1c469a9455f2d6b61be8c3711f419a3065 (accessed on 22 May 2025).

28. Nadikudhiti, M., Kovvuri, S., Dindi, S., & Bhargavi, V. (2025). Obstetric complications requiring emergency necessity of obstetric critical care unit in a rural area of Andhra Pradesh. *Global Journal for Research Analysis*. https://www.semanticscholar.org/paper/d7579e667b9158fa60b62188e9bad6c771dd0480 (accessed on 22 May 2025).

29. Padte, S., Samala Venkata, V., Mehta, P., Tawfeeq, S., Kashyap, R., & Surani, S. R. (2024). 21st century critical care medicine: An overview. *World Journal of Critical Care Medicine, 13*. https://www.semanticscholar.org/paper/8127b1ae8a3d3a3f136c365fc8a5cabe18c3e11f (accessed on 22 May 2025).

30. Pervaiz, R., Ahmed, H., & Awad, A. (2024). The use of empirical antibiotics in the critical care unit. *Pakistan Journal of Intensive Care Medicine*. https://www.semanticscholar.org/paper/37c8c585f0f6dc74b89d54576bd1a7454f500425 (accessed on 22 May 2025).

31. Pleşca, D., Spătariu, L., Bordei, L., Vlad, P., & Hurduc, V. (2017). OC-54 The role of prevention in food allergies. *Archives of Disease in Childhood, 102*, A20–A21. https://www.semanticscholar.org/paper/ca18e9ce38925a2d07c43c1d248f0a627ec7fa9b (accessed on 22 May 2025).

32. Riba, R. A., Loma-Osorio, P., Sanz-Girgas, E., Garcia-Garcia, C., Soriano, T., Sionis, A., Llaó, I., *et al.* (2024). Current post-resuscitation management of out-of-hospital cardiac arrest patients admitted to intensive cardiovascular care units. *European Heart Journal: Acute Cardiovascular Care.* https://www.semanticscholar.org/paper/99dfb3d8dfb7a051396141fae76d260f10cba125 (accessed on 22 May 2025).

33. Richardson, S., Hirsch, J. S., Narasimhan, M., Crawford, J. M., McGinn, T., Davidson, K. W., Barnaby, D. P., *et al.* (2020). Presenting characteristics, comorbidities, and outcomes among 5700 patients hospitalized with COVID-19 in the New York City area. *JAMA, 323*, 2052–2052. https://doi.org/10.1001/jama.2020.6775.

34. Russotto, V., Myatra, S. N., Laffey, J. G., Tassistro, E., Antolini, L., Bauer, P. R., Lascarrou, J. B., *et al.* (2021). Intubation practices and adverse peri-intubation events in critically ill patients from 29 countries. *JAMA, 325*, 1164–1164. https://doi.org/10.1001/jama.2021.1727.

35. Sağlam, M. F., Uğuz, E., Erdogan, K., Erçelik, H. U., Yücel, M., & Sener, E. (2025). Impact of surgeon experience on clinical outcomes in cardiovascular surgery: A retrospective analysis. *Online Türk Sağlık Bilimleri Dergisi.* https://www.semanticscholar.org/paper/d6bc3155351643263df422df5d76f069835ffe8b (accessed on 22 May 2025).

36. Sharma, V., Bhambu, S. K., & Rao, A. (2025). Diabetes mellitus prevention and management with yoga. *Journal of Ayurveda and Integrated Medical Sciences.* https://www.semanticscholar.org/paper/1099d40d02279554d6839bf644f618873d55eb2a (accessed on 22 May 2025).

37. Sooltan, I., Khan, A., Haque, R., & Bulugahapitiya, S. (2025). Enhancing emergency cardiac care delivery: Structured induction programmed improves frontline doctors' acute care competencies and reduces critical decision uncertainty. *European Heart Journal: Acute Cardiovascular Care.* https://www.semanticscholar.org/paper/60aa6791734ec340458e9200909a8e8c7bd9eee9 (accessed on 22 May 2025).

38. Steinert, J., School of Social Sciences and Technology, Heidelberg University, *et al.* (2023). The economic impact of treating hypertension in sub–Saharan Africa–A systematic review. *The European Journal of Public Health, 33.* https://www.semanticscholar.org/paper/c1dc31253734373297ec17220bb874eecdffd6f4 (accessed on 22 May 2025).

39. Vahanian, A., Beyersdorf, F., Praz, F., Milojevic, M., Baldus, S., Bauersachs, J., Capodanno, D., *et al.* (2021). 2021 ESC/EACTS guidelines for the management of valvular heart disease. *European Heart Journal, 43*, 561–632. https://doi.org/10.1093/eurheartj/ehab395.

40. Williams, B., Mancia, G., Spiering, W., Agabiti Rosei, E., Azizi, M., Burnier, M., Clement, D. L., *et al.* (2018). 2018 ESC/ESH guidelines for the management of arterial hypertension. *European Heart Journal, 39*, 3021–3104. https://doi.org/10.1093/eurheartj/ehy339.

41. Xie, L., Lan, P., Liu, M., & Zhou, K. (2024). ECMO management for severe pulmonary embolism with concurrent cerebral haemorrhage: A case report. *Frontiers in Cardiovascular Medicine, 11.* https://www.semanticscholar.org/paper/a6b50b3f77ecf99ab1d16bfd0026efcc2b6661b7 (accessed on 22 May 2025).

PHARMACOLOGY IN CRITICAL CARE

15

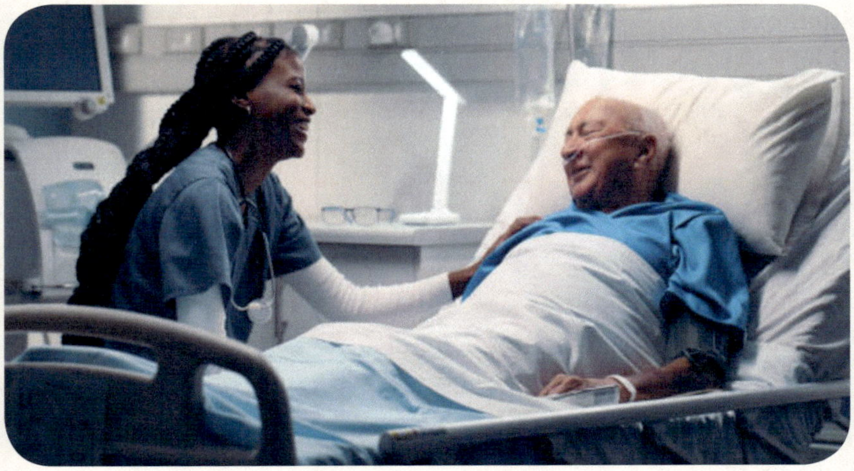

LEARNING OBJECTIVES

After studying this chapter, you will be able to:

1. Define pharmacokinetics in critical care.
2. List the common medications used in critical care..
3. Illustrate the drug interactions in critical care.
4. Describe dosing considerations in critical care.
5. Define the role of pharmacists in critical care.

Introduction

Recently, the connection between pharmacology and critical care has become more important as healthcare tries to help critically ill patients recover. Because patients in critical care often have several complex medical problems, pharmacology is essential for making clinical decisions. Giving drugs safely and effectively can help this group recover instead of experiencing adverse events. It is important to know the details of drug interactions, how much to give, and when to give them, because critical care situations require fast and accurate actions. Because pharmacological therapies are constantly advancing, it is important for critical care practitioners to stay updated to provide the best care and tailor treatments for each patient, underscoring the need for strong pharmacological training for healthcare workers in intensive care medicine. Venous thromboembolism (VTE) presents a significant risk in critical care, particularly in trauma patients. Proper use of medicines to prevent blood clots is very important in managing and preventing VTE. A recent evaluation by the Western Trauma Association highlights an algorithm focused on risk assessment and the administration of anticoagulant therapies to reduce the incidence of VTE among trauma patients (Ley *et al.*, 2020). The guidelines are developed after reviewing a large amount of literature and getting expert opinions, which show that early and uninterrupted use of prophylactic drugs can greatly reduce the risk of VTE and its complications. Thus, the importance of fast pharmacological action in acute situations highlights the key part pharmacology plays in healthcare and the importance of healthcare workers encouraging established treatment plans in the clinic. Furthermore, the COVID-19 pandemic has introduced new challenges and considerations regarding pharmacology in critical care environments, particularly for patients with opioid use disorders (Becker *et al.*, 2020). The pandemic is making it hard for people to get treatment which has made it more urgent to find new ways, such as telemedicine, in opioid agonist therapy. It demonstrates the strong link between pharmacology and public health because medicines play a key role in controlling both infectious diseases and substance use disorders. Because these challenges exist, strong pharmacological approaches will continue to be necessary in critical care practices. In the end, knowing pharmacology well helps healthcare providers make decisions and handle the challenges of patient care in the current situation.

Definition of Pharmacology

Pharmacology looks at drugs, how they act in the body, their uses in medicine, and the effects they have on the body's systems. This area of science gives the support needed for using medications safely and effectively in many healthcare areas, especially in critical care, where patients' conditions can change quickly. Pharmacology helps physicians decide on the best treatments for critical illnesses by highlighting the need for treatments that match both the drug's effects and the patient's unique body functions. Understanding pharmacodynamics and pharmacokinetics is essential, as these concepts inform clinicians about how a drug affects the body and how the body alters the drug over time, which is crucial for optimizing therapeutic outcomes in high-stakes situations (Rocca *et al.*, 2023) (Figure 15.1).

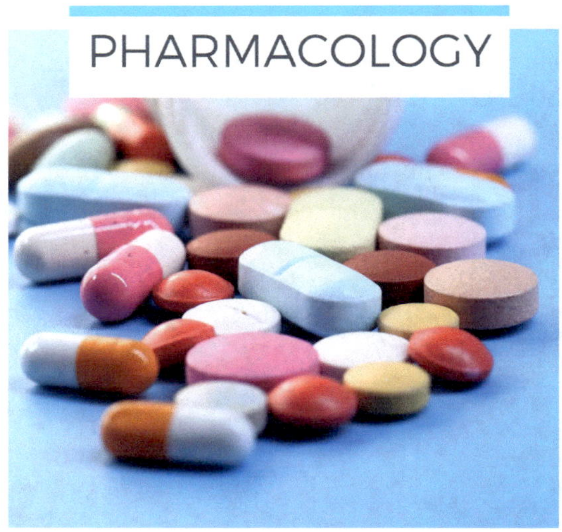

Figure 15.1. Pharmacology.

Source: https://straightanursingstudent.com/wp-content/uploads/2024/10/EP-368-FIRST-PASS-METABOLISMBLOG.png.

Pharmacology in critical care is more than giving medicines; it dramatically influences the decisions made during patient care. Intensive care units (ICUs) frequently encounter patients with multisystem failures who may be on polypharmacy regimens, necessitating a comprehensive understanding of pharmacology to minimize adverse events and optimize drug interactions. Because of this knowledge, healthcare providers can expect possible problems, adjust drug amounts, and pick alternatives that match how the patient is improving. Also, with modern monitoring tools, it is now possible to quickly check how a patient responds to drugs, which helps pharmacology and patient outcomes go hand in hand. Such a dynamic interplay signifies the vital role that pharmacology performs in enhancing the quality of care provided in critical settings (Rocca *et al.*, 2023). Pharmacology education allows healthcare professionals to choose the proper medications for patients in critical care, which can be unpredictable. This area of work helps medical staff learn about different drug types, possible side effects, situations when drugs should not be used, and how to use them in emergencies. Because medical science keeps advancing with new drugs and methods, pharmacists need to keep learning and training. Because critical care practices are constantly improving, it is important for practitioners to keep their knowledge current to manage the complexities of drugs. Thus, fostering a robust comprehension of pharmacology ultimately serves to enhance patient safety, efficacy of treatment, and overall health outcomes in critical care settings (Barbas, 2023).

Importance of Pharmacology in Critical Care

Because critical care often involves treating several severe conditions, pharmacology is fundamental due to the need to understand drugs and their effects. In these areas, healthcare providers give medications to deal with urgent and potentially fatal conditions, for example, sepsis, respiratory failure, and shock. Because patients may be very sick, medical staff have to choose, dose, and administer drugs accurately and promptly. They should also help control the main problems in the body that cause the disease, not just relieve the symptoms. Since patients in critical care react differently to medications, individualized treatment is vital for better outcomes. This points out that critical care clinicians should be aware of the latest pharmacological developments and treatment options to give the best care and improve outcomes for critically ill patients. Because new pharmacological treatments are continually being developed, managing intravenous fluids in critical care is growing more important. Fluid therapy keeps a patient alive but can lead to further problems if it is not handled properly. Earlier, it was thought that giving plenty of fluid during resuscitation was safe. However, researchers now say that too much fluid can be dangerous for patients who have increased endothelial permeability. Modern approaches prioritize a more meticulous strategy, including a dynamic model that emphasizes resuscitation, optimization, stabilization, and evacuation (R.O.S.E.). It helps to ensure patients benefit the most while the risk of adverse outcomes is reduced. Given that intravenous fluids can act similarly to pharmacological agents, a profound understanding of their pharmacological properties and impact on organ systems is essential in ensuring optimal care for critically ill patients (Malbrain *et al.*, 2020). The pharmacological management of specific conditions within the critical care spectrum, such as nonalcoholic fatty liver disease (NAFLD), further illustrates the complexity and importance of pharmacology.

Because NAFLD is a major reason for liver transplantation, it is necessary to use treatments that stop the disease and improve patients' lives. Doctors use updated guidelines for treating such diseases because the understanding of their causes and effects keeps changing. It is imperative to identify advanced fibrosis early, since it can greatly affect the treatment plan and future health of the patient. Also, the use of vitamin E and pioglitazone in critical care shows that doctors must keep researching and adapting their drug choices. This evolution highlights the importance of pharmacology not only in managing acute crises but also in addressing chronic conditions that cascade into critical care scenarios (Ando *et al.*, 2021).

Overview of Critical Care Settings

Critical care settings are key for managing patients with serious, life-threatening health problems. These environments, including ICUs, Progressive Care Units (PCUs), and High Dependency Units (HDUs), are characterized by advanced medical technology, continuous monitoring, and a multidisciplinary team of healthcare professionals. Every critical care setting is set up to handle the particular needs of patients, depending on how severe their conditions are and how much care they require. In terms of drugs, these units usually use a variety that needs to be adjusted for each patient, mainly to deal with urgent changes in body functions. So, in critical care, pharmacology covers checking for drug interactions, side effects, and the effectiveness of treatments in these serious settings. Due to the notable changes in the body of critically ill patients, managing drugs in critical care calls for a good understanding of pharmacokinetics and pharmacodynamics. Altered ways of taking up, moving through the body, and breaking down drugs play a major role in their safety and effectiveness. So, clinicians must be very careful with the dosage to avoid both giving too little and causing harm, mainly in people who already take many medicines and have other illnesses. For example, seeing how anticholinergic drugs cause xerostomia in critical care patients highlights the need to understand how drugs can change a patient's overall well-being. Research has indicated that there is a significant correlation between anticholinergic burden and xerostomia within the first 24 hours of ICU admission, underscoring the need for careful medication selection (Chung *et al.*, 2023). Also, the rise of multidrug-resistant infections in critical care makes it necessary to have strong antimicrobial stewardship in these areas. These infections, such as those caused by *Candida auris*, make treating patients more difficult and increase the risk of death for those at risk. Given the ability of *C. auris* to resist multiple antifungal agents and its propensity for rapid colonization in healthcare environments, practitioners must adopt proactive screening and infection control measures to stem outbreaks (Cristina *et al.*, 2023). It stresses that in critical care pharmacology, using an informed and planned approach to both treatment and prevention is very important. If critical care providers know the pharmacological aspects of these infections and their treatment, they can handle patient care more effectively and achieve better results in this challenging setting.

15.1. Pharmacokinetics in Critical Care

Learning Outcome

1. Define absorption of medications in critically ill patients
2. Explain the distribution of drugs in altered physiological states
3. Analyze the metabolism and elimination of drugs in critical care

Pharmacokinetics is necessary in critical care because patients usually have complicated health issues that need accurate medicine use. Physiological changes, such as problems with organs and how much fluid is in the body, can greatly influence the pharmacokinetic processes of absorption, distribution, metabolism, and excretion. Because of these factors, healthcare providers must be aware of how medications function in the body to create the right treatment plans. The way a drug works in a patient can differ a lot from what is expected, mainly in critically ill people who often have organ problems and unstable blood flow. Consequently, healthcare providers need to keep reviewing and adjusting drug doses as they watch drug levels and patient responses to get the best treatment outcomes. In the context of pharmacology in critical care, therapeutic drug monitoring (TDM) is an invaluable tool for personalizing medication regimens. TDM adjusts medication doses by looking at plasma concentrations, which helps improve both the effects and safety of the drugs. It is beneficial for patients with unpredictable drug absorption due to their critical illness, since it helps avoid the dangers of giving too much or too little medication. Although TDM is useful, it is not used as much as it could be, especially in India, which has a history of TDM but has not applied it widely. The growing recognition of TDMs' role in improving clinical outcomes underscores the need for better integration of this practice into routine pharmacologic management in critical care settings, thus heralding a new era of precision medicine in therapeutic approaches (Suneja *et al.*, 2025). Genetic traits are also essential in how drugs are used in critical care. New developments in pharmacogenetics have shown how different genes can change a person's response to drugs that cross the blood-brain barrier, which is vital for treating conditions of the brain and other critical illnesses. Pharmacogenetic profiles help clinicians foresee a patient's reaction to certain drugs, which leads to better treatment choices and fewer side effects. For example, variations in drug transporters can strongly affect how well and how easily a person can tolerate medications. Exploring these genetic influences can guide clinicians in making informed decisions regarding drug selection and dosage, thus improving patient outcomes even further in an often unpredictable clinical landscape (Skvarc *et al.*, 2024) (Figure 15.2).

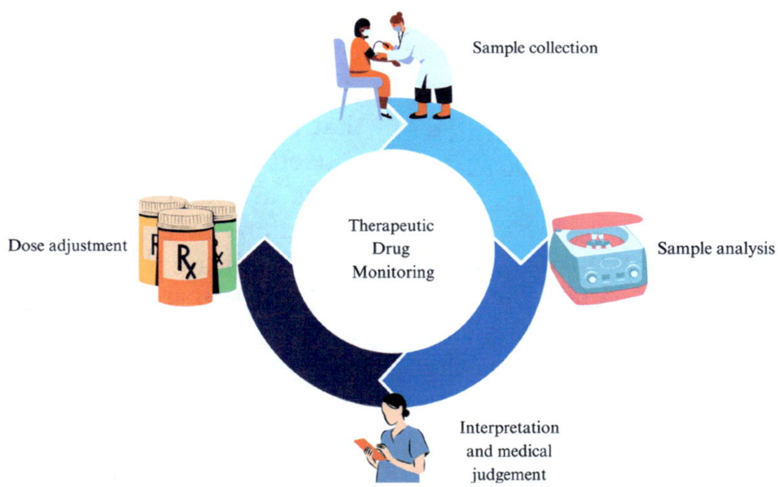

Figure 15.2. Schematization of the therapeutic drug monitoring (TDM) process.

Source: https://www.mdpi.com/1424-8247/17/5/642.

15.1.1. Absorption of Medications in Critically Ill Patients

The way medications are absorbed in critically ill patients is strongly affected by the special changes in their bodies. Factors such as altered gastrointestinal (GI) motility, changes in blood flow, and an overall compromised ability to absorb nutrients can significantly impact how drugs are absorbed. Critically ill patients might have delayed gastric emptying or a higher pH in their stomach, which can make it harder for certain orally taken medications to dissolve and be absorbed. Consequently, intravenous (IV) administration is often preferred in these scenarios to ensure rapid drug delivery and therapeutic efficacy. Also, having comorbidities or feeding tubes can make it more challenging to give medication, so healthcare providers must carefully choose how and in what form to give drugs to this group. In addition, differences in how the drug is absorbed can result in less effective treatment and more chances of side effects. The pathophysiological state of critically ill patients can alter drug pharmacokinetics, resulting in unpredictable plasma concentrations (Figure 15.3).

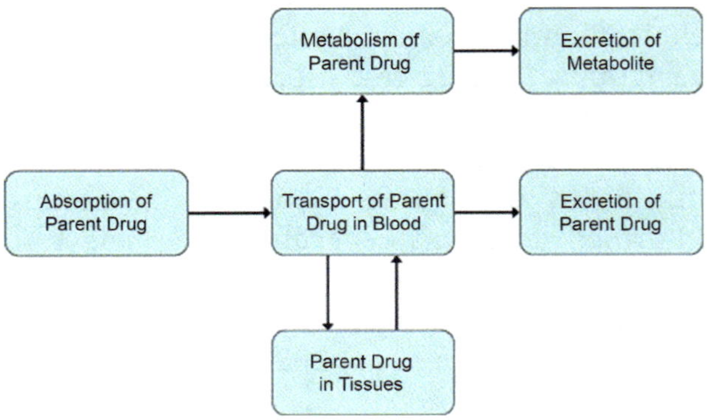

Figure 15.3. Physiologic alterations are frequently evident in critically ill patients.

Source: https://www.criticalcare.theclinics.com/article/S0749-0704%2806%2900012-1/abstract.

Many critically ill patients have hypoalbuminemia, which can cause more of some free drugs to be present in the blood. This means doctors and nurses have to change the doses to keep the drug at the right level in the blood. Also, giving nutrition through a feeding tube can create more problems, since it may influence the absorption of certain drugs that depend on acid or are quickly metabolized in the body. For this reason, knowing more about these factors helps create better medication strategies in critical care.

Being aware of the effects of other medications is very important. Since many critically ill patients receive multiple treatments, there is a chance for drugs to interact, which may affect their effectiveness. For instance, certain drug classes, such as proton pump inhibitors, can alter gastric pH and consequently the solubility and absorption of co-administered medications, a significant concern in drug regimens for conditions like COVID-19 (Bourgonje *et al.*, 2020) and cardiovascular diseases (Gheblawi *et al.*, 2020). The method of giving medications—through the mouth or a vein—can also change their bioavailability, which makes treatment more complicated. For this reason, healthcare professionals should cooperate, providing customized pharmacotherapy that considers the many changes and interactions in drug absorption, so critically ill patients receive the best possible care and their conditions are handled effectively.

15.1.2. Distribution of Drugs in Altered Physiological States

Drugs are handled differently in altered body states, and this is a major focus of pharmacology, especially in critical care. Body composition that is not normal, such as obesity or changes caused by severe illness, can affect how drugs are handled in the body. For instance, alterations in the volume of distribution (Vd) can complicate the prediction of drug behavior in obese patients, as drug-specific changes arise from various factors, including lipophilicity and tissue binding.

It may seem logical that weight gain means a person needs more medicine, but usually the link is more complicated. Clinicians should handle these drug-specific issues for each patient, mainly when the drug has a narrow therapeutic index. This complexity emphasizes the necessity for tailored pharmacotherapeutic strategies that take into account individual patient characteristics and responses to medications in critical care scenarios (Tang *et al.*, 2019). Critical care environments often involve additional challenges, particularly when managing patients undergoing extracorporeal membrane oxygenation (ECMO) (Figure 15.4).

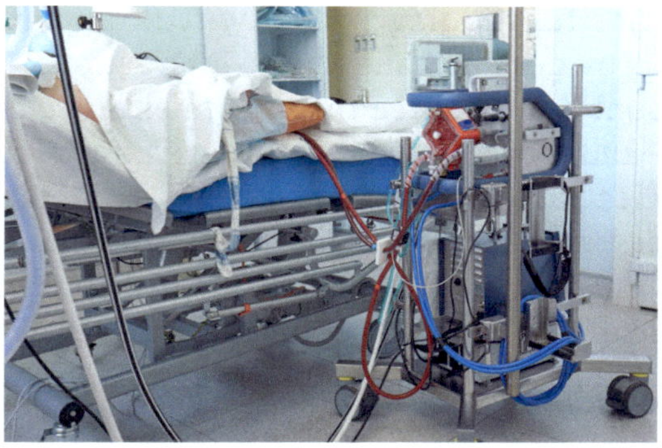

Figure 15.4. Extracorporeal membrane oxygenation (ECMO).

Source: https://heartbeatperfusion.com/wp-content/uploads/2022/07/ECMO-2.jpg.

The way drugs are handled in the body can be made more difficult by the blood flow changes and organ problems that often occur in these patients. The use of ECMO can cause different drug levels in the body because of drug sequestration and hemodilution, which may change both the volume of distribution and how quickly drugs are cleared. The way a drug is absorbed depends on its chemical form and also on the patient's age, other conditions, and genetic background. Understanding these dynamics is essential to ensure effective and safe pharmacotherapy, facilitating the optimization of dosing strategies amidst critical illness and advanced support technologies (Raffaeli *et al.*, 2019). In addition, distributing drugs to children is difficult because of their unique physiology, such as obesity. The way drugs are handled in the body changes with age, and these changes are even more noticeable during critical illness. The way children respond to drugs can be different, which can sometimes make drug disposition more challenging. It has been found that children who are obese may not clear certain drugs as well as others, which means their medication doses should be adjusted for them. The importance of more research here is high, because most available evidence is not directly applicable to clinical work. Thus, developing a comprehensive understanding of pharmacokinetics and personalized treatment plans is fundamental to managing drug therapy in critically ill pediatric patients effectively (Tang *et al.*, 2019).

15.1.3. Metabolism and Elimination of Drugs in Critical Care

It is important to know how drugs are metabolized and eliminated in critical care for better drug therapy. In patients who are critically ill, the body's functions may be altered, especially by problems with the liver and kidneys, which can change how drugs are handled. The liver, which is important for drug metabolism, includes enzymes that can make medications more or less active. When patients have hepatic failure, such as from acute or chronic liver disease, drugs that depend on the liver for metabolism are cleared more slowly. As a result, drug accumulation can occur, leading to an increased risk of adverse drug reactions and therapeutic failures, necessitating careful monitoring and appropriate dose adjustments to mitigate these risks (Diep *et al.*, 2017). Modifications in metabolic pathways may also change how drugs are removed from the body by the kidneys. The kidneys are often affected in critical care because of conditions such as acute kidney injury and multi-organ dysfunction syndrome. Drugs mainly cleared by the kidneys must be closely watched, since poor kidney function can result in high levels of medication, worsening the patient's condition, and increasing the risk of death. As an illustration, the effects of aminoglycosides and anticoagulants on the body are greatly influenced by renal function, so the amount given must be adjusted based on how well the kidneys are functioning. Close assessment of renal function parameters, such as serum creatinine and urine output, becomes essential to avoid potential drug toxicities owing to decreased elimination ratios in critical patients (Diep *et al.*, 2017). Drug interactions and variations in drug effects are also very important when managing medications in critical care. Having several comorbidities and taking several medicines can cause complex drug interactions, which can make it harder to manage the therapy. Sedatives and analgesics, which are commonly given to critically ill patients, may be cleared from the body differently if the liver or kidneys are not functioning properly. It is important for providers to take these interactions into account to guarantee that treatments are both safe and work well. Considering the profound implications of metabolism and elimination processes in critically ill patients, the formulation of individualized dosing strategies is crucial to achieving optimal clinical outcomes while minimizing adverse effects (Diep *et al.*, 2017).

Test Your Knowledge

1. How does critical illness affect the gastrointestinal absorption of medications?

What factors alter drug distribution in critically ill patients?

15.2. Common Medications Used in Critical Care

Learning Outcome

1. Define sedatives and analgesics
2. Discuss the vasopressors and inotropes
3. Explain the antibiotics and antifungals

Medication administration in critical care is detailed and important for patients to stabilize. Usually, vasopressors, sedatives, and analgesics are used, and they each play a key role in treating acute conditions. Doctors often give norepinephrine or dopamine to patients with shock or severe low blood pressure to keep their blood pressure stable. Since wrong administration may cause organ ischemia, it is vital that they work well. Nurses are responsible for making sure the drugs are given correctly, for watching for any problems, and for noticing any signs of poisoning. The emphasis on thorough pharmacological knowledge among nurses is supported by studies highlighting that medication errors greatly arise from gaps in understanding, particularly within critical care settings (Plenza *et al.*, 2025). Opioids and benzodiazepines are often given to patients in intensive care units to help with sedation during invasive procedures or to ease anxiety in seriously ill patients. It is essential to titrate these drugs properly, because they can cause serious problems such as slowed breathing and changes in blood pressure. More and more, healthcare teams rely on these drugs, which highlights the need for thorough pharmacological training. According to recent surveys, healthcare professionals recognize the need for improved access to technological tools that aid in obtaining critical dosing information and guidelines, thereby enhancing patient safety during sedation practices (Galindo *et al.*, 2025). Knowing all the possible risks from sedatives helps doctors prevent errors and improve the outcomes for patients. Along with their drug effects, using proper monitoring protocols is very important when giving common drugs in critical care. This involves monitoring the patient for any changes in their condition after medication administration, or if their health status changes. It is common for errors during administration, for example, wrong dosage, improper dilution, or scheduling, to happen more often in critical care units. So, following best practices and standard protocols is necessary to reduce these risks. In this case, nurses are the last step to prevent mistakes with medicines and should be given extra training in pharmacology to handle complicated medication routines. The intersection of pharmacological knowledge and practical administrative skills is imperative to provide safe, effective care in the critical care setting, ultimately leading to better patient outcomes (Plenza *et al.*, 2025).

15.2.1. Sedatives and Analgesics

Sedatives and analgesics are very important in critical care, since they help control pain and anxiety in patients facing serious illnesses and medical procedures. In the intensive care unit (ICU) setting, the administration of these pharmacological agents is essential to facilitate procedures, ensure patient comfort, and optimize outcomes. To induce sedation, doctors may use benzodiazepines and propofol, and opioids are usually given to manage pain. These drugs must be used with caution to avoid problems such as breathing difficulties and changes in blood pressure, which can happen in critical patients. Because the patients in critical care present unique problems, it is important for clinicians to know the pharmacology of these drugs to ensure safe and effective use of sedation and pain relief. A good example of sedative and analgesic use in critical care is ketamine, which is being used more often because of its many applications. Ketamine blocks the N-methyl-D-aspartate receptor and activates both the μ and κ opioid receptors, which causes pain relief and memory loss. Compared to most traditional sedatives, ketamine usually does not lead to low blood pressure or slow breathing, which is important for patients who need hemodynamic stability in the ICU. New research points out that ketamine works well for treating acute pain and helping patients who need to be sedated for mechanical ventilation. Nurses and clinicians must remain informed about the optimal clinical scenarios and monitoring parameters that guide the use of ketamine in the ICU, as its application can significantly impact patient management strategies (Brown *et al.*, 2020) (Figure 15.5).

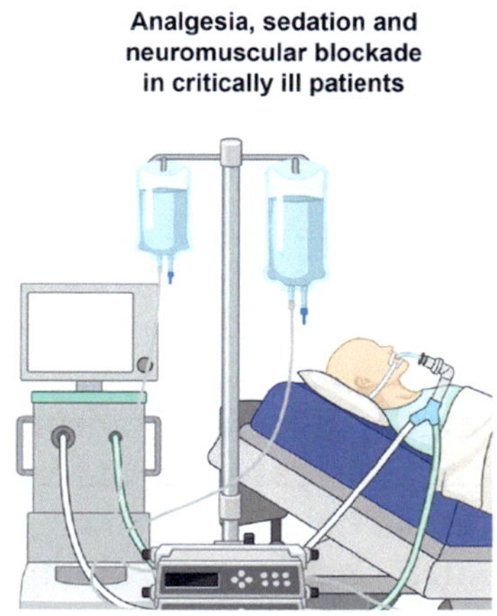

Figure 15.5. Analgesics, sedatives, and neuromuscular blockade in critically ill patients.

Source: https://healthmanagement.org/c/icu/issuearticle/analgesia-sedation-and-neuromuscular-blockade-in-critically-ill-patients.

Because of the COVID-19 pandemic, it is now more evident that sedatives and analgesics are crucial in critical care, especially for people dealing with acute respiratory distress syndrome. Because so many patients needed mechanical ventilation, there was a sudden increase in the need for medicines, which led to a lack of essential drugs such as sedatives and analgesics. Because of these challenges, clinicians started to use alternative therapies, which showed their effectiveness in treating sedation, pain, and paralysis in COVID-19 patients.

These methods, which are not commonly used in regular care, appeared to be helpful in treating critically ill patients during the pandemic. Understanding the pharmacological profiles, limitations, and potential adverse effects of these alternative treatments is vital for the ongoing management of critically ill patients, particularly in the context of future respiratory illness pandemics (Ammar *et al.*, 2020).

15.2.2. Vasopressors and Inotropes

In critical care medicine, vasopressors and inotropes are important for handling patients with severe problems related to blood pressure and heart function. These pharmacological agents are primarily employed to support blood pressure and enhance cardiac output in situations such as septic shock, cardiogenic shock, and acute respiratory distress syndrome (ARDS). Vasopressors, for example, norepinephrine and vasopressin, help by narrowing the blood vessels, which increases systemic vascular resistance and improves perfusion pressure. Alternatively, dobutamine and milrinone are used to strengthen heart contraction in people with reduced heart function because of underlying health problems. The correct and careful use of these agents helps to control blood pressure, which can impact the patient's health, so they must be chosen and monitored with care. Using vasopressors and inotropes can significantly increase the chances of survival in serious conditions like pulmonary embolism, which can cause major morbidity and mortality due to right ventricular dysfunction. If right ventricular failure occurs, it can make the heart's blood flow unstable, and giving these drugs promptly is very important. According to recent literature, prompt intervention with appropriate vasopressor therapy can reduce mortality rates associated with severe pulmonary embolism, as it directly addresses the cardiovascular collapse that can accompany this condition (Pérez-Nieto *et al.*, 2023). Moreover, studies have found that using hemodynamic support along with traditional treatments, for example, systemic thrombolysis, is a helpful way to handle these critical situations, making it clear that a variety of treatments is important in critical care. It is important to pay attention to the proper doses and monitoring of vasopressors and inotropes to ensure they work well and do not cause unnecessary side effects. Medical professionals treating people with severe acute respiratory infections, especially COVID-19, should weigh the sound effects of these drugs against the risks of arrhythmias and organ ischemia. It is also important to design individual treatment plans, since how patients respond to these drugs depends on their health problems and the severity of their condition. The World Health Organization emphasizes the importance of tailored management strategies in critical illness, reinforcing the need for thorough assessment and ongoing monitoring of hemodynamic status when deploying vasopressors and inotropes (World Health Organization, 2020). Using this method, clinicians can deal with the challenges in critical care pharmacology and help patients get the best results.

15.2.3. Antibiotics and Antifungals

Treating serious infections in the ICU depends greatly on giving antibiotics and antifungals as soon as possible. When sepsis occurs, due to the body's reaction to infection, prompt use of medications is needed to help the patient. Clinicians should start broad-spectrum antibiotics within one hour of spotting sepsis, mainly if septic shock is suspected. It is based on findings that each hour when antibiotics are not given promptly to septic patients results in higher death rates. The recommendations emphasize that early identification and treatment are crucial, aligning with the knowledge that prompt antimicrobial administration significantly contributes to reducing mortality in critically ill patients with infections (Evans *et al.*, 2021). The way these guidelines have changed highlights how important it is to respond quickly and effectively with drugs in critical care. Antibiotics are used first to treat bacterial infections, and antifungals are given to help with fungal infections, mainly in patients with weak immune systems. Because multidrug-resistant organisms are common in critical care, it is crucial to use the best possible antimicrobial regimens. Antibiograms from the area and the patient's condition should help choose the right agents. In guidelines about sepsis and septic shock management, empirical therapies must reflect a broad coverage to address both bacterial and potential fungal pathogens, particularly in patients at high risk for infection (Bhimraj *et al.*, 2020) (Figure 15.6).

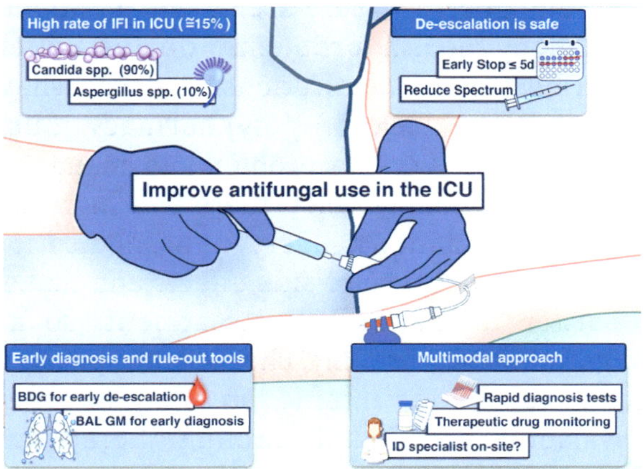

Figure 15.6. Antifungal stewardship in critically ill patients.

Source: https://media.springernature.com/lw1200/springer-static/image/art%3A10.1007%2Fs00134-023-07034-7/MediaObjects/134_2023_7034_Fig1_HTML.png.

This approach is needed for successful therapy and also to avoid more resistance by using treatments chosen based on culture results and susceptibilities. In critical care, the relationship between antibiotics and antifungals involves important points about pharmacokinetics and pharmacodynamics. When patients have septic shock, the dosing plan should make sure that enough of the drug reaches the infected area. The shift towards prolonged infusion methods for beta-lactams illustrates a trend aimed at maximizing therapeutic efficacy while minimizing toxicity (Evans *et al.*, 2021). Also, when culture results are available, reducing therapy is necessary to avoid adverse reactions and the growth of resistance. Using antibiotics and antifungals in this manner highlights the need for doctors to keep reviewing and changing treatment plans in critical care, since pharmacological management is always changing with the patient's condition.

Test Your Knowledge

1. What are the key differences between sedatives and analgesics in critical care?
2. How do vasopressors and inotropes support cardiovascular function in critically ill patients?

15.3. Drug Interactions in Critical Care

Learning Outcome

1. Define polypharmacy and its implications
2. Identify the impact of organ dysfunction on drug interactions
3. Discuss the strategies to minimize adverse interactions

Drug interactions are more complicated in critical care because patients often take many medications. In intensive care units, patients often receive multiple medications to address various acute conditions simultaneously, increasing the likelihood of drug-drug interactions (DDIs). These interactions can lead to adverse drug reactions (ADRs), which may further complicate patient management. To use pharmacological therapy well, one must understand what the drugs can do and what problems they might cause. In those who are already at risk, it is important to carefully review DDIs, since they can worsen conditions such as neurological or cardiac complications. Therefore, clinicians must continuously evaluate medication regimens to mitigate the risk of these interactions, ensuring that the benefits of drug therapies outweigh any potential harm, a critical consideration highlighted in the findings of over 52,000 medication analyses conducted in a high-stakes environment (Wolf *et al.*, 2022). In addition, situations like treating acute seizures show the importance of knowing about drug interactions in critical care pharmacology. Care of seizures in critically ill individuals requires drugs that work quickly, are safe, and do not interact with other medicines they are receiving. Intravenous brivaracetam (IV BRV), for instance, has emerged as a recommended option for treating acute seizures in hospital settings due to its favorable safety profile and efficacy. IV BRV has demonstrated that effective treatment is possible, even in situations where various medications interact and might usually make it challenging to provide the best care.

The careful evaluation of clinical studies sheds light on the administration of IV BRV, revealing not only its effectiveness but also a low incidence of behavioral side effects, making it a promising candidate for critically ill patients (Lee *et al.*, 2022). Managing drug interactions in critical care goes further than only noticing side effects; it requires using personalized drug treatments to help patients and improve treatment outcomes. Healthcare professionals must use clinical pharmacology with patient management tools to be ready for and address possible DDIs. Regular training and following the rules can help practitioners decide properly about giving medications. Suppose healthcare providers are always aware of the risks of polypharmacy; in that case they can put in place measures to ensure patients do not experience adverse effects, which leads to safer and more effective antimicrobial therapies. This proactive approach is vital to achieving successful outcomes in the high-pressure context of critical care (Wolf *et al.*, 2022).

15.3.1. Polypharmacy and Its Implications

The use of several drugs at the same time by a patient is known as polypharmacy, and it can cause important issues in pharmacology, especially in critical care areas. When patients have many health problems, doctors often prescribe several medications at once, which increases the risk of polypharmacy. Such complexity may create problems in managing medications, mainly when there is a high risk of drug interactions. Every new medication increases the chance of side effects and makes it harder to manage the treatment, so all drugs must be carefully checked for possible interactions. Such interactions may manifest in various forms, undermining therapeutic efficacy or, in some cases, precipitating serious complications, thereby heightening the need for vigilant oversight in critical care environments (Figure 15.7).

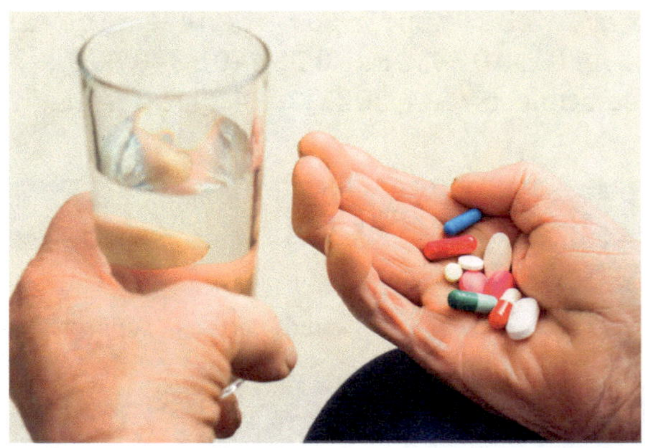

Figure 15.7. Polypharmacy.

Source: https://ceufast.com/imgs/polypharmacy-virus.jpg.

Therefore, polypharmacy can cause serious problems for patients, raising their chances of getting sick and dying. Multiple medications can disrupt how drugs interact, which may result in one drug making the other act in an unplanned way. Critical care often involves patients with cardiovascular disease or chronic kidney disease, so the risk of these interactions is much greater. It has been found that traditional clinical trials rarely investigate drug-drug interactions in depth, which leaves a knowledge gap that affects how well patients are cared for. Therefore, clinicians must remain cognizant of the potential ramifications of polypharmacy, striving to balance the necessity for comprehensive treatment against the imperative to minimize risks associated with multiple medications (Žitnik *et al.*, 2018). New tools like Decagon can provide valuable insights for predicting and managing the side effects associated with polypharmacy. This tool uses multimodal graphs to show how drugs and proteins are related and interact, which improves our awareness of polypharmacy risks. Decagon can help clinicians identify the side effects linked to different drug combinations, which should greatly improve their decision-making. The need for real-time changes and monitoring is high in critical care, so such technological progress is beneficial. As research evolves, leveraging sophisticated tools like Decagon can provide invaluable data to flag potential problematic combinations early, thereby fostering safer and more effective pharmacological management in high-stakes environments (Davies *et al.*, 2018).

15.3.2. Impact of Organ Dysfunction on Drug Interactions

The interplay between organ dysfunction and drug interactions is a critical consideration in the pharmacotherapy of patients in intensive care settings. If the organs that handle drug processing and removal do not function properly, as is common in critically ill patients, the way drugs are handled in the body may change a lot. A problem with liver function can slow the clearance of drugs, which can result in more of the drug being present in the body and a greater chance of toxicity. Also, when kidney function is impaired, it affects the way drugs are eliminated, so doctors may need to change the dosage to avoid problems. Because patients in critical care often take several medications, there is a higher chance of drugs affecting the same metabolic pathways, which can cause unexpected interactions that can influence the patient's condition. So, it is important to understand these factors when managing pharmacotherapy for these patients. Acute conditions in pharmacology tend to make existing organ issues worse, which can cause more drug interactions. Sepsis is an example where multiple organs can fail, and these failures can greatly affect drug metabolism. Drugs taken by mouth might not be adequately absorbed if the gastrointestinal tract is not working as it should, and the distribution of drugs may change because of changes in body fluids and protein levels. Because of this scenario, it is essential to use strict therapeutic drug monitoring to help with the correct dosing. There is a greater chance of adverse drug interactions, which means it is important to involve pharmacists in managing medications. For those who are critically ill and taking antiretroviral therapy, organ dysfunction is significant. Adjusting dosing regimens becomes imperative to ensure therapeutic efficacy while minimizing potential toxicities and drug interactions, underscoring the complexity of pharmacological management in critical care settings (Via *et al.*, 2025). Studies suggest that some drugs might not work the same when organ function is affected which can change the effectiveness of treatment. Acetaminophen, which is taken for its pain-relieving and fever-reducing effects, is being studied as in a this particular case. A recent study tested whether giving acetaminophen through a vein could help patients with sepsis who have organ dysfunction. While the study found that acetaminophen was safe and did not markedly enhance days alive free of organ support, it did indicate some improvement in specific secondary outcomes, such as lower SOFA scores in the treatment group (Ware *et al.*, 2024). This example shows that some drugs can still work well in the hospital, even when things are not perfect and it stresses the need to consider the setting when judging drug effectiveness in critically ill people. It is essential for clinicians to understand how drugs work differently in order to give the best treatment to their patients in the intensive care unit.

15.3.3. Strategies to Minimize Adverse Interactions

Handling polypharmacy is difficult in critical care, since patients are usually given several drugs at the same time. A good way to reduce risks is to review all a patient's medications carefully when they are admitted and at other times during their stay. When each medication is reviewed, healthcare providers can spot possible interactions, similar drugs being taken, and conditions where the drugs should not be given. Doing this improves safety for patients and also makes it possible to adjust their medications and consider various alternative treatments. Talking with patients and their caregivers about their medications can help them understand their treatment better and stick to it, which can lead to better results in critical care. Using clinical practice guidelines that are based on evidence is also very important for preventing drug interactions. Organizations such as the American College of Cardiology and the American Heart Association provide comprehensive guidelines that inform clinicians on the safe use of medications, incorporating the latest evidence to define classes of recommendations and levels of evidence for specific therapies (Whelton *et al.*, 2017). They provide a structure for deciding what to take or not, focusing on both effectiveness and safety, which lowers the risk of harmful reactions. Also, having decision support systems in electronic health records allows healthcare professionals to spot potential interactions at the time of care and act quickly when needed. When these resources are actively added to clinical work, patients are safer and their treatments are more effective. Another important approach is to watch for proper levels of drugs given in critical care to avoid harmful drug interactions. Many medications have a slight difference between safe and unsafe levels, so it is important to manage them well to avoid either problem. Regularly checking on patients helps clinicians adjust dosages according to how patients react to the drugs and any interactions that occur. For instance, drugs commonly used in critical care, such as anticoagulants and anticonvulsants, often require meticulous monitoring to ensure that drug levels remain within the desired range (Mach *et al.*, 2019). Also, being familiar with pharmacokinetic and pharmacodynamic principles is important when assessing possible drug interactions, because it allows clinicians to predict drug efficacy and safety. If healthcare teams are attentive and know about drugs, they can significantly reduce the risks of drug interactions in critically ill patients.

Test Your Knowledge

1. What are the risks associated with polypharmacy in critically ill patients?
2. How does organ dysfunction influence drug-drug interactions in the ICU?

15.4. Dosing Considerations in Critical Care

Learning Outcome

1. Explain the weight-based dosing versus fixed dosing
2. Define adjustments for renal and hepatic impairment
5. Understand the monitoring therapeutic drug levels

The need for proper dosing is essential in critical care because patients have different physiological changes during their illness. Patients in ICUs usually have changes in how their bodies handle drugs, which can influence the way a drug is absorbed, distributed, metabolized, and excreted. Organ function, the amount of fluids in the body, and other health problems should be considered. As an example, critically ill patients often have too much fluid in their bodies or different body composition, which may require changing the dose of hydrophilic medications. The function of the kidneys and liver can change a lot, which can affect how drugs are cleared from the body and may require regular checks and possible dose adjustments to prevent harm or failure of treatment. Health professionals must integrate these complexities into their dosing strategies while ensuring adherence to best practice guidelines (Mach *et al.*, 2019). It is crucial to use the right doses of sedatives and painkillers to help patients in critical care. Managing pain and agitation often starts with sedatives and analgesics, but their doses should be given with care. The use of guidelines such as the PADIS guidelines points out that pain and sedation should be managed for each patient, considering the possible dangers of drugs. In critical care, healthcare professionals may use several approaches to help patients with pain and use fewer opioids. As demonstrated in the updated evidence, the effectiveness of using adjunct medications, like acetaminophen and neuropathic pain agents, reflects an emerging paradigm in which clinicians aim to enhance analgesia while reducing side effects (Devlin *et al.*, 2018). Using this detailed and scientific approach to dosing greatly helps to improve how patients do in the short and long term. Also, using live clinical data to guide medication dosing is a developing aspect of critical care pharmacology. Because of better technology and monitoring, clinicians can now evaluate how medicines work in each patient and change the doses accordingly. Pharmacogenomics and precision medicine are being used more often which helps create drug regimens that consider differences in how genes affect drug metabolism. Also, using data to guide dosing is in line with the main goals of clinical guidelines which are patient safety and effectiveness. As critical care continues to advance, the necessity for rigorous evaluation and adaptation of dosing strategies will be paramount, ultimately contributing to the overarching goal of enhancing patient care and clinical effectiveness (Mach *et al.*, 2019).

15.4.1. Weight-Based Dosing Versus Fixed Dosing

In critical care pharmacology, the method of administering medications, whether by weight or fixed dose, is crucial for achieving optimal patient outcomes. Weight-based dosing changes the amount of medicine given based on a person's weight, which is meant to give more personalized care. This method is essential for critically ill patients, since changes in body composition can strongly affect how drugs are used in the body. In cases of sepsis and septic shock, when quick action is needed, giving the correct dose can help ensure the drug reaches the right level in the body, which can increase the patient's chances of survival. Recommendations underscore that therapeutic efficacy may be compromised when fixed dosing regimens are employed, potentially leading to subtherapeutic effects or drug toxicity, particularly in populations with diverse body morphologies and physiological conditions (Evans *et al.*, 2021). Alternatively, fixed dosing is easier to give, since it reduces the chance of making mistakes when figuring out how much medicine to give according to weight. With this approach, it is easier to follow the correct dosages, mainly when there is much activity in the ICU. Still, using the same dose for all patients can miss what is needed for those with obesity or severe malnutrition, since their drug absorption may be different. It might be best to use a mix of both methods, since this way, personalized care is possible and patients can still feel secure. The challenge lies in developing standardized dosing protocols that can adapt to both weight-based and fixed strategies without compromising treatment excellence or safety for the critically ill (Kolasinski *et al.*, 2020). The decision between weight-based and fixed dosing should depend on the patient's condition, personal characteristics, and the way the medicine acts. More research is necessary to decide when each way of giving medicine should be used. Since patient care is critical in emergency situations, the right way of giving medication can greatly affect the results. Continued education and adjustments in protocols, informed by the latest evidence, will be essential to adapt to the evolving landscape of pharmacological strategies in critical care (Evans *et al.*, 2021). Furthermore, fostering collaboration among healthcare professionals to evaluate the appropriateness of dosing strategies in real-time can enhance decision-making processes, ultimately leading to improved patient-centered care outcomes in the ICU environment (Kolasinski *et al.*, 2020).

15.4.2. Adjustments for Renal and Hepatic Impairment

It is essential to make changes in medicine dosing for kidney and liver problems when caring for critically ill patients. Impairments in the kidneys and liver can change the way many medications are handled by the body. Because of renal impairment and the subsequent decrease in glomerular filtration rate, drugs that are removed by the kidneys may build up in the body and cause toxicity. So, healthcare professionals should use caution when prescribing these drugs and adjust their dosage and how often they are given depending on the patient's current renal function. Similarly, hepatic impairment can disrupt the metabolism of drugs primarily processed by the liver, necessitating dose adjustments to avoid adverse effects associated with drug accumulation and interactions with other medications, as highlighted in the literature regarding pharmacological management in critical care settings (Rosenblat *et al.*, 2019). Renal and hepatic function must be monitored and adjusted throughout the patient's care. Clinicians typically rely on laboratory values, including serum creatinine, blood urea nitrogen (BUN), and liver enzyme levels, to evaluate renal and hepatic function. The evaluation supports the process of choosing the right dose and way to give the medication. Because patient status in critical care can change fast, these assessments should be repeated often to catch any changes early. Furthermore, understanding the pharmacodynamics of medications in conjunction with renal and hepatic function allows healthcare providers to tailor therapeutic regimens that minimize risks while maximizing therapeutic benefits, ensuring that the patient's overall health does not further deteriorate (Mach *et al.*, 2019). New studies keep stressing that tailored drug therapy is important for patients with renal and hepatic impairments, especially in critical care situations. Different people respond differently to medications because of how well their organs function, so a patient-centered approach is needed. Following the set guidelines that address renal and hepatic impairment has been linked to better results and fewer complications. When pharmacological care in critical care changes, including these adjustments, will improve patient safety and help patients stick to the prescribed treatment. Thus, the need for ongoing education and research regarding the pharmacokinetic and pharmacodynamic implications of renal and hepatic impairments remains paramount within the field (Rosenblat *et al.*, 2019).

15.4.3. Monitoring Therapeutic Drug Levels

Monitoring levels of drug in patients is crucial in critical care pharmacology, because treating critically ill patients can be very complicated. TDM means that healthcare providers can change the dosage of drugs based on the drug levels found in the patient's blood. This approach matters a lot in acute care because patients there often react differently to drugs than patients in stable conditions. By implementing TDM, practitioners can optimize drug efficacy while simultaneously minimizing the risk of adverse effects, which is vital for patient safety in critical care environments (Suneja *et al.*, 2025). The need for TDM is especially clear in the case of HIV infection in patients who are very sick. The clinical pharmacology of antiretroviral therapy (ART) is particularly complex due to factors such as altered absorption and metabolism that occur in critically ill individuals. Any changes in the body's systems, such as poor gastrointestinal function or problems with the liver or kidneys, might call for an altered medication schedule to keep drug levels safe. Also, since there is a greater chance of drug-drug interactions with polypharmacy, it is important to monitor ART to ensure both safety and effectiveness. Thus, TDM not only assists in individualizing treatment but also plays a vital role in preventing toxicities associated with high drug levels in this vulnerable patient population (Via *et al.*, 2025). Moreover, using TDM supports the use of different medical specialties in handling drug therapy in critical care units. When critical care physicians, clinical pharmacists, and infectious disease specialists work together, the success of treatment can be improved. They cooperate to examine and interpret the results of drug levels, so that immediate actions can be taken when needed. When teams collaborate, patients tend to recover better, and doctors are better able to decide on proper medication and monitoring. Moreover, the ongoing research into advanced monitoring technologies and personalized medicine opens new avenues for effective therapeutic interventions, potentially transforming the landscape of drug management in critical care (Suneja *et al.*, 2025) (Figure 15.8).

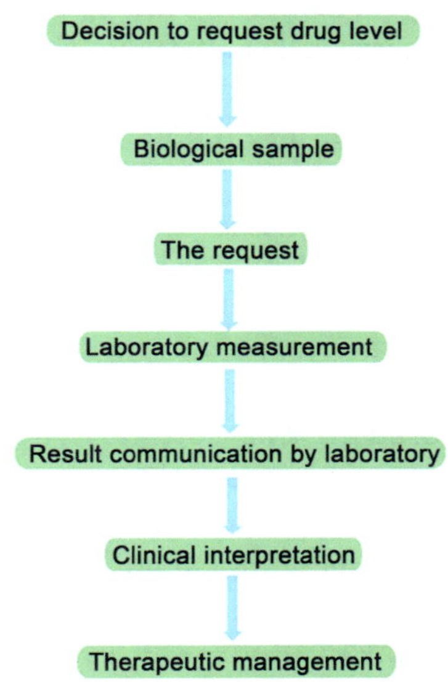

Figure 15.8. The process of monitoring therapeutic drug levels.

Source: https://www.creative-diagnostics.com/upload/image/small-molecule-drug-antibodies-and-conjugates-1.png.

Test Your Knowledge

1. When is weight-based dosing preferred over fixed dosing in critical care?
2. Why are dose adjustments necessary in patients with renal or hepatic impairment?

15.5. Role of Pharmacists in Critical Care

Learning Outcome

1. Define medication management and reconciliation
2. Discuss the participation in multidisciplinary teams
3. Explain the education and training for healthcare staff

Pharmacists are now widely seen as important members of the team that looks after patients with complicated medical conditions. Pharmacists in the ICU help improve the way medications are given by considering the special changes happening in critically ill patients. Compromised health often leads these patients to have changes in drug absorption, distribution, metabolism, and excretion. Pharmacists, physicians, and nurses collaborate to design personalized treatment plans so that the therapies used are suitable and effective. Their involvement can significantly reduce medication-related problems (MRPs), enhancing the overall safety and quality of care delivered in this setting. When clinical pharmacy services are used in critical care, everyone on the team gains from better patient outcomes, and patients spend less time in the hospital. They are responsible for overseeing the current medications and also for spotting and stopping any possible drug interactions that may occur in critical care. Because patients in ICUs are given several medications at once, the chance of adverse effects goes up a lot. Because of this environment, it is important to keep monitoring pharmaceutical interventions to guarantee they are safe and effective. Pharmacists are prepared to review all the medications a patient is on when they are admitted, moved, or discharged. They also check if the current therapies are appropriate, especially when there is organ dysfunction or renal replacement therapy is involved. In this multidimensional role, pharmacists utilize their training to make recommendations concerning therapy modifications, dosage adjustments, and drug discontinuations, ultimately leading to improved pharmacological management of critically ill patients (Naseralallah *et al.*, 2023). In addition, pharmacists can have a big impact on outcomes in critical care by using therapeutic drug monitoring. Since drug pharmacokinetics can differ greatly, using therapeutic drug monitoring, pharmacists can adjust doses according to each patient's reactions, mainly for antiretroviral drugs. Because absorption may be changed in severely ill patients, these drugs may not work as intended and thus need to be given in smaller or larger doses. It is important to watch for how well drugs are working and for any side effects, and pharmacists play a key role in this. By fostering a collaborative approach with other healthcare professionals, pharmacists can address the challenges related to drug administration in critical care, ultimately enhancing patient safety and therapeutic efficacy (Via *et al.*, 2025).

15.5.1. Medication Management and Reconciliation

Because patient cases are very complex in critical care, managing and reconciling medications is extremely important. Patients in ICUs commonly have several health issues, and their conditions can change very quickly. For this reason, medication errors happen often, which can result in adverse drug events that can increase both a patient's sickness and chances of death. A team of intensivists, clinical pharmacists, and nurses is needed to guarantee that medications are managed systematically. For example, pharmacists check the patient's medication list upon admission and discharge from the ICU, making sure the medications are right for their health, allergies, and possible interactions with other drugs. As stated in the literature, optimal interprofessional team performance hinges on efficient communication, which is vital for comprehensive medication management in critical care settings (Kleinpell *et al.*, 2021) (Figure 15.9).

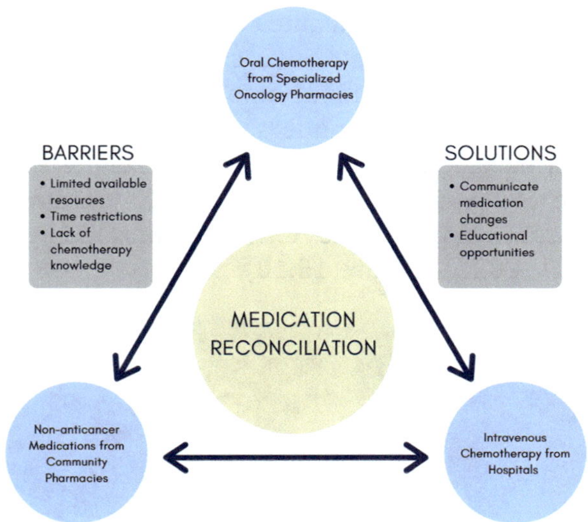

Figure 15.9. Implementing the medicines reconciliation.

Source: https://www.tandfonline.com/cms/asset/6bd985a0-442d-4b5d-b20c-d225f894d851/jppp_a_12315289_f0003.png.

Also, having a set process for medication reconciliation reduces the chances of errors when patients move from one unit or setting to another. It helps prevent mistakes with medicines and supports the ongoing care of seriously ill patients. Each time a patient is admitted, the challenge comes from their different treatment history before coming to the ICU. Talking to patients and their families about what drugs they have taken before can uncover any concerns about their previous medications. Patients in the ICU should be told about any new medications and reminded of the importance of following the instructions when they go home. A robust medication reconciliation process can significantly reduce hospital readmission rates, which is especially relevant for critically ill patients who have higher rates of complications in postoperative settings (Liu *et al.*, 2020). Regular review and updates of medication information are necessary to maintain a good approach to medication reconciliation during the patient's time in the ICU. Because the health of critical care patients can change rapidly, doctors must keep checking how well and safely the drugs are working. Having pharmacists join in on regular interdisciplinary rounds helps make changes as patients react and new guidelines are released. It is also necessary to check renal function and other lab tests to help decide on the correct dose of medicines that have a narrow range of safe doses. Ultimately, successful medication management in critical care not only safeguards against adverse drug events but also enhances overall treatment outcomes, demonstrating the importance of a cohesive interprofessional effort in the reconciliation process (Kleinpell *et al.*, 2021).

15.5.2. Participation in Multidisciplinary Teams

Having multidisciplinary teams involved in critical care helps improve patient outcomes, especially in pharmacology. In these collaborative environments, each member contributes their specialized knowledge, which can significantly decrease the incidence of drug-related problems (DRPs). Critical care pharmacists (CCPs), for instance, play a pivotal role in evaluating medication orders, often identifying potential DRPs that could lead to adverse drug events. Pharmacists joining medical rounds each day have proven to help doctors decide faster and allow patients to leave the hospital sooner because all medicines are appropriately managed. Also, when CCPs are proactive about medication reconciliation, it helps protect critically ill patients from possible problems caused by polypharmacy and incorrect medication choices. It shows how important it is for healthcare professionals to work together in critical care. In ICUs, where things move quickly, healthcare teams join forces on more than just giving medications. As an illustration, projects that help the environment, such as recycling, bring the entire critical care team together to address environmental problems in healthcare. Involving the multidisciplinary team in a project to increase the recycling of single-use plastic enteral feed bottles led to more people being aware of ecological issues. Joining forces in this way builds teamwork and a strong dedication to patients, which leads to better health results and brings the healthcare team together. Multidisciplinary involvement, according to these engagements, can encourage new ideas and positive changes in critical care. Multidisciplinary teams work well when team members can communicate openly and trust each other. In critical care settings, this is very important since fast decisions can affect a patient's life. By joining efforts, nurses, physicians, and pharmacists can handle challenging cases by thinking about all the patient's needs. It has been found that working together in this way, mainly when the focus is urgent, can reduce adverse outcomes and make care better. When team members have a good relationship and can easily communicate, they can easily share ideas, discuss issues, and work together, which promotes accountability among all team members. Participating well in multidisciplinary teams helps to improve pharmacological care and also benefits the overall health of patients in critical care.

15.5.3. Education and Training for Healthcare Staff

Training healthcare workers in critical care areas, with special attention to pharmacology, is essential for achieving the best possible results for patients. Since critical care deals with serious health issues, healthcare workers must be familiar with medicines, how much to give, what can happen if medications are combined, and what side effects to expect. When healthcare providers are trained using theory and practice, they learn to manage complicated drug treatments. Pharmacological treatments can be kept safe and effective by practicing continuous development, following up-to-date guidelines, and checking the outcomes. Furthermore, as highlighted by interprofessional collaboration in intensive care units, regular educational interactions among team members facilitate a deeper understanding of different pharmacological perspectives and strategies, thus improving patient management and monitoring practices in high-stakes environments (Kleinpell *et al.*, 2021) (Figure 15.10).

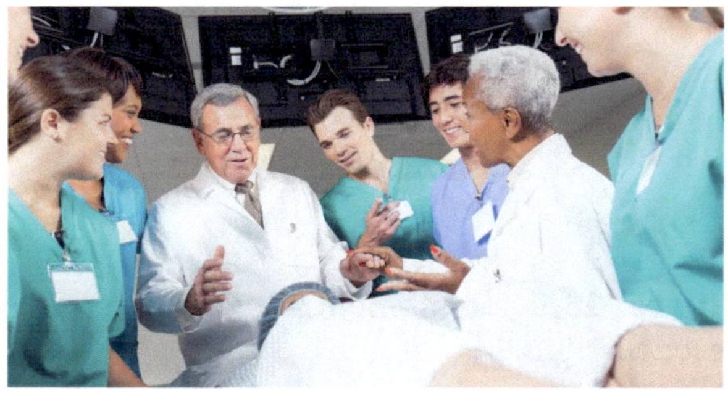

Figure 15.10. Training healthcare workers in critical care areas.

Source: https://tinehealth.com/wp-content/uploads/2017/05/Tine-Website-Photos-Articles-12.jpg.

Simulation training is very important for critical care staff in pharmacology. They make it possible for healthcare workers to practice using real-world clinical scenarios, thus helping them use pharmacology skills. For example, practicing how to give drugs during cardiac arrest or septic shock can greatly increase the ability of healthcare workers. Participating in simulations helps people practice thinking critically and learn to handle urgent pharmacological situations. In addition, these simulations help nurses work together and communicate well, which is important for carrying out complicated care plans in intensive care units and making sure drug therapies are used effectively. The incorporation of simulation in education ensures that healthcare staff remain proficient and confident in their pharmacological knowledge and application, directly impacting patient safety and care quality in critical scenarios (Kirkpatrick *et al.*, 2020). Because pharmacology keeps advancing, people in critical care need to be informed about the newest research and drug therapies. More healthcare institutions are realizing that including evidence-based pharmacology guidelines in their training programs is important. By being proactive, healthcare workers can keep up with new drug information and change their practices as needed. Along with interdisciplinary programs, encouraging healthcare professionals to keep learning in pharmacology using online courses, workshops, and journal clubs improves their ability to handle new challenges. As a result, patients receive well-informed, timely pharmacological interventions that are crucial in critical care settings, ultimately leading to improved health outcomes and enhanced recovery rates (Kleinpell *et al.*, 2021).

Test Your Knowledge

1. Why is medication reconciliation important in critical care settings?
2. What is the role of ongoing education and training in ensuring safe medication practices?

SUMMARY

A Summary in pharmacology, especially in critical care medicine, helps to gather and explain the research results and their effects on practice. Because healthcare is moving towards evidence-based care, knowing the details of critical care drugs is very important. Lately, people have pointed out that different ways of labeling and formulating norepinephrine may have a big impact on clinical practice. A task force convened by critical care specialists emphasized the need for a standardized approach to norepinephrine formulations to optimize patient safety and ensure uniformity in dosage calculations across countries (Wieruszewski *et al.*, 2024). This recommendation matters a lot since it shows how pharmacology, outcomes and research integrity are connected. Moreover, the incorporation of simulation-based learning (SBL) in medical education reflects the ongoing evolution in preparing future healthcare providers for the complexities of critical care scenarios. Studies indicate that SBL significantly enhances student satisfaction and self-confidence, thereby equipping them with essential skills to handle pharmacological interventions during critical situations (Ageel, 2024). Because medical education is changing to include these teaching methods, the benefits for critical care pharmacology are very significant. This approach to Learning helps students grasp pharmacology better, which encourages them to make wise decisions in important situations. Pharmacology in critical care points out that we should constantly be researching, standardizing, and educating. The challenges presented by varying formulations of medications, such as norepinephrine, necessitate critical examination and consensus among practitioners to enhance patient care (Wieruszewski *et al.*, 2024). Innovative strategies such as SBL, when used with other methods, are preparing pharmacology in critical care for major progress. Improving clinical practices and education simultaneously helps achieve the main goal of providing high-quality care to patients in critical situations, with nurses and physicians being ready to handle what the field requires.

Using medications is very important in the management of life-threatening illnesses in critical care. Noticing the variety in critical illnesses allows healthcare professionals to use drugs appropriately. A crucial aspect of pharmacology in this setting involves the management of acute kidney injury (AKI), which frequently arises in critically ill patients. AKI requires special care, such as renal replacement therapy, to deal with kidney-related issues that might have a big impact on patient outcomes. Consequently, healthcare providers must stay informed about the latest developments in critical care nephrology and the management options available, as detailed discussions in the literature highlight the importance of individualized treatment strategies that consider these patient's unique needs and risks (Bonilla *et al.*, 2025). The use of anticoagulants, particularly unfractionated heparin (UFH), represents a critical element in the pharmacologic management of critically ill patients. Understanding the pharmacodynamics and pharmacokinetics of UFH to prevent thrombosis and bleeding complications. Experts now believe that the usual monitoring techniques for UFH have many limitations which make it hard for clinicians to be confident about the best doses and ranges of treatment. Besides, the effects of antithrombin levels and resistance add more issues, so it is important to review current UFH administration practices. With limited validated data on optimal usage and dosing regimens, future clinical research must focus on refining UFH management strategies and enhancing anticoagulation monitoring methodologies (Gouin-Thibault *et al.*, 2024). All in all, the world of pharmacology in critical care keeps changing and growing. With the presence of AKI and the difficulties of UFH anticoagulation, clinicians need to use evidence and tailor care to each patient. Having a strong focus on both urgent issues and the details of pharmacotherapy allows healthcare teams to make major improvements for their patients. Moreover, the ongoing dialogue surrounding the challenges and advancements in critical care pharmacology will inevitably influence future research and clinical practice, ensuring a high standard of care that addresses the multifaceted nature of critical illnesses (Bonilla *et al.*, 2025; Gouin-Thibault *et al.*, 2024).

KEY TERMS FROM THIS CHAPTER

- ACE inhibitors
- Analgesics
- Antibiotics
- Anticoagulants
- Antifungals
- Antihypertensives
- Antiplatelets
- Antivirals
- Benzodiazepines
- Beta-blockers
- Calcium channel blockers
- Corticosteroids
- Critical care medications
- Diuretics
- H2 antagonists
- Inotropes
- Insulin
- Neuromuscular blockers
- Opioids
- Pharmacology
- Sedatives
- Thrombolytics
- Vasopressors

CRITICAL THINKING QUESTIONS

1. **Which of the following medications is most commonly used to manage hypertension in a critically ill patient?**
    a. Lisinopril
    b. Nitroprusside
    c. Metoprolol
    d. Amlodipine
2. **In a critically ill patient with acute respiratory distress syndrome (ARDS), which pharmacologic intervention is often used to reduce inflammation and improve oxygenation?**
    a. Steroids
    b. Diuretics
    c. Dopamine
    d. Beta-blockers
3. **Which of the following drugs is most commonly used to prevent stress ulcers in critically ill patients?**
    a. Warfarin
    b. Proton pump inhibitors (PPIs)
    c. Insulin
    d. Heparin
4. **In septic shock, the initial pharmacologic intervention after fluid resuscitation should be the use of:**
    a. Insulin
    b. Vasopressors
    c. Antibiotics
    d. Anticoagulants
5. **Which of the following medications is primarily used for sedation in intubated and mechanically ventilated ICU patients?**
    a. Propofol
    b. Atenolol
    c. Lorazepam
    d. Furosemide

Short Answer Questions

1. How do pharmacokinetics and pharmacodynamics matter for critically ill patients and how do they impact the choice of drug dosage?
2. How does organ dysfunction (e.g., liver or kidney failure) impact drug metabolism and elimination in critically ill patients?
3. What is drug half-life and how is it important for giving proper doses to critically ill patients?
4. What problems can arise from using multiple drugs in critical patients and how can risks due to drug interactions be reduced?
5. How should treatment with drugs be adjusted when septic shock is present, mainly regarding antimicrobials and vasopressors?

Answer to Critical Thinking Questions

1. (b); 2. (a); 3. (b); 4. (b); 5. (a)

REFERENCES

1. Ageel, M. (2024). Assessing the impact of simulation-based learning on student satisfaction and self-confidence in critical care medicine. *Critical Care Research and Practice, 2024*. https://www.semanticscholar.org/paper/8128e7817480ecaa7de1e2c7ec9ef0b00ad49923 (accessed on 22 May 2025).
2. Ammar, M., Sacha, G. L., Welch, S., Bass, S., Kane-Gill, S. L., Duggal, A., & Ammar, A. (2020). Sedation, analgesia, and paralysis in COVID-19 patients in the setting of drug shortages. *Journal of Intensive Care Medicine, 36*, 157–174. https://doi.org/10.1177/0885066620951426.
3. Ando, Y., & Jou, J. H. (2021). Non-alcoholic fatty liver disease and recent guideline updates. *Clinical Liver Disease, 17*, 23–28. https://doi.org/10.1002/cld.1045.
4. Barbas, C. (2023). The role of women as critical care physicians. *Revita da Associação Médica Brasileira, 69*. https://www.semanticscholar.org/paper/061b451f202c974a84023d1f78fc1cb81810b286 (accessed on 22 May 2025).
5. Becker, W. C., & Fiellin, D. A. (2020). When epidemics collide: Coronavirus disease 2019 (COVID-19) and the opioid crisis. *Annals of Internal Medicine, 173*, 59–60. https://doi.org/10.7326/m20-1210.
6. Bhimraj, A., Morgan, R. L., Shumaker, A. H., Lavergne, V., Baden, L. R., Cheng, V. C. C., Edwards, K. M., *et al.* (2020). Infectious Diseases Society of America guidelines on the treatment and management of patients with COVID-19 (April 2020). *Clinical Infectious Diseases, 78*, e83–e102. https://doi.org/10.1093/cid/ciaa478.
7. Bonilla, M. A., Koyner, J. L., & Neyra, J. A. (2025). Acute kidney injury and critical care nephrology. *Advances in Kidney Disease and Health, 32*(1), 12–23. https://www.semanticscholar.org/paper/e51d4d0bfbb7f73cef903eec0ff4d1031b9e70af (accessed on 22 May 2025).
8. Bourgonje, A. R., Abdulle, A. E., Timens, W., Hillebrands, J. L., Navis, G., Gordijn, S. J., Bolling, M. C., *et al.* (2020). Angiotensin-converting enzyme 2 (ACE2), SARS-CoV-2 and the pathophysiology of coronavirus disease 2019 (COVID-19). *The Journal of Pathology, 251*, 228–248. https://doi.org/10.1002/path.5471.
9. Brown, K., & Tucker, C. (2020). Ketamine for acute pain management and sedation. *Critical Care Nurse, 40*, e26–e32. https://doi.org/10.4037/ccn2020419.
10. Chung, J., Tjia, J., Zhang, N., & O'Connor, B. T. (2023). Anticholinergic burden and xerostomia in critical care settings. *Dimensions of Critical Care Nursing, 42*, 310–318. https://www.semanticscholar.org/paper/cd02761c9f64222a33cc705c722be5ea8797fbb2 (accessed on 22 May 2025).
11. Cristina, M. L., Spagnolo, A. M., Sartini, M., Carbone, A., Oliva, M., Schinca, E., Boni, S., *et al.* (2023). An overview on *Candida auris* in healthcare settings. *Journal of Fungi, 9*. https://www.semanticscholar.org/paper/0a37ebd753c83d1c1ed01b40982e923ef6f250e7 (accessed on 22 May 2025).
12. D'Amario, D., Arcudi, A., Narducci, M., Novelli, V., Canonico, F., Parodi, A., Dell'Era, G., *et al.* (2025). Arrhythmic risk stratification and sudden cardiac death prevention in Duchenne muscular dystrophy: A critical appraisal. *Reviews in Cardiovascular Medicine, 26*. https://www.semanticscholar.org/paper/02dc39692eb8872ba8a8122385632c9ac12575a5 (accessed on 22 May 2025).

13. Davies, M. J., D'Alessio, D. A., Fradkin, J., Kernan, W. N., Mathieu, C., Mingrone, G., Rossing, P., *et al.* (2018). Management of hyperglycemia in type 2 diabetes, 2018: A consensus report by the American Diabetes Association (ADA) and the European Association for the Study of Diabetes (EASD). *Diabetes Care, 41*, 2669–2701. https://doi.org/10.2337/dci18-0033.

14. De Rosa, S., Samoni, S., Villa, G., & Ronco, C. (2017). Management of chronic kidney disease patients in the intensive care unit: Mixing acute and chronic illness. *Blood Purification, 43*, 151–162. https://doi.org/10.1159/000452650.

15. Devlin, J. W., Skrobik, Y., Gélinas, C., Needham, D. M., Slooter, A. J. C., Pandharipande, P. P., Watson, P. L., *et al.* (2018). Executive summary: Clinical practice guidelines for the prevention and management of pain, agitation/sedation, delirium, immobility, and sleep disruption in adult patients in the ICU. *Critical Care Medicine, 46*, 1532–1548. https://doi.org/10.1097/ccm.0000000000003259.

16. Diep, U., Chudow, M., & Sunjic, K. (2017). Pharmacokinetic changes in liver failure and impact on drug therapy. *AACN Advanced Critical Care, 28*, 93–101. https://doi.org/10.4037/aacnacc2017948.

17. Dowell, D., Ragan, K., Jones, C. M., Baldwin, G., & Chou, R. (2022). CDC clinical practice guideline for prescribing opioids for pain—United States, 2022. *MMWR Recommendations and Reports, 71*, 1–95. https://doi.org/10.15585/mmwr.rr7103a1.

18. Evans, L., Rhodes, A., Alhazzani, W., Antonelli, M., Coopersmith, C. M., French, C., Machado, F. R., *et al.* (2021). Surviving Sepsis Campaign: International guidelines for management of sepsis and septic shock 2021. *Critical Care Medicine, 49*, e1063–e1143. https://doi.org/10.1097/ccm.0000000000005337.

19. Galindo, C., Bustos, R. H., Porra, M., Leon, M. X., Becerra, D., Vergara, P., Rios, F., *et al.* (2025). Sedatives and opioids best practices: An approach to the use of technological tools. *Pain Physician, 28*(2), E165–E172. https://www.semanticscholar.org/paper/b246bae94dda788a141059d04e0a2ad038efc8bd (accessed on 22 May 2025).

20. Gheblawi, M., Wang, K., Viveiros, A., Nguyen, Q., Zhong, J. C., Turner, A. J., Raizada, M. K., *et al.* (2020). Angiotensin-converting enzyme 2: SARS-CoV-2 receptor and regulator of the renin-angiotensin system. *Circulation Research, 126*, 1456–1474. https://doi.org/10.1161/circresaha.120.317015.

21. Gouin-Thibault, I., Mansour, A., Hardy, M., Gueret, P., de Maistre, E., Siguret, V., Cuker, A., *et al.* (2024). Management of therapeutic-intensity unfractionated heparin: A narrative review on critical points. *TH Open: Companion Journal to Thrombosis and Haemostasias, 8*, e297–e307. https://www.semanticscholar.org/paper/73ffff5d19bf7b6c1758cf1b54c8dee026148566 (accessed on 22 May 2025).

22. Gray, P., Gubb, S., Butler, J., & Walton, B. (2024). A recycling quality improvement project to engage the multidisciplinary team with sustainability efforts. *Nursing in Critical Care*. https://www.semanticscholar.org/paper/b23be0842e4db58bd8d48b6ee29cc4ddca8a83f3 (accessed on 22 May 2025).

23. Kirkpatrick, J. N., Mitchell, C., Taub, C., Kort, S., Hung, J., & Swaminathan, M. (2020). ASE statement on protection of patients and echocardiography service providers during the 2019 novel coronavirus outbreak: Endorsed by the American College of Cardiology. *Journal of the American Society of Echocardiography, 33*, 648–653. https://doi.org/10.1016/j.echo.2020.04.001.

24. Kleinpell, R., Grabenkort, W. R., Boyle, W. A., Vines, D., & Olsen, K. M. (2021). The Society of Critical Care Medicine at 50 years: Interprofessional practice in critical care: Looking back and forging ahead. *Critical Care Medicine, 49*, 2017–2032. https://doi.org/10.1097/ccm.0000000000005276.

25. Kolasinski, S. L., Neogi, T., Hochberg, M. C., Oatis, C. A., Guyatt, G., Block, J. A., Callahan, L. F., *et al.* (2020). 2019 American College of Rheumatology/Arthritis Foundation guideline for the management of osteoarthritis of the hand, hip, and knee. *Arthritis Care & Research, 72*, 149–162. https://doi.org/10.1002/acr.24131.

26. La Via, L., Marino, A., Cuttone, G., Nunnari, G., Deana, C., Tesauro, M., Voza, A., *et al.* (2025). Critical care pharmacology of antiretroviral therapy in adults. *European Journal of Drug Metabolism and Pharmacokinetics, 50*, 105–118. https://www.semanticscholar.org/paper/d828e064fc5332d94060006b5c5112641503aa79 (accessed on 22 May 2025).

27. Lee, K., Klein, P., Dongre, P., Choi, E., & Rhoney, D. (2022). Intravenous brivaracetam in the management of acute seizures in the hospital setting: A scoping review. *Journal of Intensive Care Medicine, 37*, 1133–1145. https://www.semanticscholar.org/paper/a23d3f0d915228339fc232b098ab200064092fac (accessed on 22 May 2025).

28. Ley, E. J., Brown, C. V. R., Moore, E. E., Sava, J., Peck, K. A., Ciesla, D. J., Sperry, J. L., *et al.* (2020). Updated guidelines to reduce venous thromboembolism in trauma patients: A Western Trauma Association critical decisions algorithm. *Journal of Trauma and Acute Care Surgery, 89*, 971–981. https://doi.org/10.1097/ta.0000000000002830.

29. Liu, K. D., Forni, L. G., Heung, M., Wu, V. C., Kellum, J. A., Mehta, R. L., Ronco, C., *et al.* (2020). Quality of care for acute kidney disease: Current knowledge gaps and future directions. *Kidney International Reports, 5*, 1634–1642. https://doi.org/10.1016/j.ekir.2020.07.031.

30. Mach, F., Baigent, C., Catapano, A. L., Koskinas, K. C., Casula, M., Badimón, L., Chapman, M. J., *et al.* (2019). 2019 ESC/EAS guidelines for the management of dyslipidemias: Lipid modification to reduce cardiovascular risk. *European Heart Journal, 41*, 111–188. https://doi.org/10.1093/eurheartj/ehz455.

31. Malbrain, M. L. N. G., Länger, T., Annane, D., Gattinoni, L., Elbers, P., Hahn, R. G., De Laet, I., *et al.* (2020). Intravenous fluid therapy in the perioperative and critical care setting: Executive summary of the International Fluid Academy (IFA). *Annals of Intensive Care, 10*. https://doi.org/10.1186/s13613-020-00679-3.

32. Naseralallah, L., Al-Badriyeh, D., Atchan, M., Abdul Rouf, P. A., Hail, M. A., El-Kassem, W., & Abushanab, D. (2023). Characteristics of the clinical pharmacists' interventions at the main general tertiary care hospital in Qatar. *Qatar Medical Journal, 2023*. https://www.semanticscholar.org/paper/4da0e9c19771971960afd56d0ed5e715d020242c (accessed on 22 May 2025).

33. Pérez-Nieto, O. R., Gómez-Oropeza, I., Quintero-Leyra, A., Kammar-García, A., Zamarrón-López, É. I., Soto Estrada, M., Morgado Villaseñor, L. A., *et al.* (2023). Hemodynamic and respiratory support in pulmonary embolism: A narrative review. *Frontiers in Medicine, 10*. https://doi.org/10.3389/fmed.2023.1123793.

34. Plenza, A. E., Gabini, S., & Ponti, L. (2025). Impact of pharmacological competencies on the reduction of medication errors in critical care units. *SCT Proceedings in Interdisciplinary Insights and Innovations*. https://www.semanticscholar.org/paper/

f65cf33c39109b72bc9191a1532be1d1969e3bcf (accessed on 22 May 2025).

35. Ponikowski, P., Voors, A. A., Anker, S. D., Bueno, H., Cleland, J. G. F., Coats, A. J. S., Falk, V., *et al.* (2016). 2016 ESC guidelines for the diagnosis and treatment of acute and chronic heart failure. *European Heart Journal, 37*, 2129–2200. https://doi.org/10.1093/eurheartj/ehw128.

36. Raffaeli, G., Pokorná, P., Allegaert, K., Mosca, F., Cavallaro, G., Wildschut, E., & Tibboel, D. (2019). Drug disposition and pharmacotherapy in neonatal ECMO: From fragmented data to integrated knowledge. *Frontiers in Pediatrics, 7*. https://www.semanticscholar.org/paper/db5ed8cbbc23e947cfcf79e4392d39690a6ca1f7 (accessed on 22 May 2025).

37. Rocca, E., Zanza, C., Longhitano, Y., Piccolella, F., Romenskaya, T., Racca, F., Savioli, G., *et al.* (2023). Lung ultrasound in critical care and emergency medicine: Clinical review. *Advances in Respiratory Medicine, 91*, 203–223. https://www.semanticscholar.org/paper/8c3da8cf7cdf07bbd60cb312f10e0bda248cb9f7 (accessed on 22 May 2025).

38. Rosenblat, J. D., Kurdyak, P., Cosci, F., Berk, M., Maes, M., Brunoni, A. R., Li, M., *et al.* (2019). Depression in the medically ill. *Australian & New Zealand Journal of Psychiatry, 54*, 346–366. https://doi.org/10.1177/0004867419888576.

39. Skvarc, D., Truong, T. T. T., Lundin, R. M., Barnes, R., Wilkes, F. A., & Singh, A. B. (2024). Pharmacogenetics and the blood–brain barrier: A whirlwind tour of potential clinical utility. *Future Pharmacology*. https://www.semanticscholar.org/paper/0eb73849110f8edefb7b8b85372915e054e332b6 (accessed on 22 May 2025).

40. Suneja, K., Patel, H., Singh, S., Dixit, R., Singh, S., & Kumar, R. (2025). Therapeutic drug monitoring in India: Why it matters and how to make it happen? *National Journal of Pharmacology and Therapeutics*. https://www.semanticscholar.org/paper/2e765341057a96d93f48d588d1a348e53a98a052 (accessed on 22 May 2025).

41. Tam, K. (2021). An ethical conundrum: Palliative care in the COVID-19 pandemic. *Palliative and Supportive Care, 19*, 127–128. https://www.semanticscholar.org/paper/5cf111800fba418327bb3072b2d162101432925f (accessed on 22 May 2025).

42. Tang, C., & Poloyac, S. (2019). A modeling-based approach to estimate fentanyl pharmacokinetics in obese critically ill children. *Pediatric Critical Care Medicine*. https://www.semanticscholar.org/paper/7f475f409e2adf0d86471b6e5efe72944bea5d9d (accessed on 22 May 2025).

43. Ware, L. B., Files, D., Fowler, A., Aboodi, M. S., Aggarwal, N. R., Brower, R. G., Chang, S. Y., *et al.* (2024). Acetaminophen for prevention and treatment of organ dysfunction in critically ill patients with sepsis: The ASTER randomized clinical trial. *JAMA*. https://www.semanticscholar.org/paper/18dc095564652f2e3b87f4b8fc9101e0d0e89ee1 (accessed on 22 May 2025).

44. Wei, C., He, J., Zhang, J., Shan, H., Jiang, A., Liu, Y., Chen, G., *et al.* (2024). The roles and patterns of critical care pharmacists: A literature review and practical operation model in China. *Frontiers in Pharmacology, 15*. https://www.semanticscholar.org/paper/59aebceb595bead530571c5517166a1f1ad7eee4 (accessed on 22 May 2025).

45. Whelton, P. K., Carey, R. M., Aronow, W. S., Casey, D. E., Collins, K. J., Himmelfarb, C. D., DePalma, S. M., *et al.* (2017). 2017 ACC/AHA/AAPA/ABC/ACPM/AGS/APhA/ASH/ASPC/NMA/PCNA guideline for the prevention, detection, evaluation, and management of high blood pressure in adults: A report of the American College of Cardiology/American Heart Association Task Force on Clinical Practice Guidelines. *Hypertension, 71*. https://doi.org/10.1161/hyp.0000000000000065.

46. Wieruszewski, P. M., Leone, M., Kaas-Hansen, B. S., Dugar, S., Legrand, M., McKenzie, C. A., Bissell Turpin, B. D., *et al.* (2024). Position paper on the reporting of norepinephrine formulations in critical care from the Society of Critical Care Medicine and European Society of Intensive Care Medicine Joint Task Force. *Critical Care Medicine, 52*, 521–530. https://www.semanticscholar.org/paper/200605ee7b80916f4604e0bb5e6dcf9ed22897f2 (accessed on 22 May 2025).

47. Wolf, U., Baust, H., Neef, R., & Steinke, T. (2022). Individual pharmacotherapy management (IPM)—IV: Optimized usage of approved antimicrobials addressing under-recognized adverse drug reactions and drug-drug interactions in polypharmacy. *Antibiotics, 11*. https://www.semanticscholar.org/paper/c5f72675c7c5a52adc7321a1385b840b0d91e05a (accessed on 22 May 2025).

48. World Health Organization. (2020). Clinical management of severe acute respiratory infection (SARI) when COVID-19 disease is suspected. Interim guidance. *Paediatric I Medicine Rodina, 16*, 9–26. https://doi.org/10.15557/pimr.2020.0003.

49. Zeppenfeld, K., Tfelt-Hansen, J., Riva, M., Winkel, B. G., Behr, E. R., Blom, N. A., Charron, P., *et al.* (2022). 2022 ESC guidelines for the management of patients with ventricular arrhythmias and the prevention of sudden cardiac death. *European Heart Journal, 43*, 3997–4126. https://doi.org/10.1093/eurheartj/ehac262.

50. Žitnik, M., Agrawal, M., & Leskovec, J. (2018). Modeling polypharmacy side effects with graph convolutional networks. *Bioinformatics, 34*, i457–i466. https://doi.org/10.1093/bioinformatics/bty294.

INDEX

E

F

G

H

N

O

P